HANDBOOK OF ORTHOPAEDIC REHABILITATION

SECOND EDITION

S. Brent Brotzman, MD

Assistant Professor
Texas A&M University System Health
  Science Center
College Station, Texas

Assistant Professor
University of Texas Health Science
  Center at San Antonio
San Antonio, Texas

Adjunct Professor
Department of Kinesiology
Texas A&M — Corpus Christi
Corpus Christi, Texas

Division I Team Physician
Department of Athletics
Texas A&M — Corpus Christi
Corpus Christi, Texas

Chief of Orthopaedic Section
North Austin Medical Center
Austin, Texas

Kevin E. Wilk, PT, DPT

Adjunct Assistant Professor
Programs in Physical Therapy
Marquette University
Milwaukee, Wisconsin

Clinical Director
Champion Sports Medicine
Birmingham, Alabama

Vice-President, Education
Benchmark Medical Inc.
Malvern, Pennsylvania

Director of Rehabilitation Research
American Sports Medicine Institute
Birmingham, Alabama

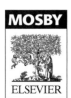

MOSBY

ELSEVIER

MOSBY
ELSEVIER

1600 John F. Kennedy Blvd.
Ste 1800
Philadelphia, PA 19103-2899

Handbook of Orthopaedic Rehabilitation
ISBN-13: 978-0-323-04405-9
ISBN-10: 0-323-04405-0

Notice

Knowledge and best practice in this field are constantly changing. As new research and experience broaden our knowledge, changes in practice, treatment, and drug therapy may become necessary or appropriate. Readers are advised to check the most current information provided (i) on procedures featured or (ii) by the manufacturer of each product to be administered, to verify the recommended dose or formula, the method and duration of administration, and contraindications. It is the responsibility of the practitioner, relying on his or her own experience and knowledge of the patient, to make diagnoses, to determine dosages and the best treatment for each individual patient, and to take all appropriate safety precautions. To the fullest extent of the law, neither the publisher nor the authors assume any liability for any injury and/or damage to persons or property arising from or related to any use of the material contained in this book.

The Publisher

Library of Congress Cataloging-in-Publication Data
Handbook of orthopaedic rehabilitation/[edited by] S. Brent Brotzman, Kevin E. Wilk.
2nd ed.
    p.;cm.
    Includes bibliographical references and index.
    ISBN-13: 978-0-323-04405-9
    ISBN-10: 0-323-04405-0
    1. People with disabilities–Rehabilitation–Handbooks, manuals, etc. 2. Orthopaedics–Handbooks, manuals, etc. I. Brotzman, S. Brent. II. Wilk, Kevin E. III. Title: Orthopaedic rehabilitation.
    [DNLM: 1. Orthopaedic Procedures–methods–Handbooks. 2. Orthopaedic Procedures–rehabilitation–Handbooks. WE 39 H2365 2007]
RD799.H36 2007
617.4′ 7–dc22
                                                                        2006023634

Publishing Director: Kim Murphy
Developmental Editor: Boris Ginsburgs
Publishing Services Manager: Tina Rebane
Design Direction: Louis Forgione
Cover Designer: Louis Forgione

Printed in the United States of America

Last digit is the print number: 9 8 7 6 5 4 3 2 1

Working together to grow
libraries in developing countries
www.elsevier.com | www.bookaid.org | www.sabre.org

ELSEVIER   BOOK AID International   Sabre Foundation

To my wife Cynthia,
whose patience, love, and understanding
throughout this long process have provided
continued inspiration and encouragement.
To my parents,
whose love and sacrifice over the years
have opened countless opportunities.
And finally to my three beautiful children,
who make me want to be
the best surgeon, educator, and
father I can be.

S. Brent Brotzman, MD

CONTRIBUTORS

David W. Altchek, MD
Associate Professor of Clinical Surgery
(Orthopaedics)
Weill Medical College of Cornell
University
New York, New York

Associate Attending Surgeon
The Hospital for Special Surgery
New York, New York

James R. Andrews, MD
Clinical Professor
Orthopaedics and Sports Medicine
University of Virginia School of Medicine
Charlottesville, Virginia

Clinical Professor of Surgery
School of Medicine, Division of
Orthopaedic Surgery
University of Alabama at Birmingham
Birmingham, Alabama

Medical Director
American Sports Medicine Institute
Birmingham, Alabama

Orthopaedic Surgeon
Alabama Sports Medicine &
Orthopaedic Center
Birmingham, Alabama

Bernard R. Bach, Jr., MD
Professor
Department of Orthopaedic Surgery
Director
Sports Medicine Section
Rush Medical College
Chicago, Illinois

Champ L. Baker, Jr., MD
Orthopaedic Surgeon
Hughston Clinic
Columbus, Georgia

Clinical Assistant Professor
Department of Orthopaedics
Tulane University
New Orleans, Louisiana

Team Physician
Columbus State University
Columbus RedStixx
Columbus Cottonmouths
Columbus, Georgia

Mark Baker, PT
Hughston Sports Medicine
Foundation
Columbus, Georgia

Mark Bohling, MS, ATC, LAT
Head Athletic Trainer/Instructor
Texas A&M University
Corpus Christi, Texas

S. Brent Brotzman, MD
Assistant Professor
Texas A&M University System Health
Science Center
College Station, Texas

Assistant Professor
University of Texas Health Science
Center at San Antonio
San Antonio, Texas

Adjunct Professor
Department of Kinesiology
Texas A&M—Corpus Christi
Corpus Christi, Texas

Division I Team Physician
Department of Athletics
Texas A&M—Corpus Christi
Corpus Christi, Texas

Chief of Orthopaedic Section
North Austin Medical Center
Austin, Texas

Gae Burchill, MHA, OTR/L, CHT
Clinical Specialist
Occupational Therapy—Hand and
Upper Extremity Services
Massachusetts General Hospital
Boston, Massachusetts

Dann C. Byck, MD
Attending Physician
Department of Orthopaedic Surgery
McKay-Dee Hospital
Ogden, Utah

James H. Calandruccio, MD
Instructor
University of Tennessee—Campbell
    Clinic
Department of Orthopaedic Surgery
Memphis, Tennessee

Staff Orthopaedic Surgeon
Campbell Clinic
Memphis, Tennessee

**Donna Ryan Callamaro,
    OTR/L, CHT**
Senior Occupational Therapist
Occupational Therapy—Hand and
    Upper Extremity Services
Massachusetts General Hospital
Boston, Massachusetts

Hugh Cameron, MD
Associate Professor
Department of Surgery, Pathology, and
    Engineering
University of Toronto
Toronto, Canada

Staff Orthopaedic Surgeon
SunnyBrook Women's Hospital
Toronto, Canada

Mark M. Casillas, MD
Clinical Assistant Professor
University of Texas Health Sciences
    Center
San Antonio, Texas

Thomas O. Clanton, MD
Professor and Chairman
Department of Orthopaedics
University of Texas—Houston Medical
    School

Team Physician
Rice University Department of
    Athletics
Houston, Texas

Brian S. Cohen, MD
Attending Orthopaedic Surgeon
Center for Advanced Orthopaedics
    and Sports Medicine
Adena Regional Medical Center
Chillicothe, Ohio

Mark R. Colville, MD
Assistant Professor
Portland State University

Orthopaedic Surgeon
Team Physician
Portland Winterhawks Hockey
    Team
Portland, Oregon

**Jenna Deacon Costella,
    MA, ATC**
Assistant Athletic Trainer
Instructor
Department of Kinesiology
Texas A&M University
Corpus Christi, Texas

Kevin J. Coupe, MD
Assistant Professor of
    Orthopaedics
Program Director
University of Texas–Houston
Houston, Texas

Michael J. D'Amato, MD
Team Physician
Shawnee State University
Portsmouth, Ohio

Adjunct Clinical Consultant
Ohio University
Athens, Ohio

Larry D. Field, MD
Partner
Mississippi Sports Medicine and
    Orthopaedic Center
Jackson, Mississippi

Brett R. Fink, MD
Foot and Ankle Specialist
Orthopaedic Surgeon
Community Hospitals
Indianapolis, Indiana

G. Kelley Fitzgerald, PT, PhD, OCS
Assistant Professor
Department of Physical Therapy
School of Health and Rehabilitation
  Sciences
University of Pittsburgh
Pittsburgh, Pennsylvania

Robert C. Greenberg, MD
Associate Clinical Professor
Department of Orthopaedic
  Surgery
Berkshire Medical Center
Pittsfield, Massachusetts

James J. Irrgang, PhD, PT, ATC
Assistant Professor
Vice Chairman for Clinical Services
University of Pittsburgh
Pittsburgh, Pennsylvania

Margaret Jacobs, PT
Physical Therapist
Orthopaedic Store
San Antonio, Texas

Stan L. James, MD
Courtesy Professor
Department of Exercise and
  Movement Science
University of Oregon
Eugene, Oregon

Orthopaedic Surgeon
Orthopaedic Healthcare
  Northwest
Eugene, Oregon

Jesse B. Jupiter, MD
Professor
Department of Orthopaedic
  Surgery
Harvard Medical School
Cambridge, Massachusetts

Director
Orthopaedic Hand Service
Massachusetts General Hospital
Boston, Massachusetts

W. Ben Kibler, MD
Medical Director
Lexington Clinic Sports Medicine
  Center
Lexington, Kentucky

Michael L. Lee, MD
University Sports Medicine
  Associates
Corpus Christi, Texas

Michael Levinson, PT
Clinical Supervisor
Sports Medicine Rehabilitation
  Department
Hospital for Special Surgery
New York, New York

John McMullen, MS, ATC
Manager, Sports Medicine and
  Physical Therapy
Sports Medicine Center
Lexington Clinic
Lexington, Kentucky

Steven J. Meyers, MD
Assistant Professor, Pediatrics
Texas A&M University Health Science
  Center
College Station, Texas

Team Physician
Department of Athletics
Texas A&M University—
  Corpus Christi
Corpus Christi, Texas

Mark S. Mizel, MD
Professor
Department of Orthopaedics and
  Rehabilitation
University of Miami School of
  Medicine
Miami, Florida

Kenneth J. Mroczek, MD
Assistant Professor
Department of Orthopaedic Surgery
New York University School of
  Medicine
New York, New York

Kyle C. Phillips, PA-C, BHS
Clinical Instructor
Health Science
University of North Texas
Fort Worth, Texas

Physician Assistant
Allied Health
Spohn Hospital
Corpus Christi, Texas

Bruce Reider, MD
Professor of Surgery
Section of Orthopaedic Surgery and
  Rehabilitation Medicine
Department of Surgery
The University of Chicago
Chicago, Illinois

Director of Sports Medicine
The University of Chicago Hospitals
Chicago, Illinois

David Ring, MD
Instructor of Orthopaedics
Department of Orthopaedic Surgery
Harvard Medical School
Boston, Massachusetts

Anthony A. Romeo, MD
Associate Professor
Department of Orthopaedic Surgery
Rush Medical College
Chicago, Illinois

Melvin P. Rosenwasser, MD
Director
Orthopaedic Hand and Trauma
  Service
New York Presbyterian Hospital,
  Columbia Campus
New York, New York

Robert E. Carroll Professor of
  Orthopaedic Surgery
College of Physicians and Surgeons
Columbia University
New York, New York

Charles L. Saltzman, MD
Professor
Department of Orthopaedic Surgery
Department of Biomedical
  Engineering
University of Iowa
Iowa City, Iowa

Felix H. Savoie III, MD
Partner
Mississippi Sports Medicine and
  Orthopaedic Center
Jackson, Mississippi

Kenneth A. Stephenson, MD
Attending Surgeon
Covenant Medical Center
Lubbock, Texas

Attending Surgeon
Northstar Surgical Center
Lubbock, Texas

Teresa Triche, M Ed
Exercise Physiologist
Certified Aquatic Specialist
Personal Trainer
San Antonio, Texas

Kevin E. Wilk, PT, DPT
Adjunct Assistant Professor
Programs in Physical Therapy
Marquette University
Milwaukee, Wisconsin

Clinical Director
Champion Sports Medicine
Birmingham, Alabama

Vice-President, Education
Benchmark Medical, Inc.
Malvern, Pennsylvania

Director of Rehabilitation Research
American Sports Medicine Institute
Birmingham, Alabama

Anna Williams, PT
Director of Physical Therapy
Crossroads Home Health
Port Lavaca, Texas

PREFACE

Our goal in preparing the *Handbook of Orthopaedic Rehabilitation* was to widen the scope of available information for the musculoskeletal practitioner. The expanded material should prove relevant to physical therapists, orthopaedic surgeons, family practitioners, athletic trainers, chiropractors, and others who treat musculoskeletal disorders.

We have attempted to provide sound examination techniques, classification systems, differential diagnoses, treatment options, and rehabilitation protocols for common musculoskeletal problems. With this material the clinician who suspects de Quervain's tenosynovitis of the wrist, for example, may easily look up the appropriate examination, differential diagnosis, treatment options, and rehabilitation protocol.

Although the literature describing orthopaedic surgery techniques and acute fracture care is sound and comprehensive, there has been a relative paucity of information concerning nonoperative and postoperative rehabilitative care. This void exists even though rehabilitative therapy often has as much or greater impact as the initial surgery does on the long-term results. A technically superb surgery may be compromised by improper postoperative rehabilitative techniques that allow scar formation, stiffness, rupture of incompletely healed tissue, or loss of function.

Many of the current rehabilitation protocols are empirically based. They have been shaped by years of trial and error with a large number of patients. Changes in rehabilitation protocols will be improved in the future by more clinical research and biomechanical studies. At present, however, the principles outlined in this text are those accepted by most orthopaedic surgeons and therapists.

We hope that the practitioner will find this text to be a concise, easy-to-use guide for performing precise examinations, formulating effective treatment options, and achieving successful rehabilitation of orthopaedic injuries.

S. Brent Brotzman, MD

CONTENTS

CHAPTER 6
THE ARTHRITIC LOWER EXTREMITY   647
Hugh Cameron, MD • S. Brent Brotzman, MD

CHAPTER 7
SPECIAL TOPICS   699
Thomas Clanton, MD • Stan L. James, MD • S. Brent Brotzman, MD

1 Hand and Wrist Injuries

S. BRENT BROTZMAN, MD •
JAMES H. CALANDRUCCIO, MD • JESSE B. JUPITER, MD

Metacarpophalangeal Joint Arthroplasty	Triangular Fibrocartilage Complex Injury
Thumb Carpometacarpal Joint Arthroplasty	De Quervain's Tenosynovitis
Wrist Disorders	Intersection Syndrome of the Wrist
Scaphoid Fractures	Dorsal and Volar Carpal Ganglion Cysts
Fractures of the Distal Radius	

Findings in Common Conditions of the Hand and Wrist

DEGENERATIVE ARTHRITIS OF THE FINGERS

- Heberden's nodes (most common)
- Bouchard's nodes (common)
- Mucous cysts (occasional)
- Decreased motion at involved interphalangeal (IP) joints
- Instability of involved joints (occasional)

BASILAR JOINT ARTHRITIS OF THE THUMB

- Swelling and tenderness of the basilar joint (carpometacarpal [CMC] joint)
- Subluxation of the basilar joint (shuck test) (more severe cases)
- Reduced motion at the basilar joint (palmar abduction, opposition)
- Weakened opposition and grip strength
- Abnormal compression grind test
- Hyperextension of the first metacarpophalangeal (MCP) joint (more severe cases)

CARPAL TUNNEL SYNDROME

- Median nerve compression and Phalen test abnormal (most sensitive tests)
- Tinel's sign over the median nerve (frequent)
- Abnormal sensation (two-point discrimination) in the median nerve distribution (more severe cases). This distribution is the palmar surface of the thumb, index, and long fingers
- Thenar eminence softened and atrophied (more severe cases)
- Weakened or absent thumb opposition (more severe cases)

DE QUERVAIN'S STENOSING TENOSYNOVITIS

- Tenderness and swelling over the first dorsal compartment at the radial styloid
- Pain aggravated by the Finkelstein test

WARTENBERG'S SYNDROME (ENTRAPMENT OF THE SENSORY BRANCH OF THE RADIAL NERVE)

- Pain in the sensory distribution of the superficial sensory branch of the radial nerve
- Nerve entrapped or compressed as it exits its submuscular position from below the brachioradialis

Findings in Common Conditions of the Hand and Wrist   *Continued*

GANGLION

- Palpable mass (may be firm or soft)
- Most common locations: volar surface of the hand at the web flexion crease of the digits or the transverse palmar crease, dorsal surface of the wrist near the extensor carpi radialis longus (ECRL) and extensor carpi radialis brevis (ECRB) tendons, volar surface of the wrist near the radial artery
- Mass transilluminates (larger ganglia)

DUPUYTREN'S DISEASE

- Palpable nodules and pretendinous cords in the palmar aponeurosis, most commonly affecting the ring or the little finger
- Secondary flexion contracture of the MCP and, occasionally, the proximal interphalangeal (PIP) joints

RHEUMATOID ARTHRITIS

- Boggy swelling of multiple joints (MCP joints and wrist joint most commonly involved)
- Boggy swelling of the tenosynovium of the extensor tendons over the dorsum of the wrist and the hand (common)
- Boggy swelling of the tenosynovium and the flexor tendons on the volar surface of the wrist (common)
- Secondary deformities in more severe cases, such as ulnar deviation of the MCP joints and swan neck and boutonnière deformities
- Secondary rupture of the extensor or flexor tendons (variable)

FLEXOR TENDON SHEATH INFECTION

- Cardinal signs of Kanavel present
- Finger held in a flexed position at rest
- Swelling along the volar surface of the finger
- Tenderness on the volar surface of the finger along the course of the flexor tendon sheath
- Pain exacerbated by passive extension of the involved finger

INJURY TO THE ULNAR COLLATERAL LIGAMENT OF THE METACARPOPHALANGEAL JOINT OF THE THUMB (SKIER'S OR GAMEKEEPER'S THUMB)

- Swelling and tenderness over the ulnar aspect of the thumb MCP joint
- Pain exacerbated by stress of the ulnar collateral ligament (UCL) (valgus stressing of the thumb)
- Increased laxity of the thumb UCL (more severe injuries)
- Mechanism is that of thumb being forcibly abducted away from the wrist (e.g., falling on a ski pole and abducting a thumb)

ULNAR NERVE ENTRAPMENT AT THE WRIST

- Compression of the ulnar nerve at Guyon's canal reproduces symptoms (most sensitive test)
- Abnormal Tinel's sign over Guyon's canal (variable)
- Weakness of the intrinsic muscles (finger abduction or adduction) (most severe cases)

Findings in Common Conditions of the Hand and Wrist   *Continued*

ULNAR NERVE ENTRAPMENT AT THE WRIST—CONT'D

- Atrophy of the interossei and the hypothenar eminence (most severe cases)
- Abnormal sensation in the little finger and the ulnar aspect of the ring finger (variable)
- Abnormal Froment's sign (variable)

SCAPHOLUNATE INSTABILITY

- Swelling over the radial aspect of the wrist. Radiographs show an increased scapholunate gap on a clenched-fist view (>1 mm)
- Tenderness on the dorsal surface of the wrist over the scapholunate ligament
- Scaphoid shift test produces abnormal popping and reproduces the patient's pain

MALLET FINGER

- Flexed or dropped posture of the finger at the distal interphalangeal (DIP) joint
- History of a jamming injury (e.g., impact of a thrown ball)
- Inability to actively extend or straighten the DIP joint

JERSEY FINGER (FLEXOR DIGITORUM PROFUNDUS [FDP] AVULSION)

- Mechanism is hyperextension stress applied to a flexed finger (e.g., grabbing a player's jersey)
- Patient lacks active flexion at the DIP joint (FDP function lost)
- Swollen finger often assumes a position of relative extension in comparison to the other, more flexed fingers

Modified from Reider B: The Orthopaedic Physical Examination. Philadelphia, WB Saunders, 1999.

Flexor Tendon Injuries

IMPORTANT POINTS FOR REHABILITATION AFTER FLEXOR TENDON INJURY OR REPAIR

- Researchers have demonstrated that repaired flexor tendons stressed through an early mobilization program heal faster, gain tensile strength faster, and have fewer adhesions and better excursion than unstressed repairs do (Hunter et al. 2002)
- The A2 and A4 pulleys are the most important to mechanical function of the finger. Loss of a substantial portion of either may diminish digital motion and power or lead to flexion contractures of the IP joints.
- The flexor digitorum superficialis (FDS) tendons lie on the palmar side of the FDP until they enter the A1 entrance of the digital sheath. The FDS then splits (at Camper's chiasma) and terminates into the proximal half of the middle phalanx.
- As much as 9 cm of flexor tendon excursion is required to produce composite wrist and digital flexion. Only 2.5 cm of excursion is required for full digital flexion when the wrist is stabilized in the neutral position.

- Three millimeters to 5 mm of tendon excursion is necessary to prevent the formation of flexor tendon adhesions (Hunter et al. 2002).
- Tendons in the hand have both intrinsic and extrinsic capabilities for healing.
- Factors that influence the formation of excursion-restricting adhesions around repaired flexor tendons include
  - The amount of initial trauma to the tendon and its sheath
  - Tendon ischemia
  - Tendon immobilization
  - Gapping at the repair site
  - Disruption of the vincula (blood supply), which decreases the recovery of tendon excursion
- Lacerations of the palmar aspect of the finger will almost always injure the FDP before severing the FDS.
- Delayed primary repair results (within the first 10 days) are equal to or better than immediate repair of the flexor tendon.
- Immediate (primary) repair is **contraindicated** in patients with
  - Severe multiple tissue injuries to the fingers or palm
  - Wound contamination
  - Significant skin loss over the flexor tendons
- Despite the use of early controlled tendon mobilization, adhesion formation remains the most common complication after flexor tendon surgery. Surgical tenolysis is the treatment of choice if an appropriate period of therapy has failed (3 to 6 months). Tendon rupture after primary repair is uncommon (Hunter et al. 2002).
- Although rupture can occur late, it is usually noted around the 7th to 10th post-operative day.

REHABILITATION RATIONALE AND BASIC PRINCIPLES OF TREATMENT AFTER FLEXOR TENDON INJURY OR REPAIR

Timing

The timing of flexor tendon repair influences the rehabilitation and outcome of flexor tendon injuries.
- *Primary repair* is done within the first 12 to 24 hours after injury.
- *Delayed primary repair* is done within the first 10 days after injury.

If primary repair is not performed, delayed primary repair should be performed as soon as there is evidence of wound healing without infection.

- *Secondary repair* is done 10 to 14 days after injury.
- *Late secondary repair* is done more than 4 weeks after injury.

After 4 weeks, it is extremely difficult to deliver the flexor tendon through the digital sheath, which usually becomes extensively scarred. However, clinical situations in which the tendon repair is of secondary importance often make late repair necessary, especially for patients with massive crush injuries, inadequate soft tissue coverage, grossly contaminated or infected wounds, multiple fractures, or untreated injuries. If the sheath is not scarred or destroyed, single-stage tendon grafting, direct repair, or tendon transfer can be performed. If extensive disturbance and scarring have occurred, two-stage tendon grafting with a Hunter rod should be performed.

TABLE 1-1	Boyes' Preoperative Classification
Grade	**Preoperative Conditions**
1	Good: minimal scar with mobile joints and no trophic changes
2	Cicatrix: heavy skin scarring because of injury or previous surgery; deep scarring as a result of failed primary repair or infection
3	Joint damage: injury to the joint with restricted range of motion
4	Nerve damage: injury to the digital nerves resulting in trophic changes in the finger
5	Multiple damage: involvement of multiple fingers with a combination of the above problems

Before tendons can be secondarily repaired, the following requirements must be met:

- Joints must be supple and have useful passive range of motion (ROM) (Boyes' grade 1 or 2, Table 1-1). Restoration of passive ROM is aggressively achieved with rehabilitation before secondary repair is performed.
- Skin coverage must be adequate.
- The surrounding tissue in which the tendon is expected to glide must be relatively free of scar tissue.
- Wound erythema and swelling must be minimal or absent.
- Fractures must have been securely fixed or healed with adequate alignment.
- Sensation in the involved digit must be undamaged or restored, or it should be possible to repair damaged nerves at the time of tendon repair directly or with nerve grafts.
- The critical A2 and A4 pulleys must be present or have been reconstructed. Secondary repair is delayed until these pulleys are reconstructed. During reconstruction, Hunter (silicone) rods are useful to maintain the lumen of the tendon sheath while the grafted pulleys are healing.

Anatomy

The anatomic zone of injury of the flexor tendons influences the outcome and rehabilitation of these injuries. The hand is divided into five distinct flexor zones (Fig. 1-1):

- *Zone 1*—from the insertion of the profundus tendon at the distal phalanx to just distal to the insertion of the sublimus
- *Zone 2*—Bunnell's "no man's land": the critical area of pulleys between the insertion of the sublimus and the distal palmar crease
- *Zone 3*—"area of lumbrical origin": from the beginning of the pulleys (A1) to the distal margin of the transverse carpal ligament
- *Zone 4*—area covered by the transverse carpal ligament
- *Zone 5*—area proximal to the transverse carpal ligament

As a rule, repair of tendons injured outside the flexor sheath produces much better results than does repair of tendons injured inside the sheath (zone 2).

It is essential that the A2 and A4 pulleys (Fig. 1-2) be preserved to prevent tendon bowstringing. In the thumb, the A1 and oblique pulleys are the most important. The thumb lacks a vinculum for blood supply.

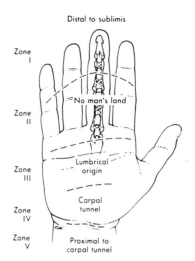

Figure 1–1 Flexor tendon zones. (From Canale ST [ed]: Campbell's Operative Orthopaedics, 9th ed. St Louis, CV Mosby, 1998.)

Tendon Healing

The exact mechanism of tendon healing is still unknown. Healing probably occurs through a combination of extrinsic and intrinsic processes. *Extrinsic* healing depends on the formation of adhesions between the tendon and the surrounding tissue to provide a blood supply and fibroblasts, but unfortunately, adhesions also prevent the tendon from gliding. *Intrinsic* healing relies on synovial fluid for nutrition and occurs only between the tendon ends.

Flexor tendons in the distal sheath have a dual source of nutrition via the vincular system and synovial diffusion. Diffusion appears to be more important than perfusion in the digital sheath (Green, 1993).

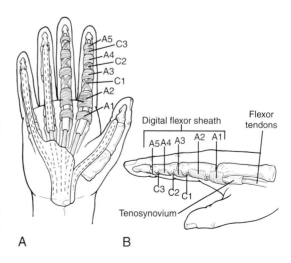

Figure 1–2 **A**, Uninvolved hand showing the position of the pulleys and synovial sheaths of the fingers. **B**, Normal anatomy of the pulley system. (Adapted from Idler RS: Anatomy and biomechanics of the digital flexor tendons. Hand Clin 1:6, 1985; and Idler RS: Helping the patient who has wrist or hand tenosynovitis. J Musculoskel Med 14[2]:21, 1997.)

Several factors have been reported to affect tendon healing:

- Age—The number of vincula (blood supply) decreases with age.
- General health—Cigarettes, caffeine, and poor general health delay healing. The patient should refrain from caffeine and cigarettes during the first 4 to 6 weeks after repair.
- Scar formation—The remodeling phase is not as effective in patients in whom heavy keloid or scar develops.
- Patient motivation and compliance—Motivation and the ability to follow the postoperative rehabilitation regimen are critical factors in outcome.
- Level of injury—Zone 2 injuries are more apt to form limiting adhesions from the tendon to the surrounding tissue. In zone 4, where the flexor tendons lie in close proximity to each other, injuries tend to form tendon-to-tendon adhesions that limit differential glide.
- Trauma and extent of injury—Crushing or blunt injuries promote more scar formation and cause more vascular trauma, thereby impairing function and healing. Infection also impedes the healing process.
- Pulley integrity—Pulley repair is important in restoring mechanical advantage (especially A2 and A4) and maintaining tendon nutrition through synovial diffusion.
- Surgical technique—Improper handling of tissues (such as forceps marks on the tendon) and excessive postoperative hematoma formation trigger adhesion formation. Suture strength is critical as well.

The two most frequent causes of failure of primary tendon repair are the formation of adhesions and rupture of the repaired tendon.

Through experimental and clinical observation, Duran and Houser (1975) determined that 3 to 5 mm of tendon glide is sufficient to prevent motion-limiting tendon adhesions. Exercises are thus designed to achieve this motion.

Treatment of Flexor Tendon Lacerations

- Partial lacerations involving less than 25% of the tendon substance can be treated by beveling the cut edges.
- Lacerations between 25% and 50% can be repaired with 6-0 running nylon suture in the epitenon.
- Lacerations involving more than 50% should be considered complete and repaired with a core suture and an epitenon suture.
- FDP lacerations should be repaired directly or advanced and reinserted into the distal phalanx with a pull-out wire, but they should not be advanced more than 1 cm to avoid the quadriga effect (a complication of a single digit with limited motion causing limitation of excursion and motion of the uninvolved digits). This limited excursion of the remaining FDP tendons occurs because the FDP tendons share a common muscle belly. Thus, an FDP repair should not be advanced more than 1 cm or excursion of the remaining FDP tendons will be limited.

REHABILITATION AFTER FLEXOR TENDON REPAIR

There are two basic types of early passive mobilization protocols for flexor tendon repairs of the hand. One approach is that of Duran and Houser; the other is based on the work of Kleinert.

In both approaches a forearm-based dorsal blocking splint (DBS), applied in surgery, blocks the MCP joints and wrist in flexion to place the flexor tendons on slack, and the IP joints are left free or allowed to extend to neutral within the splint.

The splint allows passive flexion of the digits but does not allow extension beyond the limits of the splint. Dynamic traction maintains the fingers in flexion to further relax the flexor tendon and prevent inadvertent active flexion. Dynamic traction may be provided by rubber bands, elastic threads, springs, and other devices. The traction is applied to the fingernail by gluing a dress hook to the fingernail, Velcro, a suture through the nail, or other means (Hunter et al. 2002).

Duran and Houser determined through clinical and experimental observation that 3 to 5 mm of glide was sufficient to prevent the formation of firm tendon adhesions. Thus, exercises are designed with six to eight repetitions twice a day to prevent firm adhesion.

With the MCP and PIP joints flexed, the DIP joint is passively extended, thus moving the FDP repair distally, away from the FDS repair. Then, with the DIP and MCP joints flexed, the PIP joint is extended; both repairs glide distally away from the site of repair and surrounding scar tissue (Hunter et al. 2002).

The rehabilitation protocol chosen depends on the *timing* of the repair (delayed primary or secondary), the *location* of the injury (zones 1 through 5), and the *compliance* of the patient (early mobilization for compliant patients and delayed mobilization for noncompliant patients and children younger than 7 years).

REHABILITATION PROTOCOL   *After Immediate or Delayed Primary Repair of Flexor Tendon Injury in Zones 1, 2 and 3*
Modified Duran Protocol (Cannon)

PREREQUISITES

- Compliant patient
- Clean or healed wound
- Repair within 14 days of injury

1-3 DAYS TO 4.5 WEEKS

- Remove the bulky compressive dressing and apply light compressive dressing.
- Use digital-level fingersocks or a Coban wrap for edema control.
- Fit a DBS to the wrist and digits for continual wear with the following positions:
  - Wrist—20 degrees flexion
  - MCP joints—50 degrees flexion
  - DIP and PIP joints—full extension
- Initiate controlled passive mobilization exercises, including passive flexion/extension exercises for the DIP and PIP joints individually.
- Composite passive flexion/extension exercises for the MCP, PIP, and DIP joints of digits (modified Duran program). Active extension should be within the restraints of the DBS. If full flexion is not obtained, the patient may begin prolonged flexion stretching with a Coban wrap or taping.

Continued

REHABILITATION PROTOCOL: *After Immediate or Delayed Primary Repair of Flexor Tendon Injury in Zones 1, 2 and 3* *Continued*

1-3 DAYS TO 4.5 WEEKS—cont'd

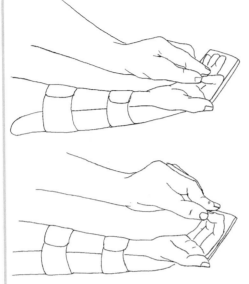

Figure 1–3 Passive flexion and extension exercises of the proximal interphalangeal joint in a dorsal blocking splint.

Figure 1–4 Passive flexion and extension exercises of the distal interphalangeal joint in a dorsal blocking splint.

- Eight repetitions each of isolated passive flexion/extension exercises of the PIP, DIP, and MCP joints within the DBS (Figs. 1-3 to 1-5).

4.5 WEEKS

- Continue the exercises and begin active ROM for finger and wrist flexion, with active wrist extension allowed to neutral or 0 degrees of extension only.
- The patient should perform hourly exercise with the splint removed, including composite fist, wrist flexion and extension to neutral, and composite finger flexion with the wrist immobilized (Fig. 1-6).
- Have the patient perform a fist to hook fist (intrinsic minus position) to extended fingers exercise (Fig. 1-7).
- Watch for PIP joint flexion contractures. If an extension lag is present, add protected passive extension of the PIP joint with the MCP joint held in flexion. This should be done only by reliable patients or therapists. The PIP joint should be blocked to 30 degrees of flexion for 3 weeks if a concomitant distal nerve repair is performed.

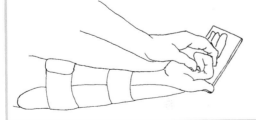

Figure 1–5 Combined passive flexion and extension exercises of the metacarpophalangeal, proximal interphalangeal, and distal interphalangeal joints.

REHABILITATION PROTOCOL: *After Immediate or Delayed Primary Repair of Flexor Tendon Injury in Zones 1, 2 and 3*   *Continued*

1-3 DAYS TO 4.5 WEEKS—cont'd

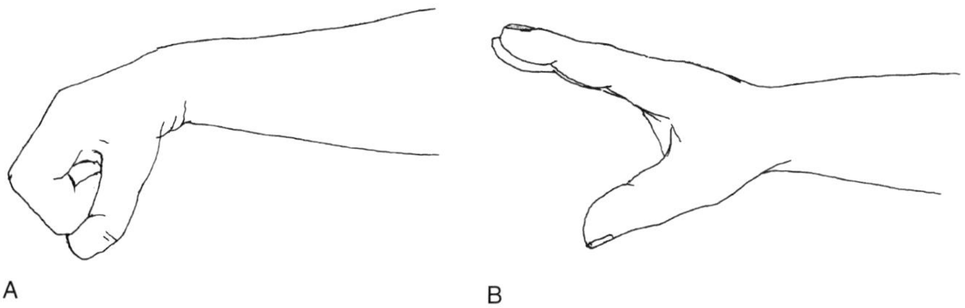

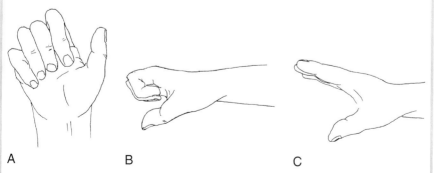

Figure 1–6   The wrist is bent in flexion with a composite fist (**A**), and then the wrist and fingers are extended (**B**).

- Patients may reach a plateau in ROM 2 months after surgery, but maximal motion is usually achieved by 3 months after surgery.

5 WEEKS

- Functional electrical stimulation (FES) can be used to improve tendon excursion. Consider the quality of the primary repair, the nature of the injury, and the patient's medical history before initiating FES.

5.5 WEEKS

- Add blocking exercises for the PIP and DIP joints to the previous home program.
- Discontinue the DBS.
- Focus on gaining full passive ROM for flexion. Do not begin passive extension stretching at this time. A restraining extension splint can be used and positioned in the available range if tightness is noted.

6 WEEKS

- Begin passive extension exercises of the wrist and digits.
- Fit an extension resting pan splint in maximal extension if extrinsic flexor tendon tightness is significant; frequently, the patient may need only an extension gutter splint for night wear.

Figure 1–7   The patient makes a fist (**A**) and then straightens the metacarpophalangeal joints ("back knuckles") (**B**). The fingers are then straightened with the wrist in neutral (**C**).

Continued

REHABILITATION PROTOCOL: *After Immediate or Delayed Primary Repair of Flexor Tendon Injury in Zones 1, 2 and 3*   *Continued*

8 WEEKS

- Begin resistive exercises with sponges or a Nerf ball and progress to putty and a hand-helper.
- Allow use of the hand in light work activities, but no lifting or heavy use of the hand.

10-12 WEEKS

- Allow full use of the hand in all daily activities.
- Use a work stimulator or strengthening program to improve hand strength.
   The greatest achievement in total motion is seen between 12 and 14 weeks after surgery. It is not uncommon for the patient's ROM to plateau between 6 and 8 weeks.
   Patients with associated digital nerve repair and some degree of tension at the nerve site should be fitted with a separate digital DBS in 30 degrees of PIP joint flexion. This splint is worn for 6 weeks and is progressively adjusted into increased extension during that time frame (see the section on digital nerve repair).

(Many of the rehabilitation protocols in this chapter are taken from *Diagnosis and Treatment Manual for Physicians and Therapists*, third edition., by Nancy Cannon, OTR, The Hand Rehabilitation Clinic of Indiana, PC. We highly recommend this manual as a detailed reference text for hand therapy.)

REHABILITATION PROTOCOL   *Early Mobilization after Immediate or Delayed Primary Repair of Flexor Tendon Injuries in Zones 4 and 5*
Modified Duran Protocol (Cannon)

PREREQUISITES

- Compliant patient
- Clean or healed wound
- Repair within 14 days of injury

7-10 DAYS

- Remove the bulky compressive dressing and apply a light compressive dressing.
- Use digital-level fingersocks or a Coban wrap for edema control.
- Fit a DBS to the wrist and digits for continual wear with the following positions:
  - Wrist—30 degrees palmar flexion
  - MCP joints—50 degrees flexion
  - DIP and PIP joints—full extension
- Begin hourly passive ROM exercises in flexion and extension within the restraints of the DBS (see Figs. 1-3 to 1-5).

3 WEEKS

- Begin active ROM exercises (including blocking) 10 to 15 minutes each hour; exercises can be done within the restraints of the DBS.
- FES or electrical muscle stimulation (EMS) can be initiated to improve tendon excursion within 2 days of initiation of active ROM.

REHABILITATION PROTOCOL: *Early Mobilization after Immediate or Delayed Primary Repair of Flexor Tendon Injuries in Zones 4 and 5* *Continued*

3 WEEKS—cont'd

- Begin scar massage, scar retraction, and scar remodeling techniques to remodel scar tissue and minimize subcutaneous adhesions.

4.5 WEEKS

- Begin active ROM exercises of the wrist and digits outside the DBS. If nerve repair has been done at the wrist level, ROM exercises are performed within the splint to alleviate additional stress at the nerve repair site (see the digital nerve repair section).

6 WEEKS

- Discontinue the DBS.
- Begin passive ROM exercises of the wrist and digits.
- A full-extension resting pan splint or a long dorsal outrigger with a lumbrical bar can be used if extrinsic flexor tightness is present. Generally, this type of splinting is necessary with this level of repair.
- Do not allow lifting or heavy use of the hand.
- Begin gentle strengthening with a Nerf ball or putty.

7 WEEKS

- May progress strengthening to include the use of a hand-helper.

10-12 WEEKS

- Allow full use of the injured hand.

   Once active ROM exercise is initiated at 3 weeks, it is important to emphasize blocking exercises along with the composite active ROM exercises. If the patient is having difficulty regaining active flexion, it is important to carefully monitor progress and request frequent patient visits to maximize flexion. *The first 3 to 7 weeks after surgery are critical for restoring tendon excursion.*

REHABILITATION PROTOCOL

After Immediate or Delayed Primary Repair of Flexor Tendon Injuries in Zones 1, 2, and 3
Modified Early Motion Program (Cannon)

PREREQUISITES

- Compliant, motivated patient
- Good repair
- Healing wound

1-3 DAYS

- Remove the bulky compressive dressing and apply a light compressive dressing.
- Use digital-level fingersocks or a Coban wrap for edema control.
- Fit a DBS to the wrist and digits for continual wear with the following positions:
  - Wrist—20 degrees palmar flexion
  - MCP joints—50 degrees flexion
  - DIP and PIP joints—full extension

Continued

REHABILITATION PROTOCOL: *After Immediate or Delayed Primary Repair of Flexor Tendon Injuries in Zones 1, 2, and 3*   *Continued*

1-3 DAYS—cont'd

- Begin hourly passive ROM exercises in flexion and extension within the restraints of the DBS (refer to the Modified Duran Protocol earlier in this chapter).

3 WEEKS

- Begin active ROM exercises in flexion and extension within the restraints of the DBS four to six times a day, in addition to the Modified Duran Protocol.

4.5 WEEKS

- Begin hourly active ROM exercises of the wrist and digits outside the DBS.
- The patient should wear the DBS between exercise sessions and at night.

5.5 WEEKS

- Begin blocking exercises of the DIP and PIP joints, as outlined in the Modified Duran Protocol (see Figs. 1-3 and 1-4).

6 WEEKS

- Discontinue the DBS.
- Begin passive ROM exercises of the wrist and digits in extension as needed.
- Begin extension splinting if extrinsic flexor tendon tightness or PIP joint contracture is present.

8 WEEKS

- Begin progressive strengthening.
- Do not allow lifting or heavy use of the hand.

10-12 WEEKS

- Allow full use of the hand, including sports.
    This protocol differs from the Modified Duran Protocol in that the patient can begin active ROM exercises within the restraints of the DBS at 3 weeks instead of exercising out of the splint at 4.5 weeks.

REHABILITATION PROTOCOL   *Delayed Mobilization after Flexor Tendon Injury in Zones 1 through 5 in Noncompliant Patients*
Cannon

INDICATIONS

- Crush injury
- Younger than 11 years
- Poor compliance and/or intelligence
- Soft tissue loss, wound management problems

3 WEEKS

- Remove the bulky compressive dressing and apply a light compressive dressing.
- Fit a DBS to the wrist and digits for continual wear with the following positions:
    - Wrist—30 degrees palmar flexion
    - MCP joints—50 degrees flexion
    - DIP and PIP joints—full extension

REHABILITATION PROTOCOL: *Delayed Mobilization after Flexor Tendon Injury in Zones 1 through 5 in Noncompliant Patients* Continued

3 WEEKS—cont'd

- Begin hourly active and passive ROM exercises within restraints of the DBS; blocking exercises of the PIP and DIP joints may be included.
- Active ROM is initiated earlier than in other protocols because of longer (3 weeks) immobilization in the DBS.

4.5 WEEKS

- Begin active ROM exercises of the digits and wrist outside the DBS; continue passive ROM exercises within the restraints of the DBS.
- Use FES or EMS to improve tendon excursion.
- If an associated nerve repair is under a degree of tension, continue exercises within the DBS that are appropriate for the level of nerve repair for 6 weeks.

6 WEEKS

- Discontinue the DBS.
- Begin passive ROM exercises of the wrist and digits in extension.
- Use an extension resting pan splint for extrinsic flexor tendon tightness or joint stiffness.
- Do not allow lifting or heavy use of hand.

8 WEEKS

- Begin progressive strengthening with putty and a hand-helper.

10-12 WEEKS

- Allow full use of the hand.
  This delayed mobilization program for digital-level to forearm-level flexor tendon repairs is reserved primarily for significant crush injuries, which may include severe edema or wound problems. This program is best used for patients whose primary repair may be somewhat "ragged" because of the crushing or bursting nature of the wound. It is also indicated for young children who cannot comply with an early motion protocol, such as the Modified Duran Program. *It is not indicated for patients who undergo a simple primary repair.*

REHABILITATION PROTOCOL
Early Mobilization after Injury of the Flexor Pollicis Longus of the Thumb
Cannon

PREREQUISITES

- Compliant patient
- Clean or healed wound

1-3 DAYS TO 4.5 WEEKS

- Remove the bulky compressive dressing and apply a light compressive dressing.
- Use fingersocks or a Coban wrap on the thumb for edema control.
- Fit a DBS to the wrist and digits for continual wear with the following positions:
  - Wrist—20 degrees palmar flexion
  - Thumb MCP and IP joints—15 degrees flexion at each joint
  - Thumb CMC joint—palmar abduction

Continued

REHABILITATION PROTOCOL: *Early Mobilization after Injury of the Flexor Pollicis Longus of the Thumb* *Continued*

1-3 DAYS TO 4.5 WEEKS—cont'd

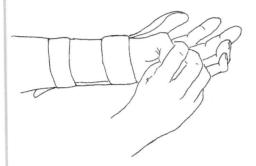

Figure 1–8 Passive flexion and extension of the thumb metacarpophalangeal joint.

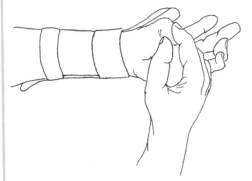

Figure 1–9 Passive flexion and extension of the thumb interphalangeal joint.

It is important to ensure that the thumb IP joint is in 15 degrees of flexion and not extended. When the IP joint is left in a neutral position, restoration of IP joint flexion can be difficult.

- Begin an hourly controlled passive mobilization program within the restraints of the DBS:
  - Eight repetitions of passive flexion and extension of the MCP joints (Fig. 1-8)
  - Eight repetitions of passive flexion and extension of the IP joints (Fig. 1-9)
  - Eight repetitions of passive flexion and extension of the MCP and IP joints in the composite manner (Fig. 1-10)

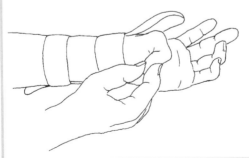

Figure 1–10 Passive flexion and extension of the metacarpophalangeal and interphalangeal joints in the composite manner.

REHABILITATION PROTOCOL: *Early Mobilization after Injury of the Flexor Pollicis Longus of the Thumb*   *Continued*

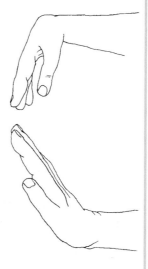

Figure 1–11   Active flexion and extension of the wrist.

4.5 WEEKS

- Remove the DBS each hour to allow the following exercises to be performed:
  - Ten repetitions of active flexion and extension of the wrist (Fig. 1-11)
  - Ten repetitions of active flexion and extension of the thumb (Fig. 1-12)
- Continue passive ROM exercises.
- The patient should wear the DBS between exercise sessions and at night.

5 WEEKS

- Use FES or EMS within the restraints of the DBS to improve tendon excursion.

5.5 WEEKS

- Discontinue the DBS.

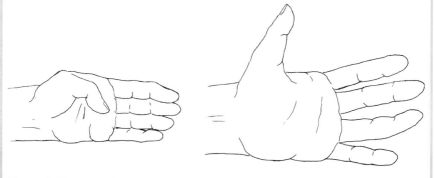

Figure 1–12   Active flexion and extension of the thumb.

Continued

REHABILITATION PROTOCOL: *Early Mobilization after Injury of the Flexor Pollicis Longus of the Thumb* *Continued*

5.5 WEEKS—cont'd

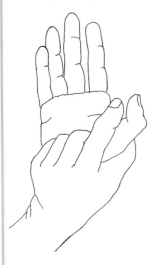

Figure 1–13 Blocking exercises of the thumb interphalangeal joint.

- Begin hourly active ROM exercises:
  - Twelve repetitions of blocking of the thumb IP joint (Fig. 1-13)
  - Twelve repetitions of composite active flexion and extension of the thumb
- Continue passive ROM exercises as necessary.

6 WEEKS

- Begin passive ROM exercises of the wrist and thumb in extension.
- If needed for extrinsic flexor tendon tightness in the flexor pollicis longus (FPL), a wrist and thumb static splint can be used to hold the wrist and thumb in extension. Often, a simple extension gutter splint in full extension can be used for night wear.

8 WEEKS

- Begin progressive strengthening with a Nerf ball and progress to a hand-helper.
- Do not allow lifting or heavy use of the hand.

10-12 WEEKS

- Allow full use of the hand for most activities, including sports.
- ROM generally begins to plateau at approximately 7 to 8 weeks after surgery.
- If an associated digital nerve repair is under tension, position the thumb in 30 degrees of flexion at the MCP and IP joints.
- If passive flexion is limited, taping or dynamic flexion splinting may be used.
- Scar management, including scar retraction, scar massage, and the use of Otoform or Elastomer, may be initiated 2 weeks after surgery.

REHABILITATION PROTOCOL	*Delayed Mobilization after Injury of the Flexor Pollicis Longus of the Thumb* Cannon

INDICATIONS

- Crush injury
- Younger than 7 years
- Poor compliance and/or intelligence
- Soft tissue loss, wound management problems

3 WEEKS

- Remove the bulky compressive dressing and apply a light compressive dressing.
- Use a fingersock or Coban wrap on the thumb as needed for edema control.
- Fit a DBS to the wrist and digits for continual wear with the following positions:
  - Wrist—30 degrees palmar flexion
  - Thumb MCP and IP joints—15 degrees flexion at each joint
  - Thumb CMC joint—palmar abduction
- Begin hourly active and passive ROM exercises within the restraints of the DBS, including blocking exercises.
- If passive flexion of the thumb is limited, taping or dynamic flexion splinting may be used.
- Begin scar massage and scar management techniques.

4.5 WEEKS

- Begin hourly active ROM exercises of the wrist and thumb outside the DBS.
- May use FES or EMS to improve tendon excursion of the FPL.

6 WEEKS

- Discontinue the DBS.
- Begin passive ROM exercises of wrist and thumb in extension.
- If extrinsic flexor tendon tightness of the FPL is present, a wrist and thumb static splint may be used as needed; the patient should wear the splint between exercise sessions and at night.
- Do not allow lifting or heavy use of the hand.

8 WEEKS

- Begin progressive strengthening with a Nerf ball or putty.

10-12 WEEKS

- Allow full use of the hand for most activities.
- If an associated digital nerve repair is under tension, position the thumb MCP and IP joints in 30 degrees flexion to minimize tension at the repair site.
- Composite active flexion of the thumb tends to reach a plateau between 9 and 10 weeks after surgery.

Delayed mobilization of FPL repairs is best reserved for patients with crush injuries, soft tissue loss, and wound management problems and those in whom end-to-end repair was difficult.

REHABILITATION PROTOCOL	*After Two-Stage Reconstruction for Delayed Tendon Repair*
	Cannon

STAGE 1 (HUNTER ROD)

Before Surgery

- Maximize passive ROM of the digit with manual passive exercises, digital-level taping, or dynamic splinting.
- Use scar management techniques to improve the suppleness of soft tissues, including scar massage, scar retraction, and the use of Otoform or Elastomer silicone molds.
- Begin strengthening exercises of the future donor tendon to improve postoperative strength after the stage 2 procedure.
- If needed for protection or assistance with ROM, use buddy taping of the involved digit.

After Surgery

5-7 Days

- Remove the bulky dressing and apply a light compressive dressing; use digital-level fingersocks or a Coban wrap.
- Begin active and passive ROM exercises of the hand for approximately 10 minutes, six times a day.
- Fit an extension gutter splint that holds the digit in full extension to wear between exercise sessions and at night.
- If pulleys have been reconstructed during stage 1, use taping for about 8 weeks during the postoperative phase.

3-6 Weeks

- Gradually wean the patient from the extension gutter splint; continue buddy taping for protection.
  The major goals during stage 1 are to maintain passive ROM and to obtain supple soft tissues before tendon grafting.

STAGE 2 (FREE TENDON GRAFT)

After Surgery

Follow the instructions for the early motion program for injuries in zones 1 through 3 (Modified Duran Protocol earlier in this chapter) or the delayed mobilization program for injuries in zones 1 through 5.

For most patients, the Modified Duran Program is preferable to the delayed mobilization program because it encourages greater excursion of the graft and helps maintain passive ROM through the early mobilization exercises.

Do not use FES before 5 to 5.5 weeks after surgery because of the initial avascularity of the tendon graft. Also consider the reasons for failure of the primary repair.

Trigger Finger (Stenosing Flexor Tenosynovitis)

Steven J. Meyers, MD • Michael L. Lee, MD

Background

Trigger finger is a painful snapping phenomenon that occurs as the finger flexor tendons suddenly pull through a tight **A1 pulley** portion of the flexor sheath. The underlying pathophysiology of trigger finger is an inability of the two flexor tendons of the finger (FDS and FDP) to slide smoothly under the A1 pulley, thus resulting in a need for increased tension to force the tendon to slide and a sudden jerk as the tendon nodule suddenly pulls through the constricted pulley (triggering). The triggering can occur with flexion or extension of the finger or with both. Whether this pathologic state arises primarily from the A1 pulley becoming stenotic or from a thickening of the tendon remains controversial, but both elements are usually found at surgery.

Clinical History and Examination

Trigger finger most commonly occurs in the thumb, middle finger, or ring finger of postmenopausal women and is more common in patients with diabetes or rheumatoid arthritis, Dupuytren's contracture, and other tendinitis (de Quervain's tendinitis or lateral epicondylitis ["tennis elbow"]). Patients have clicking, locking, or popping in the affected finger that is often painful, but not necessarily so.

Patients often have a **palpable nodule** in the area of the thickened A1 pulley (which is at the level of the distal palmar crease) (Fig. 1-14). This nodule can be felt to move with the tendon and is usually painful with deep palpation.

To induce the triggering during examination, it is necessary to **have the patient make a full fist** and then completely extend the fingers because the patient may avoid triggering by only partially flexing the fingers.

Treatment

Spontaneous long-term resolution of trigger finger is rare. If left untreated, a trigger finger will remain a painful nuisance; however, if the finger should become locked, permanent joint stiffness may develop. Historically, conservative treatment included splinting of the finger in extension to prevent triggering, but such treatment has been abandoned because of stiffening and poor results.

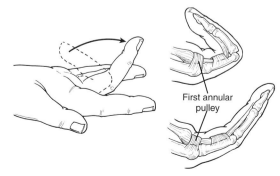

Figure 1–14 A nodule or thickening in the flexor tendon strikes the proximal pulley and makes finger extension difficult. (Adapted from Idler RS: Helping the patient who has hand tenosynovitis. J Musculoskel Med 14[2]:62, 1997.)

First annular pulley

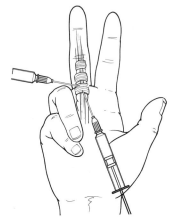

Figure 1–15 A midline palmar approach can be used for injection of corticosteroid into the flexor tendon sheath in patients with trigger finger; however, an approach from the lateral base of any digit (except the thumb) is much less painful. (Adapted from Idler RS: Helping the patient who has wrist or hand tenosynovitis. Part 2. Managing trigger finger, de Quervain's disease. J Musculoskel Med 14[2]: 68, 1997.)

Currently, *nonoperative treatment* involves the injection of corticosteroids with local anesthetic into the flexor sheath. The authors' preference is 0.5 ml lidocaine, 0.5 ml bupivacaine, and 0.5 ml methylprednisolone acetate (Depo-Medrol) (Fig. 1-15). A single injection can be expected to relieve triggering in about 66% of patients. Multiple injections can relieve triggering in 75% to 85% of patients.

About a third of patients will have lasting relief of symptoms with fewer than three injections, which means that about two thirds will require surgical intervention.

Surgery for trigger finger is a relatively simple outpatient procedure done with the patient under local anesthesia. The surgery involves a 1- to 2-cm incision in the palm to identify and completely divide the A1 pulley.

Pediatric Trigger Thumb

Pediatric trigger thumb is a congenital condition in which stenosis of the A1 pulley of the thumb in infants causes locking of the IP joint in flexion (inability to extend the joint). It is often bilateral. There is usually no pain or clicking because the thumb remains locked. About 30% of children have spontaneous resolution by 1 year. The rest require surgical intervention to release the tight A1 pulley by about 2 to 3 years of age to prevent permanent joint flexion contracture.

REHABILITATION PROTOCOL | *After Trigger Finger Cortisone Injection or Release*

AFTER INJECTION

Physical therapy is not usually necessary for motion because most patients are able to regain motion once the triggering resolves.

AFTER TRIGGER RELEASE SURGERY

0-4 days	Gentle active MCP/PIP/DIP joint ROM (avoid gapping of the wound)
4 days	Remove the bulky dressing and cover the wound with a Band-Aid.
4-8 days	Continue ROM exercises. Remove the sutures at 7-9 days.
8 days-3 weeks	Active/active-assisted ROM/passive ROM of the MCP/PIP/DIP joints
3 weeks +	Aggressive ROM and strengthening. Return to unrestricted activities.

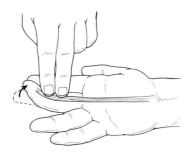

Figure 1–16 With avulsion of the flexor digitorum profundus, the patient is unable to flex the distal interphalangeal joint, shown here. (Adapted from Regional Review Course in Hand Surgery. Rosemont, IL, American Society of Surgery of the Hand, 1991.)

Flexor Digitorum Profundus Avulsion ("Jersey Finger")

S. Brent Brotzman, MD • Steven J. Meyers, MD

Background

Avulsion of the FDP (**"jersey finger"**) can occur in any digit, but it is most common in the ring finger. This injury usually occurs when an athlete grabs an opponent's jersey and feels sudden pain as the distal phalanx of the finger is forcibly extended while it is actively flexed (hyperextension stress applied to a flexed finger).

Lack of active flexion of the DIP joint (FDP function) must be specifically checked to make the diagnosis (Fig. 1-16). Often the swollen finger assumes a position of extension relative to the other, more flexed fingers. The level of retraction of the FDP generally denotes the force of the avulsion.

Leddy and Packer (1977) described *three types of FDP avulsion* based on where the avulsed tendon retracts. The treatment is based on the anatomy of the injury.

Classification of Jersey Finger Injury (Flexor Digitorum Profundus Avulsion)

TYPE I INJURY

The avulsed FDP tendon retracts into the palm (no bony fragment).
Both vincula are avulsed, thereby disrupting the blood supply.
Early reattachment at the distal phalanx (<10 days) gives the best results. After 2 weeks, tendon elasticity decreases, thus preventing the tendon from reaching the distal phalanx.

TYPE II INJURY

The most common type of FDP avulsion.
The avulsed tendon retracts to the point where the tendon is trapped by the FDS decussation and held by the vincula.
The vincula are intact.
The avulsion may or may not involve a bone fragment from the distal phalanx.
Successful surgical repair may be delayed up to 3 months, if needed, because of adequate tendon nutrition (vincula).
Early repair is the treatment of choice to avoid impaired DIP joint motion and tendon gliding.

Continued

Classification of Jersey Finger Injury (Flexor Digitorum Profundus Avulsion)   Continued

TYPE III INJURY

A large bony fragment (from the distal phalanx) prevents retraction past the level of the A1 pulley (middle phalanx).

The FDP blood supply remains intact, and the tendon is nourished within the sheath.

Treatment involves reduction and stabilization of the bony avulsion (suture anchors or pull-out wires).

Treatment

Treatment of FDP avulsion is primarily surgical. The success of treatment depends on the acuteness of the diagnosis, the rapidity of surgical intervention, and the level of retraction. Tendons with minimal retraction usually have significant bone fragments, which may be reattached in a bone-to-bone manner as late as 6 weeks. Tendons with a large amount of retraction often have no bone fragment along with disruption of the vascular supply (vinculum), thus making surgical repair more than 10 days after injury difficult because of retraction, the longer healing time of weaker non–bone-to-bone fixation, and limited blood supply to the repair.

Surgical salvage procedures for late repair include DIP joint arthrodesis, tenodesis, and staged tendon reconstructions.

REHABILITATION PROTOCOL   *After Surgical Repair of Jersey Finger*
Brotzman and Lee

WITH SECURE BONY REPAIR

0-10 Days

- Place the wrist in a DBS at 30 degrees flexion, the MCP joint at 70 degrees flexion, and the PIP and DIP joints in full extension
- Gentle passive DIP and PIP joint flexion to 40 degrees within the DBS
- Suture removal at 10 days

10 Days-3 Weeks

- Place the wrist in a removable DBS in neutral position and the MCP joint at 50 degrees flexion
- Gentle passive DIP joint flexion to 40 degrees, PIP joint flexion to 90 degrees within the DBS
- Active MCP joint flexion to 90 degrees
- Active finger extension of the IP joints within the DBS, 10 repetitions per hour

3-5 Weeks

- Discontinue the DBS (5-6 weeks)
- Active/assisted MCP/PIP/DIP joint ROM exercises
- Begin place-and-hold exercises

5 Weeks +

- Strengthening/power grasping
- Progress activities

REHABILITATION PROTOCOL: *After Surgical Repair of Jersey Finger*   *Continued*

WITH SECURE BONY REPAIR—cont'd

- Begin tendon gliding exercises
- Continue passive ROM, scar massage
- Begin active wrist flexion/extension
- Composite fist and flex wrist, then extend the wrist and fingers

WITH PURELY TENDINOUS REPAIR OR POOR BONY REPAIR

0-10 Days

- Place the wrist in a DBS at 30 degrees flexion and the MCP joint at 70 degrees flexion
- Gentle passive DIP and PIP joint flexion to 40 degrees within the DBS
- Suture removal at 10 days

10 Days-4 Weeks

- Place the wrist in a DBS at 30 degrees flexion and the MCP joint at 70 degrees flexion
- Gentle passive DIP joint flexion to 40 degrees, PIP joint flexion to 90 degrees within the DBS, passive MCP joint flexion to 90 degrees
- Active finger extension within the DBS
- Remove pull-out wire at 4 weeks

4-6 Weeks

- Place the wrist in a DBS in neutral position and the MCP joint at 50 degrees flexion
- Passive DIP joint flexion to 60 degrees, PIP joint to 110 degrees, MCP joint to 90 degrees
- Gentle place-and-hold composite flexion
- Active finger extension within the DBS
- Active wrist ROM out of the DBS

6-8 Weeks

- Discontinue daytime splinting; night splinting only
- Active MCP/PIP/DIP joint flexion and full extension

8-10 Weeks

- Discontinue night splinting
- Assisted MCP/PIP/DIP joint ROM
- Gentle strengthening

10 Weeks +

- More aggressive ROM
- Strengthening/power grasping
- Unrestricted activities

Extensor Tendon Injuries

ANATOMY

Extensor mechanism injuries are grouped into eight anatomic zones according to Kleinert and Verdan (1983). Odd-numbered zones overlie the joint levels, so zones 1, 3, 5, and 7 correspond to the DIP, PIP, MCP, and wrist joint regions, respectively (Figs. 1-17 and 1-18; Table 1-2).

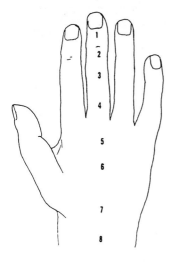

Figure 1–17 Extensor tendon zones.

Normal extensor mechanism activity relies on concerted function between the intrinsic muscles of the hand and the extrinsic extensor tendons. Even though PIP and DIP joint extension is normally controlled by the intrinsic muscles of the hand (interossei and lumbricals), the extrinsic tendons may provide satisfactory digital extension when MCP joint hyperextension is prevented.

An injury at one zone typically produces compensatory imbalance in neighboring zones; for example, a closed mallet finger deformity may be accompanied by a more striking secondary swan neck deformity at the PIP joint.

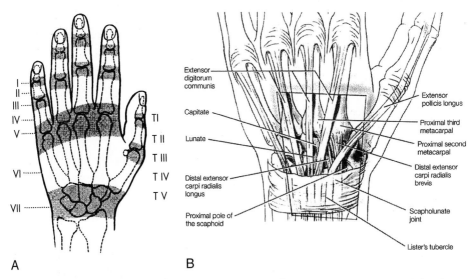

Figure 1–18 **A** and **B**, Extensor anatomy and extensor tendon zones. (From Kleinert HE, Schepel S, Gill T: Flexor tendon injuries. Surg Clin North Am 61:267, 1981.)

TABLE 1–2	Zones of Extensor Mechanism Injury	
Zone	Finger	Thumb
1	DIP joint	IP joint
2	Middle phalanx	Proximal phalanx
3	Apex PIP joint	MCP joint
4	Proximal phalanx	Metacarpal
5	Apex MCP joint	
6	Dorsal hand	
7	Dorsal retinaculum	Dorsal retinaculum
8	Distal forearm	Distal forearm

DIP, distal interphalangeal; IP, interphalangeal; MCP, metacarpophalangeal; PIP, proximal interphalangeal.

From Kleinert HE, Verdan C: Report of the committee on tendon injuries (International Federation of Societies for Surgery of the Hand). J Hand Surg [Am] 8:794, 1983.

Disruption of the terminal slip tendon allows the extensor mechanism to migrate proximally and exert a hyperextension force at the PIP joint by the central slip attachment. Thus, extensor tendon injuries cannot be considered simply static disorders.

EXTENSOR TENDON INJURIES IN ZONES 1 AND 2

These injuries **in children** should be considered Salter-Harris type II or III physeal injuries. Splinting of extremely small digits is difficult, and fixing the joint in full extension for 4 weeks produces satisfactory results. Open injuries are especially difficult to splint, and the DIP joint may be transfixed with a 22-gauge needle (also see the mallet finger section).

REHABILITATION PROTOCOL — *Treatment and Rehabilitation of Chronic Extensor Tendon Injuries in Zones 1 and 2*

TENODERMODESIS

Tenodermodesis is a simple procedure used in relatively young patients who are unable to accept a mallet finger disability. With the use of a local anesthetic, the DIP joint is fully extended and the redundant pseudotendon is excised so that the edges of the tendon coapt. A Kirschner wire may be used temporarily to fix the DIP joint in full extension.

3-5 Days

- Remove the postoperative splint and fit the DIP joint with an extension splint. A pin protection splint may be necessary if the pin is left exposed; however, some patients have their pins buried to allow unsplinted use of the finger.
- PIP joint exercises are begun to maintain full PIP joint motion.

5 Weeks

- Remove the Kirschner wire and begin active DIP motion with interval splinting.
- Continue nightly splinting for an additional 3 weeks.

Continued

REHABILITATION PROTOCOL: *Treatment and Rehabilitation of Chronic Extensor Tendon Injuries in Zones 1 and 2*   *Continued*

CENTRAL SLIP TENOTOMY (FOWLER)

With the use of a local anesthetic, the insertion of the central slip is sectioned at the point where it blends with the PIP joint dorsal capsule. The combined lateral band and the extrinsic contribution should be left undisturbed. Proximal migration of the dorsal apparatus improves the extensor force at the DIP joint. A 10- to 15-degree extensor lag at the PIP joint may occur.

0-2 Weeks

- The postoperative dressing maintains the PIP joint at 45 degrees of flexion and the DIP joint at 0 degrees.

2-4 Weeks

- Allow active DIP joint extension and flexion.
- Allow full extension of the PIP joint from 45 degrees of flexion.

4 Weeks

- Begin full finger motion exercises.

OBLIQUE RETINACULAR LIGAMENT

Reconstruction of the oblique retinacular ligament is done for correction of a chronic mallet finger deformity and secondary swan neck deformity. A free tendon graft, such as the palmaris longus tendon, is passed from the dorsal base of the distal phalanx and volar to the axis of the PIP joint. The graft is anchored to the contralateral side of the proximal phalanx at the fibro-osseous rim. Kirschner wires temporarily fix the DIP joint in full extension and the PIP joint in 10 to 15 degrees of flexion.

3 Weeks

- Remove the bulky postoperative dressing and sutures.
- Withdraw the PIP joint pin.
- Begin active flexion and extension exercises of the PIP joint.

4-5 Weeks

- Remove the DIP joint K-wire.
- Begin full active and passive PIP and DIP joint exercises.
- Supplement home exercises with a supervised program over the next 2-3 weeks to achieve full motion.
- Continue internal splinting of the DIP joint in full extension until 6 weeks after the operation.

EXTENSOR TENDON INJURIES IN ZONES 4, 5, AND 6

Normal function is usually possible after unilateral injuries to the dorsal apparatus, and splinting and immobilization are not recommended. Complete disruptions of the dorsal expansion and central slip lacerations are repaired.

REHABILITATION PROTOCOL — *After Surgical Repair of Extensor Tendon Injuries in Zones 4, 5, and 6*

0-2 WEEKS

- Allow active and passive PIP joint exercises; keep the MCP joint in full extension and the wrist in 40 degrees of extension.

2 WEEKS

- Remove the sutures and fit the patient with a removable splint.
- Keep the MCP joints in full extension and the wrist in neutral position.
- Continue PIP joint exercises and remove the splint for scar massage and hygienic purposes only.

4-6 WEEKS

- Begin MCP and wrist joint active flexion exercises with interval and night splinting and the wrist in neutral position.
- Over the next 2 weeks, begin active-assisted and gentle passive flexion exercises.

6 WEEKS

- Discontinue splinting unless an extensor lag develops at the MCP joint.
- Use passive wrist flexion exercises as necessary.

Zone 5 Extensor Tendon Subluxation

Zone 5 extensor tendon subluxations rarely respond to a splinting program. The affected MCP joint can be splinted in full extension and radial deviation for 4 weeks, with the understanding that surgical intervention will probably be required. Painful popping and swelling, in addition to a problematic extensor lag with radial deviation of the involved digit, usually require prompt reconstruction.

Acute injuries can be repaired directly, and chronic injuries can be reconstructed with local tissue. Most reconstructive procedures use portions of the juncturae tendinum or extensor tendon slips anchored to the deep transverse metacarpal ligament or looped around the lumbrical tendon.

REHABILITATION PROTOCOL — *After Surgical Repair of Zone 5 Extensor Tendon Subluxation*

2 WEEKS

- Remove the postoperative dressing and sutures.
- Keep the MCP joints in full extension.
- Fashion a removable volar short arm splint to maintain the operated finger MCP joint in full extension and radial deviation.
- Allow periodic splint removal for hygienic purposes and scar massage.
- Allow full PIP and DIP joint motion.

Continued

REHABILITATION PROTOCOL: *After Surgical Repair of Zone 5 Extensor Tendon*
Subluxation   *Continued*

4 WEEKS

- Begin MCP joint active and active-assisted exercises hourly with interval daily and full-time night splinting.
- At week 5, begin gentle passive MCP joint motion if necessary to gain full MCP joint flexion.

6 WEEKS

- Discontinue splinting during the day and allow full activity.

EXTENSOR TENDON INJURIES IN ZONES 7 AND 8

Extensor tendon injuries in zones 7 and 8 usually result from lacerations, but attritional ruptures secondary to remote distal radial fractures and rheumatoid synovitis may occur at the wrist level. These injuries may require tendon transfers, free tendon grafts, or side-by-side transfers rather than direct repair. The splinting program for these injuries, however, is identical to that for penetrating trauma.

Repairs performed 3 weeks or more after the injury may weaken the extensor pollicis longus (EPL) muscle sufficiently for electrical stimulation to become necessary for tendon glide. The EPL is selectively strengthened by thumb retropulsion exercises performed against resistance with the palm held on a flat surface.

REHABILITATION PROTOCOL   *After Surgical Repair of Extensor Tendon Injuries in Zones 7 and 8*

0-2 WEEKS

- Maintain the wrist in 30 to 40 degrees of extension with a postoperative splint.
- Encourage hand elevation and full PIP and DIP joint motion to reduce swelling and edema.
- Treat any significant swelling by loosening the dressing and elevating the extremity.

2-4 WEEKS

- At 2 weeks, remove the postoperative dressing and sutures.
- Fashion a volar splint to keep the wrist in 20 degrees of extension and the MCP joints of the affected finger or fingers in full extension.
- Continue full PIP and DIP joint motion exercises and initiate scar massage to improve skin-tendon glide during the next 2 weeks.

4-6 WEEKS

- Begin hourly wrist and MCP joint exercises, with interval and nightly splinting over the next 2 weeks.
- From week 4 to 5, hold the wrist in extension during the MCP joint flexion exercises and extend the MCP joints during the wrist flexion exercises.

REHABILITATION PROTOCOL: *After Surgical Repair of Extensor Tendon Injuries in Zones 7 and 8*   *Continued*

4-6 WEEKS—cont'd

- Composite wrist and finger flexion from the fifth week forward. An MCP joint extension lag of more than 10 to 20 degrees requires interval daily splinting.
- The splinting program can be discontinued at 6 weeks.

6-7 WEEKS

- Begin gentle passive ROM.
- Begin resistive extension exercises.

REHABILITATION PROTOCOL   *After Repair of an Extensor Pollicis Longus Laceration (Thumb)*

After repair of thumb extensor tendon lacerations, regardless of the zone of injury, apply a thumb spica splint with the wrist in 30 degrees of extension and the thumb in 40 degrees of radial abduction with full retroposition.

0-2 WEEKS

- Allow activity as comfortable in the postoperative splint.
- Edema control measures include elevation and motion exercises of the uninvolved digits.

2-4 WEEKS

- At 2 weeks after repair, remove the splint and sutures. Refit a thumb spica splint with the wrist and thumb positioned to minimize tension at the repair site as before.
- Fit a removable splint for reliable patients and permit scar massage.
- The vocational interests of some patients are best suited with a thumb spica cast.
- Continue edema control measures.

4-6 WEEKS

- Fit a removable thumb spica splint for night use and interval daily splinting between exercises.
- During the next 2 weeks, the splint is removed for hourly wrist and thumb exercises.
- Between weeks 4 and 5, thumb IP, MCP, and CMC joint flexion and extension exercises should be done with the wrist held in extension.
- Alternately, wrist flexion and extension motion is regained with the thumb extension.
- After the fifth week, composite wrist and thumb exercises are performed concomitantly.

6 WEEKS

- Discontinue the splinting program unless an extensor lag develops.
- Treat an extensor lag at the IP joint of more than 10 degrees with intermittent IP extension splinting in addition to nightly thumb spica splinting.
- Problematic MCP and CMC joint extension lag requires intermittent thumb spica splinting during the day and night for an additional 2 weeks or until acceptable results are obtained.
- It may be necessary to continue edema control measures for 8 weeks or longer.
- Use taping to gain full composite thumb flexion.
- Use electrical stimulation for lack of extensor pull-through.

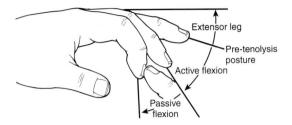

Figure 1–19 A passive supple digit with an **extensor lag** is an indication for possible extensor tenolysis. (Adapted from Strickland JW: The Hand: Master Techniques in Orthopaedic Surgery. Philadelphia, Lippincott-Raven, 1998.)

EXTENSOR TENOLYSIS

Indications

- Digital active or passive motion has reached a plateau after injury.
- Restricted isolated or composite active or passive flexion of the PIP or DIP joint
- Otherwise passively supple digit that exhibits an extensor lag (Fig. 1-19)

Treatment

Surgical intervention for extension contractures frequently follows an extensive period of presurgical therapy. Patients who have been active in their rehabilitation are more apt to appreciate that an early and postsurgical program is vital to their final outcome. Presurgical patient counseling should always be attempted to delineate the immediate postsurgical tenolysis program. The quality of the extensor tendon, bone, and joint encountered at surgery may alter the intended program, and the surgeon relays this information to the therapist and the patient. Ideally, the surgical procedures are performed with the patient under local anesthesia or awakened from general anesthesia near the end of the procedure. The patient can then see the gains achieved, and the surgeon can evaluate active motion, tendon glide, and the need for additional releases. Unusual circumstances may be well served by having the therapist observe the operative procedure.

Frequently, MCP and PIP joint capsular and ligament releases are necessary to obtain the desired joint motion. Complete collateral ligament resection may be required, and special attention may be necessary in the early postoperative period for resultant instability.

REHABILITATION PROTOCOL   *After Extensor Tenolysis*

0-24 HOURS

- Apply a light compressive postoperative dressing to allow as much digital motion as possible. Anticipate bleeding through the dressing, and implement exercises hourly in 10-minute sessions to achieve as much of the motion noted intraoperatively as possible.

1 DAY-4 WEEKS

- Remove the surgical dressings and drains at the first therapy visit. Apply light compressive sterile dressings.
- Edema control measures are critical at this stage.

REHABILITATION PROTOCOL: *After Extensor Tenolysis*   *Continued*

1 DAY-4 WEEKS—cont'd

- Continue active and passive ROM exercises hourly for 10- to 15-minute sessions. Poor IP joint flexion during the first session is an indication for flexor FES. Extensor FES should be used initially with the wrist, MCP, PIP, and DIP joints passively extended to promote maximal proximal tendon excursion. After several stimulations in this position, place the wrist, MCP, and PIP joints in more flexion and continue FES.
- Remove the sutures at 2 weeks; dynamic flexion splints and taping may be required.
- Use splints to keep the joint in question in full extension between exercises and at night for the first 4 weeks. Extensor lags of 5 to 10 degrees are acceptable and are not indications to continue splint wear after this period.

4-6 WEEKS

- Continue hourly exercise sessions during the day for 10-minute sessions. Emphasis is on achieving MCP and IP joint flexion.
- Continue passive motion with greater emphasis during this period, especially for the MCP and IP joints.
- Continue extension night splinting until the sixth week.

6 WEEKS

- Encourage the patient to resume normal activity.
- Edema control measures may be required. Intermittent Coban wrapping of the digits may be useful in conjunction with an oral anti-inflammatory agent.
- Banana splints (foam cylindrical digital sheaths) can also be effective for edema control.
  The therapist must have acquired some critical information regarding the patient's tenolysis. Specific therapeutic program and anticipated outcomes depend on the following:
- The quality of the tendon or tendons undergoing tenolysis.
- The condition of the joint that the tendon acts about.
- The stability of the joint that the tendon acts about.
- The joint motions achieved during the surgical procedure. Passive motions are easily achieved; however, active motions in both extension and flexion are even more beneficial for meeting patient therapy goals.
  Achieving maximal MCP and PIP joint flexion during the first 3 weeks is essential. Significant gains after this period are uncommon.

Extensive tenolyses may require analgesic dosing before and during therapy sessions. Indwelling catheters may also be needed for the instillation of local anesthetics for this purpose.

MALLET FINGER (EXTENSOR INJURY—ZONE 1)

Background

Avulsion of the extensor tendon from its distal insertion at the dorsum of the DIP joint produces an **extensor lag** at the DIP joint. The tendon avulsion may occur with or without avulsion of a bony fragment from the dorsum of the distal phalanx. This condition is termed a *mallet finger of bony origin* or a *mallet finger of tendinous origin*, respectively (Figs. 1-20 and 1-21). The hallmark finding of a mallet finger is a flexed or dropped posture of the DIP joint (Fig. 1-22) and an inability to actively extend or straighten the DIP joint. The mechanism is typically forced flexion of the fingertip, often from the impact of a thrown ball.

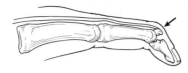

Figure 1–20 Mallet finger of bony origin with detachment of the extensor mechanism.

Classification of Mallet Finger

Doyle (1993) described four types of mallet injury:
- Type I—extensor tendon avulsion from the distal phalanx
- Type II—laceration of the extensor tendon
- Type III—deep avulsion injuring the skin and tendon
- Type IV—fracture of the distal phalanx with three subtypes:
  - Type IV A—transepiphyseal fracture in a child
  - Type IV B—less than half of the articular surface of the joint involved with no subluxation
  - Type IV C—more than half of the articular surface involved and may include volar subluxation

Treatment

Abound and Brown (1968) found that several factors are likely to lead to a **poor prognosis** after mallet finger injury:
- Age older than 60 years
- Delay in treatment of more than 4 weeks

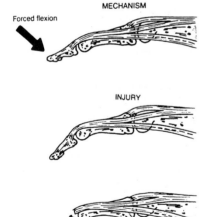

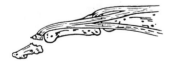

Figure 1–21 **A**, Stretching of the common extensor mechanism. **B**, Mallet finger of tendinous origin (complete disruption of the extensor tendon). **C**, Mallet finger of bony origin. (From DeLee J, Drez D [eds]: Orthopaedic Sports Medicine. Philadelphia, WB Saunders, 1994, p 1011.)

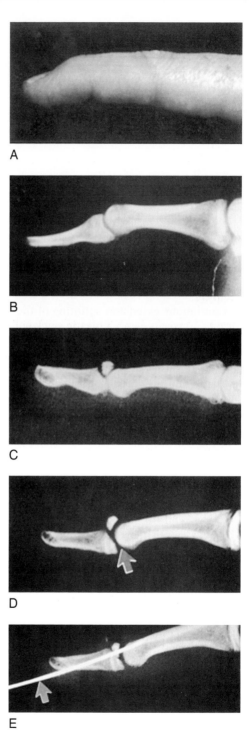

Figure 1–22 **A**, Mild mallet finger deformity (extensor lag at the distal interphalangeal [DIP] joint with an inability to extend the DIP joint) seen as a flexed DIP joint. It is important to treat this acute injury before further tearing of the extensor tendon and stretching of new scar tissue lead to greater deformity. **B**, No bony injury is seen on the radiograph. After 6 weeks in a splint, the finger was nearly normal. **C**, Note that the palmar fragment is concentrically reduced with the middle phalanx. Despite a large dorsal fragment, which makes up more than a third of the articular surface, continuous splinting for 8 weeks resulted in pain-free function with only a trivial decrease in range of motion. **D**, A mallet finger with a subluxated palmar fragment may need surgical reduction and internal fixation. The *arrow* points to loss of concentricity of the joint surfaces. **E**, Intraoperative radiograph showing reduction and pinning (*arrow*) through a dorsal-ulnar approach without sectioning of the extensor tendon. Note the restored concentricity of the joint surface. (From Vetter WL: How I manage mallet finger. Physician Sports Med 17[3]:17-24, 1989.)

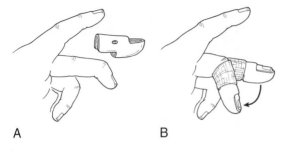

Figure 1–23 **A**, Use of a stack splint at the distal interphalangeal (DIP) joint for closed treatment of a mallet finger (note the extension lag). The splint is held in place with paper or adhesive tape. **B**, Active range-of-motion exercises of the proximal interphalangeal joint to keep the joint from stiffening during DIP joint immobilization. (Adapted from Regional Review Course in Hand Surgery. Memphis, TN, American Society of Surgery of the Hand, 1991.)

- Initial extensor lag of more than 50 degrees
- Too short a period of immobilization (<4 weeks)
- Short, stubby fingers
- Peripheral vascular disease or associated arthritis

The results of mallet finger treatment are not universally good by any method of treatment.

Continuous extension splinting of the DIP joint, with the PIP joint left free for 6 to 10 weeks (with a plastic stack splint), is the typical treatment of mallet fingers of tendinous origin (Fig. 1-23). If no extensor lag is present at 6 weeks, night splinting is used for 3 weeks and splinting during sports activities for an additional 6 weeks.

The patient must work on active ROM of the MCP and PIP joints to avoid stiffening of these uninvolved joints. At no point during the healing process is the DIP joint allowed to drop into flexion, or the treatment must be repeated from the beginning. During skin care or washing, the finger must be held continuously in extension with the other hand while the splint is off.

Treatment of Mallet Finger (Fig. 1-24)

TYPE I: TENDINOUS AVULSION

- Continuous extension splinting of the DIP joint (stack splint) for 4 weeks
- Bedtime splinting for another 6 weeks
- Sports splinting for another 6 weeks
- Active ROM of the MCP and PIP joints

TYPE II: LACERATION OF THE EXTENSOR TENDON

- Surgical repair of the tendon laceration
- See type I protocol

TYPE III: DEEP AVULSION OF THE SKIN AND TENDON

- Skin grafting
- Surgical repair of the tendon laceration
- See type I protocol

Treatment of Mallet Finger   Continued

TYPE III: DEEP AVULSION OF THE SKIN AND TENDON—cont'd

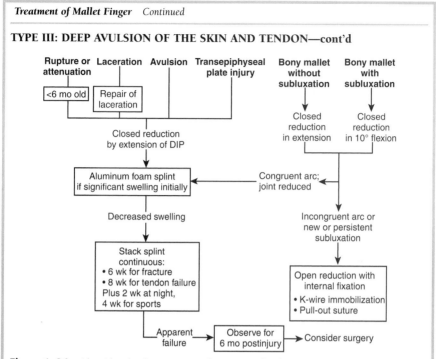

Figure 1–24   Algorithm for the treatment of various mallet finger conditions. DIP, distal interphalangeal. (Adapted from Damron TA, Lange RW, Engber WD: Mallet fingers: A review and treatment algorithm. Int J Orthop Trauma 1:105, 1991.)

TYPE IV: BONY ORIGIN

- Type IV A—reduction of the fracture and splinting for 6 weeks, night splinting for 6 weeks
- Type IV B—reduction and splinting for 6 weeks, night splinting for 6 weeks
- Type IV C—(controversial) splinting versus open reduction and internal fixation (ORIF) with splinting versus percutaneous pinning with splinting for 6 weeks

Fractures and Dislocations of the Hand

STABILITY WITH REQUIRED REHABILITATION MOTION

Fractures and dislocations involving the hand are classified as stable or unstable injuries to determine the appropriate treatment. *Stable* fractures are those that would not displace if some degree of early digital motion were allowed. *Unstable* fractures are those that displace to an unacceptable degree if early digital motion is allowed. Although some unstable fractures can be converted to stable fractures with closed reduction, it is very difficult to predict which of these fractures will maintain their stability throughout the early treatment phase. For this reason, *most unstable fractures should undergo closed reduction and percutaneous pinning or ORIF to allow early protected digital motion and thus prevent stiffness.*

Fractures that often require surgical intervention also include
- Open fractures
- Comminuted displaced fractures
- Fractures associated with joint dislocation or subluxation
- Displaced spiral fractures
- Displaced intra-articular fractures, especially around the PIP joint
- Fractures in which there is loss of bone
- Multiple fractures

Because of the hand's propensity to quickly form a permanently stiffening scar, unstable fractures must be surgically converted to stable fractures (e.g., by pinning) to allow early ROM exercises. Failure to initiate early ROM will result in a stiff hand with poor function regardless of bony healing.

METACARPAL AND PHALANGEAL FRACTURES

Nondisplaced Metacarpal Fractures

Nondisplaced metacarpal fractures are stable injuries that are treated with the application of an anterior-posterior splint in the **position of function**: the wrist in 30 to 60 degrees of extension, the MCP joints in 70 degrees of flexion, and the IP joints in 0 to 10 degrees of flexion. In this position, the important ligaments of the wrist and hand are maintained in maximal tension to prevent contractures (Fig. 1-25).

Allowing early PIP and DIP joint motion is essential. Motion prevents adhesions between the tendons and the underlying fracture and controls edema. The dorsal fiberglass splint should extend from below the elbow to the fingertips of all the **involved** digits and one adjacent digit. The anterior splint should extend from below the elbow to the distal aspect of the proximal phalanx (Fig. 1-26A) to allow the patient to resume PIP and DIP joint active flexion and extension exercises immediately (see Fig. 1-26B).

Comminuted Phalangeal Fractures

Comminuted phalangeal fractures, especially those that involve diaphyseal segments with thick cortices, may be slow to heal and could require fixation for up to 6 weeks (Fig. 1-27).

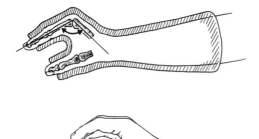

Figure 1–25 The position of immobilization of the hand involves splinting the wrist in approximately 30 degrees of extension, the metacarpophalangeal joints in 60 to 80 degrees of flexion, and the interphalangeal joints in full extension. (From DeLee J, Drez D [eds]: Orthopaedic Sports Medicine. Philadelphia, WB Saunders, 1994.)

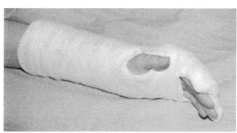

A

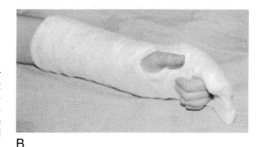

B

Figure 1–26 **A**, Anterior and posterior fiberglass splints typically used to treat metacarpal and proximal phalangeal fractures. **B**, Proximal and distal interphalangeal joint flexion and extension are allowed. The anterior splint should extend 2 cm distal to the level of the fracture.

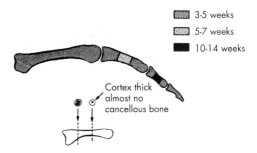

3-5 weeks
5-7 weeks
10-14 weeks

Figure 1–27 The time required for fracture healing varies, depending on the ratio of cortical to cancellous bone at the fracture site. Healing is slowest where the ratio of cortical to cancellous bone is highest. (Redrawn from Wilson RE, Carter MS: Management of hand fractures. In Hunter JM, Schneider LH, Mackin EJ, Callahan AD [eds]: Rehabilitation of the Hand. St Louis, CV Mosby, 1990, p 290.)

Cortex thick
almost no
cancellous bone

REHABILITATION PROTOCOL *After Metacarpal or Phalangeal Fracture*

0-4 WEEKS

- Before pin removal, begin active ROM exercises while the therapist supports the fracture site.

4-6 WEEKS

- Active and active-assisted intrinsic stretching exercises (i.e., simultaneous MCP joint extension and IP joint flexion) are recommended.
- Prevent PIP joint flexion contractures by ensuring that the initial splint immobilizes the PIP joint in an almost neutral position.

> **REHABILITATION PROTOCOL:** *After Metacarpal or Phalangeal Fracture* *Continued*
>
> **4-6 WEEKS—cont'd**
>
>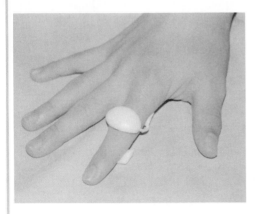
>
> **Figure 1–28** Dynamic proximal interphalangeal joint extension splint (LMB, or Louise M. Barbour).
>
> - When the fracture is considered solid on radiographs, a dynamic splinting program can be started. The LMB dynamic splint and the Capner splint are quite useful. They should be worn for 2-hour increments, 6 to 12 hours a day (Fig. 1-28), and alternated with dynamic flexion strapping (Fig. 1-29).
> - Therapy may be prolonged for up to 3 to 6 months after injury.
>
>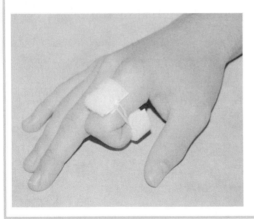
>
> **Figure 1–29** Flexion strap used to help regain proximal and distal interphalangeal joint motion.

PROXIMAL INTERPHALANGEAL JOINT INJURIES (FIG. 1-30; TABLE 1-3)

Volar PIP joint dislocations are less common than dorsal dislocations and are often difficult to reduce by closed techniques because of entrapment of the lateral bands around the flare of the proximal phalangeal head. If not treated properly, these injuries may result in a boutonnière deformity (combined PIP joint flexion and DIP joint extension contracture). Usually, the joint is stable after closed or open reduction;

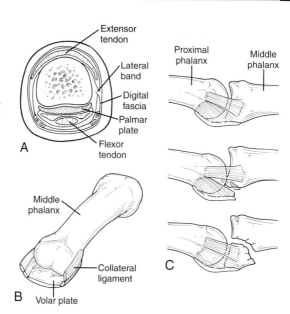

Figure 1–30 **A**, The skeleton of the proximal phalanx is surrounded by gliding structures that are crucial for digital function. **B**, The proximal interphalangeal (PIP) joint is stabilized by a "three-dimensional ligament-box complex" consisting of collateral ligaments and a thick volar or palmar plate. **C**, PIP joint in its normal anatomy (*top*). A tear in the three-dimensional ligament-box complex (*middle*) results in a stable injury. An unstable PIP fracture-dislocation (*bottom*) occurs when stabilizers remain attached to a fragment that contains more than 40% of the articular surface.

TABLE 1–3	Managing Proximal Interphalangeal Joint Injuries of the Hand	
Injury	**Clinical Manifestation or Special Considerations**	**Treatment**
Sprain	Stable joint with active and passive motion; negative radiographs; pain and swelling only	Buddy tape for comfort; begin early ROM exercises, ice, NSAIDs
Open dislocation	Dislocated exposed joint	Irrigation, débridement, and antibiotics; treat as for any open fracture or dislocation
Dorsal PIP Dislocation		
Type 1	Hyperextension, volar plate avulsion, minor collateral ligament tear	Reduction; very brief immobilization, 3-5 days, followed by ROM exercises with buddy taping and close radiographic follow-up
Type 2	Dorsal dislocation, volar plate avulsion, major collateral ligament tear	Same as type 1
Type 3	Stable fracture-dislocation: <40% of the articular arc on the fracture fragment	Extension block splint; *refer to hand surgeon*

Continued

TABLE 1–3	Managing Proximal Interphalangeal Joint Injuries of the Hand—cont'd	

Injury	Clinical Manifestation or Special Considerations	Treatment
Dorsal PIP Dislocation—cont'd		
	Unstable fracture dislocation: >40% of the articular arc on the fracture fragment	Extension block splint; *open reduction with internal fixation if closed treatment impossible; refer to hand surgeon*
Lateral dislocation	Secondary to collateral ligament injury and avulsion and/or rupture of the volar plate; angulation >20 degrees indicates complete rupture	Same as dorsal dislocation types 1 and 2 above if the joint is stable and congruous through active ROM
Volar PIP Dislocation		
Straight volar dislocation	Proximal condyle causes significant injury to the central extensor slip (may reduce easily, but the extensor tendon may be seriously injured; requires careful examination)	*Refer to a hand surgeon* experienced in these rare injuries; closed reduction and traction with the metatarsophalangeal and PIP joints flexed and the wrist extended; full-extension immobilization of the PIP joint if postreduction radiographs show no subluxation; if closed reduction is not achieved or subluxation persists, surgery recommended
Ulnar or radial volar displacement	Condyle often buttonholes through the central slip and lateral band; reduction often extremely difficult	Same as straight volar PIP dislocation (above)

NSAIDs, nonsteroidal anti-inflammatory drugs; PIP, proximal interphalangeal; ROM, range of motion.
From Laimore JR, Engber WD: Serious, but often subtle finger injuries. Physician Sports Med 26(6):226, 1998.

however, static PIP joint extension splinting is recommended for 6 weeks to allow healing of the central slip.

Avulsion fractures involving the dorsal margin of the middle phalanx occur at the insertion of the central slip. These fractures may be treated by closed technique; however, if the fragment is displaced more than 2 mm proximally with the finger splinted in extension, ORIF of the fragment is indicated.

REHABILITATION PROTOCOL	*After Volar Proximal Interphalangeal Joint Dislocation or Avulsion Fracture*

AFTER CLOSED REDUCTION

- An extension gutter splint is fitted for continuous wear with the PIP joint in neutral position.
- The patient should perform active and passive ROM exercises of the MCP and DIP joints approximately six times a day.
- PIP joint motion is not allowed for 6 weeks.
- Begin active ROM exercises at 6 weeks in conjunction with intermittent daytime splinting and continuous night splinting for an additional 2 weeks.

AFTER ORIF

- The transarticular pin is removed between 2 and 4 weeks after the wound has healed.
- Continuous splinting in an extension gutter splint is continued for a total of 6 weeks.
- The remainder of the protocol is similar to that after closed reduction.

  Extension splinting is continued as long as an extensor lag is present, and passive flexion exercises are avoided as long as an extension lag of 30 degrees or more is present.

Dorsal fracture-dislocations of the PIP joint are much more common than volar dislocations. If less than 50% of the articular surface is involved, these injuries are usually stable after closed reduction and protective splinting.

REHABILITATION PROTOCOL	*After Dorsal Fracture-Dislocation of the Proximal Interphalangeal Joint*

- If the injury is believed to be stable after closed reduction, a DBS is applied with the PIP joint in 30 degrees of flexion. This allows full flexion but prevents the terminal 30 degrees of extension.
- After 3 weeks, the DBS is adjusted at weekly intervals to increase PIP joint extension by about 10 degrees each week.
- The splint should be in neutral position by the sixth week, then discontinued.
- An active ROM program is begun, and dynamic extension splinting is used as needed.
- Progressive strengthening exercises are begun at 6 weeks.

Dorsal fracture-dislocations involving more than 40% of the articular surface may be unstable, even with the digit in flexion, and may require surgical intervention. The Eaton volar plate advancement is probably the most common procedure used (Fig. 1-31). The fracture fragments are excised, and the volar plate is advanced into the remaining portion of the middle phalanx. The PIP joint is usually pinned in 30 degrees of flexion.

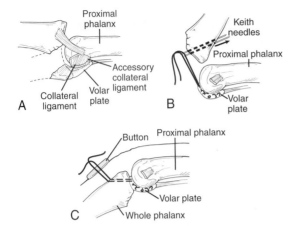

Figure 1–31 **A**, Pathology of injury demonstrating loss of collateral ligament support to the joint and producing marked instability. **Eaton volar plate arthroplasty** is commonly used when more than 40% comminution or impaction of the inferior aspect of the middle phalanx of the proximal interphalangeal (PIP) joint is present. **B**, Sutures are passed through the lateral margins of the defect and exit dorsally. The comminuted fragment has been excised, and the volar plate is being advanced. **C**, Sutures are tied over a padded button to draw the volar plate into the defect and simultaneously reduce the PIP joint. (Adapted from Strickland JW: The Hand: Master Techniques in Orthopaedic Surgery. Philadelphia, Lippincott-Raven, 1999.)

REHABILITATION PROTOCOL	*After Dorsal Fracture-Dislocation of the Proximal Interphalangeal Joint Involving More Than 40% of the Articular Surface*

- At 3 weeks after surgery, the pin is removed from the PIP joint and a DBS is fitted with the PIP joint in 30 degrees of flexion for continuous wear.
- Active and active-assisted ROM exercises are begun within the restraints of the DBS.
- At 5 weeks, the DBS is discontinued and active and passive extension exercises are continued.
- At 6 weeks, dynamic extension splinting may be necessary if full passive extension has not been regained.

Flexion contractures are not uncommon after this procedure. Agee (1987) described the use of external fixation combined with rubber bands to allow early active ROM of the PIP joint in unstable fracture-dislocations while maintaining reduction. The bulky hand dressing is removed 3 to 5 days after surgery, and active ROM exercises are carried out for 10-minute sessions every 2 hours. Pins should be cleansed twice daily with cotton swabs and hydrogen peroxide and the base of the pin protected with gauze. The external fixator can be removed between 3 and 6 weeks, at which time an unrestricted active and passive ROM exercise program is started.

Dorsal dislocations of the PIP joint without associated fractures are usually stable after closed reduction. Stability is tested after reduction under digital block, and if the joint is believed to be stable, buddy taping (Fig. 1-32; Table 1-4) for 3 to 6 weeks, early active ROM exercises, and edema control are necessary. If instability is present with passive extension of the joint, a DBS similar to that used for fracture-dislocations should be applied.

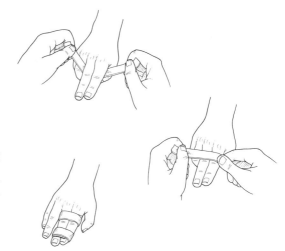

Figure 1–32 Fingers are taped after a dislocation, fracture, or sprain. "Buddy taping" of the injured finger to the adjacent finger provides the best support for the joint. (Adapted from Idler RS: Treatment of common hand injuries. J Musculoskel Med 17:73, 1996.)

BASE OF THUMB FRACTURES

Intra-articular fractures involving the base of the thumb metacarpal are classified as either *Bennett fractures* (if a single volar ulnar fragment exists) or *Rolando fractures* (if there is a T-condylar fracture pattern). These fractures often displace because of the proximal pull of the abductor pollicis longus on the base of the proximal thumb metacarpal.

Nondisplaced Bennett fractures are treated in a short arm thumb spica cast, which can be removed at 6 weeks if the fracture has healed clinically. Active and gentle passive ROM exercises are begun. At that time the patient is also fitted with a removable thumb spica splint. This splint should be used between exercise sessions and at night for an additional 2 weeks. Strengthening exercises using silicone putty are then started. The patient generally returns to normal activity between 10 and 12 weeks. If there is persistent joint subluxation after the application of a short arm cast with the thumb positioned in palmar and radial abduction, closed reduction plus percutaneous pinning is carried out. After pinning, the thumb is placed in a thumb spica splint and protected for 6 weeks. After the pin is removed, therapy progresses as described for nondisplaced fractures.

Rolando fractures have a poor prognosis. The choice of treatment usually depends on the severity of comminution and the degree of displacement. If large fragments are present with displacement, ORIF with Kirschner wires or a mini-fragment plate is used. If severe comminution is present, manual molding in palmar abduction and immobilization in a thumb spica cast for 3 to 4 weeks are recommended. After stable internal fixation, motion can be started at 6 weeks in a manner similar to that for Bennett fractures.

TABLE 1–4	Materials for Taping an Injured Finger
1-inch white zinc oxide tape or elastic tape	
Tape-adherent spray	

Fifth Metacarpal Neck Fracture (Boxer's Fracture)

Steven J. Meyers, MD • Michael L. Lee, MD

Background

Metacarpal neck fractures are among the most common fractures in the hand. Fracture of the fifth metacarpal is by far the most frequent and has been termed a *boxer's fracture* because the usual mechanism is a glancing punch that does not land on the stronger second and third metacarpals.

Clinical History and Examination

Patients usually have pain, swelling, and loss of motion about the MCP joint. Occasionally, a rotational deformity is present. Careful examination should be performed to ensure that there is no malrotation of the finger when the patient makes a fist (Fig. 1-33), no significant prominence of the distal fragment (palmarly displaced) in the palm, and no extensor lag of the involved finger.

Radiographic Examination

On a lateral radiograph, the angle of the metacarpal fracture is determined by drawing lines down the shafts of the metacarpal and measuring the resultant angle with a goniometer.

Treatment

Treatment is based on the degree of displacement, as measured on a true lateral radiograph of the hand (Fig. 1-34). Metacarpal neck fractures are usually impacted and angulated, with the distal fragment displacing palmarly because of the pull of the

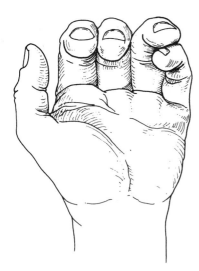

Figure 1–33   Malrotation of a fracture (and thus the finger).

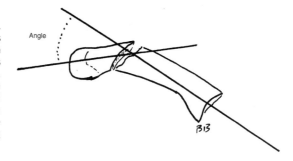

Figure 1–34 "Boxer's" fracture. On a lateral radiograph, a line is drawn down the middle of each fracture fragment and the angles are measured with a goniometer. More than 40 degrees of angulation of the more mobile fifth metacarpal neck fracture requires reduction (maneuver of Jahss). If the fracture is unstable, percutaneous pinning is often required.

intrinsic muscles. Excessive angulation results in loss of the MCP joint knuckle and may cause the palmar metacarpal head to be prominent in the palm during activities. *Only about 10 degrees of angulation can be accepted in second and third metacarpal neck fractures, whereas up to 30 degrees in the fourth metacarpal and 50 degrees in the fifth metacarpal can be accepted because of greater mobility in the fourth and fifth CMC joints* (DeLee and Drez 2003).

If the displacement is unacceptable, closed reduction can be attempted with wrist block anesthesia via the maneuver credited to Jahss (1938), in which the proximal phalanx is flexed to 90 degrees and used to apply a dorsally directed force to the metacarpal head (Fig. 1-35). The hand is then splinted in an ulnar gutter splint for about 3 weeks with the MCP joint at 80 degrees of flexion, the PIP joint straight, and the DIP joint free (Fig. 1-36).

Rapid mobilization of the fingers is required to avoid scarring, adhesions, and stiffness unrelated to the fracture itself but rather to the propensity of an immobilized hand to quickly stiffen.

Operative treatment of boxer's fracture is indicated if
- Fracture alignment remains unacceptable (>50 degrees displacement).
- Late redisplacement occurs in a previously reduced fracture.
- There is any malrotation of the finger.

Operative fixation usually involves percutaneous pinning of the fracture, but ORIF may be required.

Fractures stabilized operatively still require splinting for stability and ROM exercise.

Figure 1–35 Maneuver of Jahss. **A**, The proximal interphalangeal joint is flexed 90 degrees, and the examiner stabilizes the metacarpal proximal to the neck fracture and then pushes the finger to dorsally displace the volar-angulated boxer's fracture to "straight." **B**, The splint is molded in reduced position with the ulnar gutter in the position of function. (Adapted from Regional Review Course in Hand Surgery. Rosemont, IL, American Society for Surgery of the Hand, 1991.)

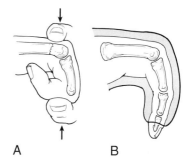

A   B

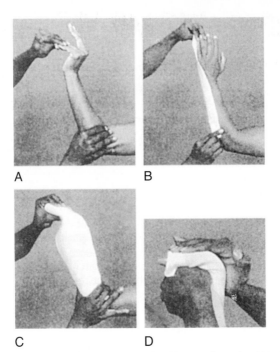

A   B

C   D

Figure 1–36 **A**, For application of a gutter splint, the patient's elbow should be flexed 90 degrees and the wrist dorsiflexed 10 to 15 degrees. Only the fourth and fifth fingers are included in the splint. **B**, The splint should extend from the end of the fifth finger to within two to four finger-breadths of the antecubital space. **C**, The splinting material should be wide enough to cover half the circumference of the patient's wrist. The moistened splint is molded to the patient's hand and wrist and secured with an elastic wrap. Wrapping should be done in a distal-to-proximal direction so that edema can be pushed up and out of the extremity. Padding (Webril) is wrapped around the fingers, wrist, and forearm under the splint to avoid skin pressure. **D**, After the splint has been secured, the hand must be positioned properly: 10 to 15 degrees of dorsiflexion at the wrist, as close as possible to 90 degrees of dorsiflexion at the metacarpophalangeal joints, and 10 to 15 degrees of flexion at the proximal interphalangeal joints. (From Petrizzi MJ: Making an ulnar gutter splint for a boxer's fracture. Physician Sports Med 27[1]:111, 1999.)

REHABILITATION PROTOCOL	*After a Boxer's Fracture* Brotzman and Lee

AFTER CLOSED TREATMENT (NONOPERATIVE)

0-1 Week

- Elevation of the hand, icing, ulnar gutter splint with the MCP joints at 80 degrees flexion; the DIP joints are free
- Active motion of the nonimmobilized thumb, index finger, and long finger
- Radiographs at 6-8 days (three views of the hand)

1-2 Weeks

- Continue active finger ROM of the nonimmobilized joints
- Radiographs at 2 weeks

2-3 Weeks

- Remove the ulnar gutter splint at 3 weeks and x-ray
- Apply a short arm cast (that allows active motion of the fourth and fifth DIP, PIP, and MCP joints) for 3 more weeks

---

REHABILITATION PROTOCOL: *After a Boxer's Fracture*   *Continued*

AFTER CLOSED TREATMENT (NONOPERATIVE)—cont'd

3-5 Weeks

- Active/gentle-assisted ROM of the fourth and fifth fingers
- Passive extension

5-7 Weeks

- Active/aggressive-assisted/passive ROM of the fourth and fifth fingers
- Strengthening
- Unrestricted activities
- Radiographs at 6 weeks

AFTER OPERATIVE TREATMENT (K-WIRE, ORIF)

0-1.5 Weeks

- Elevate, ice
- Splinted with the PIP joints and DIP joints *free*
- Gentle active ROM of the PIP and DIP joints
- Active ROM of the uninvolved fingers and thumb
- Remove sutures at 10-14 days if ORIF performed

1.5-3 Weeks

- Continue splinting with the PIP and DIP joints free
- Gentle active ROM of the PIP and DIP joints
- Active ROM of the uninvolved fingers and thumb
- Remove the splint at 3 weeks
- Remove the pins at 3-6 weeks

3-5 Weeks

- Buddy taping
- Active/assisted/passive ROM of the fourth and fifth fingers
- Passive extension of all joints

5-7 Weeks

- Active/aggressive-assisted/passive ROM of the fourth and fifth fingers
- Strengthening
- Unrestricted activities

Injuries to the Ulnar Collateral Ligament of the Thumb Metacarpophalangeal Joint (Skier's Thumb)

S. Brent Brotzman, MD

Background

The classic chronic **"gamekeeper's thumb"** was first described in Scottish gamekeepers. **"Skier's thumb"** was coined by Schultz, Brown, and Fox in 1973, with skiing being

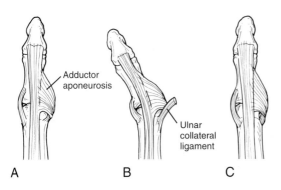

Figure 1–37 **A**, In the thumb metacarpophalangeal joint, the adductor aponeurosis covers the ulnar collateral ligament. **B**, When thumb angulation is sufficient, the ligament can rupture and displace. **C**, If the ligament becomes trapped outside the aponeurosis, a Stener lesion results. A trapped ligament that is not surgically repaired leads to chronic instability. (Adapted from Lairmore JR, Engber WD: Serious, but often subtle, finger injuries. Physician Sports Med 26[6]:57, 1998.)

the most common cause of **acute** rupture (e.g., after a fall causing the ski pole to stress the UCL of the thumb). The typical **mechanism of injury** is an extreme valgus stress to the thumb (e.g., falling on an abducted thumb).

Stability of the thumb on the ulnar side is maintained by four structures: the adductor aponeurosis, the adductor pollicis muscle, the proper and accessory UCL, and the volar plate. The UCL provides resistance to radially applied forces (e.g., pinching or holding large objects). A torn UCL weakens the key pinch grip strength and allows volar subluxation of the proximal phalanx. With prolonged instability, the MCP joint frequently degenerates.

The amount of valgus laxity of "normal" thumbs varies widely. In full MCP joint extension, valgus laxity averages 6 degrees, and in 15 degrees of MCP joint flexion, it increases to an average of 12 degrees.

The adductor aponeurosis (when torn and pulled distally) occasionally entraps the UCL and therefore prevents anatomic reduction or healing of the UCL (**Stener lesion**) (Fig. 1-37).

Evaluation

Patients typically have a history of a valgus injury to the thumb followed by pain, swelling, and frequently ecchymosis at the ulnar aspect of the thumb MCP joint. Palpation of the ulnar aspect of the MCP joint may reveal a small lump, which is usually indicative of a Stener lesion or avulsion fracture.

In addition to plain radiographs (three views of the thumb and carpus), valgus stress testing radiographs should be obtained. Because acutely injured patients will guard from pain, 1% lidocaine should be injected into the joint before stress testing. The integrity of the proper (ulnar collateral) ligament is **assessed by valgus stress testing with the MCP joint of the thumb flexed in 30 degrees of flexion**. This test can be done clinically or with radiographic documentation. There is some variation in the literature regarding the degree of angulation on valgus stressing that is compatible with complete rupture of the UCL. **Thirty to 35 degrees of radial deviation of the thumb on valgus stressing indicates a complete UCL rupture and is an indication for surgical correction**. With complete ruptures (>30 degrees of opening), the likelihood of UCL displacement (a Stener lesion) is greater than 80%.

Treatment of Skier's Thumb

Stable Thumb on Valgus Stressing (No Stener Lesion)

- The ligament is only partially torn, and healing will occur with nonoperative treatment.
- The thumb is immobilized for 4 weeks in a short arm spica cast or thermoplastic splint (molded), usually with the thumb IP joint free.
- Active and passive thumb motion is begun at 3 to 4 weeks, but valgus is avoided.
- If ROM is painful at 3 to 4 weeks, re-evaluation by a physician is indicated.
- The thermoplastic splint is removed several times a day for active ROM exercises.
- Grip-strengthening exercises are begun at 6 weeks after injury. A brace is worn for protection in contact situations for 2 months.

Unstable Thumb on Valgus Stressing (>30 Degrees)

- Direct operative repair with a suture anchor is required (Fig. 1-38).
- Because 80% of patients with a complete rupture are found to have a Stener lesion (thus obtaining a poor healing result if treated nonoperatively), it is critical to make the correct diagnosis of stable versus unstable gamekeeper's thumb.

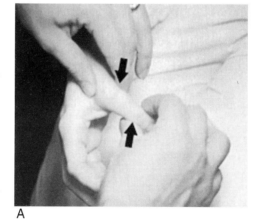

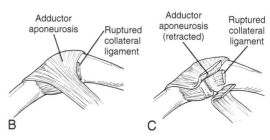

Figure 1–38 A, During stress examination of a skier's thumb, the physician stabilizes the metacarpal to prevent rotation and then applies radial stress (*arrows*) to the distal end of the phalanx. With the thumb in 30 degrees of flexion, a valgus stress is applied. Test both thumbs for symmetry, congenital laxity, and other abnormalities. **B,** When complete rupture of the ulnar collateral ligament occurs, the distal end of the torn ligament is usually displaced proximal and superficial to the proximal edge of the intact adductor aponeurosis. **C,** Division of the adductor aponeurosis is required for repair of the ligament. (**A,** From Wadsworth LT: How I manage skiers thumb. Physician Sports Med 20[3]:69, 1992; **B** and **C,** adapted from Heyman P: Injuries to the ulnar collateral ligament of the thumb MCP joint. J Am Acad Orthop Surg 5:224, 1997.)

REHABILITATION PROTOCOL	*After Repair or Reconstruction of the Ulnar Collateral Ligament of the Thumb Metacarpophalangeal Joint*

3 WEEKS

- Remove the bulky dressing.
- Remove the MCP joint pin (K-wire) if used for joint stabilization.
- Fit with a wrist and thumb static splint for continual wear.

6 WEEKS

- Begin active and gentle passive ROM exercises of the thumb for 10 minutes each hour.
- *Avoid any lateral stress to the MCP joint of the thumb.*
- Begin dynamic splinting if necessary to increase passive ROM of the thumb.

8 WEEKS

- Discontinue splinting. A wrist and thumb static splint or short opponens splint may be useful during sports-related activities or heavy lifting.
- Begin progressive strengthening.

12 WEEKS

- Allow the patient to return to unrestricted activity.

Nerve Compression Syndromes

Carpal Tunnel Syndrome

S. Brent Brotzman, MD

Background

Carpal tunnel syndrome (CTS) is relatively common (the most common peripheral neuropathy) and affects 1% of the general population. It occurs most frequently during middle or advanced age, with 83% of 1215 study patients being older than 40 years with a mean age of 54 years. Women are affected twice as frequently as men.

The carpal tunnel is a rigid, confined fibro-osseous space that physiologically acts as a "closed compartment." CTS is caused by compression of the median nerve at the wrist. The clinical syndrome is characterized by pain, numbness, or tingling in the distribution of the median nerve (the palmar aspect of the thumb, index finger, and long finger). These symptoms may affect all or a combination of the thumb, index, long, and ring fingers. Pain and **paresthesias at night** in the palmar aspect of the hand (median nerve distribution) are common symptoms.

Prolonged flexion or extension of the wrists under the patient's head or pillow during sleep is believed to contribute to the prevalence of nocturnal symptoms. Conditions that alter fluid balance (pregnancy, use of oral contraceptives, hemodialysis) may predispose to CTS. CTS associated with **pregnancy** is transitory and typically resolves spontaneously. Therefore, surgery should be avoided during pregnancy.

Types of Carpal Tunnel Syndrome

ACUTE ETIOLOGY

Sudden trauma
Wrist fracture
Crush injury
Burns
Gunshot wound

CHRONIC ETIOLOGY (USUALLY IDIOPATHIC; OTHER CAUSES INCLUDE)

Extrinsic causes

Constrictive casts (must be released quickly and the wrist taken out of flexion and placed into neutral)
Handcuffs
Tight gloves
Repetitive and forceful gripping and/or power vibrating tools

Intrinsic causes

Anatomic anomalies such as hypertrophy or proximal location of the lumbricals, palmaris longus, or palmaris profundus
Inflammatory proliferative tenosynovium
Perineural scarring from previous carpal tunnel release

OCCUPATIONAL ETIOLOGY (CONTROVERSIAL AND INCONCLUSIVE)

Repetitive wrist flexion/extension
Intense gripping
Awkward (poor ergonomics) wrist flexion
Computer keyboards
Power vibratory tools

Typical Clinical Findings

Paresthesias, pain, and numbness or tingling in the palmar surface of the hand in the distribution of the median nerve (Fig. 1-39) (i.e., the palmar aspect of the three and one-half radial digits) are the most common symptoms. Nocturnal pain is also common. Activities of daily living (such as driving a car, holding a cup, and typing)

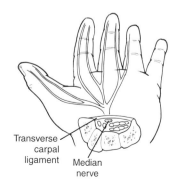

Figure 1–39 Sensory symptoms of carpal tunnel syndrome localize to the sensory distribution of the median nerve. They most commonly consist of pain, numbness, and burning or tingling of the palmar surfaces of the thumb, index finger, middle finger, and radial half of the ring finger. (Adapted from Steyers CM, Schelkuns PH: Practical management of carpal tunnel. Physician Sports Med 23[1]: 83, 1995.)

Transverse
carpal
ligament   Median
nerve

often aggravate the pain. Pain and paresthesias are sometimes relieved by the patient massaging or shaking the hand.

Provocative Testing Maneuvers (Table 1-5)

Phalen's Maneuver (Fig. 1-40)

- The patient's wrists are placed in complete (but not forced) flexion.
- If paresthesias in the median nerve distribution occur during the 60-second test, the test is positive for CTS.
- Gellman and associates (1986) found this to be the most sensitive (sensitivity, 75%) of the provocative maneuvers in their study of CTS.

Tinel's Sign (Median Nerve Percussion)

- Tinel's sign may be elicited by lightly tapping the patient's median nerve at the wrist while moving in a proximal-to-distal direction.
- The sign is positive if the patient complains of tingling or an electric shock–like sensation in the distribution of the median nerve.

Sensory Testing of the Median Nerve Distribution

Decreased sensation may be tested by
- Threshold tests: Semmes-Weinstein monofilament; vibrometry perception of a 256-cps tuning fork
- Innervation density tests: two-point discrimination

Sensory loss and thenar muscle weakness are often *late findings*.

Electrodiagnostic Tests

- Electrodiagnostic studies are a useful adjunct to clinical evaluation, but they do not supplant the need for a careful history and physical examination.
- These tests are indicated when the clinical picture is ambiguous or there is suspicion of other neuropathies.

The criteria for a positive electrodiagnostic test are a motor latency greater than 4.0 m/sec and a sensory latency greater than 3.5 m/sec.

The interpretation of findings in patients with CTS is classified in Table 1-6.

Special Tests for Evaluation

- Phalen's maneuver (60 seconds)
- Tinel's sign at the carpal tunnel (percussion test)
- Direct compression of the carpal tunnel (60 seconds)
- Semmes-Weinstein monofilament sensory testing
- Palpation of the pronator teres/Tinel's (rule out pronator syndrome)
- Spurling test of the neck (to rule out cervical radiculopathy) (see Chapter 3, Shoulder Injuries)
- Radicular testing (motor, sensory, reflexes) of the involved extremity (to rule out radiculopathy)
- Inspection for weakness or atrophy of the thenar eminence (a *late* finding of CTS)
- Exploration for possible global neuropathy (e.g., diabetic) on history and examination

TABLE 1–5		Available Tests Used to Diagnose Carpal Tunnel Syndrome		
No.	Test	Method	Condition Measured	Positive Result	Interpretation of Positive Result
1*	Phalen maneuver	Patient holds the wrist in marked flexion for 30-60 sec	Paresthesias in response to position	Numbness or tingling on radial-side digits	Probable CTS (sensitivity, 0.75; specificity, 0.47); Gellman found it to have the best sensitivity of provocative tests
2*	Percussion test (Tinel's sign)	Examiner lightly taps along the median nerve at the wrist in a proximal-to-distal direction	Site of nerve lesion	Tingling response in the fingers	Probable CTS if the response is at the wrist (sensitivity, 0.60; specificity, 0.67)
3*	Carpal tunnel compression	Direct compression of the median nerve by the examiner	Paresthesias in response to pressure	Paresthesias within 30 sec	Probable CTS (sensitivity, 0.87; specificity, 0.90)
4	Hand diagram	Patient marks sites of pain or altered sensation on an outline	Patient's perception of the site of the nerve deficit	Pain depiction on the palmar side of the radial digits without depiction of the palm	Probable CTS (sensitivity, 0.96; specificity, 0.73; negative predictive value of a negative test, 0.91
5	Hand volume stress test	Measure hand volume by water displacement; repeat after 7-min stress test and 10-min rest	Hand volume	Hand volume increased by ≥10 ml	Probable dynamic CTS

Continued

TABLE 1-5	Available Tests Used to Diagnose Carpal Tunnel Syndrome—cont'd			
No.	Test	Method	Condition Measured	Positive Result	Interpretation of Positive Result
6	Static two-point discrimination	Determine the minimum separation of two points perceived as distinct when lightly touched on the palmar surface of the digit	Innervation density of slowly adapting fibers	Failure to discriminate points <6 mm apart	Advanced nerve dysfunction (late finding)
7	Moving two-point discrimination	As above, but with the points moving	Innervation density of slowly adapting fibers	Failure to discriminate points <5 mm apart	Advanced nerve dysfunction (late finding)
8	Vibrometry	Vibrometer head is placed on the palmar side of the digit; amplitude at 120 Hz increased to the threshold of perception; compare the median and ulnar nerves in both hands	Threshold of quickly adapting fibers	Asymmetry in the contralateral hand or between the radial and ulnar digits	Probable CTS (sensitivity, 0.87)

9*	Semmes-Weinstein monofilament test	Monofilaments of increasing diameter touched to the palmar side of the digit until the patient can tell which digit is untouched	Threshold of slowly adapting fibers	Value >2.83 in radial digits	Median nerve impairment (sensitivity, 0.83)
10*	Distal sensory latency and conduction velocity	Orthodromic stimulus and recording across the wrist	Latency and conduction velocity of sensory fibers	Latency >3.5 ms or asymmetry >0.5 ms in comparison to the contralateral hand	Probable CTS
11*	Distal motor latency conduction	Orthodromic stimulus and recording across the wrist	Latency and conduction velocity of the motor fibers of the median nerve	Latency >4.5 ms or asymmetry >1 ms	Probable CTS
12	Electromyography	Needle electrodes placed in muscle	Denervation of t the henar muscles	Fibrillation potentials, sharp waves, increased insertional activity	Very advanced motor median nerve compression

*Most common tests/methods used in our practice.
CTS, carpal tunnel syndrome.
Adapted from Szabo RM, Madison M: Carpal tunnel syndrome. Orthop Clin North Am 1:103, 1992.

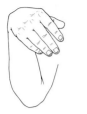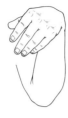

Figure 1–40   Phalen test. When the patient holds the wrists flexed for 60 seconds, numbness and tingling along the distribution of the median nerve indicate carpal tunnel syndrome. (Adapted from Slade JF, Mahoney JD, Dailinger JE, Boxamsa TH: Wrist injuries in musicians. J Musculoskel Med 16:548, 1999.)

- If gray area, electromyographic/nerve conduction velocity testing of the *entire* involved upper extremity to exclude cervical radiculopathy versus CTS versus pronator syndrome

Evaluation

- Patients with **systemic peripheral neuropathies** (e.g., diabetes, alcoholism, hypothyroidism) typically have a sensory abnormality distribution that is not solely isolated to the median nerve distribution.
- More proximal compressive neuropathies (e.g., C6 **cervical radiculopathy**) will produce sensory deficits in the C6 distribution (well beyond the median nerve distribution), plus weakness in the C6 innervated muscles (biceps) and an abnormal biceps reflex.
- Electrodiagnostic tests are helpful in distinguishing local compressive neuropathies (such as CTS) from peripheral systemic neuropathies (such as diabetic neuropathy).

TABLE 1–6	Interpreting Findings in Patients with Carpal Tunnel Syndrome
Degree of CTS	**Findings**
Dynamic	Symptoms primarily activity induced; patient otherwise asymptomatic; no detectable physical findings
Mild	Patient has intermittent symptoms; decreased light-touch sensibility; digital compression test usually positive, but Tinel's sign, as well as positive result on Phalen's maneuver, may or may not be present
Moderate	Frequent symptoms; decreased vibratory perception in the median nerve distribution; positive Phalen's maneuver and digital compression test; Tinel's sign present; increased two-point discrimination; weakness of the thenar muscles
Severe	Symptoms are persistent; marked increase in or absence of two-point discrimination; thenar muscle atrophy

CTS, carpal tunnel syndrome.

Differential Diagnosis of Carpal Tunnel Syndrome

Thoracic outlet syndrome (TOS)

> TOS exhibits a positive Adson test (see Chapter 3, Shoulder Injuries), costoclavicular maneuver, Roos test, etc.

Cervical radiculopathy (CR)

> CR has a positive Spurling test of the neck (see Chapter 3, Shoulder Injuries), *proximal* arm/neck symptoms, dermatomal distribution, occasional neck pain.

Brachial plexopathy

Pronator teres syndrome (PTS)

> Median nerve compression in the *proximal* part of the forearm (PTS) rather than the wrist (CTS) produces similar median nerve symptoms.

> PTS is usually associated with activity-induced *daytime* paresthesias rather than nighttime paresthesias (CTS).

> **Tenderness and the Tinel sign are palpable in the forearm at the pronator teres, not at the carpal tunnel.**

> PTS (more proximal) involves the median nerve–innervated extrinsic forearm motors *and* the palmar cutaneous nerve branch of the median nerve (unlike CTS).

> Perform the provocation test for PTS (see Fig. 1-43).

Digital nerve compression (bowler's thumb)

> Caused by direct pressure applied to the palm or digits (base of the thumb in bowler's thumb).

> Tenderness and the Tinel sign are localized to the thumb digit at the irritated digital nerve rather than the carpal tunnel.

Neuropathy (systemic)

> Alcohol, diabetes, hypothyroidism—more diffuse neuropathy findings noted.

Tenosynovitis (rheumatoid arthritis)

Reflex sympathetic dystrophy (RSD)

> RSD is manifested as skin color alteration, temperature changes, hyperesthesias, etc.

Treatment

- All patients should undergo **initial conservative management**, unless the symptoms are acute and associated with trauma (such as CTS associated with an acute swollen distal radius fracture).
- All patients with **acute CTS** associated with a fracture should have the wrist taken out of flexion in the cast and placed in neutral (see the section on distal radius fractures).

- Circumferential casts should be removed or bivalved, and icing and elevation of the extremity above the heart should be initiated.
- Close serial observation should be performed to check for a possible requirement for "emergency" carpal tunnel release if the symptoms do not improve.
- Some authors recommend measurement of wrist compartment pressure.

Nonoperative Management

- All pregnant women are treated nonoperatively because of spontaneous resolution after delivery of the baby.
- Nonoperative treatment may include
  - The use of a **prefabricated wrist splint** with the wrist placed in a neutral position and worn at night; daytime splinting is used if the patient's job allows. Intratunnel carpal tunnel pressures vary with position. Burke found that intratunnel pressures were lowest with the wrist near neutral, most specifically with 2 degrees of flexion and 3 degrees of ulnar deviation. Burke recommends this position for wrist control splinting.
  - **Activity modification** (discontinuing the use of vibratory machinery or placing a support under unsupported arms at the computer).
  - **Cortisone injection** into the carpal tunnel (Fig. 1-41) (**not** the actual median nerve). Studies have shown that less than 25% of patients who had cortisone injected into the carpal tunnel were symptom free at 18 months after injection. As many as 80% of patients do have *temporary relief* with cortisone injection and splinting. Green found that symptoms typically recurred 2 to 4 months after cortisone injection and led to operative treatment in 46% of patients.
- The technique for injection is shown in Figure 1-41. If injection creates paresthesias in the hand (nerve injection), the needle should be immediately withdrawn and redirected; the injection **should not** be directed into the median nerve.

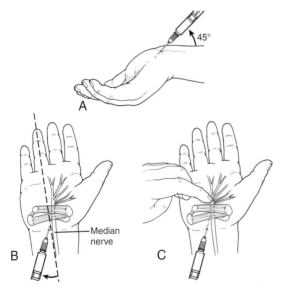

Figure 1–41 **A,** During carpal tunnel injection, a 25- or 27-gauge needle is used to introduce a mixture of dexamethasone and lidocaine into the carpal canal. **B,** The needle is aligned with the ring finger and directed 45 degrees dorsally and 30 degrees radially as it is advanced slowly beneath the transverse carpal ligament into the tunnel. **C,** After injection, lidocaine is dispersed. Injection into the nerve should be avoided. If any paresthesias occur during injection, the needle is immediately withdrawn and redirected. (Adapted from Royan GM: Understanding and managing carpal tunnel syndrome. J Musculoskel Med 16:661, 1999.)

- Vitamin B_6 has not been shown in clinical trials to have any therapeutic effect on CTS, but it may help in patients with "missed" neuropathies (pyridoxine deficiency).
- Nonsteroidal anti-inflammatory drugs (NSAIDs) can be used for control of inflammation.
- Any underlying systemic disease (such as diabetes, rheumatoid arthritis, or hypothyroidism) must be controlled.

Surgical Treatment

Indications for surgical treatment of CTS include
- Thenar atrophy or weakness
- Sensation loss on objective measures
- Fibrillation potentials on electromyelograms
- Symptoms that persist more than a year despite appropriate conservative measures

The goals of carpal tunnel release are
- Decompression of the nerve
- Improvement of nerve excursion
- Prevention of progressive nerve damage

Our recommendation is **open carpal tunnel release** (complication rate of 10% to 18%) rather than endoscopic release (complication rate up to 35% in some studies). In our experience, the time to return to work and sporting activities has not been different enough between the two procedures to warrant the difference in complication rates (dramatically increased frequency of digital nerve lacerations with the endoscopic technique).

REHABILITATION PROTOCOL *After Open Release for Carpal Tunnel Syndrome*

0-7 DAYS

- Encourage gentle wrist extension and flexion exercises and full finger flexion and extension exercises immediately after surgery in the postsurgical dressing.

7 DAYS

- Remove the dressing.
- Prohibit the patient from submerging the hand in liquids, but permit showering.
- Discontinue the wrist splint if the patient is comfortable.

7-14 DAYS

- Permit the patient to use the hand for activities of daily living as pain allows.

2 WEEKS

- Remove the sutures and begin ROM and gradual strengthening exercises. Scar tenderness is the most common complication after open carpal tunnel release. Do not take the sutures out before the wound has gained adequate tensile strength.
- Achieve initial scar remodeling by using Elastomer or a silicone gel-sheet scar pad at night and deep scar massage.
- If scar tenderness is intense, use desensitization techniques such as applying various textures to the area with light pressure and progressing to deep pressure. Textures include cotton, velour, wool, and Velcro.
- Control pain and edema with the use of Isotoner gloves or electrical stimulation.

Continued

REHABILITATION PROTOCOL: *After Open Release for Carpal Tunnel Syndrome* *Continued*

2-4 WEEKS

- Advance the patient to more rigorous activities; allow the patient to return to work if the pain permits. The patient can use a padded glove for tasks that require pressure to be applied over the tender palmar scars.
- Begin pinch/grip strengthening with Baltimore Therapeutic Equipment work-simulator activities.

PRONATOR SYNDROME

A less common cause of median nerve entrapment occurs in the proximal part of the forearm where the median nerve is compressed by either the pronator teres, the flexor superficialis arch, or the lacertus fibrosus in a condition referred to as *pronator syndrome* (Fig. 1-42). In addition to dysesthesias in the thumb and the index, middle, and ring fingers, there may be a sensory disturbance of the volar base of the thenar eminence because of involvement of the palmar cutaneous branch of the medial nerve.

Physical findings include marked proximal forearm tenderness; a proximal median nerve compression test will reproduce the symptoms. The most common cause of this disorder is entrapment of the median nerve by the fascia of the pronator teres proximally, which can be tested by resisted pronation with gradual extension of the elbow (Fig. 1-43). A positive resisted middle finger flexion test may suggest median nerve entrapment by the FDS arch, and resisted supination with the elbow flexed may suggest entrapment by the lacertus fibrosus, a fascial extension of the biceps tendon.

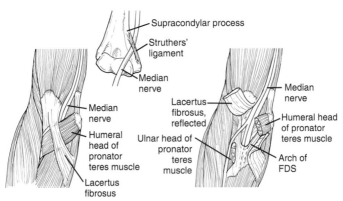

Figure 1–42 Anatomy of the antecubital fossa and structures overlying the course of the median nerve. The *inset* shows the supracondylar process that is occasionally present. F.D.S., flexor digitorum superficialis. (Adapted from Idler RS, Strickland JW, Creighton JJ Jr: Hand clinic: Pronator syndrome. Indiana Med 84:124, 1991.)

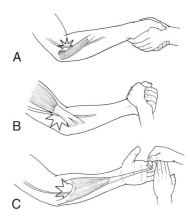

Figure 1–43 Provocative tests for pronator syndrome. **A**, Pronator teres: resisted forearm pronation with the elbow relatively extended. **B**, Lacertus fibrosus: resisted elbow flexion with the forearm supinated. **C**, Flexor digitorum superficialis: resisted middle finger extension. (Adapted from Idler RS, Strickland JW, Creighton JJ Jr: Hand clinic: Pronator syndrome. Indiana Med 84:124, 1991.)

Treatment

Nonoperative management of this disorder includes minimizing resisted pronation activities and performing repetitive gripping and squeezing. A long arm splint with the elbow at 90 degrees and the forearm in neutral rotation, in addition to anti-inflammatory medications and vitamin B, may be beneficial. Conservative management of this disorder is often ineffective, and surgery is usually required.

REHABILITATION PROTOCOL	*After Surgical Decompression for Pronator Teres Syndrome*

0-7 DAYS

- Keep a soft, light compressive dressing in place to allow full elbow, forearm, and wrist motion.

7 DAYS

- Remove the dressing and encourage activities as tolerated, including light manual labor.
- Begin ROM of the wrist and elbow, including gripping in extension with putty.

2 WEEKS

- Remove the sutures and encourage progressive strengthening and use of the upper extremity.

4 WEEKS

- Allow moderate to heavy work.

6 WEEKS

- Allow full, unprotected use of the arm.
    Discomfort after surgical decompression of the median nerve in the proximal part of the forearm is less than after decompression of the median nerve at the wrist level, and desensitization techniques are unnecessary.

Dupuytren's Contracture

The manifestations of Dupuytren's disease are variable and may be confined to a single digit, but palmar digital involvement of the ring and small fingers is more common. Diffuse involvement of the first web space and thumb in addition to the fingers is less common.

No exact criteria exist for surgical intervention in Dupuytren's disease. Some patients who have severe MCP and PIP joint contractures have surprisingly few complaints of functional disability, whereas other patients with pretendinous cords and nodules without contractures desire surgical intervention.

Guidelines for surgical intervention include
- 30 degrees of MCP joint contracture
- 15 degrees of PIP joint contracture
- Inability to place the hand in a pocket, lay it flat on a table, or bring it together with the opposite hand (as in prayer)

Regardless of the criteria used for surgical intervention, the PIP joint contracture is the most difficult to correct and warrants early intervention.

Surgical procedures used in the treatment of Dupuytren's contracture include subcutaneous fasciotomy, partial selective fasciectomy, complete fasciectomy, fasciectomy with skin grafting, and amputation.

SUBCUTANEOUS FASCIOTOMY

In elderly patients with an MCP joint contracture, subcutaneous fasciotomy is ideal, regardless of whether one or two digits are involved. This procedure may be done in the office with local anesthesia.

Technique of Subcutaneous Fasciotomy

With the palm anesthetized, a No. 15 blade is introduced across the palm between the skin and the pretendinous cord. The finger is extended and the knife blade is gently pressed onto the taut cord. An abrupt release of the MCP joint contracture follows when transection of the cord is complete. Manipulation of the fingers may result in some tearing of the palmar skin; however, such tearing is usually minor, and the wound can be left open and covered with a sterile dressing.

Surgical procedures other than cordotomy for Dupuytren's disease require considerable dissection, and subsequent palmar and finger hematomas become more likely. Small suction drain systems may be incorporated to prevent these hematomas.

REHABILITATION PROTOCOL	*Dupuytren's Contracture, Subcutaneous Fasciotomy*

0-7 DAYS
- Encourage the patient to work on stretching exercises immediately after surgery. Maintain digital extension with a resting pan splint with Velcro straps.
- Have the patient wear the splint during the day between exercises and at night for the first week.
- Continue night splints for 6 weeks after surgery.

Arthroplasty

PROXIMAL INTERPHALANGEAL JOINT ARTHROPLASTY

PIP joint arthroplasty is primarily indicated for patients who are relatively free of disease at the MCP joints. This usually precludes patients with rheumatoid arthritis and significant MCP joint involvement. The best treatment option for these patients is MCP joint arthroplasty and either soft tissue procedures for correction of the soft tissue deformities or PIP joint fusion. Patients with osteoarthritis may benefit from isolated PIP joint arthroplasty, other than the index finger.

A volar approach for placement of the implant may be used when the extensor mechanism does not require repair or corrective surgery. Active flexion and extension exercises may be started immediately after surgery.

Rehabilitation after PIP joint arthroplasty depends on whether the arthroplasty is performed for a stiff IP joint, for reconstruction with lateral deviation, or to correct a boutonnière deformity.

REHABILITATION PROTOCOL · *Proximal Interphalangeal Joint Arthroplasty for Joint Stiffness*

0-3 WEEKS

- Begin active flexion and extension exercises at 3-5 days after surgery.
- Have the patient use a padded aluminum splint between hourly exercises to maintain full PIP joint extension.

3-6 WEEKS

- Continue interval PIP joint splinting during the day for 6 weeks.

6 WEEKS

- Begin resistive exercises.
- Continue interval splinting to correct any angular deviation and extensor lag of more than 20 degrees.
- Have the patient wear a protective splint at night for 3 months after surgery.
  The ideal ROMs obtained are 0-70 degrees of flexion in the ring and small fingers, 60 degrees of flexion in the middle finger, and 45 degrees of flexion in the index finger.

REHABILITATION PROTOCOL · *Proximal Interphalangeal Joint Arthroplasty for Lateral Deviation*

The central slip and collateral ligaments are reconstructed in this deformity.

2-3 WEEKS

- Use an extension splint and gutter splints to correct residual angular deformities.
- Perform active exercises three to five times a day with taping or radial outriggers.
- Have the patient wear splints for 6-8 weeks after surgery.

6-8 WEEKS

- Continue night splinting for 3-6 months.

METACARPOPHALANGEAL JOINT ARTHROPLASTY

MCP joint arthroplasty is indicated primarily for patients with rheumatoid arthritis, although unusual post-traumatic or osteoarthritic conditions may require implant arthroplasty. Correction of radial deviation of the metacarpals, as well as intrinsic imbalance, is necessary for acceptable results. The procedure increases the range of functional motion of the fingers, although grip and pinch strength do not improve significantly.

REHABILITATION PROTOCOL   *Metacarpophalangeal Joint Arthroplasty*

0-7 DAYS

- Remove drains 2 days after surgery.
- Use a postoperative splint to maintain the MCP joints in full extension and neutral to slight radial deviation.

7 DAYS

- Fashion a dynamic extension outrigger splint and resting hand splints.
- Begin active MCP joint exercises.
- Apply a supinator tab to the index finger.

2-4 WEEKS

- Remove the sutures. Continue the night resting pan splint.
- Continue the dynamic extension outrigger splint for daily use.

4 WEEKS

- Allow light hand use and activities of daily living.
- Continue night splinting for 4 months to help reduce extensor lag.

  Note: If MCP joint motion is not obtained in 2 weeks, the PIP joint should be splinted in full extension and flexion force concentrated at the MCP joint level. Careful follow-up is necessary during the first 3 weeks, when the desired motion should be achieved. At 3 weeks, the capsular structures are significantly tight, and no further ROM should be expected. Dynamic flexion may be necessary to regain early MCP joint flexion.

THUMB CARPOMETACARPAL JOINT ARTHROPLASTY

An arthritic basilar joint of the thumb offers another clear example that the radiographic appearance has no correlation with the severity of clinical symptoms. Radiographic evidence of advanced arthritic change may be an incidental finding, whereas a radiographically normal thumb may have significant disability. Treatment regimens consisting of steroid injection, splinting, and NSAIDs should be exhausted before surgical intervention.

Total joint arthroplasty, implant arthroplasty, interposition arthroplasty, suspension arthroplasty, and CMC joint fusion have been used to alleviate pain and restore function in the diseased basilar joint of the thumb.

Interposition and Sling Suspension Arthroplasty

Trapezial excision techniques combined with soft tissue interposition or sling suspension arthroplasty have similar postsurgical protocols. Sling suspension arthroplasties are designed to prevent thumb osteoarticular column shortening and provide stability beyond that afforded by simple trapezial excision.

REHABILITATION PROTOCOL — *Interposition and Sling Suspension Arthroplasty*

2 WEEKS

- Remove the surgical thumb spica splint and sutures. Apply a short arm thumb spica cast for an additional 2 weeks.

4 WEEKS

- Begin active, active-assisted, and passive ROM exercises with interval splinting.
- Ideally, the splint or cast should include only the CMC joint, with the MCP or IP joint left free for ROM.

6 WEEKS

- Begin gentle strengthening exercises.

8 WEEKS

- Encourage light to moderate activity.
- The wrist and thumb static splint may be discontinued in the presence of a pain-free and stable joint.

3 MONTHS

- Allow normal activity.
  Discomfort frequently lasts for 6 months after surgery. The function and strength of the thumb will improve over a 6- to 12-month period.

Wrist Disorders

Scaphoid Fractures

S. Brent Brotzman, MD • Steven J. Meyers, MD •
Michael L. Lee, MD

Background

The scaphoid (carpal navicular) is the most commonly fractured of the carpal bones and is often difficult to diagnose and treat. Complications include nonunion and malunion, which alter wrist kinematics and can lead to pain, decreased ROM, decrease in strength, and early radiocarpal arthrosis.

The scaphoid blood supply is precarious. The radial artery branches enter the scaphoid on the dorsum, distal third, and lateral volar surfaces. The **proximal third**

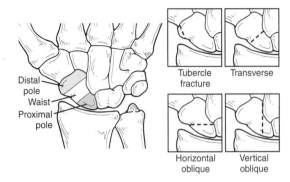

Distal pole
Waist
Proximal pole

Tubercle fracture
Transverse
Horizontal oblique
Vertical oblique

Figure 1–44 A dorsal view of the scaphoid bone demonstrates various fracture orientations. Determining the orientation on radiographs is important because the orientation helps guide treatment decisions.

of the scaphoid receives its blood supply solely from the interosseous circulation in about a third of cases and thus is **at high risk for avascular necrosis**.

Scaphoid fractures are usually **classified by location of the fracture: proximal third, middle third (or waist), distal third, or tuberosity** (Fig. 1-44). Fractures of the middle third are most common, and distal third fractures are very rare.

Clinical History and Examination

Scaphoid fractures usually occur after a fall with hyperextension and radial flexion of the wrist, most often in young active male patients. Patients generally have **tenderness in the anatomic snuffbox** (Fig. 1-45) (between the first and third dorsal compartments), less commonly on the distal scaphoid tuberosity volarly, and may have increased pain with axial compression of the thumb metacarpal. *Scaphoid* is derived from the Greek word for boat, and it is often difficult to evaluate radiographically because of its oblique orientation in the wrist.

Initial radiographs should include posteroanterior (PA), oblique, lateral, and ulnar deviation PA. If there is any question clinically, magnetic resonance imaging (MRI) is extremely sensitive in detecting scaphoid fractures as early as 2 days after injury.

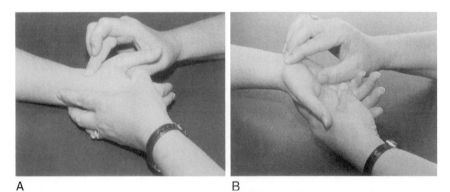

A   B

Figure 1–45 Evaluation of scaphoid fractures. **A,** Scaphoid tenderness can be identified by palpation dorsally within the anatomic snuffbox. **B,** Tenderness may also be identified palmarly at the scaphoid tuberosity radial to the flexor carpi radialis tendon and the proximal wrist crease (the wrist should be extended). (From Zabinski SJ: Investigating carpal injuries. Sports Med Update, 1999.)

A B C

D E F

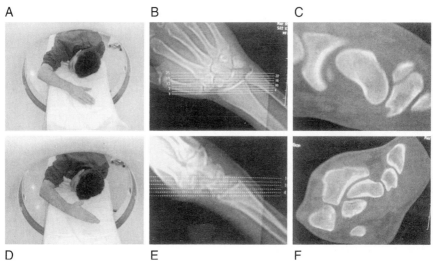

Figure 1–46 A computed tomography scan of the scaphoid is easier to interpret if the images are obtained in planes defined by the long axis of the scaphoid. To achieve this, the patient lies prone on the table with the arm overhead. **A**, For sagittal plane images, the forearm is held pronated (palm down) and the hand lies flat on the table. The forearm crosses the gantry at an angle of approximately 45 degrees (roughly in line with the abducted thumb metacarpal). **B**, Scout images are obtained to confirm the appropriate orientation and ensure that the entire scaphoid is imaged. Sections are obtained at 1-mm intervals. **C**, Images obtained in the sagittal plane are best for measuring the intrascaphoid angle. **D**, For coronal plane images, the forearm is in neutral position. **E**, Scout images demonstrate alignment of the wrist through the gantry of the scanner. **F**, Interpretation of the images obtained in the coronal plane is straightforward. (From Ring D, Jupiter JB, Herndon JH: Acute fractures of the scaphoid. J Am Acad Orthop Surg 8:225, 2000.)

If MRI is unavailable, patients with snuffbox tenderness should be immobilized for 10 to 14 days and then return for repeat radiographs out of the splint. If the diagnosis still remains questionable, a bone scan is indicated.

Assessment of scaphoid fracture displacement is crucial for treatment and is often best assessed with thin-section (1-mm) computed tomography (CT) scans (Fig. 1-46). Displacement is defined as a fracture gap of more than 1 mm, a lateral scapholunate angle greater than 60 degrees (Fig. 1-47), a lateral radiolunate angle greater than 15 degrees, or an intrascaphoid angle greater than 35 degrees.

Treatment

- Truly nondisplaced fractures can be treated in closed fashion and nearly always heal with thumb spica cast immobilization.
- Above- or below-elbow casting is still the subject of controversy. The authors prefer 6 weeks of sugar-tong (long arm) thumb spica casting, followed by a minimum of 6 weeks of short arm thumb spica casting.
- Scaphoid union is verified with a thin-section CT scan.
- **Surgical treatment is indicated for** nondisplaced fractures in which the complications of prolonged immobilization (wrist stiffness, thenar atrophy, and delayed return to heavy labor or sports) would be intolerable, scaphoid fractures that were previously unrecognized or untreated, all displaced scaphoid fractures (see earlier for displacement criteria), and scaphoid nonunion.

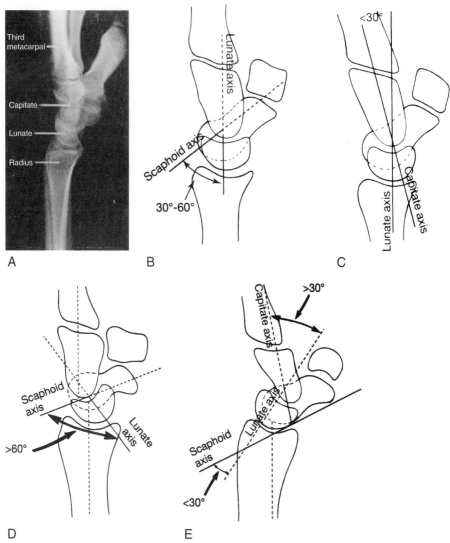

Figure 1–47   **A**, Lateral radiograph showing the normal collinear relationship of the radius, lunate, capitate, and third metacarpal. **With normal carpal alignment, the scapholunate angle is between 30 and 60 degrees (B) and the capitolunate angle is less than 30 degrees (C).** Note that the scaphoid axis can be drawn through the center of the scaphoid, but it is also adequate and may be easier to draw a line along the inferior pole as shown in **C**. **D**, Dorsiflexion instability—**dorsal intercalary segment instability (DISI)**—is suspected when dorsal tilting of the lunate and volar tilting of the scaphoid are present with a resulting increase in the scapholunate angle to more than 60 degrees. **E**, Palmar flexion instability—**volar intercalary segment instability (VISI)**—is suspected with volar tilting of the lunate that results in a scapholunate angle of less than 30 degrees or a capitolunate angle of more than 30 degrees, or both. (**A**, From Honing EW: Wrist injuries. Part 2: Spotting and treating troublemakers. Physician Sports Med 26[10]:62, 1996; **B-E**, from Mann FA, Gilula LA: Post-traumatic wrist pain and instability: A radiographic approach to diagnosis. In Lichtman DM, Alexander AH [eds]: The Wrist and Its Disorders, 2nd ed. Philadelphia, WB Saunders, 1997, p 105;)

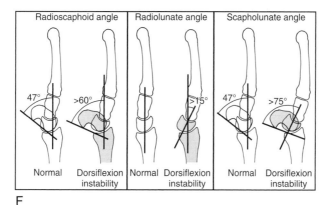

F

Figure 1–47 Cont'd.   F, DISI parameters for radioscaphoid, radiolunate, and scapholunate angles. **F,** adapted from Regional Review Course in Hand Surgery. Rosemont, IL, American Society for Surgery of the Hand, 1991, p 12.)

- For nondisplaced fractures, percutaneous fixation with cannulated screws has recently become an accepted treatment.
- For fractures with displacement, ORIF is mandatory.

REHABILITATION PROTOCOL	*Treatment and Rehabilitation for Scaphoid Fractures*

FOR FRACTURES TREATED IN CLOSED FASHION (NONOPERATIVE), TREATMENT IN A THUMB SPICA CAST

0-6 Weeks

- Sugar-tong thumb spica cast
- Active shoulder ROM
- Active second through fifth MCP/PIP/DIP joint ROM

6-12 Weeks (Bony Union)

- Nontender to palpation, painless ROM with the cast off
- Short arm thumb spica cast
- Continue shoulder and finger exercises
- Begin active elbow flexion/extension/supination/pronation

12 Weeks

- CT scan to confirm union. If ununited, continue the short arm thumb spica cast (Fig. 1-48)

12-14 Weeks

- Assuming union at 12 weeks, removable thumb spica splint
- Begin home exercise program
  - Active/gentle-assisted wrist flexion/extension ROM
  - Active/gentle-assisted wrist radial/ulnar flexion ROM
  - Active/gentle-assisted thumb MCP/IP joint ROM
  - Active/gentle-assisted thenar cone exercise

Continued

REHABILITATION PROTOCOL: *Treatment and Rehabilitation for*
Scaphoid Fractures *Continued*

FOR FRACTURES TREATED IN CLOSED FASHION (NONOPERATIVE), TREATMENT IN A THUMB SPICA CAST—cont'd

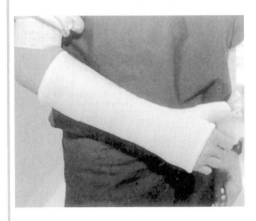

Figure 1–48 Thumb spica cast. (From Zabinski JJ: Investigating carpal tunnel. Sports Med Update, 1999.)

14-18 Weeks

- Discontinue all splinting
- Formalized occupational therapy
  - Active/aggressive-assisted wrist flexion/extension ROM
  - Active/aggressive-assisted wrist radial/ulnar flexion ROM
  - Active/aggressive-assisted thumb MCP/IP joint ROM
  - Active/aggressive-assisted thenar cone exercise

18 Weeks +

- Grip strengthening, aggressive ROM
- Unrestricted activities

FOR SCAPHOID FRACTURES TREATED WITH ORIF

0-10 Days

- Elevate the sugar-tong thumb spica splint, ice
- Shoulder ROM
- MCP/PIP/DIP joint active ROM exercises

10 Days-4 Weeks

- Suture removal
- Sugar-tong thumb spica cast (immobilizing the elbow)
- Continue hand/shoulder ROM

4-8 Weeks

- Short arm thumb spica cast
- Elbow active/assisted extension, flexion/supination/pronation; continue active ROM in fingers 2 through 5 and shoulder active ROM

8 Weeks

- CT scan to verify union of the fracture

FOR SCAPHOID FRACTURES TREATED WITH ORIF—cont'd

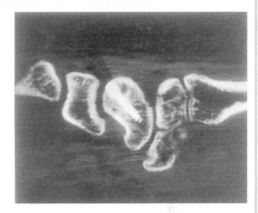

Figure 1–49 Computed tomography scan showing union without avascular necrosis or loss of anatomic reduction. (From Zabinski JJ: Investigating carpal tunnel. Sports Med Update, 1999.)

8-10 Weeks (assuming union) (Fig. 1-49)

- Removable thumb spica splint
- Begin home exercise program
  - Active/gentle-assisted wrist flexion and extension ROM
  - Active/gentle-assisted wrist radial/ulnar flexion ROM
  - Active/gentle-assisted thumb MCP/IP joint ROM
  - Active/gentle-assisted thenar cone exercise

10-14 Weeks

- Discontinue all splinting
- Formalized occupational therapy
  - Active/aggressive-assisted wrist flexion/extension ROM
  - Active/aggressive-assisted wrist radial/ulnar flexion ROM
  - Active/aggressive-assisted thumb MCP/IP joint ROM
  - Active/aggressive-assisted thenar cone exercise

14 Weeks +

- Grip strengthening
- Aggressive ROM
- Unrestricted activities

Fractures of the Distal Radius

David Ring, MD • Gae Burchill, OT •
Donna Ryan Callamaro, OT • Jesse B. Jupiter, MD

Background

Successful treatment of a distal radial fracture must respect the soft tissues while restoring anatomic alignment of the bones (Fig. 1-50). The surgeon must choose a treatment method that maintains bony alignment without relying on tight casts or

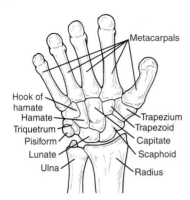

Figure 1–50 Bones of the wrist.

restricting the gliding structures that control the hand. **MCP joint motion must remain free. The wrist should not be distracted or placed in a flexed position** because these abnormal positions diminish the mechanical advantage of the extrinsic tendons, increase pressure in the carpal canal, exacerbate carpal ligament injury, and contribute to stiffness. Recognition and prompt treatment of median nerve dysfunction (e.g., CTS as a result of swelling within the tight fibro-osseus tunnel) and avoidance of injury to branches of the radial sensory nerve are also important. **Special attention should be given to limiting swelling of the hand. Swelling can contribute to stiffness and even contracture of the intrinsic muscles of the hand.** Mobilization and functional use of the hand, wrist, and forearm complete the rehabilitation of the fractured wrist.

The keys to successful treatment of distal radial fractures include restoration of articular congruity, radial length, and proper volar inclination; avoidance of stiffness; and early motion of a stable construct.

Clinical Background

Fractures of the distal end of the radius are common in older persons, particularly women, because they have weaker bones and are more susceptible to falls. Older persons are healthier, more active, and more numerous than ever, and treatment decisions cannot be based on patient age alone but must consider the possibility of poor bone quality.

Considerable energy is required to fracture the distal radius of a younger adult, and most such fractures occur in motor vehicle accidents, falls from heights, or sports. Displaced fractures in younger adults are more likely to be associated with concomitant carpal fractures and ligament injuries, acute compartment syndrome, and multitrauma.

The distal end of the radius has two important functions: it is both the primary support of the carpus and part of the forearm articulation. When a distal radial fracture heals with malalignment, the surface pressure on the articular cartilage may be elevated and uneven, the carpus may become malaligned, the ulna may impact with the carpus, or the distal radioulnar joint (DRUJ) may be incongruent. These conditions can produce pain, loss of motion, and arthrosis.

Distal radial alignment is monitored by radiographic measurements to define alignment in three planes. Distal radial shortening is measured best as the offset between the ulnar head and the lunate facet of the distal radius on the PA view—**the ulnar variance.** Alignment of the distal radius in the sagittal plane is evaluated by measuring the inclination of the distal radial articular surface on the PA radiograph—**the ulnar inclination.**

Figure 1–51 Impaction (loss of length). **A,** A normal radius is usually level with or within 1 to 2 mm distal or proximal to the distal ulnar articular surface. **B,** With a Colles fracture, significant loss of radial length causes loss of congruency with the distal radioulnar joint. (Adapted from Newport ML: Colles fractures. J Musculoskel Med 17[1]:292, 2000.)

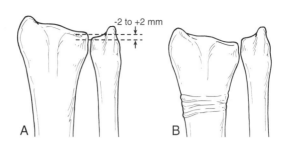

Distal radial alignment in the coronal plane is evaluated by measuring the inclination of the distal radial articular surface on the lateral radiograph. Studies of normal volunteers have determined that the articular surface of the distal radius is usually oriented about 11 degrees palmar and 22 degrees ulnar and has neutral ulnar variance.

Loss of Radial Length (Distal Radial Impaction)

Loss of radial length or height is a result of impaction of the fracture. Normally, the radial articular surface is level with or within 1 to 2 mm distal (ulnar positive) or proximal (ulnar negative) to the distal ulnar articular surface (Fig. 1-51). Colles fractures tend to lose significant height, which causes loss of congruency with the DRUJ and difficulties with wrist rotation.

Dorsal Angulation (Loss of Volar Inclination)

Normally, the distal end of the radius has a volar inclination of 11 degrees on the lateral view (Fig. 1-52). A Colles fracture often reverses that volar inclination. Dorsal inclination of **20 degrees or more** significantly affects the congruency of the DRUJ and may cause compensatory changes in carpal bone alignment.

Dorsal Displacement

Dorsal displacement contributes significantly to increased instability of the distal fragment by decreasing the contact area between fragments (Fig. 1-53).

Radial Displacement (Lateral Displacement)

Radial displacement occurs when the distal radial fragment displaces away from the ulna (Fig. 1-54).

Loss of Radial Inclination

The radius normally has a radial-to-ulnar inclination of approximately 22 degrees, measured from the tip of the radial styloid to the ulnar corner of the radius and compared with a longitudinal line along the length of the radius (Fig. 1-55). Loss of inclination can cause hand weakness and fatigability after the fracture.

Figure 1–52 Dorsal angulation. **A,** In a *normal radius*, volar inclination averages 11 degrees. **B,** A *Colles fracture* can reverse the inclination. Dorsal inclination of 20 degrees or greater significantly affects the congruency of the distal radioulnar joint and may alter carpal alignment. (Adapted from Newport ML: Colles fracture. J Musculoskel Med 17[1]:292, 2000.)

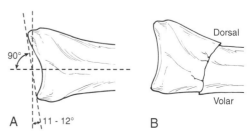

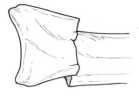

Figure 1–53   Dorsal displacement in a Colles fracture contributes to instability of the distal fragment. (Adapted from Newport ML: Colles fracture. J Musculoskel Med 17[1]:296, 2000.)

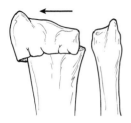

Figure 1–54   Radial (or lateral) displacement. In a displaced Colles fracture, it is possible for the distal fragment to slide away from the ulna. (Adapted from Newport ML: Colles fracture. J Musculoskel Med 17[1]:294, 2000.)

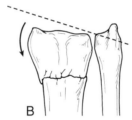

Figure 1–55   Loss of radial inclination. **A**, In a normal radius, the radial-to-ulnar inclination averages 22 degrees as measured from the tip of the radial styloid to the ulnar corner of the radius and compared with a vertical line along the midline of the radius. **B**, With a Colles fracture, radial inclination is lost because of imbalances in force on the radial versus the ulnar side of the wrist. (Adapted from Newport ML: Colles fracture. J Musculoskel Med 17[1]:296, 2000.)

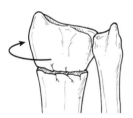

Figure 1–56   Supination of the distal fragment of a Colles fracture creates instability. A supination deformity is not usually visible on a radiograph and is best appreciated during open reduction of the fracture. (Adapted from Newport ML: Colles fracture. J Musculoskel Med 17[1]:298, 2000.)

Unrecognized supination of the distal radial fragment also creates fracture instability (Fig. 1-56).

Classification

Successful treatment of distal radial fractures requires accurate identification of certain injury characteristics and an understanding of their importance (Table 1-7). Although a number of classification systems have been described, most of the important injury elements are captured in the **system of Fernandez** (Fig. 1-57), **which distinguishes bending fractures (type 1), shearing fractures (type 2), compression fractures (type 3), fracture-dislocations (type 4), and high-energy fractures combining multiple types (type 5).**

TABLE 1–7	Treatment-Based Classification of Distal Radial Fractures	
Type	Description	Management
I	Undisplaced, extra-articular	Splinting or casting with the wrist in a neutral position for 4-6 wk. The splint chosen depends on the patient and the patient's condition and compliance, as well as on physician preference
II	Displaced, extra-articular	Fracture reduced under local or regional anesthesia
A	Stable	Splint, then cast
B	Unstable, reducible*	Remanipulation, with possible percutaneous pinning for improved stability
C	Unreducible	Open reduction and internal fixation
III	Intra-articular, undisplaced	Immobilization and possible percutaneous pinning for stability
IV	Intra-articular, displaced	
A	Stable, reducible	Adjunctive fixation with percutaneous pinning and, sometimes, external fixation
B	Unstable, reducible	Percutaneous pinning and, probably, external fixation to improve rigidity and immobilization. Dorsal comminution contributes to instability, so a bone graft may be necessary
C	Unreducible	Open reduction and internal fixation, often external fixation
D	Complex, significant soft tissue injury, carpal injury, distal ulnar fracture, or comminuted metaphyseal-diaphyseal area of the radius	Open reduction and pin or plate fixation, often supplemented with external fixation

*Instability becomes evident when radiographs show a change in position of the fracture fragments. Patients should be seen 3, 10, and 21 days after injury to check for any change in fracture position.

From Cooney WP: Fractures of the distal radius: A modern treatment-based classification. Orthop Clin North Am 24:211, 1993.

Type 1, or bending-type fractures, are extra-articular, metaphyseal fractures. Dorsally displaced fractures are commonly referred to by the eponym *Colles fracture*. Volarly displaced bending fractures are often called *Smith fractures*. **Type 2**, or articular shearing fractures, include volar and dorsal Barton fractures, shearing fracture of the radial styloid (the so-called chauffeur's fracture), and shearing fractures of the lunate facet. **Type 3**, or compression fractures, include fractures that split the articular surface of the distal radius. There is a progression of injury with greater injury force—separation of the scaphoid and lunate facets occurring first, with progression

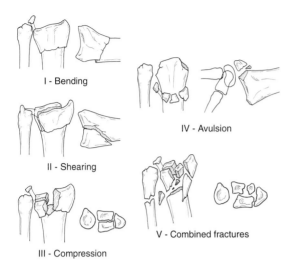

I - Bending

IV - Avulsion

II - Shearing

V - Combined fractures

III - Compression

Figure 1–57 Classification of distal radius fractures based on the mechanism of injury (Fernandez): bending (I), shearing (II), compression (III), avulsion (IV), and combined (V) mechanisms. This classification is useful because the mechanism of injury influences management of the injury. (Adapted from Fernandez DL: Fractures of the distal radius: Operative treatment. Instr Course Lect 42:74, 1993.)

to coronal splitting of the lunate or scaphoid facets and then further fragmentation. **Type 4**, radiocarpal fracture-dislocations, feature dislocation of the radiocarpal joint with small ligamentous avulsion fractures. **Type 5** fractures may combine features of all the other types and may also include forearm compartment syndrome, an open wound, or associated injury to the carpus, forearm, or elbow.

Another classification used by orthopaedic surgeons is the universal classification system (Fig. 1-58).

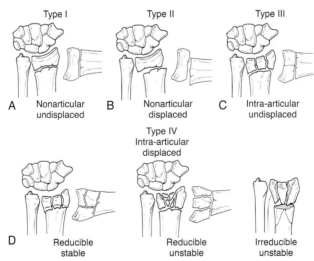

Type I

Type II

Type III

A   Nonarticular undisplaced

B   Nonarticular displaced

C   Intra-articular undisplaced

Type IV
Intra-articular displaced

D   Reducible stable

Reducible unstable

Irreducible unstable

Figure 1–58 Universal classification of distal radial fractures. **A**, Type I, nonarticular, undisplaced. **B**, Type II, nonarticular, displaced. **C**, Type III, intra-articular, undisplaced. **D**, Type IV, intra-articular, displaced. (Adapted from Cooney WP, Agee JM, Hastings H, et al: Symposium: Management of intraarticular fractures of the distal radius. Contemp Orthop 21:71, 1990.)

Diagnosis and Treatment

The wrist often appears deformed with the hand dorsally displaced. This is called a "silver fork" deformity because of the resemblance to a dinner fork when viewed from the side. The distal ulna may also be prominent. The wrist is swollen and tender, and palpation may elicit crepitus.

Patients with substantially displaced fractures should undergo rapid closed manipulation under anesthesia to reduce pressure on the soft tissues, including the nerves and skin, and to help define the pattern of injury. Closed manipulation and sugar-tong splints provide definitive treatment in many patients. This is most often accomplished with a so-called hematoma block anesthetic. Five milliliters to 10 ml of 1% lidocaine anesthetic without epinephrine is injected into the fracture site. Consideration should be given to injecting the DRUJ and an ulnar styloid fracture in some patients. Injection of the fracture site is easiest from the volar-radial aspect of the wrist in the more common dorsally displaced fractures. Manipulation is performed manually. The use of finger traps is cumbersome, limits the surgeon's ability to correct all three dimensions of the deformity, and will not help maintain length in injuries with metaphyseal impaction or fragmentation.

Radiographs taken after closed reduction may need to be supplemented by CT scanning to precisely define the pattern of injury. In particular, it can be difficult to tell whether the lunate facet of the distal radial articular surface is split in the coronal plane.

Bending fractures are extra-articular (metaphyseal) fractures. They may displace in either a dorsal or a volar direction. Dorsal displacement—known eponymically as a **Colles fracture**—is much more common. Many dorsally displaced bending fractures can be held reduced in a cast or splint. **In older patients, more than 20 degrees of dorsal angulation of the distal radial articular surface on a lateral radiograph taken before manipulative reduction usually indicates substantial fragmentation and impaction of dorsal metaphyseal bone. Many such fractures require operative fixation to maintain reduction.** Dorsally displaced fractures are reduced under a hematoma block and splinted with either a sugar-tong or a Charnley type of splint. The reduction maneuver consists of traction, flexion, ulnar deviation, and pronation. **The wrist should be splinted in an ulnar-deviated position, but without wrist flexion.** Circumferential casts and tight wraps should not be used (Fig. 1-59). **Great care must be taken to ensure that motion of the MCP joints is not restricted.**

Options for the treatment of **unstable dorsal bending fractures** include external fixation that crosses the wrist, so-called nonbridging external fixation that gains hold

Figure 1–59 A, A sugar-tong splint is made from approximately 10 thicknesses of 4-inch-wide plaster. Four layers of cast padding are used over the splint on the skin side. The splint goes from the palm, reaches around the elbow, and ends on the dorsum of the hand. The fingers are free to actively exercise. **B,** The metacarpophalangeal joints must not be restricted.

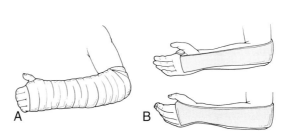

of the distal fracture fragment and does not cross the wrist, percutaneous Kirschner wire fixation, and internal plate fixation. External fixation that crosses the wrist should be used with great care. **The wrist should not be left in a flexed position, and there should be no distraction across the wrist.** Usually, this means that Kirschner wires are needed in conjunction with the external fixator. Plate fixation is generally reserved for fractures with incipient callus formation that are resistant to closed manipulation (this can occur as early as 2 weeks after injury) and fractures with fragmentation of the volar as well as the dorsal metaphysis. All these methods place the radial sensory nerve at risk. Great care must be taken to protect this nerve and its branches.

Volarly displaced bending fractures (or **Smith fractures**) are subclassified as *transverse, oblique,* or *fragmented.* Oblique and fragmented fractures will not be stable in a cast and require operative fixation. Fixation of the distal radius with a plate applied to its volar surface is straightforward and associated with few problems. Therefore, unstable volar bending fractures are best treated by internal plate fixation.

Shearing fractures may involve the volar or dorsal articular margin (so-called **Barton fractures**), the radial styloid, or the lunate facet of the distal radius. These partial articular fractures are inherently unstable. Failure to securely realign the fragment risks subluxation of the carpus. For this reason, shearing fractures are most predictably treated by open reduction and plate and screw fixation.

Many simple **compression articular fractures** can be treated by closed manipulation, external fixation, and percutaneous Kirschner wire fixation. When the lunate facet is split in the coronal plane, the volar lunate facet fragment is usually unstable and can be held only by a plate or tension band wire applied through a small volar-ulnar incision.

Radiocarpal fracture-dislocations and high-energy fractures require ORIF, in some cases supplemented by external fixation. One must also be extra vigilant regarding the potential for forearm compartment syndrome and acute CTS with these fractures.

For all these fracture types, the stability of the DRUJ should be evaluated after the distal radius has been fixed. Instability of the distal ulna merits treatment of the ulnar side of the wrist. A large ulnar styloid fracture contains the origin of the triangular fibrocartilage complex (TFCC), and ORIF of such a fragment will restore stability. Similarly, unstable ulnar head and neck fractures may benefit from internal fixation. If the DRUJ is unstable in the absence of an ulnar fracture, the radius should be pinned or casted in midsupination (45 degrees supination) for 4 to 6 weeks to enhance stability of the DRUJ.

Indications for operative treatment of distal radial fractures include an unstable fracture, an irreducible fracture, more than 20 degrees of dorsal angulation of the distal fragment, intra-articular displacement or incongruity of 2 mm or more of the articular (joint) fragments, and radial (lateral) displacement (Table 1-8).

Rehabilitation after Distal Radial Fractures

Rehabilitation after fracture of the distal radius is nearly uniform among various fracture types, provided that the pattern of injury has been identified and appropriately treated. The stages of rehabilitation can be divided into early, middle, and late.

After Distal Radial Fracture
Ring, Jupiter, Burchill, and Calamaro

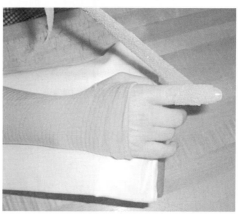

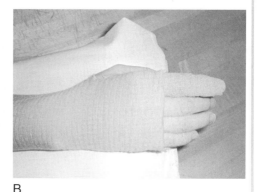

Figure 1–60 Compressive dressings can help eliminate swelling of the fingers, hand, and wrist. **A**, Self-adhesive elastic tape should be applied by rolling the tape out and laying it on while applying a safe and limited amount of compression. **B**, The hand and wrist are compressed by an elastic stocking.

EARLY PHASE (0-6 WEEKS)

The critical part of the early phase of rehabilitation is limitation of swelling and stiffness in the hand.

- Swelling can be limited and reduced by encouraging elevation of the hand above the level of the heart, by encouraging frequent active mobilization, and by wrapping the digits and hand with self-adhesive elastic tape (e.g., Coban, 3M, St. Paul, Minn) and applying a compressive stocking to the hand and wrist (Fig. 1-60).
- Stiffness can be limited by teaching the patient an aggressive program of active and passive digit ROM exercises (Fig. 1-61).
- The use of an external fixator as a splint to protect percutaneous or internal fixation is helpful to avoid the use of restrictive circumferential dressings in the early postoperative period.
- Stable fractures and fractures with internal fixation can be supported with a light, removable thermoplastic splint. We use an Austin wrist splint, which is a

Continued

TABLE 1–8   Palmar Treatment Algorithm for Distal Radius Fractures

Fracture Type		Treatment Protocol
Nondisplaced fracture		Group 1 (physiologically young and/or active) STS—3 wk SAC—3 wk Splint (R)—3 wk Closed reduction X-ray findings
Displaced fracture		
Acceptable reduction		
	Unacceptable reduction (>2 mm radial shortening) (>2 mm displacement of articular fragment) (>15 degrees dorsiflexion of radius)	Group 2 (physiologically old and/or inactive) STS—2 wk SAC—2 wk Splint (R)—3 wk Closed reduction 1. STS—2 wk 2. SAC—3 wk Splint (R)—3 wk 3. Late-distal ulna resection

Stable fracture
STS—3 wk
LAC—3 wk
Splint (R)—3 wk

Unstable fracture
1. External fixation with supplemental percutaneous pins
   Ex. fix—6 wk
   Pins—8 wk
   Splint (R)—3 wk

2. ORIF (plate)
   SAS—10 days
   Splint (R)—5 wk

3. Percutaneous pins
   STS—3 wk
   SAC—3 wk
   Pins—6 wk
   Splint (R)—3 wk

→

1. External fixation with fragment elevation (pins optional) and iliac crest bone graft—5 wk

2. ORIF (K-wire) with iliac crest bone graft
   Ex. fix—6 wk
   Pins—6 wk
   SAS—6 wk
   Splint (R)—4 wk

Our protocol of the treatment of nondisplaced and displaced distal radial fractures in the physiologically young and/or active (group 1) and the physiologically old and/or inactive (group 2). Nondisplaced fractures are easily treated with immobilization alone in both groups. Displaced fractures require reduction in both groups, but only in group 1 do we recommend further treatment. Based on the reduction and whether the fracture is stable, immobilization is recommended with or without operative treatment. Fractures in which the reduction is unacceptable require reduction of the fragments with external fixation and/or internal fixation and bone grafting.

Ex., external; LAC, long arm cast; ORIF, open reduction and internal fixation; R, removable; SAC, short arm cast; SAS, short arm splint; STS, sugar-tong splint.

From Palmar AK: Fractures of the distal radius. In Green D (ed): Operative Hand Surgery, 3rd ed. New York, Churchill Livingstone, 1993.

REHABILITATION PROTOCOL: *After Distal Radial Fracture*   *Continued*

EARLY PHASE (0-6 WEEKS)—cont'd

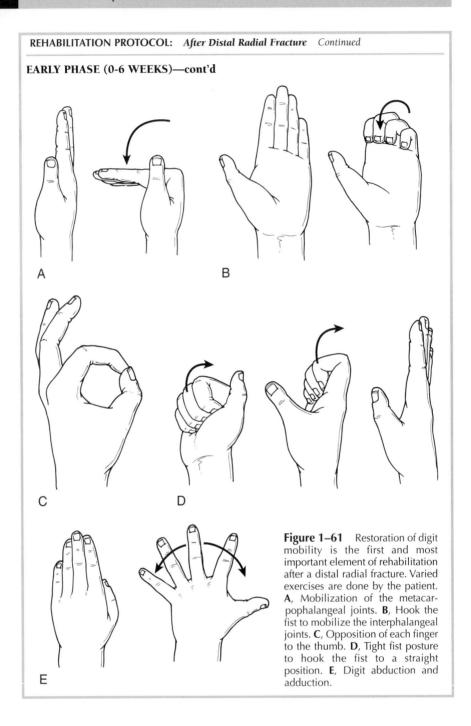

A

B

C

D

E

Figure 1–61   Restoration of digit mobility is the first and most important element of rehabilitation after a distal radial fracture. Varied exercises are done by the patient. **A**, Mobilization of the metacarpophalangeal joints. **B**, Hook the fist to mobilize the interphalangeal joints. **C**, Opposition of each finger to the thumb. **D**, Tight fist posture to hook the fist to a straight position. **E**, Digit abduction and adduction.

REHABILITATION PROTOCOL: *After Distal Radial Fracture* Continued

EARLY PHASE (0-6 WEEKS)—cont'd

well-padded thermoplastic brace that comes "off the shelf" but is custom moldable to each patient.

- A well-padded sugar-tong splint is used initially for stable, nonoperatively treated distal radial fractures. Eventually, the elbow is "freed" from the sugar-tong splint (to avoid elbow stiffness) when the fracture looks sticky (approximately 3-4 weeks).

Another critical part of the early rehabilitation phase is functional use of the hand. Many of these patients are older and have a diminished capacity to adapt to their wrist injury.

- Appropriate treatment should be sufficiently stable to allow functional use of the hand for light activities (i.e., <5 pounds of force).
- When the hand is used to assist with daily activities such as dressing, feeding, and toileting, it will be more quickly incorporated back into the patient's physical role and may be less prone to becoming dystrophic.
- Functional use also helps restore mobility and reduce swelling.
- Most fractures are stable with forearm rotation. Supination, in particular, can be very difficult to regain after fracture of the distal radius. Initiation of active and gentle-assisted forearm rotation exercises in the early phase of rehabilitation may speed and enhance the recovery of supination (Fig. 1-62).
- Some methods of treatment (e.g., nonbridging external fixation and plate fixation) offer the potential to initiate wrist flexion/extension and radial/ulnar deviation during

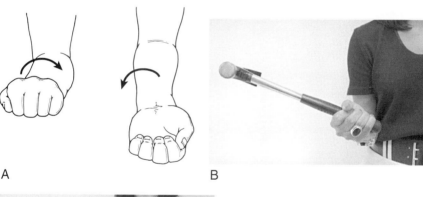

A   B

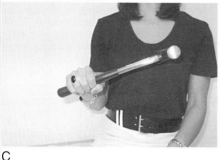

C

Figure 1–62 Forearm range of motion (ROM) is part of the early phase of rehabilitation of most distal radial fractures. **A**, Active forearm ROM is done with the elbow stabilized at the side to avoid "cheating" by moving the shoulder rather than the forearm. **B**, Gentle assistive stretch can be provided by using either the other hand or the weight of a mallet grasped in the hand. **C**, A mallet can be used to assist pronation.

Continued

REHABILITATION PROTOCOL: *After Distal Radial Fracture*   *Continued*

EARLY PHASE (0-6 WEEKS)—cont'd

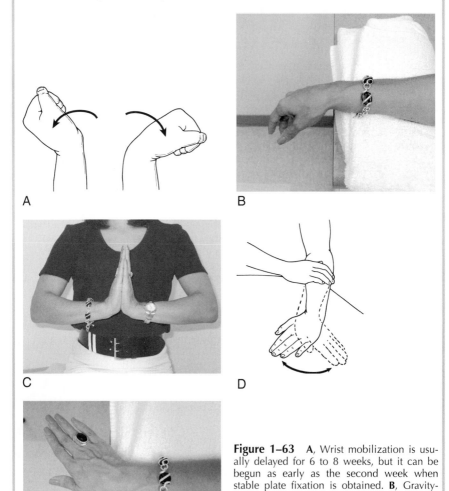

Figure 1–63 **A**, Wrist mobilization is usually delayed for 6 to 8 weeks, but it can be begun as early as the second week when stable plate fixation is obtained. **B**, Gravity-assisted wrist flexion—hanging the hand off a towel. **C**, Wrist extension exercises. **D**, Radial and ulnar deviation. **E**, Wrist and ulnar deviation.

the early phase of healing. Provided that fixation of the fragments is secure, we usually allow wrist mobilization at the time of suture removal (10-14 days after the operation) (Fig. 1-63).

- Scar massage may help limit adhesions in the area of incisions. In some patients with raised or hypertrophic scars, we recommend Otoform (Dreve-Otoplastik GMBH, Unna, Germany) application to help flatten and diminish the scar (Fig. 1-64).

REHABILITATION PROTOCOL: *After Distal Radial Fracture*   *Continued*

EARLY PHASE (0-6 WEEKS)—cont'd

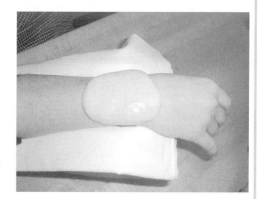

Figure 1–64 Conforming plastics can be applied with pressure (such as under a Coban wrap) to help diminish the prominence of the scar.

- Active motion of the ipsilateral shoulder and elbow is recommended to avoid a frozen shoulder or elbow throughout the postoperative rehabilitation.

MIDDLE PHASE (6-8 WEEKS)

- Once early healing of the fracture is established (between 6 and 8 weeks after the injury or operation), the pins and external fixation can be removed and the patient weaned from external support.
- Radiographs should guide this transition because some very fragmented fractures may require support for longer than 8 weeks.
- Active-assisted forearm and wrist mobilization exercises are used to maximize mobility (see Figs. 1-65 and 1-66). *There is no role for passive manipulation in the rehabilitation of fractures of the distal radius.*
- Dynamic splinting may help improve motion. In particular, if supination is slow to return, a dynamic supination splint can be used intermittently (Fig. 1-65).

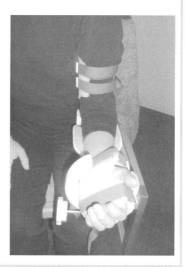

Figure 1–65 A supination splint provides a constant stretching force that is useful when stiffness is resistant to simple active-assisted exercises.

Continued

REHABILITATION PROTOCOL: *After Distal Radial Fracture* *Continued*

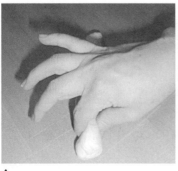
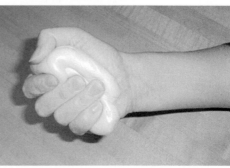

A   B

Figure 1–66 Digit strengthening can be accomplished by exercises incorporating the manipulation of putty. Separate exercises emphasize manipulation with the fingertips (**A**) and in a clenched fist (**B**).

LATE PHASE (8-12 WEEKS)

- Once healing is well established (between 6 and 12 weeks after the injury or operation), strengthening exercises can be initiated while active-assisted mobilization is continued.
- The wrist and hand have been rested for a number of months from the time of the injury and will benefit from focused strengthening exercises, including digit strengthening with Theraputty (Smith and Nephew, Memphis, TN) (Fig. 1-66), the use of small weights (Fig. 1-67), and the use of various machines (Fig. 1-68).

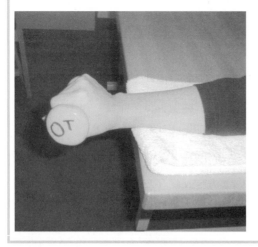

Figure 1–67 Wrist-strengthening exercises are part of the final phase of rehabilitation. Small weights can be used.

REHABILITATION PROTOCOL: *After Distal Radial Fracture* Continued

LATE PHASE (8-12 WEEKS)—cont'd

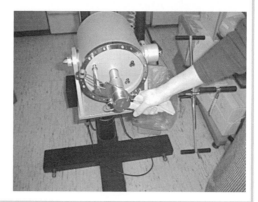

Figure 1–68 More sophisticated machines, such as this one made by Baltimore Therapeutic Equipment, can provide more controlled and quantifiable methods of strengthening.

Conclusions

Rehabilitation after fracture of the distal radius focuses first on preventing a problem with the wrist from creating a problem with the hand; second, on restoring functional mobility quickly; and finally, on optimizing the function of the wrist after injury. Any method of treatment that contributes to excessive swelling or restriction of digit motion or tendon gliding should be abandoned. For instance, if a cast that is molded tightly to maintain fracture reduction increases edema, the surgeon should consider changing to percutaneous pinning and external fixation to avoid a constrictive dressing. Once effective treatment is administered, the rehabilitation program is straightforward.

Triangular Fibrocartilage Complex Injury

Dan C. Byck, MD • Felix H. Savoie III, MD • Larry D. Field, MD

Clinical Background

The TFCC is an arrangement of several structures. **The primary structure is the triangular fibrocartilage or meniscal disk, which is a relatively avascular disklike structure that provides a cushion effect between the distal articular surface of the ulna and the proximal carpal row, primarily the triquetrum.** Much like the menisci in the knee, vascular studies have demonstrated poor central vascularity, whereas the peripheral 15% to 20% has the arterial inflow required for healing. In addition, there is no vascular contribution from the radial base of the TFCC. **Thus, central defects or tears tend to have difficulty healing, and more peripheral injuries heal at a much higher rate**.

The disk is a biconcave structure with a radial attachment that blends with the articular cartilage of the radius. The ulnar attachment lies at the base of the ulnar styloid. There are superficial and deep layers of the TFCC that attach separately at the base

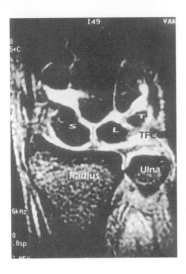

Figure 1–69 The scaphoid (S) and lunate (L) articulate with the distal articular surface of the radius, and the ulnar head articulates with the sigmoid notch. The triangular fibrocartilage complex (TFCC) is interposed between the ulnar carpus and the ulnar head. T, triquetrum.

of the ulna styloid (Fig. 1-69). The anterior and posterior thickenings of the TFCC are confluent with the anterior and posterior radioulnar capsule and are called the *palmar* and *dorsal radioulnar ligaments*. These structures are placed under tension as the forearm is pronated and supinated and provide the primary stabilization of the DRUJ (Fig. 1-70). The TFCC itself is under maximal tension in neutral rotation. Additional attachments to the lunate, triquetrum, hamate, and the base of the fifth metacarpal have been described. These structures, combined with the extensor carpi ulnaris subsheath, make up the TFCC. Normal function of the DRUJ requires a normal relationship of these anatomic structures. Tear, injury, or degeneration of any one structure leads to pathophysiology of the DRUJ and abnormal kinesis of the wrist and forearm. When evaluating **ulnar-sided wrist pain** or painful forearm rotation, several entities should be considered.

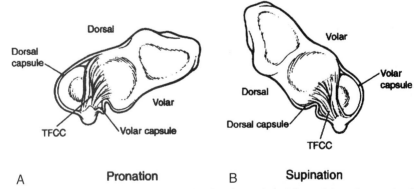

Figure 1–70 **A**, Right wrist in pronation. The dorsal capsule is tight, and the volar margin of the triangular fibrocartilage complex (TFCC; the volar radioulnar ligament) is tight. **B**, Right wrist in supination. The volar distal radioulnar joint capsule is tight, and the dorsal margin of the TFCC (dorsal radioulnar ligament) is tight as the dorsal margin of the radius moves farther away from the base of the ulnar styloid.

Classification

The most widely accepted classification system of TFCC injuries is that developed by Palmer (1989). ***TFCC tears are divided into two categories: traumatic and degenerative.*** The system uses clinical, radiographic, anatomic, and biomechanical data to define each tear. Rehabilitation of these lesions is based on the type of procedure performed. For **class 1A or 2A lesions**, the central portion of the disk is débrided, and in this case, rehabilitation consists of return to activities as tolerated after wound healing has taken place. For most other TFCC lesions, a more extensive immobilization period followed by aggressive physical therapy is required.

Classification of Triangular Fibrocartilage Complex Lesions (Palmer)

CLASS 1: TRAUMATIC

A. Central perforation
B. Ulnar avulsion
   With ulnar styloid fracture
   Without ulnar styloid fracture
C. Distal avulsion
D. Radial avulsion
   With sigmoid notch fracture
   Without sigmoid notch fracture

CLASS 2: DEGENERATIVE (ULNOCARPAL ABUTMENT SYNDROME)

A. TFCC wear
B. TFCC wear
   With lunate or ulnar chondromalacia
C. TFCC perforation
   With lunate or ulnar chondromalacia
D. TFCC perforation
   With lunate or ulnar chondromalacia
   With lunotriquetral ligament perforation
E. TFCC perforation
   With lunate or ulnar chondromalacia
   With lunotriquetral ligament perforation
   With ulnocarpal arthritis

Diagnosis

A thorough history is critical to the diagnosis of TFCC lesions. Factors such as onset and duration of symptoms, type and force of trauma, eliciting activities, recent changes in symptoms, and past treatment attempts should be noted. Most TFCC injuries are caused by a fall on an outstretched hand, rotational injuries, or repetitive axial loading. ***Patients complain of ulnar-sided wrist pain and clicking and often crepitation with forearm rotation, gripping, or ulnar deviation of the wrist.*** Tenderness is often present on either the dorsal or palmar side of the TFCC. Instability of the DRUJ or clicking may or may not be elicited. Care should be taken to rule out extensor carpi ulnaris tendon subluxation and radial-sided wrist injuries as well.

Provocative maneuvers are often helpful in differentiating TFCC injuries from lunotriquetral pathology. First, however, the pisotriquetral joint should be tested to rule out disease at this joint. With the wrist in neutral rotation, the triquetrum is firmly compressed against the lunate. The "**shuck test**" described by Reagan and coworkers (1984) is a more sensitive test of the lunotriquetral joint. The lunotriquetral joint is grasped between the thumb and the index finger while the wrist is stabilized with the other hand, and the lunotriquetral joint is "shucked" in a dorsal-to-palmar direction. Kleinman and Graham (1996) suggested that the most sensitive test to elicit lunotriquetral pathology is the **shear test**. In this test, one thumb is placed against the pisiform and the other thumb stabilizes the lunate on its dorsal surface. As the examiner's thumbs are forced toward the carpus, a shear force is created in the lunotriquetral joint. Lester and colleagues (1995) described a **press test** to diagnose TFCC tears. They did not differentiate the region of the tear but stated that the test was 100% sensitive for tears. In the press test, the patient grasps both sides of a chair seat while sitting in the chair. The patient then presses the body weight directly upward, and if the pain replicates the ulnar-sided pain, the test is considered positive.

Once a normal lunotriquetral joint is established, the TFCC is then evaluated. The **TFCC grind test** is very sensitive in eliciting tears in the TFCC and DRUJ instability. With the wrist in neutral rotation and ulnarly deviated, it is rolled palmarly and then dorsally. Pain or a click suggests a TFCC tear. When done with the forearm fully pronated, the dorsal radioulnar ligaments are tested. With the forearm fully supinated, the volar radioulnar ligaments are assessed.

The **piano key test** evaluates DRUJ stability. With the forearm fully pronated, the distal ulna is balloted in a dorsal-to-volar direction. This test correlates with the "piano key sign" seen on lateral wrist radiographs.

Diagnostic Studies

Radiographs of the wrist include PA, lateral, and oblique views taken with the shoulder abducted to 90 degrees, the elbow flexed to 90 degrees, and the forearm flat on the table. *When indicated, specialty views such as a supination-pronation, a clenched-fist PA, and a 30-degree supination view to assess the pisotriquetral joint may be obtained.*

Arthrography may be used as a confirmatory test. Radiopaque contrast material is injected directly into the radiocarpal joint. If a tear is present, the dye will extravasate into the region of the tear. More recent reports suggest that three-compartment (radiocarpal, DRUJ, and midcarpal) injections are a more accurate method of assessing TFCC lesions. Care must be taken when interpreting wrist arthrograms because a high frequency of false-negative readings has been reported. An asymptomatic TFCC, interosseous ligament tears, and details of the exact tear location may also appear on wrist arthrography, although adjacent soft tissue structures or articular surfaces are not well delineated.

MRI of the wrist has evolved into a useful resource for diagnosing TFCC lesions. Although an experienced radiologist is imperative, the coils and techniques are now approaching arthroscopy in sensitivity and predictive value for TFCC tears. *Potter and associates (1997) reported that MRI had a sensitivity of 100%, specificity of 90%, and accuracy of 97% in 57 wrists with arthroscopically verified TFCC lesions*. The advantage of MRI over arthrography lies in its ability to identify the location of the lesion. Potter and associates reported a sensitivity of 100%, specificity of 75%, and accuracy of 92% in locating the structure injured. Gadolinium-enhanced MR arthrograms are no longer necessary to produce significant results.

The "gold standard" in diagnosing wrist injuries is arthroscopy. No other technique is as accurate or reliable in locating the lesion. In addition, arthroscopy allows the surgeon to palpate and observe every structure in the wrist, thus making it easier to treat all possible components of the injury. Arthroscopy also avoids the complications associated with open wrist surgery and allows speedier rehabilitation after immobilization.

Differential Diagnosis of Ulnar-Sided Wrist Pain

Radial shortening (e.g., comminuted distal radial fracture)

TFCC tear (central versus peripheral)

Degenerative joint disease

Lunotriquetral arthritis

Extensor carpi ulnaris instability or tendinitis

Fracture of the hook of the hamate

Flexor carpi ulnaris calcific tendinitis

Pisotriquetral arthritis

Ulnar artery stenosis

Guyon's canal syndrome

Ulnar styloid fracture

Congenital positive ulnar variance

Ulnar nerve disease

Treatment

Surgical intervention for TFCC injuries is indicated only after a full course of non-operative measures.

Initially, the wrist is **braced** for 4 to 6 weeks. NSAIDs are prescribed, and occasionally a **corticosteroid injection** may be beneficial. After **immobilization, physical therapy** is initiated. First, active-assisted and passive ROM exercises are begun. Aggressive motion exercises and resisted strengthening rehabilitation are then added, followed by plyometric and sports-specific therapy. Most patients with TFCC tears respond well to bracing and therapy.

If nonoperative care fails and symptoms persist, surgery is indicated. In athletes, surgery may be performed earlier because of competitive and seasonal considerations. Though a controversial issue, delaying surgical treatment of TFCC tears may adversely affect the outcome.

Surgical intervention is predicated on the type of TFCC tear. Treatment of some tears remains controversial, whereas treatment of others is more widely accepted.

For **type 1A** tears, débridement of the central tear is usually preferred if there is no DRUJ instability. Up to two thirds of the central disk can be removed without significantly altering the biomechanics of the wrist. Care must be taken to avoid violating the volar or dorsal radioulnar ligaments to prevent DRUJ instability.

Type 1B tears affect the periphery of the TFCC. This is recognized by loss of the "trampoline" effect of the central portion of the disk. Repairs of these tears usually heal because of the adequate blood supply.

Type 1D tears fall in the controversial category. Traditional treatment has been débridement of the tear, followed by early motion. Several authors, however, have reported improved results with surgical repair of these tears. In our clinic, repair of radial-sided tears of the sigmoid notch of the radius is preferred.

Type 2 tears are degenerative by definition and often occur in athletes who stress their wrists (gymnastics, throwing and racquet sports, wheelchair sports). Nonoperative treatment should be continued for at least 3 months before arthroscopy. Most of these lesions occur in patients with an ulna neutral or positive wrist. In these patients, débridement of the central degenerative disk tear is followed by an extra-articular ulnar shortening procedure such as the wafer procedure.

REHABILITATION PROTOCOL   *After TFCC Débridement*
Byrk, Savoie, and Field

The protocol initially focuses on tissue healing and early immobilization.
When TFCC *repair* is performed, the wrist is immobilized for 6-8 weeks and forearm pronation/supination is prevented for the same period with the use of a Münster cast.

PHASE 1: 0-7 DAYS

• Soft dressing to encourage wound healing and decrease soft tissue edema

PHASE 2: 7 DAYS-VARIABLE

• ROM exercises encouraged
• Return to normal activities as tolerated

PHASE 3: WHEN PAIN FREE

• Resisted strengthening exercises, plyometrics, and sport-specific rehabilitation (see later)

REHABILITATION PROTOCOL   *After Repair of a TFCC Tear (with or without Lunotriquetral Pinning)*
Byrk, Savoie, and Field

PHASE 1

0-7 Days

• The immediate postoperative period focuses on decreasing the soft tissue edema and joint effusion. Maintaining an immobilized wrist and elbow is important, and a combination of ice or cold therapy and elevation is desired. The upper extremity is placed in a sling.

REHABILITATION PROTOCOL: *After Repair of a TFCC Tear (with or without Lunotriquetral Pinning)* Continued

PHASE 1—cont'd

- Finger flexion/extension exercises are initiated to prevent possible tenodesis and decrease soft tissue edema.
- Active-assisted and passive shoulder ROM exercises are instituted to prevent loss of motion in the glenohumeral joint. These exercises are performed at home.

7 Days-2 Weeks

- During the first office visit, the sutures are removed and a Münster cast is applied. Once again, the wrist is completely immobilized and elbow flexion/extension is encouraged.
- Hand and shoulder ROM exercises are continued.
- The sling is removed.

PHASE 2

4-8 Weeks

- The Münster cast is removed and a removable Münster cast is applied. Elbow flexion and extension are continued, but forearm rotation is avoided.
- Gentle wrist flexion/extension exercises are initiated.
- Progression to a squeeze ball is begun.
- Hand and shoulder exercises are continued.

PHASE 3

8 Weeks

- The Münster cast is removed and a neutral wrist splint is used as needed.
- The lunotriquetral wires are removed in the office.

3 Months

- Progressive active and passive ROM exercises are instituted in the six planes of wrist motion (see the section on distal radial fractures).
- Once pain-free ROM exercises are accomplished, strengthening exercises are begun.
  1. Weighted wrist curls in six planes of wrist motion with small dumbbells or elastic tubing. This includes the volar, dorsal, ulnar, radial, pronation, and supination directions. Once strength returns, the Cybex machine may be used to further develop pronation-supination strength.
  2. Four-way diagonal upper extremity patterns using dumbbells, cable weights, or elastic tubing.
  3. Flexor-pronator forearm exercises. The wrist begins in extension, supination, and radial deviation, and with a dumbbell used as resistance, the wrist is brought into flexion, pronation, and ulnar deviation.
  4. Resisted finger extension/flexion exercise with hand grips and elastic tubing.
  5. Upper extremity plyometrics are instituted. Once wall-falling/push-off is accomplished (see 6A), weighted medicine ball exercises are begun. Initially, a 1-pound ball is used; then the weight of the ball is progressed as indicated.
  6. The plyometric exercises are tailored to the patient's activity interests. If the patient is an athlete, sports-specific exercises are added.
     A. Wall-falling in which a patient stands 3-4 feet from a wall. The patient falls into the wall, catches on hands, and rebounds to the starting position.

Continued

REHABILITATION PROTOCOL: *After Repair of a TFCC Tear (with or without Lunotriquetral Pinning)*   *Continued*

PHASE 3—cont'd

   B. Medicine ball throw in which a medicine ball is grasped with both hands in the overhead position. The ball is thrown to a partner or trampoline. On return, the ball is taken into the overhead position.
   C. Medicine ball throw in which a medicine ball is grasped with both hands in the chest position. The ball is push-passed to a partner or trampoline. On return, the ball is taken into the chest position.
   D. Medicine ball throw in which a medicine ball is push-passed off a wall and rebounded in the chest position.
   E. Medicine ball throw in which the ball is grasped in one hand in the diagonal position and thrown to a partner or trampoline. The rebound is taken in the diagonal position over the shoulder. This may be performed across the body or with both hands.
   F. Medicine ball throw in which the patient is lying supine with the upper extremity unsupported, abducted to 90 degrees, and externally rotated to 90 degrees. A medicine ball weighing 8 ounces to 2 pounds is dropped by a partner from a height of 2-3 feet. When the ball is caught, it is returned to the partner in a throwing motion as rapidly as possible.
   G. Medicine ball push-up with wrist in palmar flexion, dorsiflexion, radial deviation, and ulnar deviation. This may be performed with the knees on the ground to begin with and progress to weight on toes as strength returns.
- Sports-specific exercises are designed to emulate the biomechanical activity encountered during play. For overhead and throwing athletes, the following program should be instituted:
  - Initially, ROM exercises establish pain-free motion. All aforementioned exercises are instituted and developed.
  - A weighted baton is used to re-create the motion of throwing, shooting, or racquet sports. This is progressed to elastic resistance. Ball-free batting practice is likewise begun.
  - Finally, actual throwing, shooting, or overhead racquet activities are begun.
  - Contact athletes, such as football linemen, will begin bench presses and bench flies. Initially, the bars are unweighted. Painless weight progression and repetition progression as tolerated are performed.
- Work-hardening tasks such as using a wrench and pliers to tighten nuts and bolts. A screwdriver may be used to tighten/loosen screws.

PHASE 4

3 Months

- Minimum time for splint-free return to sports.

De Quervain's Tenosynovitis

S. Brent Brotzman, MD • Steven J. Meyers, MD • Kyle Phillips, PA-C

Background

This disorder is the most common overuse injury involving the wrist and often occurs in individuals who regularly use a forceful grasp coupled with ulnar deviation of the wrist (such as in a tennis serve).

Injury occurs because of inflammation around the tendon sheath of the abductor pollicis longus (APL) and extensor pollicis brevis (EPB) in the first dorsal compartment (Fig. 1-71A). Pain and tenderness localized over the radial aspect of the wrist (over the first dorsal compartment) are the typical symptoms.

The **Finklestein test** is diagnostic for de Quervain's tenosynovitis (Fig. 1-71B). This test places stress on the APL and EPB by placing the thumb into the palm of a "fist" and then ulnarly deviating the wrist. Mild de Quervain's tenosynovitis may cause pain only on resisted thumb MCP joint extension.

Other possible causes of pain in the "radial dorsal pain" category include
- CMC arthritis of the thumb—pain and crepitance are present with the thumb "crank and grind test." This test is performed by applying axial pressure to the thumb while palpating the first CMC joint. (The crank and grind test is positive only with CMC arthritis of the thumb. Both de Quervain's tenosynovitis and CMC arthritis may have a "positive" Finklestein test and pain on thumb motion; however, the crank and grind test will be positive *only* in patients with arthritis of the basal joint [CMC] of the thumb.)
- Scaphoid fracture—tender in the anatomic snuffbox.
- Chauffeur's fracture—radial styloid fracture.
- Intersection syndrome—more proximal pain and tenderness (see later in this chapter).

Figure 1–71 **A,** Anatomic arrangement of the first dorsal extensor compartment. The tunnel contains the extensor pollicis brevis tendon and one or more slips of the abductor pollicis longus tendon. **B,** Finkelstein test: flexion and ulnar deviation of the wrist with the fingers flexed over the thumb. Pain over the first compartment strongly suggests de Quervain's stenosing tenosynovitis. (Adapted from Idler RS: Helping the patient who has wrist or hand tenosynovitis. J Musculoskel Med 14[2]:183, 1997.)

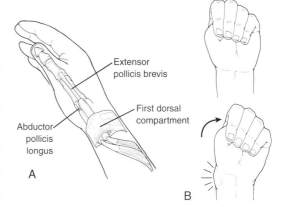

Extensor pollicis brevis

First dorsal compartment

Abductor pollicis longus

A

B

- Wartenberg's syndrome (entrapment of the sensory branch of the radial nerve) causes pain in the sensory distribution of the superficial sensory branch of the radial nerve because of entrapment or compression at the point where the nerve exits its submuscular position below the brachioradialis.

Conservative Management

A thumb spica splint is used to immobilize the first dorsal compartment tendons. A commercially available splint or, depending on the patient's comfort, a custom-molded Orthoplast device can be used. The splint maintains the wrist in 15 to 20 degrees of extension and the thumb in 30 degrees of radial and palmar abduction. The IP joint is left free, and motion at this joint is encouraged. The patient wears the splint during the day for the first 2 weeks and at night until the next office visit, generally at 6 to 8 weeks. Splinting may continue longer, depending on the response to treatment. The splint can be discontinued during the day if symptoms permit and if daily activities are gradually resumed. Workplace activities are advanced accordingly. Other considerations include the following:

- A **corticosteroid sheath injection** can be offered to patients with moderate to marked pain or with symptoms lasting more than 3 weeks. The injection should individually distend the APL and EPB sheaths. Discomfort after injection is variable, and a 2- to 3-day supply of mild analgesic is recommended.
- A systemic **NSAID** (e.g., Celebrex) is commonly prescribed for the initial 6 to 8 weeks of treatment.
- Thumb use is restricted so that the first dorsal compartment tendons are at relative rest. Activities that require prolonged thumb IP joint flexion, pinch, or repetitive motions are avoided.
- Distal-to-proximal thumb Coban wrapping, retrograde application of lotion, or ice massage over the radial styloid.
- Phonophoresis with 10% hydrocortisone can be used for edema control.
- Gentle active and passive thumb and wrist motion is encouraged 5 minutes every hour to prevent joint contracture and tendon adhesions.

Operative Management

Symptoms are often temporarily relieved and the patient elects to repeat the management outlined previously. Unsatisfactory symptom reduction or symptom persistence requires surgical decompression.

Multiple separate compartments for the APL (which typically has two to four tendon slips) and the EPB require decompression. Extreme caution in the approach will spare the sensory branches of the lateral antebrachial cutaneous nerve and dorsal sensory branches of the radial nerve. Before decompression, the encasing circular retinacular fibers that arc across the radial styloid should be exposed. The floor of this compartment is the tendinous insertion of the brachioradialis tendon, which sends limbs to the volar and dorsal margins of the compartment. The APL and EPB tendons may be difficult to differentiate, especially in the absence of septation. When this Y tendinous floor is identified, it can serve as a landmark to indicate decompression of the first dorsal compartment.

Intersection Syndrome of the Wrist

S. Brent Brotzman, MD

Background

Intersection syndrome is tendinitis or tenosynovitis of the first and second dorsal compartments of the wrist (Fig. 1-72). The muscles and tendons of these two compartments traverse each other at a 60-degree angle, three fingerbreadths proximal to the wrist joint on the dorsal aspect (several centimeters proximal to Lister's tubercle). **This area is *proximal* to the location of de Quervain's tenosynovitis**.

This overuse syndrome most often occurs in rowing, skiing, racquet sports, canoeing, and weightlifting. In skiers, the mechanism of injury is repetitive dorsiflexion and radial deviation of the wrist as the skier withdraws the planted ski pole

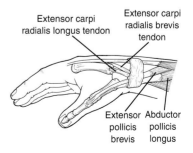

Figure 1–72 Wrist anatomy. The tendinitis of intersection syndrome occurs in the area shown. (Adapted from Servi JT: Wrist pain from overuse. Physician Sports Med 25[12]:41, 1997.)

from the resistance of deep snow. Weightlifters who overuse their radial extensors of the wrist and perform excessive curling are subject to intersection syndrome.

Physical Examination

- Examination reveals point tenderness to palpation on the dorsum of the wrist, three fingerbreadths proximal to the wrist joint.
- Crepitation or "squeaking" may be noted with passive or active motion of the involved tendons, and swelling (tenosynovitis) may be visible along the two compartments.
- Pain is present on wrist flexion or extension (dorsally), rather than on radial and ulnar deviation as in de Quervain's tenosynovitis (e.g., the Finklestein test is positive in de Quervain's tenosynovitis; Table 1-9).

TABLE 1–9	Distinctive Clinical Findings in Common Forms of Tenosynovitis (Hand and Wrist)	
Tenosynovitis	**Findings**	**Differential Diagnosis**
Intersection syndrome	Edema, swelling, and crepitation in the intersection area; pain over the **dorsum** of the wrist that is exacerbated by wrist flexion and extension, unlike the pain of de Quervain's tenosynovitis, which is exacerbated by radial and ulnar deviation; pain extends less radially than it does in de Quervain's tenosynovitis	Wartenberg's syndrome, de Quervain's tenosynovitis
de Quervain's	Pain along the radial aspect of the wrist that worsens with radial and ulnar wrist deviation; pain on performing the Finkelstein maneuver is pathognomonic	Arthritis of the first carpometacarpal joint, scaphoid fracture and nonunion, radiocarpal arthritis, Wartenberg's syndrome, intersection syndrome
Sixth dorsal compartment	Pain over the ulnar dorsum of the wrist that is worsened by ulnar deviation and wrist extension; other planes of motion may also be painful; tenderness over the sixth dorsal compartment; instability of the extensor carpi ulnaris is shown by having the patient circumduct the wrist while rotating the forearm from pronation to supination	Extensor carpi ulnaris instability, triangular fibrocartilage complex tears, lunotriquetral ligament tears, ulnocarpal abutment syndrome, distal radioulnar joint arthritis, traumatic rupture of the subsheath that normally stabilizes this tendon to the distal ulna

TABLE 1–9	Distinctive Clinical Findings in Common Forms of Tenosynovitis (Hand and Wrist)—cont'd	
Tenosynovitis	**Findings**	**Differential Diagnosis**
Flexor carpi radialis tunnel	Pain, swelling, and erythema around the *palmar* radial aspect of the wrist at the flexor carpi radialis tunnel; pain exacerbated by resisted wrist flexion	Retinacular ganglion; scaphotrapezial arthritis, first carpometacarpal arthritis; scaphoid fracture/nonunion; radial carpal arthritis; injury to the palmar cutaneous branch of the median nerve; Lindberg's syndrome (tendon adhesions between the flexor pollicis longus and the flexor digitorum profundus)
Trigger finger	Pain on digital motion, with or without associated triggering or locking at the interphalangeal joint of the thumb or proximal interphalangeal joint of other fingers; may be crepitus or a nodular mass near the first annular pulley that moves with finger excursion.	Connective tissue disease, partial tendon laceration, retained foreign body, retinacular ganglion, infection, extensor tendon subluxation

From Idler RS: Helping the patient who has wrist or hand tenosynovitis. J Musculoskel Med 14(2): 62, 1997.

Prevention

Skiers should be instructed in proper powder skiing pole techniques, such as avoiding deep pole planting and pole dragging. Decreasing ski pole length by 2 inches and decreasing the basket diameter to 2 inches may help prevent intersection syndrome.

Treatment

- Exacerbating activities (e.g., rowing) are avoided for several weeks.
- A removable commercial thumb spica splint (wrist in 15 degrees of extension) is used to immobilize and support the thumb for 3 to 6 weeks.
- Training modifications are made on resumption of activity (e.g., avoid curling with excessive weight).
- Cryotherapy is used several times a day (ice massage with frozen water from a peeled-away Styrofoam cup).
- NSAIDs are given, and corticosteroid injection of the compartment may be effective (avoid injection of the actual tendon).
- Gentle ROM exercises of the wrist and hand are begun, and wrist extensor strengthening is initiated after the patient is asymptomatic for 2 to 3 weeks to avoid repetitive "overuse" of relatively "weak" musculotendinous units.

REHABILITATION PROTOCOL	*After Surgical Decompression of Intersection Syndrome*

0-14 DAYS

- Keep the wrist in neutral position within the surgical plaster splint.
- Encourage digital, thumb, and elbow motion as comfort allows.
- Remove the sutures at 10-14 days after surgery.

2-4 WEEKS

- Maintain the presurgical splint until the patient can perform activities of daily living with little pain.
- Active and active-assisted wrist extension and flexion exercises should attain full preoperative values by 4 weeks after surgery.

4-6 WEEKS

- Advance the strengthening program.
- Anticipate full activities at the end of the sixth week after surgery.
- Use the splint as needed.
- Scar desensitization techniques may be necessary, including the use of a transcutaneous electric nerve stimulation (TENS) unit if the scar region is still tender 6 weeks after surgery.

Dorsal and Volar Carpal Ganglion Cysts

S. Brent Brotzman, MD • Anna Williams, PT

Background

Dorsal carpal ganglion cysts rarely originate from sites other than near the scapholunate interval. These cysts may decompress into the EPL or common extensor tendon sheaths and may appear to arise from sites remote from their origin (Fig. 1-73).

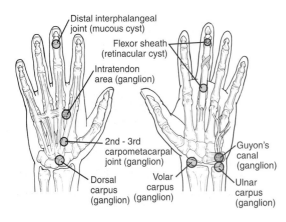

Figure 1–73 Common sites for the development of ganglia. (Adapted from Kozin SH, Urban MA, Bishop AT, Dobyns SH: Wrist ganglia: Diagnosis and treatment. J Musculoskel Med 10[1]:21, 1993.)

A dorsal transverse incision in a Langer line over the scapholunate interval clearly exposes the pathology through a window bounded by the second and third dorsal compartments radially, the fourth compartment ulnarly, the dorsal intercarpal ligament distally, and the dorsal radiocarpal ligament proximally.

Volar carpal ganglion cysts originate from the flexor carpi radialis tendon sheath or from articulations between the radius and the scaphoid, the scaphoid and the trapezium, or the scaphoid and the lunate. Excision of these cysts, as with dorsal carpal ganglion cysts, should include a generous capsulectomy at the site of the cyst origin.

Physical Examination (Fig. 1-74)

- Dorsal ganglion cysts are most visible with the wrist flexed.
- Palpation may produce mild discomfort, and provocation motion (extremes of wrist flexion and wrist extension) often increases the pain.
- For a volar wrist ganglion, the differential diagnosis includes vascular lesions, and an Allen test should be performed to check vascular patency.

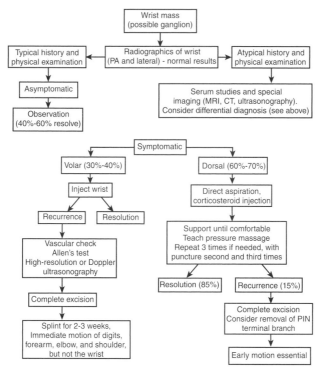

Figure 1–74 Management of wrist ganglia. CT, computed tomography; MRI, magnetic resonance imaging; PA, posteroanterior; PIN, posterior interosseus nerve. (From Kozin SH, Urban MA, Bishop AT, Dobyns SH: Wrist ganglia: Diagnosis and treatment. J Musculoskel Med 10[1]:21, 1993.)

Differential Diagnosis of Wrist Ganglia

Non-neoplastic masses
  Extraskeletal
    Aneurysm/arteriovenous malformation
    Anomalous muscle and other anomalous structure
    Bursa
    Displaced tendon
    Foreign body granulomas
    Hypertrophic structure
    Nerve entrapment
    Nerve ganglion
    Periarticular calcaneal
    Post-traumatic (neuroma, tendon remnant)
    Repetitive use fibrosis
    Scar
    Tendon entrapment
    Tuberous sclerosis
  Skeletal
    Arthritic residuum
    Pigmented villonodular synovitis
    Post-traumatic residuum: subluxated scaphoid
Neoplastic masses
    Soft tissue
    Benign tumor (chondroma, fibroma, giant cell tumor of the tendon
      sheath, hemangioma, lipoma, neuroma)
    Malignant tumor (epithelioid sarcoma, malignant fibrous histiocytoma,
      metastasis, synovial sarcoma)
    Skeletal
    Benign tumor (cyst, chondroma, giant cell tumor, collagen
      osteochondroma, osteoid osteoma)
    Malignant tumor (chondrosarcoma, metastasis, osteosarcoma)
    Infectious
    Fungus, mycobacteria, pyogen, tuberculosis
    Disease/Metabolic

Continued on following page

> Rheumatoid arthritis and disease, rheumatoid nodule, synovial cyst, tenosynovitis
>
> Gout and pseudogout
>
> Neuritis (posterior interosseous nerve), vasculitis, amyloidosis

From Kozin SH, Urban MA, Bishop AT, Dobyns JH: Wrist ganglia: Diagnosis and treatment. J Musculoskel Med 10(1):21, 1993.

Treatment

- Conservative treatment, which may include aspiration and corticosteroid injection, is tried first.
- If symptoms persist, excision of the ganglion may be indicated.
- Postoperative resolution is usual for both volar and dorsal ganglia (greater than 90% with the ideal technique), but recurrence or even new formation of a ganglion or pain is possible.

REHABILITATION PROTOCOL   *After Excision of a Wrist Ganglion*

2 WEEKS

- Remove the short arm splint and sutures.
- Initiate active and active-assisted wrist extension and flexion.
- Continue interval splint wear during the day between exercises and at night.

2-4 WEEKS

- Advance ROM exercises to resistive and gradual strengthening exercises.
- Discontinue the splint at 4 weeks.

4-6 WEEKS

- Allow normal activities to tolerance.

6 WEEKS

- Allow full activity.

Bibliography

FLEXOR TENDON INJURIES

Boyes JH: Flexor tendon grafts in the fingers and thumb: An evaluation of end results. J Bone Joint Surg Am 32:489, 1950.

Bunnell S: Surgery of the Hand, 3rd ed. Philadelphia, JB Lippincott, 1956.

Cannon NM: Diagnosis and Treatment Manual for Physicians and Therapists, 3rd ed. Indianapolis, IN, The Hand Rehabilitation Center of Indiana, PC, 1991.

Creighton JJ, Idler RS, Strickland JW: Hand clinic, trigger finger and thumb. Indiana Med 83:260, 1990.

Dinham JM, Meggitt BF: Trigger thumbs in children: A review of the natural history and indications for treatment in 105 patients. J Bone Joint Surg Br 56:153, 1974.

Duran RJ, Houser RG: Controlled passive motion following flexor tendon repair in zones 2 and 3. AAOS Symposium on Tendon Surgery in the Hand. St Louis, Mosby, 1975, p 105.

Fahey JJ, Bollinger JA: Trigger finger in adults and children. J Bone Joint Surg Am 36:1200, 1954.

Green D: Operative Hand Surgery, 3rd ed. New York, Churchill Livingstone, 1993.

Hunter JH: Rehabilitation of the Hand, 3rd ed. St Louis, CV Mosby, 1992.

Hunter JH, Mackin EJ, Callahan AD: Rehabilitation of the Hand and Upper Extremity, 5th ed. St Louis, CV Mosby, 2002.

Idler RS: Anatomy and biomechanics of the digital flexor tendons. Hand Clin 1:3, 1985.

Leddy JP, Packer JW: Avulsion of the profundus tendon insertion in athletes. J Hand Surg [Am] 1:66, 1977.

Rhoades CE, Gelberman RH, Manjarris JF: Stenosing tenosynovitis of the fingers and thumbs. Clin Orthop 190:236, 1984.

EXTENSOR TENDON INJURIES

Mallet Finger

Abound JM, Brown H: The treatment of mallet finger: The results in a series of consecutive cases and a review of the literature. Br J Surg 9:653, 1968.

Bowers WH, Hurst LC: Chronic mallet finger: The use of Fowler's central slip release. J Hand Surg [Am] 3:373, 1978.

Doyle JR: Extensor tendons—acute injuries. In Green D (ed): Operative Hand Surgery, 3rd ed. New York, Churchill Livingstone, 1993.

Fess EE, Gettle KS, Strickland JW: Hand Splinting Principles and Methods. St Louis, CV Mosby, 1981.

Hillman FE: New technique for treatment of mallet fingers and fractures of the distal phalanx. JAMA 161:1135, 1956.

Iselin F, Levame J, Godoy J: A simplified technique for treating mallet fingers: Tenodermodesis. J Hand Surg [Am] 2:118, 1977.

Kleinert HE, Verdan C: Report of the committee on tendon injuries (International Federation of Societies for Surgery of the Hand). J Hand Surg [Am] 5:794, 1983.

Kleinman WB, Peterson DP: Oblique retinacular ligament reconstruction for chronic mallet finger deformity. J Hand Surg [Am] 9:399, 1984.

McCoy FJ, Winsky AJ: Lumbrical loop for luxation of the extensor tendons of the hand. Plast Reconstr Surg 44:142, 1969.

Stark HH, Gainor BJ, Ashworth CR, et al: Operative treatment of intraarticular fractures of the dorsal aspect of the distal phalanx of digits. J Bone Joint Surg Am 69:892, 1987.

Stern PJ, Kastrup JJ: Complications and prognosis of treatment of mallet finger. J Hand Surg [Am] 13:329, 1988.

Wehbe MA, Schneider LH: Mallet fractures. J Bone Joint Surg Am 66:658, 1984.

Wood VE: Fractures of the hand in children. Orthop Clin North Am 7:527, 1976.

FRACTURES AND DISLOCATIONS

Agee JM: Unstable fracture-dislocations of the proximal interphalangeal joint: Treatment with the force couple splint. Clin Orthop 214:101, 1987.

Cannon NM: Diagnosis and Treatment Manual for Physicians and Therapists, 3rd ed. Indianapolis, IN, The Hand Center of Indiana, 1991.

Crenshaw AH: Campbell's Operative Orthopaedics, 8th ed. St Louis, CV Mosby, 1992.

DeLee JC, Drez D: Orthopaedic Sports Medicine, 2nd ed. Philadelphia, WB Saunders, 2003.

Greene D: Operative Hand Surgery, 3rd ed. New York, Churchill Livingstone, 1993.

Hunter JM: Rehabilitation of the Hand: Surgery and Therapy, 3rd ed. St Louis, CV Mosby, 1990.

Jahss SA: Fractures of the metacarpals: A new method of reduction and immobilization. J Bone Joint Surg 20:278, 1938.

Jobe MT: Fractures and dislocations of the hand. In Gustilo RB, Kyle RK, Templeman D (eds): Fractures and Dislocations. St Louis, CV Mosby, 1993.

Kaukonen JP, Porras M, Karaharju E: Anatomical results after distal forearm fractures. Ann Chir Gynaecol 77:21, 1988.

Knirk JL, Jupiter JB: Intra-articular fractures of the distal end of the radius in young adults. J Bone Joint Surg Am 63:647, 1986.

Moberg E: Emergency Surgery of the Hand. Edinburgh, Churchill Livingstone, 1968.

Putnam MD: Fractures and dislocations of the carpus including the distal radius. In Gustillo RB, Kyle RF, Templeman D (eds): Fractures and Dislocations. St Louis, CV Mosby, 1993.

Ryu J, Watson HK, Burgess RC: Rheumatoid wrist reconstruction utilizing a fibrous nonunion and radiocarpal arthrodesis. J Hand Surg [Am] 10:830, 1985.

Schultz RJ, Brown V, Fox JM: Gamekeeper's thumb: Results of skiing injuries. N Y State J Med 73:2329, 1973.

NERVE COMPRESSION SYNDROMES

Carpal Tunnel Syndrome

Burke DT: Splinting for carpal tunnel syndrome. Arch Phys Med Rehabil 75:1241, 1994.

Gellman H, Gelberman RH, Tan AM, Botte MJ: Carpal tunnel syndrome: An evaluation of provocative diagnostic tests. J Bone Joint Surg Am 5:735, 1986.

Green D: Operative Hand Surgery, 3rd ed. New York, Churchill Livingstone, 1993.

Szabo RM, Madison M: Carpal tunnel syndrome. Orthop Clin North Am 1:103, 1992.

Pronator Syndrome

Gainor BJ: The pronator compression test revisited. Orthop Rev 19:888, 1990.

Hartz CR, Linscheid RL, Gramse RR, Daube JR: The pronator teres syndrome; compressive neuropathy of the median nerve. J Bone Joint Surg Am 63:885, 1981.

Idler RS, Strickland JW, Creighton JJ: Pronator Syndrome. Indianapolis Hand Clinic, Indiana Center for Surgery and Rehabilitation of the Hand and Upper Extremity, 1999.

ARTHROPLASTY

Finger Arthroplasty

Bieber EJ, Weiland AJ, Volenec-Dowling S: Silicone-rubber implant arthroplasty of the metacarpophalangeal joints for rheumatoid arthritis. J Bone Joint Surg Am 68:206, 1986.

Blair WF, Shurr DG, Buckwalter JA: Metacarpophalangeal joint implant arthroplasty with a Silastic spacer. J Bone Joint Surg Am 66:365, 1984.

Cannon NM: Diagnosis and Treatment Manual for Physicians and Therapists, 3rd ed. Indianapolis, IN, The Hand Rehabilitation Center of Indiana, PC, 1991.

Eaton RG, Malerich MM: Volar plate arthroplasty of the proximal interphalangeal joint: A review of ten years' experience. J Hand Surg [Am] 5:260, 1980.

Swanson AB: Silastic HP 100 Swanson finger joint implant for metacarpophalangeal and proximal interphalangeal joint arthroplasty and Dow Corning Wright Swanson finger joint Grommet II for metacarpophalangeal implant arthroplasty. Grand Rapids, MI, Dow Corning Wright, 1988.

Swanson AB: Flexible implant arthroplasty for arthritic finger joints. J Bone Joint Surg Am 54:435, 1972.

Swanson AB, Leonard JB, deGroot Swanson G: Implant resection arthroplasty of the finger joints. Hand Clin 2:107, 1986.

Swanson AB, Maupin BK, Gajjar NV, Swanson GD: Flexible implant arthroplasty in the proximal interphalangeal joint of the hand. J Hand Surg [Am] 10:796, 1985.

Thumb Carpometacarpal Joint Arthroplasty

Burton RI, Pellegrini VD: Surgical management of basal joint arthritis of the thumb. II. Ligament reconstruction with tendon interposition arthroplasty. J Hand Surg [Am] 11:324, 1986.

Cannon NM: Diagnosis and Treatment Manual for Physicians and Therapists, 3rd ed. Indianapolis, IN, The Hand Rehabilitation Center of Indiana, PC, 1991.

Creighton JJ, Steichen JB, Strickland JW: Long-term evaluation of Silastic trapezial arthroplasty in patients with osteoarthritis. J Hand Surg [Am] 16:510, 1991.

Dell PC, Brushart TM, Smith RJ: Treatment of trapeziometacarpal arthritis: Results of resection arthroplasty. J Hand Surg [Am] 3:243, 1978.

Eaton RG, Littler JW: Ligament reconstruction for the painful thumb carpometacarpal joint. J Bone Joint Surg Am 55:1655, 1973.

Kleinman WB, Eckenrode JF: Tendon suspension sling arthroplasty for thumb trapeziometacarpal arthritis. J Hand Surg [Am] 16:983, 1991.

Hofammann DY, Ferlic DC, Clayton ML: Arthroplasty of the basal joint of the thumb using a silicone prosthesis. J Bone Joint Surg Am 69:993, 1987.

Pellegrini VD, Burton RI: Surgical management of basal joint arthritis of the thumb. I. Long-term results of silicone implant arthroplasty. J Hand Surg [Am] 11:309, 1986.

WRIST AND DISTAL RADIOULNAR JOINT DISORDERS

Radius Fractures

Alffram PA, Bauer GCH: Epidemiology of fractures of the forearm: A biomechanical investigation of bone strength. J Bone Joint Surg Am 44:158, 1962.

Anderson DD, Bell AL, Gaffney MB, Imbriglia JE: Contact stress distributions in malreduced intraarticular distal radius fractures. J Orthop Trauma 10:331, 1996.

Fernandez DL: Smith Frakturen. Z Unfallmed Berusfskrankheiten 3:110, 1980.

Fernandez DL: Fractures of the distal radius: Operative treatment. Instr Course Lect 42:73, 1993.

Fernandez DL: Acute and chronic derangement of the distal radio ulnar joint after fractures of the distal radius. EFORT 41, 1999.

Fernandez DL, Geissler WB: Treatment of displaced articular fractures of the radius. J Hand Surg [Am] 16:375, 1991.

Fernandez DL, Jupiter JB: Fractures of the Distal Radius. A Practical Approach to Management. New York, Springer-Verlag, 1995.

Friberg S, Lundstrom B: Radiographic measurements of the radiocarpal joint in normal adults. Acta Radiol Diagn 17:249, 1976.

Gartland JJ, Werley CW: Evaluation of healed Colles' fractures. J Bone Joint Surg Am 33:895, 1951.

Gelberman RH, Szabo RM, Mortensen WW: Carpal tunnel pressures and wrist position in patients with Colles' fractures. J Trauma 24:747, 1984.

Kaempffe FA, Wheeler DR, Peimer CA, et al: Severe fractures of the distal radius: Effect of amount and duration of external fixator distraction on outcome. J Hand Surg [Am] 18:33, 1993.

Kozin SH: Early soft-tissue complications after fractures of the distal part of the radius. J Bone Joint Surg Am 75:144, 1993.

Melone CP: Articular fractures of the distal radius. Orthop Clin North Am 15:217, 1984.

Melone CP: Open treatment for displaced articular fractures of the distal radius. Clin Orthop 202:103, 1988.

Newport ML: Colles fracture: Managing a common upper extremity injury. J Musculoskel Med 17:292, 2000.

Pattee GA, Thompson GH: Anterior and posterior marginal fracture-dislocation of the distal radius. Clin Orthop 231:183, 1988.

Short WH, Palmer AK, Werner FW, Murphy DJ: A biomechanical study of distal radius fractures. J Hand Surg [Am] 12:529, 1987.

Simpson NS, Jupiter JB: Delayed onset of forearm compartment syndrome: A complication of distal radius fracture in young adults. J Orthop Trauma 9:411, 1995.

Talesnick J, Watson HK: Midcarpal instability caused by malunited fractures of the distal radius. J Hand Surg [Am] 9:350, 1984.

Trumble T, Glisson RR, Seaber AV, Urbaniak JR: Forearm force transmission after surgical treatment of distal radioulnar joint disorders. J Hand Surg [Am] 12:196, 1987.

Viegas SF, Tencer AF, Cantrell J, et al: Load transfer characteristics of the wrist. Part II. Perilunate instability. J Hand Surg [Am] 12:978, 1987.

TRIANGULAR FIBROCARTILAGE COMPLEX TEARS

Adams BD: Partial excision of the triangular fibrocartilage complex articular disc: Biomechanical study. J Hand Surg [Am] 18:919, 1993.

Bednar M, Arnoczky S, Weiland A: The microvasculature of the triangular fibrocartilage complex: Its clinical significance. J Hand Surg [Am] 16:1101, 1991.

Bowers WH, Zelouf DS: Treatment of chronic disorders of the distal radioulnar joint. In Lichtman DM, Alexander AH (eds): The Wrist and Its Disorders, 2nd ed. Philadelphia, WB Saunders, 1997, p 475.

Byrk FS, Savoie FH III, Field LD: The role of arthroscopy in the diagnosis and management of cartilaginous lesions of the wrist. Hand Clin 15:423, 1999.

Chidgey LK, Dell PC, Bittar ES, Spanier SS: Histologic anatomy of the triangular fibrocartilage complex. J Hand Surg [Am] 16:1084, 1991.

Cooney WP, Linscheid RL, Dobyns JH: Triangular fibrocartilage tears. J Hand Surg [Am] 19:143, 1994.

Corso SJ, Savoie FH, Geissler WB, et al: Arthroscopic repair of peripheral avulsions of the triangular fibrocartilage complex of the wrist: A multicenter study. Arthroscopy 13:78, 1997.

Feldon P, Terrono AL, Belsky MR: Wafer distal ulna resection for triangular fibrocartilage tears and/or ulna impaction syndrome. J Hand Surg [Am] 17:731, 1992.

Fellinger M, Peicha G, Seibert FJ, Grechenig W: Radial avulsion of the triangular fibrocartilage complex in acute wrist trauma: A new technique for arthroscopic repair. Arthroscopy 13:370, 1997.

Jantea CL, Baltzer A, Ruther W: Arthroscopic repair of radial-sided lesions of the fibrocartilage complex. Hand Clin 11:31, 1995.

Johnstone DJ, Thorogood S, Smith WH, Scott TD: A comparison of magnetic resonance imaging and arthroscopy in the investigation of chronic wrist pain. J Hand Surg [Br] 22:714, 1997.

Kleinman WB, Graham TJ: Distal ulnar injury and dysfunction. In Peimer CA (ed): Surgery of the Hand and Upper Extremity, vol 1. New York, McGraw-Hill, 1996, p 667.

Lester B, Halbrecht J, Levy IM, Gaudinez R: "Press test" for office diagnosis of triangular fibrocartilage complex tears of the wrist. Ann Plast Surg 35:41, 1995.

Levinsohn EM, Rosen ID, Palmer AK: Wrist arthrography: Value of the three-compartment injection method. Radiology 179:231, 1991.

Lichtman DM: The Wrist and Its Disorders. Philadelphia, WB Saunders, 1988.

Loftus JB, Palmer AK: Disorders of the distal radioulnar joint and triangular fibrocartilage complex: An overview. In Lichtman DM, Alexander AH (eds): The Wrist and Its Disorders, 2nd ed. Philadelphia, WB Saunders, 1997, p 385.

Mikic ZDJ: Age changes in the triangular fibrocartilage in the wrist joint. J Anat 126:367, 1978.

Palmer AK: Triangular fibrocartilage complex lesions: A classification. J Hand Surg [Am] 14:594, 1989.

Palmer AK, Glisson RR, Werner FW: Ulnar variance determination. J Hand Surg [Am] 7:376, 1982.

Palmer AK, Werner FW: The triangular fibrocartilage complex of the wrist: Anatomy and function. J Hand Surg [Am] 6:153, 1981.

Palmer AK, Werner FW: Biomechanics of the distal radial ulnar joint. Clin Orthop 187:26, 1984.

Palmer AK, Werner FW, Glisson RR, Murphy DJ: Partial excision of the triangular fibrocartilage complex. J Hand Surg [Am] 13:403, 1988.

Pederzini L, Luchetti R, Soragni O, et al: Evaluation of the triangular fibrocartilage complex tears by arthroscopy, arthrography and magnetic resonance imaging. Arthroscopy 8:191, 1992.

Peterson RK, Savoie FH, Field LD: Arthroscopic treatment of sports injuries to the triangular fibrocartilage. Sports Med Orthop Rev 6:262, 1998.

Potter HG, Asnis-Ernberg L, Weiland AJ, et al: The utility of high-resolution magnetic resonance imaging in the evaluation of the triangular fibrocartilage complex of the wrist. J Bone Joint Surg Am 79:1675, 1997.

Reagan DS, Linscheid RL, Dobyns JH: Lunotriquetral sprains. J Hand Surg [Am] 9:502, 1984.

Roth JH, Haddad RG: Radiocarpal arthroscopy and arthrography in the diagnosis of ulnar wrist pain. Arthroscopy 2:234, 1986.

Sagerman SD, Short W: Arthroscopic repair of radial-sided triangular fibrocartilage complex tears. Arthroscopy 12:339, 1996.

Savoie FH: The role of arthroscopy in the diagnosis and management of cartilaginous lesions of the wrist. Hand Clin 11:1, 1995.

Savoie FH, Grondel RJ: Arthroscopy for carpal instability. Orthop Clin North Am 26:731, 1995.

Savoie FH, Whipple TL: The role of arthroscopy in athletic injuries of the wrist. Clin Sports Med 15:219, 1996.

Thuri-Pathi RG, Ferlic DC, Clayton ML, McLure DC: Arterial anatomy of the triangular fibrocartilage of the wrist and its surgical significance. J Hand Surg [Am] 11:258, 1986.

Trumble TE, Gilbert M, Bedder N: Arthroscopic repair of the triangular fibrocartilage complex. Arthroscopy 12:588, 1996.

Viegas SF, Patterson RM, Hokanson JA, et al: Wrist anatomy: Incidence, distribution and correlation of anatomic variations, tears and arthrosis. J Hand Surg [Am] 18:463, 1993.

De Quervain's Disease

Edwards EG: deQuervain's stenosing tendo-vaginitis at the radial styloid process. South Surg 16:1081, 1950.

Jackson WT, Viegas SF, Coon TM, et al: Anatomical variations in the first extensor compartment of the wrist. J Bone Joint Surg Am 68:923, 1986.

Minamikawa Y, Peimer CA, Cox WL, Sherwin FS: deQuervain's syndrome: Surgical and anatomical studies of the fibroosseous canal. Orthopaedics 14:545, 1991.

Strickland JW, Idler RS, Creighton JC: Hand clinic deQuervain's stenosing tenovitis. Indiana Med 83:340, 1990.

Totten PA: Therapist's management of deQuervain's disease. In Hunter JM (ed): Rehabilitation of the Hand, Surgery and Therapy. St Louis, CV Mosby, 1990.

Intersection Syndrome

Grundberg AB, Reagan DS: Pathologic anatomy of the forearm: Intersection syndrome. J Hand Surg [Am] 10:299, 1985.

Wrist Ligament Injury

Blatt G: Capsulodesis in reconstructive hand surgery. Hand Clin 3:81, 1987.

Lavernia CJ, Cohen MS, Taleisnik J: Treatment of scapholunate dissociation by ligamentous repair and capsulodesis. J Hand Surg [Am] 17:354, 1992.

Watson HK, Ballet FL: The SLAC wrist: Scapholunate advanced collapse pattern of degenerative arthritis. J Hand Surg [Am] 9:358, 1984.

2 | Elbow Injuries

KEVIN E. WILK, PT • JAMES R. ANDREWS, MD

Findings in Common Conditions of the Elbow and Forearm

VALGUS EXTENSION OVERLOAD SYNDROME

- Tenderness around the tip of the olecranon (posterior of the elbow)
- Pain with forced passive elbow extension
- Increased valgus laxity (variable)

CUBITAL TUNNEL SYNDROME

- Tenderness over the course of the ulnar nerve
- Abnormal Tinel's sign over the ulnar nerve as it passes through the cubital tunnel (at the elbow medially)
- Ulnar nerve compression test abnormal
- Elbow flexion test abnormal (variable)
- Abnormal sensation (two-point discrimination or light touch) of the little finger (fifth finger), ulnar aspect of the ring finger (fourth finger), and ulnar aspect of the hand (variable)

Continued

Findings in Common Conditions of the Elbow and Forearm   *Continued*

CUBITAL TUNNEL SYNDROME—CONT'D

- Weakness and atrophy of the ulnar-innervated intrinsic muscles of the hand (variable)
- Weakness of the flexor digitorum profundus to the little finger (variable)
- Signs of concomitant ulnar nerve instability, elbow instability, or elbow deformity (occasionally)

LATERAL EPICONDYLITIS (EXTENSOR ORIGIN TENDINITIS)

- Tenderness at the lateral epicondyle and at the origin of the involved tendons
- Pain produced by resisted wrist extension (see the section "Lateral Epicondylitis [tennis elbow]")
- Pain with passive flexion of the fingers and the wrist with the elbow fully extended (variable)

RADIAL TUNNEL SYNDROME

- Tenderness in the extensor muscle mass of the forearm at the arcade of Frohse (distal to the lateral epicondyle)
- Long finger extension test reproduces familiar pain
- Weakness of the finger and thumb extensors and extensor carpi ulnaris (unusual); (see text)

PRONATOR TERES SYNDROME

- Tenderness in the proximal part of the forearm over the pronator teres
- Abnormal sensation (two-point discrimination or light touch) in the thumb, index finger, long finger, and radial side of the ring finger (variable)
- Prolonged resisted pronation reproduces symptoms
- Weakness of the median innervated muscle (variable)
- Rare, but **often incorrectly diagnosed as carpal tunnel syndrome**
- Resisted elbow flexion with forearm supination reproduces symptoms (compression at the lacertus fibrosus)
- Resisted long finger proximal interphalangeal joint flexion reproduces symptoms (compression by the flexor digitorum superficialis)
- Weakness of the median innervated muscles (variable)

ANTERIOR INTEROSSEOUS NERVE SYNDROME

- Weakness of the flexor pollicis longus and flexor digitorum profundus to the index finger (O sign)
- Weakness of the pronator quadratus (variable)

MEDIAL EPICONDYLITIS (FLEXOR-PRONATOR TENDINITIS)

- Tenderness over the common flexor origin
- Resisted wrist flexion test reproduces pain
- Resisted forearm pronation reproduces pain
- Differentiate this from ulnar collateral ligament (UCL) tear and/or cubital tunnel syndrome (ulnar nerve)

DISTAL BICEPS TENDON RUPTURE

- Swelling
- Ecchymosis
- Palpable gap in the biceps tendon
- Weak or absent supination and elbow flexion

Findings in Common Conditions of the Elbow and Forearm *Continued*

ULNAR COLLATERAL LIGAMENT STRAIN OR TEAR

- Medial elbow joint pain in a thrower
- Complete tears open on valgus stress testing with the elbow flexed at 25 degrees (versus the uninvolved side)
- Incomplete tears are tender on palpation of the UCL but do not open on valgus stressing
- Differentiate a UCL strain or tear from a flexor-pronator strain or medial epicondylitis (see text).

NURSEMAID'S ELBOW (PULLED ELBOW SYNDROME)

- Mean age is 2 to 3 years.
- History of longitudinal traction on an extended elbow
- Partial slippage of the annular ligament over the head of the radius and into the radiocapitellar joint
- History is critical to making diagnosis
- Child typically holds the arm at the side with the hand pronated (palm down)
- Closed reduction is highly successful (86% to 98%). First supinate (palm up) the forearm. Then hyperflex the elbow
- Keep the examiner's thumb over the radial head laterally to feel the snap of the ligament reduction

LITTLE LEAGUER'S ELBOW

- Term encompasses a spectrum of pathologies about the elbow joint in young, developing (pediatric) throwers with open physes
- Four distinct areas vulnerable to throwing stress: (1) medial elbow tension overload, (2) lateral articular surface compression overload, (3) posterior medial shear forces, and (4) extension overload of the lateral restraints
- May be manifested as Panner's disease (necrosis of the capitellum), osteochondritis dissecans, medial epicondylar fracture, medial apophysitis, medial ligament rupture, and posterior osteophyte formation at the tip of the olecranon
- This subset of pediatric throwing athletes should be evaluated by a pediatric orthopaedic surgeon.

OSTEOARTHRITIS

- Restricted flexion or extension
- Effusion (variable)

Modified from Reider B: The Orthopaedic Physical Examination. Philadelphia, WB Saunders, 1999.

▌Evaluation

We typically take an anatomically oriented approach to identifying and treating elbow injuries. With few exceptions, pain in a particular area of the elbow is caused by the surrounding or underlying physical structures (Fig. 2-1). Injuries should also be classified into **acute** (such as a radial head fracture or posterior elbow dislocation) or **progressive overuse** with repetitive microtrauma. The athlete should be able to localize the primary symptoms into one of five areas.

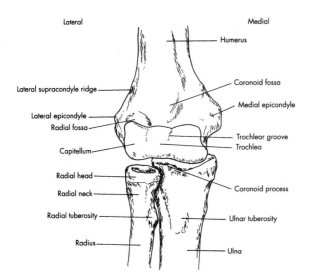

Lateral

Medial

Humerus

Lateral supracondyle ridge

Coronoid fossa

Medial epicondyle

Lateral epicondyle

Radial fossa

Capitellum

Trochlear groove

Trochlea

Radial head

Radial neck

Coronoid process

Radial tuberosity

Ulnar tuberosity

Radius

Ulna

Figure 2–1 Osseous structures of the humeroradial and humeroulnar joints.

Differential Diagnosis of Elbow Pain According to Symptom Location (Figs. 2-2 to 2-5)

Location	Possible Disorders
Anterior	Anterior capsular strain
	Distal biceps tendon rupture/tendinitis
	Dislocation of the elbow
	Pronator syndrome (throwers)
Medial	Medial epicondylitis
	UCL injury (medial collateral ligament [MCL])
	Ulnar neuritis or ulnar nerve subluxation
	Flexor pronator muscle strain
	Fracture
	Little leaguer's elbow in skeletally immature throwers
	Valgus extension overload/overuse symptoms
Posteromedial	Olecranon tip stress fracture
	Posterior impingement in throwers
	Trochlear chondromalacia
Posterior	Olecranon bursitis
	Olecranon process stress fracture
	Triceps tendinitis
Lateral	Capitellum fracture
	Lateral epicondylitis
	Lateral collateral injury

Continued on following page

Osteochondral degenerative changes

Osteochondritis dissecans (Panner's disease)

Posterior interosseous nerve syndrome

Radial head fracture

Radial tunnel syndrome

Synovitis

Cervical radiculopathy—referred pain

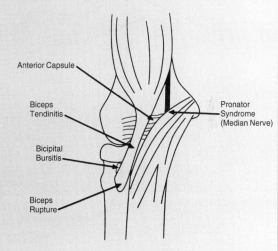

Figure 2–2 Anterior elbow pain. (From Mellion MB, Walsh WM, Shelton GL: The Team Physician's Handbook, 3rd ed. Philadelphia, Hanley & Belfus, 2000, p 419.)

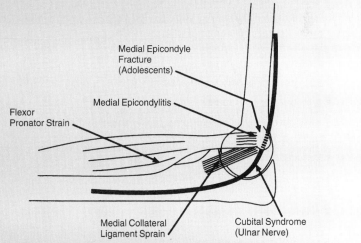

Figure 2–3 Medial elbow pain. (From Mellion MB, Walsh WM, Shelton GL: The Team Physician's Handbook, 3rd ed. Philadelphia, Hanley & Belfus, 2002, p 419.)

Continued on following page

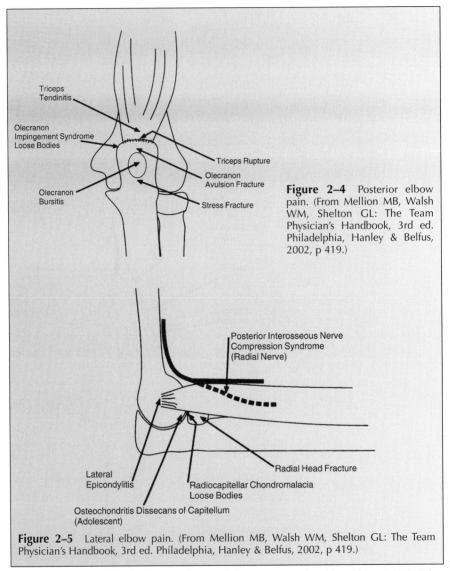

Figure 2–4 Posterior elbow pain. (From Mellion MB, Walsh WM, Shelton GL: The Team Physician's Handbook, 3rd ed. Philadelphia, Hanley & Belfus, 2002, p 419.)

Figure 2–5 Lateral elbow pain. (From Mellion MB, Walsh WM, Shelton GL: The Team Physician's Handbook, 3rd ed. Philadelphia, Hanley & Belfus, 2002, p 419.)

Modified from Conway JE: Clinical evaluation of elbow injuries in the athlete. J Musculoskel Med 10(3):20, 1988.

THROWER'S HISTORY

In a throwing athlete, the examiner should seek out details, including
- Acute versus progressive injury
- Intensity of symptoms
- Duration of symptoms
- Throwing schedule
  - Frequency of throwing
  - Intensity
  - Duration
- Delivery style (sidearm versus overhead—the former more injurious to the elbow)
- Types and proportions of throws delivered (e.g., curves are more deleterious than fastballs)
- Rest periods taken
- Warm-up and cool-down regimens used
- Phase of throwing in which the pain occurs (e.g., early cocking, acceleration, follow-through)
- Restriction of motion (posterior capsular contracture)
- Locking or checkrein-type symptoms

Common Complaints in Throwing Athletes

Medial elbow pain from UCL valgus overload (UCL injury) may be felt as an acute "pop" or progressive medial elbow discomfort after heavy throwing. These athletes complain of losing significant speed of their throw. Ulnar nerve signs (including numbness and paresthesias radiating into the ulnar two fingers) often occur with UCL injury (in up to 40% of athletes). Instability of the ligament allows traction injury of the ulnar nerve.

Posterior elbow pain is often present with **valgus extension overload syndrome**.

Lateral elbow pain in throwers is produced by excess **compression** and subsequent lesions of the radial head or capitellum or resultant loose bodies (e.g., little leaguer's elbow).

PHYSICAL EXAMINATION

Physiologic/pathologic changes often noted in throwers include
- Flexion contracture of elbow (loss of extension)
- Cubitus valgus
- Flexor-pronator muscular hypertrophy
- Anterior capsular contracture
- Olecranon hypertrophy
- Posterior or anterior compartment loose bodies

Medial Joint Examination

- Point tenderness at the medial epicondyle or musculoskeletal junction indicates a flexor-pronator strain (rarely a defect is noted and indicates a tear).
- Tenderness on palpation of the anterior band of the UCL **differentiates pathology of the UCL from that of the flexor-pronator group (medial epicondyle)**.

- Pain or asymmetrical laxity on valgus stress testing of the UCL should be noted. Valgus stress testing is performed by flexing the elbow 20 to 30 degrees to unlock the olecranon and comparing the affected with the asymptomatic elbow. This test can be performed in the supine, prone, or seated position.
- The **valgus extension snap maneuver** is performed by placing a firm valgus stress on the elbow and then snapping the elbow into extension. Reproduction of pain during this test is indicative of **valgus extension overload syndrome of the elbow**.
- The posteromedial ulnohumeral joint is palpated for tenderness or osteophytes found in the valgus extension overload syndrome.
- Inflammation of the ulnar nerve can be identified by a Tinel examination.
- An attempt is made to sublux the ulnar nerve in its cubital tunnel.
- The fifth finger and ulnar half of the ring finger are checked for paresthesias or sensory loss associated with ulnar nerve neurapraxia.

Lateral Joint Examination

- The radiocapitellar joint is palpated to check for osteophytes.
- Joint effusion may be palpable at the posterolateral aspect of the joint.
- The stability of the lateral ligament complex is tested with varus stressing.
- The lateral epicondyle is palpated for possible lateral epicondylitis or "tennis elbow," typically from a late or mechanically poor backhand.

Posterior Joint Examination

- The olecranon is palpated for spurs, fractures, or loose bodies.
- The triceps insertion into the olecranon is palpated for tendinitis or a partial tear.

Anterior Joint Examination

- Anterior capsulitis produces poorly localized tenderness that can be identified by palpation.
- The biceps tendon and brachialis are palpated for tendinitis or a partial tear.
- The "checkrein phenomenon" may produce symptoms and coronoid hypertrophy anteriorly.

REHABILITATION RATIONALE FOR THROWERS

Repetitive throwing results in muscular and bony hypertrophic changes about the elbow. Slocum was one of the first to classify throwing injuries of the elbow into medial tension and valgus compression overload injuries. *Valgus stress plus forced extension is the major pathologic mechanism of a thrower's elbow. Tension* (Fig. 2-6) is produced on the medial aspect of the elbow during throwing. *Compression* is produced on the lateral aspect of the elbow.

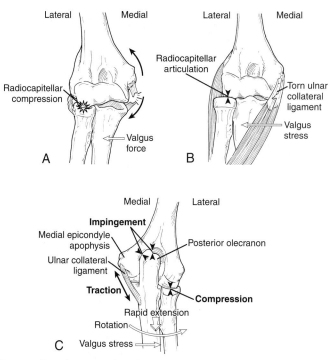

Figure 2–6 **A**, Valgus forces at the elbow injure the ulnar collateral ligament (UCL) and compress the radiocapitellar joint. **B**, Patients who have medial elbow instability with throwing are subject to lateral compression forces (*arrowheads*) on the radiocapitellar articulation and medial valgus stress (*arrow*), which can lead to a torn UCL. **C**, **Valgus extension overload syndrome**. Rapid elbow extension with valgus stress and rotation causes medial traction, lateral compression, and intra-articular posterior impingement. Such stress can injure the UCL, medial epicondyle apophysis, lateral compartment, and posterior olecranon. (Adapted from Nirsahl RP, Kraushaar BS: Assessment and treatment guidelines for elbow injuries. Physician Sports Med 24[5]:230, 1996; Harding WG: Use and misuse of the tennis elbow strap. Physician Sports Med 20[8]:430, 1992; and Fox GM, Jebson PT, Orwin JF: Over-use injuries of the elbow. Physician Sports Med 23[8]:58.)

Classification of Injuries of the Elbow in Throwing Athletes

MEDIAL STRESS

- Flexor muscle strain or tear
- Avulsion of the medial epicondyle
- Attenuation or tear of the MCL
- Ulnar nerve traction

LATERAL COMPRESSION

- Hypertrophy of the radial head and capitellum
- Avascular necrosis of the capitellum
- Osteochondral fractures of the radial head or capitellum

Continued

Classification of Injuries of the Elbow in Throwing Athletes   *Continued*

FORCED EXTENSION
- Olecranon osteophyte formation on the tip of the olecranon process
- Loose body formation
- Scarring and fibrous tissue deposition in the olecranon fossa

---

General Rehabilitation Principles

Rehabilitation of the elbow complex in a throwing athlete requires a carefully directed program to ensure full restoration of motion and function. Frequently after surgery, motion is lost as a result of the elbow's high degree of joint congruency, capsular anatomy, and soft tissue changes. To obtain full function without complications, a sequential, progressive treatment program must be developed. Such a program requires that specific criteria be met at each stage before advancement to the next one. The final goal is to return the athlete to the sport as quickly and as safely as possible.

Several key principles should be considered during rehabilitation of a throwing athlete with an elbow disorder. **(1) The effects of immobilization must be minimized. (2) Healing tissue must never be overstressed. (3) The patient must fulfill specific criteria before progressing from one phase to the next during the rehabilitation process. (4) The rehabilitation program must be based on current clinical and scientific research. (5) The rehabilitation program should be adaptable to each patient and the patient's specific goals**. Finally, these basic treatment principles should be followed throughout the rehabilitation process.

Elbow rehabilitation in throwing athletes generally follows a **four-phase progression**. It is important that certain criteria be met at each level before advancement to the next stage. This allows athletes to progress at their own pace in accordance with tissue-healing constraints.

Phase 1: Regaining Motion

The first phase involves *regaining motion* lost during immobilization after surgery. Pain, inflammation, and muscle atrophy are also treated. Common regimens for inflammation and pain involve modalities such as cryotherapy, high-voltage galvanic stimulation (HVGS), ultrasound, and whirlpool. Joint mobilization techniques can also be used to help minimize pain and promote motion.

To minimize muscular atrophy, submaximal isometric exercises for the elbow flexors and extensors, as well as for the forearm pronators and supinators, are started early. Strengthening of the shoulder should also begin relatively early to prevent functional weakness. **Care should be taken early in the rehabilitation program to restrict shoulder external rotation movements that may place valgus stress on the medial structures of the elbow**.

Elbow flexion contracture is common after an elbow injury or surgery when range of motion (ROM) is not treated appropriately. **Fifty percent of baseball pitchers have been found to have flexion contractures of the elbow**, and 30% have cubitus valgus deformities. Prevention of these contractures is the key. Early ROM is vital to nourish the articular cartilage and promote proper collagen fiber alignment.

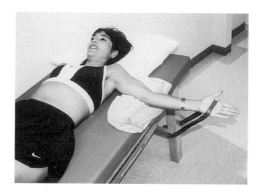

Figure 2–7 Low-load, long-duration stretching of the elbow for restoration of full elbow extension.

A gradual increase in and early restoration of full passive elbow extension are essential to prevent flexion contracture. Several popular techniques to improve limited ROM are joint mobilization, contract-relax stretching, and low-load, long-duration stretching for the restoration of full elbow extension.

Joint mobilization exercises can be performed on the humeroulnar, humeroradial, and radioulnar joints. Limited elbow extension tends to respond to posterior glide of the ulna on the humerus. The grade of mobilization depends on the phase of rehabilitation in effect.

Another technique to restore full elbow extension is **low-load, long-duration stretching** (Fig. 2-7). A good passive overpressure stretch can be achieved by having the patient hold a 2- to 4-pound weight or use an elastic band with the upper extremity resting on a fulcrum just proximal to the elbow joint to allow greater extension. This stretch should be performed for 10 to 12 minutes to incorporate a long-duration, low-intensity stretch. Stretching of this magnitude has been found to elicit a plastic collagen tissue response that results in permanent soft tissue elongation. It is important to note that if the intensity of this stretch is too great, pain and/or a protective muscle response may result, which could inhibit collagen fiber elongation.

Phase 2: Regaining Strength and Endurance

The **intermediate phase** consists of improving the patient's overall *strength, endurance,* and *elbow mobility*. To progress to this phase, the patient must demonstrate full elbow ROM (0 to 135 degrees), minimal or no pain or tenderness, and a "good" (4/5) muscle grade for the elbow flexor and extensor groups. During this phase, isotonic strengthening exercises are emphasized for the entire arm and shoulder complex.

Phase 3: Return to Functional Participation

The third phase is the advanced strengthening phase. The primary goal in this phase is to prepare the athlete for *return to functional participation* and initiation of throwing activities. A total arm-strengthening program is used to improve the power, endurance, and neuromuscular control of the entire limb. Advancement to phase 3 requires demonstration of full, pain-free ROM, no pain or tenderness, and 70% strength in comparison to the contralateral side.

Plyometric exercises are most beneficial in this phase; these drills closely simulate functional activities, such as throwing and swinging, and are performed at higher speed. They also teach the athlete to transfer energy and stabilize the involved area. Plyometrics use a stretch-shortening cycle of muscle, thus involving the use of eccentric/concentric muscle extension. For instance, greater emphasis is placed on the biceps musculature in this phase of rehabilitation because it plays a vital role eccentrically during the deceleration and follow-through phases of the throwing motion by preventing hyperextension. One specific plyometric activity involves exercise tubing. Starting with the elbow flexed and the shoulder in 60 degrees of flexion, the patient releases the isometric hold and initiates an eccentric phase. As full extension is approached, the athlete quickly flexes the elbow again and goes into a concentric phase. The eccentric activity produces a muscular stretch, thus activating the muscle spindles and producing greater concentric contraction.

The primary targets for strengthening in this phase are the biceps, triceps, and wrist flexor/pronator muscles. The biceps and wrist flexors and pronators greatly reduce valgus stress on the elbow during the throwing motion. Other key muscle groups stressed in this phase are the triceps and rotator cuff. The triceps is used in the acceleration phase of the throwing motion, whereas attention to the rotator cuff helps establish the goal of total arm strengthening.

To improve shoulder strength, the throwing athlete is introduced to a set of exercises known as the "**Thrower's Ten**" program, discussed later in this chapter.

Rehabilitation of an injured elbow is different from any other rehabilitation program for throwing athletes. Initially, elbow extension ROM must be obtained to prevent elbow flexion contracture. Next, valgus stress needs to be minimized through conditioning of the elbow and wrist flexors, as well as the pronator muscle group. Finally, the shoulder, especially the rotator cuff musculature, must be included in the rehabilitation process. The rotator cuff is vital to the throwing pattern and, if not strengthened, can lead to future shoulder problems.

Phase 4: Return to Activity

The final stage of the rehabilitation program for a throwing athlete is *return to activity*. This stage uses a progressive interval throwing program to gradually increase the demands on the upper extremity by controlling throwing distance, frequency, and duration.

| REHABILITATION PROTOCOL | *Posterior Rehabilitation after Elbow Arthroscopy (Posterior Compartment or Valgus Extension Overload Surgery)* |

PHASE I: IMMEDIATE MOTION PHASE

Goals

- Improve or regain full ROM
- Decrease pain or inflammation
- Retard muscular atrophy

REHABILITATION PROTOCOL: *Posterior Rehabilitation after Elbow Arthroscopy (Posterior Compartment or Valgus Extension Overload Surgery)* *Continued*

PHASE I: IMMEDIATE MOTION PHASE—CONT'D

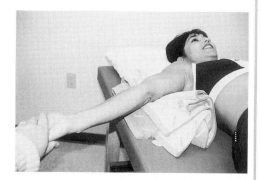

Figure 2–8 Gentle elbow overpressure into extension.

Days 1-4

- ROM to tolerance (extension-flexion and supination-pronation). Often, full elbow extension is not possible because of pain
- Gentle overpressure into extension (Fig. 2-8)
- Wrist flexion-extension stretches
- Gripping exercises with putty
- Isometrics, wrist extension-flexion
- Isometrics, elbow extension-flexion
- Compression dressing, ice four to five times daily

Days 5-10

- ROM exercises to tolerance (at least 20-90 degrees)
- Overpressure into extension
- Joint mobilization to re-establish ROM
- Wrist flexion-extension stretches
- Continue isometrics
- Continue use of ice and compression to control swelling

Days 11-14

- ROM exercises to tolerance (at least 10-100 degrees)
- Overpressure into extension (three to four times daily)
- Continue joint mobilization techniques
- Initiate light dumbbell program (progressive resistance exercise [PRE] for the biceps, triceps, and wrist flexors, extensors, supinators, and pronators)
- Continue use of ice after exercise

PHASE II: INTERMEDIATE PHASE

Goals

- Improve strength, power, and endurance
- Increase ROM
- Initiate functional activities

Continued

REHABILITATION PROTOCOL: *Posterior Rehabilitation after Elbow Arthroscopy (Posterior Compartment or Valgus Extension Overload Surgery)* Continued

PHASE II: INTERMEDIATE PHASE—CONT'D

Weeks 2-4

- Full ROM exercises (four to five times daily)
- Overpressure into elbow extension
- Continue PRE program for the elbow and wrist musculature
- Initiate shoulder program (external rotation and rotator cuff)
- Continue joint mobilization
- Continue ice after exercise

Weeks 5-7

- Continue all exercises listed above
- Initiate light upper body program
- Continue use of ice after activity

PHASE III: ADVANCED STRENGTHENING PROGRAM

Goals

- Improve strength, power, and endurance
- Gradual return to functional activities

Criteria to Enter Phase III

- Full, nonpainful ROM
- Strength 75% or greater of contralateral side
- No pain or tolerance

Weeks 8-12

- Continue PRE program for the elbow and wrist
- Continue shoulder program
- Continue stretching of the elbow and shoulder
- Initiate interval throwing program and gradually return to sports activities

From Wilk KE, Arrigo CA, Andrews JR, Azar FM: Rehabilitation following elbow surgery in the throwing athlete. Oper Tech Sports Med 4:114, 1996.

Medial Collateral Ligament (Ulnar Collateral Ligament) Injuries

David W. Altchek, MD • Michael Levinson, PT

Important Rehabilitation Points

- The MCL (or UCL) of the elbow has been clearly documented as a frequent site of serious injury in overhead throwers.
- Pitching generates a large valgus force at the elbow. This force peaks at the medial aspect of the elbow during the late cocking and early acceleration phases of throwing as the elbow moves from flexion to extension, at speeds that have been estimated to reach 3000 degrees/sec.

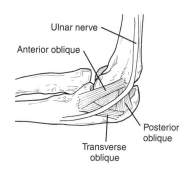

Figure 2–9 The ulnar collateral ligament complex of the elbow consists of three bundles: anterior, posterior, and transverse oblique. (Adapted from Wilk KE, Arrigo CA, Andrews JR: Rehabilitation of the elbow in the throwing athlete. J Orthop Sports Phys Ther 17:305, 1993.)

- Dillman and coworkers have estimated that the typical fastball thrown by an elite pitcher produces a load that approaches the actual tensile strength of the MCL.

Anatomy and Biomechanics

The **MCL** has two bundles of primary importance, **anterior and posterior** (Fig. 2-9). These bundles tighten in reciprocal fashion as the elbow is flexed and extended. The anterior bundle tightens in extension and loosens in flexion. The posterior bundle tightens in flexion and loosens in extension.

Most MCL tears cause pain during the acceleration phase of throwing.

Treatment

- The anterior bundle of the MCL is the primary focus of MCL reconstruction.
- The most common graft is the ipsilateral palmaris longus; other options are the gracilis or semitendinosus or the plantaris tendon.
- Altchek recently described a "docking procedure" for MCL reconstruction. The reconstruction is done through a muscle-splitting approach that preserves the flexor-pronator origin. This technique generally avoids ulnar nerve transposition and minimizes the number of bony tunnels required.

Rehabilitation after MCL reconstruction emphasizes early, controlled ROM to avoid excessive stretching. The patient is encouraged to wear the postoperative brace at all times to prevent any chance of valgus stress being placed on the graft. Passive stretching by the therapist should also be avoided.

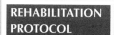

Conservative Treatment of Medial (Ulnar) Collateral Sprains
Wilk, Arrigo, and Andrews

PHASE 1: IMMEDIATE MOTION PHASE

Goals

- Increase ROM
- Promote healing of the UCL
- Retard muscular atrophy
- Decrease pain and inflammation

Continued

REHABILITATION PROTOCOL: *Conservative Treatment of Medial (Ulnar)*
Collateral Sprains   Continued

PHASE 1: IMMEDIATE MOTION PHASE—CONT'D

Range of Motion

- Brace (optional), nonpainful ROM (20-90 degrees)
- Active-assisted ROM, passive ROM of the elbow and wrist (nonpainful range)

Exercises

- Isometrics—wrist and elbow musculature
- Shoulder strengthening (no external rotation strengthening)

Ice and Compression

PHASE 2: INTERMEDIATE PHASE

Goals

- Increase ROM
- Improve strength and endurance
- Decrease pain and inflammation
- Promote stability

Range of Motion

- Gradually increase motion 0-135 degrees (increase 10 degrees/wk)

Exercises

- Initiate isotonic exercises
  - Wrist curls
  - Wrist extension
  - Pronation-supination
  - Biceps-triceps
  - Dumbbells: external rotation of the deltoid, supraspinatus, rhomboids; internal rotation

Ice and Compression

PHASE 3: ADVANCED PHASE

Criteria for Progression to Phase 2

- Full ROM
- No pain or tenderness
- No increase in laxity
- Strength of elbow flexors-extensors

Goals

- Improve strength, power, and endurance
- Improve neuromuscular control

Exercises

- Initiate exercise tubing, shoulder program
- "Thrower's Ten" program
- Biceps-triceps program
- Supination-pronation
- Wrist extension-flexion

REHABILITATION PROTOCOL: *Conservative Treatment of Medial (Ulnar) Collateral Sprains* *Continued*

PHASE 4: RETURN-TO-ACTIVITY PHASE

Criteria for Progression to Return to Throwing

- Full, nonpainful ROM
- No increase in laxity
- Isokinetic test fulfills criteria
- Satisfactory clinical examination

Exercises

- Initiate interval throwing
- Continue "Thrower's Ten" program
- Continue plyometrics

REHABILITATION PROTOCOL

Postoperative Rehabilitation Protocol after Ulnar Collateral Ligament Reconstruction with an Autogenous Palmaris Longus Graft

IMMEDIATE POSTOPERATIVE PHASE (0-3 WEEKS)

Goals

- Protect healing tissue
- Decrease pain/inflammation
- Retard muscular atrophy
- Protect graft site to allow healing

Postoperative Week 1

Brace

- Posterior splint at 90 degrees elbow flexion

Range of Motion

- Wrist active ROM extension/flexion immediately postoperatively
- Knee ROM on day 1

Dressings

- Elbow postoperative compression dressing (5-7 days)
- Wrist (graft site) compression dressing 7-10 days as needed

Exercises

- Gripping exercises
- Wrist ROM
- Shoulder isometrics (no shoulder external rotation)
- Biceps isometrics

Cryotherapy

- To elbow joint and to graft site at the wrist

Continued

REHABILITATION PROTOCOL: *Postoperative Rehabilitation Protocol after Ulnar Collateral Ligament Reconstruction with an Autogenous Palmaris Longus Graft*   Continued

IMMEDIATE POSTOPERATIVE PHASE (0-3 WEEKS)—CONT'D

Postoperative Week 2

Brace

- Elbow ROM 25-100 degrees
- Gradually increase ROM—5 degrees extension/10 degrees flexion per week)

Exercises

- Continue all exercises listed above
- Elbow ROM in brace (30-105 degrees)
- Initiate elbow extension isometrics
- Continue wrist ROM exercises
- Initiate light scar mobilization over distal incision (graft)

Cryotherapy

- Continue to ice the elbow and graft site

Postoperative Week 3

Brace

- Elbow ROM 15-115 degrees

Exercises

- Continue all exercises listed above
- Elbow ROM in brace
- Initiate active ROM of the wrist and elbow (no resistance)
- Initiate light wrist flexion stretching
- Initiate active ROM of the shoulder:
  - Full can
  - Lateral raises
  - External/internal rotation tubing
  - Elbow flexion/extension
- Initiate light scapular strengthening exercises
- May incorporate bicycle for lower extremity strength and endurance

INTERMEDIATE PHASE (WEEKS 4-7)

Goals

- Gradual increase to full ROM
- Promote healing of repaired tissue
- Regain and improve muscular strength
- Restore full function of graft site

Week 4

Brace

- Elbow ROM 0-125 degrees

REHABILITATION PROTOCOL: *Postoperative Rehabilitation Protocol after*
Ulnar Collateral Ligament Reconstruction with an Autogenous Palmaris
Longus Graft   *Continued*

INTERMEDIATE PHASE (WEEKS 4-7)—CONT'D

Exercises

- Begin light resistance exercises for the arm (1 pound)
  - Wrist curls, extension, pronation, supination
  - Elbow extension/flexion
- Progress the shoulder program to emphasize rotator cuff and scapular strengthening
- Initiate shoulder strengthening with light dumbbells

Week 5

- Elbow ROM 0-135 degrees
- Discontinue brace
- Continue all exercises; progress all shoulder and upper extremity exercises (progress weight 1 pound)

Week 6

Active ROM

- 0-145 degrees without brace or full ROM

Exercises

- Initiate "Thrower's Ten" program
- Progress elbow-strengthening exercises
- Initiate shoulder external rotation strengthening
- Progress shoulder program

Week 7

- Progress "Thrower's Ten" program (progress weights)
- Initiate proprioceptive neuromuscular facilitation (PNF) diagonal patterns (light)

ADVANCED STRENGTHENING PHASE (WEEKS 8-14)

Goals

- Increase strength, power, and endurance
- Maintain full elbow ROM
- Gradually initiate sporting activities

Week 8

Exercises

- Initiate eccentric elbow flexion/extension
- Continue isotonic program: forearm and wrist
- Continue shoulder program—"Thrower's Ten" program
- Manual resistance diagonal patterns
- Initiate plyometric exercise program (two-hand plyometric exercises close to the body only)
  - Chest pass
  - Side throw close to the body
- Continue stretching the calf and hamstrings

Continued

REHABILITATION PROTOCOL: *Postoperative Rehabilitation Protocol after*
Ulnar Collateral Ligament Reconstruction with an Autogenous Palmaris
Longus Graft   Continued

ADVANCED STRENGTHENING PHASE (WEEKS 8-14)—CONT'D

Week 10

Exercises

- Continue all exercises listed above
- Progress plyometrics to two-hand drills away from the body
  - Side-to-side throws
  - Soccer throws
  - Side throws

Weeks 12-14

- Continue all exercises
- Initiate isotonic machine strengthening exercises (if desired)
  - Bench press (seated)
  - Lateral pull-down
- Initiate golf, swimming
- Initiate interval hitting program

RETURN-TO-ACTIVITY PHASE (WEEKS 14-32)

Goals

- Continue to increase strength, power, and endurance of the upper extremity musculature
- Gradual return to sport activities

Week 14

Exercises

- Continue strengthening program
- Emphasis on elbow and wrist strengthening and flexibility exercises
- Maintain full elbow ROM
- Initiate one-hand plyometric throwing (stationary throws)
- Initiate one-hand wall dribble
- Initiate one-hand baseball throws into a wall

Week 16

Exercises

- Initiate interval throwing program (phase I) (long toss program)
- Continue "Thrower's Ten" program and plyometrics
- Continue to stretch before and after throwing

Weeks 22-24

Exercises

- Progress to phase II throwing (once phase I successfully completed)

Weeks 30-32

Exercises

- Gradually progress to competitive throwing/sports

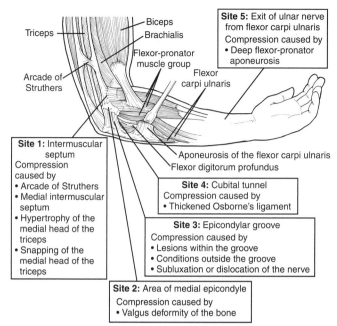

Site 5: Exit of ulnar nerve from flexor carpi ulnaris
Compression caused by
• Deep flexor-pronator aponeurosis

Triceps

Biceps
Brachialis
Flexor-pronator muscle group
Flexor carpi ulnaris

Arcade of Struthers

Site 1: Intermuscular septum
Compression caused by
• Arcade of Struthers
• Medial intermuscular septum
• Hypertrophy of the medial head of the triceps
• Snapping of the medial head of the triceps

Aponeurosis of the flexor carpi ulnaris
Flexor digitorum profundus

Site 4: Cubital tunnel
Compression caused by
• Thickened Osborne's ligament

Site 3: Epicondylar groove
Compression caused by
• Lesions within the groove
• Conditions outside the groove
• Subluxation or dislocation of the nerve

Site 2: Area of medial epicondyle
Compression caused by
• Valgus deformity of the bone

Figure 2–10   The five sites of potential ulnar nerve compression and the causes of compression at each site. (Adapted from Amadio PC: Anatomical basis for a technique of ulnar nerve transposition. Surg Radiol Anat 8:155, 1986.)

Ulnar Nerve Injury at the Elbow (Cubital Tunnel) (Fig. 2-10)

Repetitive valgus stress on the elbow during throwing often produces medial traction on the ulnar nerve. Ulnar nerve injury results from repetitive traction combined with elbow ligament laxity, recurrent subluxation or dislocation of the nerve outside the ulnar groove, compression of the nerve, or direct trauma.

Deficiency or laxity of the anterior bundle of the UCL of the elbow commonly causes stress on the ulnar nerve, and in throwers, these conditions are frequently found to coexist. Throwers often have a hypertrophied forearm flexor mass (attaching to the medial epicondyle) that compresses the nerve during muscle contraction.

Initial treatment of ulnar nerve symptoms in throwers is relative rest, cryotherapy, nonsteroidal anti-inflammatory drugs (NSAIDs), and modification of biomechanical throwing errors. Surgical transposition of the nerve may eventually be required (use of a fasciodermal sling) for recalcitrant symptoms.

The physician must examine for concomitant elbow pathology (unstable UCL) in throwers with ulnar nerve symptoms. If found, these other pathologies must be addressed.

| REHABILITATION PROTOCOL | *After Ulnar Nerve Transposition* |

PHASE 1: IMMEDIATE POSTOPERATIVE PHASE (WEEKS 1-2)

Goals

- Allow soft tissue healing of the relocated nerve
- Decrease pain and inflammation
- Retard muscular atrophy

Week 1

- Posterior splint at 90 degrees elbow flexion with the wrist free for motion (sling for comfort)
- Compression dressing
- Exercises: gripping exercises, wrist ROM, shoulder isometrics

Week 2

- Remove the posterior splint for exercise and bathing
- Progress elbow ROM (passive ROM of 15-120 degrees)
- Initiate elbow and wrist isometrics
- Continue shoulder isometrics

PHASE 2: INTERMEDIATE PHASE (WEEKS 3-7)

Goals

- Restore full pain-free ROM
- Improve strength, power, and endurance of the upper extremity musculature
- Gradually increase functional demands

Week 3

- Discontinue the posterior splint
- Progress elbow ROM, with emphasis on full extension
- In itiate flexibility exercises for
  - Wrist extension-flexion
  - Forearm supination-pronation
  - Elbow extension-flexion
- Initiate strengthening exercises for
  - Wrist extension-flexion
  - Forearm supination-pronation
  - Elbow extension-flexion
  - Shoulder program

Week 6

- Continue all exercises listed above
- Initiate light sport activities

PHASE 3: ADVANCED STRENGTHENING PHASE (WEEKS 8-11)

Goals

- Increase strength, power, and endurance
- Gradually initiate sporting activities

Week 8

- Initiate eccentric exercise program
- Initiate plyometric exercise drills
- Continue shoulder and elbow strengthening and flexibility exercises
- Initiate interval throwing program

REHABILITATION PROTOCOL: *After Ulnar Nerve Transposition* Continued

PHASE 4: RETURN-TO-ACTIVITY PHASE (WEEKS 12-16)

Goals

- Gradual return to sporting activities

Week 12

- Return to competitive throwing
- Continue "Thrower's Ten" program

From Wilk KE, Arrigo CA, Andrews JR, Azar FM: Rehabilitation following elbow surgery in the throwing athlete. Oper Tech Sports Med 4:114, 1996.

Treating Flexion Contracture (Loss of Extension) in Throwing Athletes

- Gelinas and colleagues reported that 50% of the professional baseball pitchers they tested had a flexion contracture (loss of extension) of the elbow.
- Typically, a loss of up to 10 degrees of extension is unnoticed by the athlete and is not required for "functional" elbow ROM.
- Joint mobilization and **low-load, long-duration stretching** (see Fig. 2-7) are advocated for restoration of extension.
- High-intensity, short-duration stretching is **contraindicated** for limited elbow ROM (may produce myositis ossificans).
- Initial treatment includes moist heat and ultrasound, dynamic splinting at night during sleep (low-load, long-duration stretching), joint mobilization, and ROM exercises at end ranges, done several times a day.
- If nonoperative measures fail in the rare patient with *loss of functional motion*, arthroscopic arthrolysis may be required.
- Accelerated rehabilitation after this surgery is required, but overly aggressive rehabilitation must be avoided to prevent inflammation (and thus reflex splinting and stiffening) of the elbow.

REHABILITATION PROTOCOL *After Arthroscopic Arthrolysis of the Elbow*

PHASE 1: IMMEDIATE MOTION PHASE

Goals

- Improve ROM
- Re-establish full passive extension
- Retard muscular atrophy
- Decrease pain/inflammation

Days 1-3

- ROM to tolerance (elbow extension-flexion) (two sets of 10/hr)
- Overpressure into extension (at least 10 degrees)

Continued

REHABILITATION PROTOCOL: *After Arthroscopic Arthrolysis of the Elbow*   *Continued*

PHASE 1: IMMEDIATE MOTION PHASE—CONT'D

- Joint mobilization
- Gripping exercise with putty
- Isometrics for the wrist and elbow
- Compression and ice hourly

Days 4-9

- ROM extension-flexion (at least 5-120 degrees)
- Overpressure into extension—5-pound weight, elbow in full extension (four to five times daily)
- Joint mobilization
- Continue isometrics and gripping exercises
- Continue use of ice

Days 10-14

- Full passive ROM
- ROM exercises (two sets of 10/hr)
- Stretch into extension
- Continue isometrics

PHASE 2: MOTION MAINTENANCE PHASE

Goals

- Maintain full ROM
- Gradually improve strength
- Decrease pain/inflammation

Weeks 2-4

- ROM exercises (four to five times daily)
- Overpressure into extension—stretch for 2 minutes (three to four times daily)
- Initiate PRE program (light dumbbells)
  - Elbow extension-flexion
  - Wrist extension-flexion
- Continue use of ice after exercise

Weeks 4-6

- Continue all exercises listed above
- Initiate interval sport program

From Wilk KE, Arrigo CA, Andrews JR, Azar FM: Rehabilitation following elbow surgery in the throwing athlete. Oper Tech Sports Med 4:114, 1996.

A Basic Elbow Exercise Program (Performed Three Times a Day)

Kevin Wilk, PT

1. **Deep Friction Massage**

   Deep transverse friction across the area of the elbow that is sore; 5 minutes, several times daily (not shown).

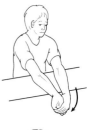

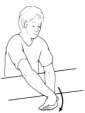

Figure 2–11 Flexor stretching. (Adapted from Wilk KE: Elbow Exercises. HealthSouth Handout, 1993.)

2. **Grip**

Grip an apparatus, putty, small rubber ball, or the like. Use as continuously as possible all day long (not shown).

3. **Stretch Flexors** (Fig. 2-11)

Straighten the elbow completely. With the palm facing up, grasp the middle of the hand and thumb. Pull the wrist down as far as possible. Hold for 10 counts. Release and repeat 5 to 10 times before and after each exercise session.

4. **Stretch Extensors**

Straighten the elbow completely. With the palm facing down, grasp the back of the hand and pull the wrist down as far as possible. Hold for a 10 count. Release and repeat 5 to 10 times, before and after each exercise session.

PROGRESSIVE RESISTANCE ELBOW EXERCISES

Begin each PRE with one set of 10 repetitions without weight and progress to five sets of 10 repetitions as tolerable. When you are able to easily perform five sets of 10 repetitions, you may begin adding weight. Begin each PRE with one set of 10 repetitions with 1 pound and progress to five sets of 10 as tolerable. When you are able to easily perform five sets of 10 repetitions with 1 pound, you may begin to progress your weight in the same manner.

In a preventive elbow maintenance program (excluding specific rotator cuff exercises), it is permissible to advance weight as tolerable with strengthening exercises while taking care to emphasize proper lifting technique.

5. **Wrist Curls** (Fig. 2-12)

The forearm should be supported on a table with the hand off the edge; the palm should face upward. Using a weight or hammer, lower that hand as far as possible and then curl it up as high as possible. Hold for a two count.

6. **Reverse Wrist Curls** (Fig. 2-13)

The forearm should be supported on a table with the hand off the edge; the palm should face downward. Using a weight or hammer, lower the hand as far as possible and then curl the wrist up as high as possible. Hold for a two count.

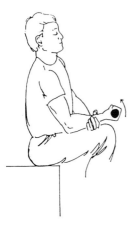

Figure 2–12   Wrist curls. (From Andrews JR, Wilk KE: The Athlete's Shoulder. New York, Churchill Livingstone, 1994, p 707.)

7. **Neutral Wrist Curls** (Fig. 2-14)

The forearm should be supported on a table with the wrist in neutral position and the hand off the edge. Using a weight or hammer held in a normal hammering position, lower the wrist into ulnar deviation as far as possible. Then bring the wrist into radial deviation as far as possible. Hold for a two count. Relax.

8. **Pronation** (Fig. 2-15)

The forearm should be supported on a table with the wrist in neutral position. Using a weight or hammer held in a normal hammering position, roll the wrist and bring the hammer into pronation as far as possible. Hold for a two count. Raise back to the starting position.

9. **Supination** (Fig. 2-16)

The forearm should be supported on the table with the wrist in neutral position. Using a weight or hammer held in a normal hammering position, roll the wrist and bring the hammer into full supination. Hold for a two count. Raise back to the starting position.

10. **Broomstick Curl-up** (Fig. 2-17A)

Use a 1- to 2-foot broom handle with a 4- to 5-foot cord attached in the middle and a 1- to 5-pound weight tied in the center.
   ○ Extensors (see Fig. 2-17B)

   Grip the stick on either side of the rope with the palms down. Curl the cord up by turning the stick toward you (the cord is on the side of the stick, away from you). Once the weight is pulled to the top, lower the weight by unwinding the stick, rotating it away from you. Repeat three to five times.
   ○ Flexors

Same as above exercise (extensors), but have the palms facing upward.

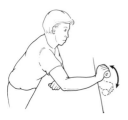

Figure 2–13   Reverse wrist curls. (Adapted from Wilk KE: Elbow exercises. HealthSouth Handout, 1993.)

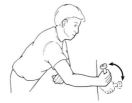

Figure 2–14   Neutral wrist curls. (Adapted from Wilk KE: Elbow exercises. HealthSouth Handout, 1993.)

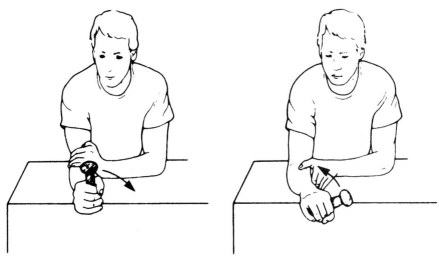

Figure 2–15   Pronation exercises. (From Andrews JR, Wilk KE: The Athlete's Shoulder. New York, Churchill Livingstone, 1994, p 387.)

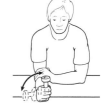

Figure 2–16   Supination exercises. (Adapted from Wilk KE: Elbow exercises. HealthSouth Handout, 1993.)

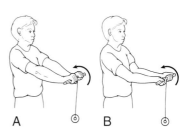

Figure 2–17   Broomstick curl-up. (Adapted from Wilk KE: Elbow exercises. HealthSouth Handout, 1993.)

A   B

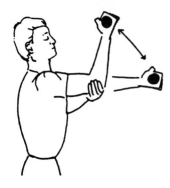

Figure 2–18 Biceps curl. (From Andrews JR, Wilk KE: The Athlete's Shoulder. New York, Churchill Livingstone, 1994, p 706.)

11. **Bicep Curl** (Fig. 2-18)
    Support the arm on the opposite hand. Bend the elbow to full flexion, and then straighten the arm completely.
12. **French Curl** (Fig. 2-19)
    Raise the arm overhead. Take the opposite hand and give support at the elbow. Straighten the elbow over the head; hold for a two count.

ECCENTRIC ELBOW PRONATION (FIG. 2-20)

Holding a hammer in the hand (tied to a rubber band), start with the hand supinated and pronate against the rubber band. Then slowly allow the rubber band to overpower the wrist into supination.

ECCENTRIC ELBOW SUPINATION (FIG. 2-21)

Holding a hammer in pronation (tied to a rubber band), supinate against the rubberband resistance. Then slowly allow the rubber band to overpower the wrist into pronation.

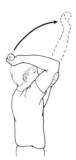

Figure 2–19 French curl. (Adapted from Wilk KE: Elbow exercises. HealthSouth Handout, 1993.)

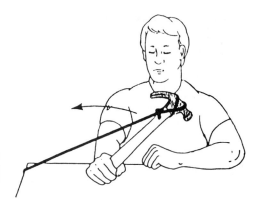

Figure 2–20 Eccentric elbow pronation exercise. (From Andrews JR, Wilk KE: The Athlete's Shoulder. New York, Churchill Livingstone, 1994, p 708.)

Treatment and Rehabilitation of Elbow Dislocations

Kevin Wilk, PT • James R. Andrews, MD

Rehabilitation Considerations

- Elbow dislocations account for 10% to 25% of all injuries to the elbow.
- Ninety percent of elbow dislocations produce posterior or posterolateral displacement of the forearm relative to the distal humerus.
- Fractures associated with elbow dislocations most frequently involve the radial head and the coronoid process of the elbow.
- The distal radioulnar joint (wrist) and the interosseous membrane of the forearm should be examined for tenderness and stability to rule out a possible Essex-Lopresti injury.
- When intra-articular fractures of the radial head, olecranon, or coronoid process occur with elbow dislocation, the condition is termed a **complex dislocation**.

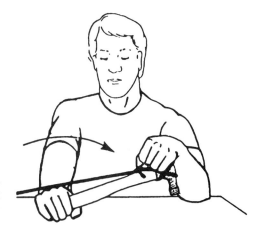

Figure 2–21 Eccentric elbow supination exercise. (From Andrews JR, Wilk KE: The Athlete's Shoulder. New York, Churchill Livingstone, 1994, p 708.)

- Associated neurologic injury is very uncommon, with the ulnar nerve being the most commonly injured (stretch neurapraxia).
- A minor (but permanent) **loss of terminal elbow extension** (5 to 15 degrees) **is the most common sequela after posterior elbow dislocation**.
- Pronation and supination are characteristically unaffected after this injury.
- Elbow flexion returns first, with maximal improvement usually taking 6 to 12 weeks. Elbow extension returns more slowly and may continue to improve for 3 to 5 months.

Prolonged rigid immobilization has been associated with the least satisfactory arc of elbow motion and should be avoided.

- Heterotopic ossification (calcification) is common after elbow dislocation (up to 75% of patients) but rarely limits motion (less than 5% of patients). The most common sites of periarticular calcification are the anterior elbow region and the collateral ligaments.
- Mechanical testing confirms a 15% average loss of elbow strength after elbow dislocation.
- Approximately 60% of patients do not believe that the injured elbow is as "good" as the uninvolved elbow at the end of treatment.

Classification

The traditional classification of elbow dislocation divides injuries into **anterior** (2%) and **posterior** dislocation. *Posterior* dislocation is further subdivided according to the final resting position of the olecranon in relation to the distal end of the humerus: **posterior, posterolateral (most common), posteromedial (least common), and pure lateral**.

Morrey makes a clinical distinction between complete dislocation and **perched** dislocation (Fig. 2-22). Because perched dislocations are associated with less

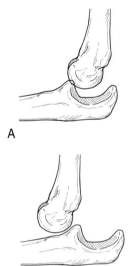

A

B

Figure 2–22 Simplified classification of elbow dislocation with prognostic implications. **A**, Perched (subluxed). **B**, Complete (dislocated). (Adapted from Morrey BF: Biomechanics of the elbow and forearm. Orthop Sports Med 17:840, 1994.)

ligament tearing, recovery and rehabilitation are more rapid. For a complete elbow dislocation, the anterior capsule must be disrupted. The brachialis must also be torn or significantly stretched.

Many elbow dislocations are accompanied by some type of UCL involvement. More specifically, the anterior oblique band of the UCL is affected. Tullos and colleagues found that the anterior oblique band of the UCL was torn in 34 of 37 patients who had previously experienced a posterior elbow dislocation. Repair of this ligament is sometimes indicated in athletes if the injury occurs in the dominant arm. Such repair optimizes the chance for full return to the athlete's previous level of competition.

Evaluation, Work-up, and Reduction

- Swelling and deformity are noted on initial inspection.
- Concomitant upper extremity injuries should be ruled out by palpation of the shoulder and wrist.
- Complete neurovascular examinations should be performed before and after reduction.
- For posterior dislocations

    The player is removed from the field with the arm supported.

    A neurovascular examination is performed with the patient placed prone and the arm flexed 90 degrees over the edge of the table (Fig. 2-23).

    Any medial or lateral translation of the proximal ulna is gently corrected.

    The physician grasps the wrist and applies traction and slight supination of the forearm to distract and unlock the coronoid process from the olecranon fossa.

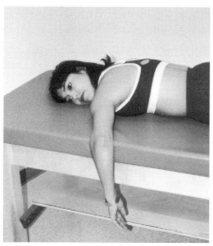
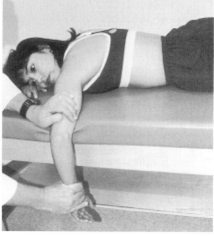

A   B

Figure 2–23 **A**, Reduction of a simple posterior elbow dislocation can be done with the patient lying prone and the injured elbow flexed about 90 degrees over the edge of the table. **B**, After correcting any medial or lateral translation of the proximal end of the ulna, the clinician applies downward traction to the forearm and gentle pressure to the olecranon.

An assistant places countertraction on the arm. Pressure is applied to the olecranon while the arm is pronated (i.e., palm down) to complete the reduction.

An obvious "clunk" indicates reduction.

The neurovascular examination is repeated and elbow instability is evaluated by placing the elbow through gentle ROM while watching for instability as the elbow is extended. Instability noted at a certain degree of extension (e.g., 20 degrees) should be documented and conveyed to the therapist.

The arm is placed in a sling (at 90 degrees) and iced and elevated.

If an immediate on-the-field reduction cannot be performed, muscle relaxation in the emergency department is of great importance.

Radiographs (anteroposterior and lateral) of the elbow, forearm, and wrist are obtained to ensure that no associated fractures are present.

Surgical Indications

- For acute elbow dislocations when flexion of the elbow beyond 50 to 60 degrees is required to maintain reduction
- When the dislocation is associated with an unstable fracture about the joint
- Irreducible dislocation

Recurrent Instability after Elbow Dislocation

- Recurrent elbow instability is extremely rare and occurs in less than 1% to 2% of patients.
- The MCL has been identified as the primary stabilizer of the elbow joint. Examination and repair of the MCL complex and flexor-pronator musculo-tendinous origin are recommended.
- The lateral elbow ligaments play a role in stability by keeping the elbow from subluxing posteriorly and rotating away (posterolateral rotatory instability).

Important Rehabilitation Points

- **Early *active* mobilization (within the first 2 to 3 weeks) is needed to avoid post-traumatic stiffness (*not passive mobilization*).**
- Dynamic elbow splints or patient-adjusted progressive static splints should be used if motion is not steadily improving at 4 to 6 weeks after injury.
- **Valgus stressing should be avoided during rehabilitation because it can lead to instability or repeat dislocation.**
- Excessive early passive ROM should be avoided because it increases swelling and inflammation.
- Beginning at week 1, a hinged ROM elbow brace preset at 30 to 90 degrees is worn.
- Each week, motion in the brace is increased by 5 degrees of extension and 10 degrees of flexion.
- **Forced terminal extension should be avoided.** Full elbow extension is less critical for a nonthrowing patient and is preferable to recurrent instability.

REHABILITATION PROTOCOL	*After Elbow Dislocation* Wilk and Andrews

PHASE 1 (DAYS 1-4)

- Immobilization of the elbow at 90 degrees of flexion in a well-padded posterior splint for 3-4 days
- Begin light gripping exercises (putty or tennis ball)
- **Avoid any passive ROM** (patient to perform active ROM when the posterior splint is removed and replaced with a hinged elbow brace or sling)
- Avoid valgus stress on the elbow
- Use cryotherapy and HVGS

PHASE 2 (DAYS 4-14)

- Replace the posterior splint with a hinged elbow brace initially set at 15-90 degrees
- Wrist and finger active ROM in all planes
- Active elbow ROM (*avoid* valgus stress)
  - Flexion-extension-supination-pronation
- Multiangle flexion isometrics
- Multiangle extension isometrics (*avoid* valgus stress)
- Wrist curls/reverse wrist curls
- Light biceps curls
- Shoulder exercises (**avoid external rotation of the shoulder because it places valgus stress on the elbow**). The elbow is stabilized during shoulder exercises.

PHASE 3 (WEEKS 2-6)

- Hinged brace at settings of 0 degrees to full flexion
- PRE progression of elbow and wrist exercises
- Okay to initiate some gentle low-load, long-duration stretching (see Fig. 2-7) around 5-6 weeks for the patient's loss of extension
- Gradual progression of weight with curls, elbow extension, and so on
- Sport-specific exercises and drills initiated
- External rotation and internal rotation exercises of the shoulder may be incorporated at 6-8 weeks
- Around 8 weeks in an asymptomatic patient, start interval throwing program
- No return to play until strength is 85% to 90% that of the uninvolved limb

Lateral and Medial Epicondylitis

Champ L. Baker, Jr., MD • Mark Baker, PT

Lateral Epicondylitis (Tennis Elbow)

Background

Lateral epicondylitis (tennis elbow) is defined as a pathologic condition of the wrist extensor muscles at their origin on the lateral humeral epicondyle. The tendinous origin of the extensor carpi radialis brevis (ECRB) is the area of most pathologic change. Changes can also be found in the musculotendinous structures of the extensor carpi radialis longus, extensor carpi ulnaris, and extensor digitorum

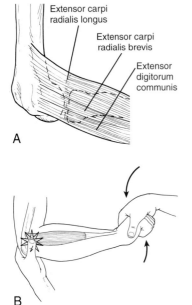

Extensor carpi
radialis longus

Extensor carpi
radialis brevis

Extensor
digitorum
communis

A

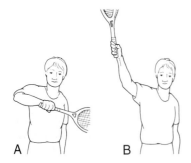

B

Figure 2–24 **A**, Lateral extensor wad. **B**, A patient with lateral epicondylitis (tennis elbow) has local tenderness and pain directly over the midpoint of the lateral epicondyle when the wrist is extended against resistance. (Adapted from Tullos H, Schwab G, Bennett JB, Woods GW: Factors influencing elbow instability. Instr Course Lect 30:185, 1981; and Shaffer B, O'Mara J: Common elbow problems, part 2: Management specifics. J Musculoskel Med 14[4]:30, 1997.)

communis (Fig. 2-24A). Overuse or repetitive trauma in this area causes fibrosis and microtears in involved tissues. Nirschl referred to microtears and vascular ingrowth of the involved tissues as **angiofibroblastic hyperplasia**. He also suggested that the degenerative process should be termed *tendinosis* rather than *tendinitis*.

Most patients with lateral epicondylitis are between the ages of 30 and 55 years, and many have poorly conditioned muscles. Ninety-five percent of cases of tennis elbow occur in *non*-tennis players. Ten percent to 50% of regular tennis players experience tennis elbow symptoms of varying degree at some time in their tennis lives. The most common cause of tennis elbow in tennis players is a "late," mechanically poor backhand (Fig. 2-25) that places excess force across the extensor wad; that is, the elbow "leads" the arm. Other contributing factors include incorrect grip size or string tension, poor racquet "dampening," and underlying weak muscles of the shoulder, elbow, and arm. Tennis grips that are too small often exacerbate or cause tennis elbow.

Figure 2–25 **A**, A "late" backhand or "leading with the elbow" causes excessive repetitive force across the extensor wad of the elbow that results in lateral epicondylitis (tennis elbow). **B**, In the correct position, the arm strikes the ball early, in front of the body, and the arm is raised and extended in follow-through. (Adapted from Harding WG: Use and misuse of the tennis elbow strap. Physician Sports Med 20[8]:40, 1992.)

A   B

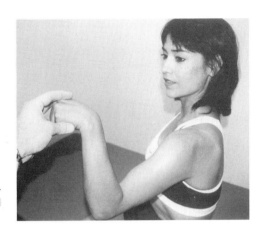

Figure 2–26 Mill test. Pain occurs over the lateral epicondyle when the wrist and fingers are completely flexed.

More often a history of repetitive flexion-extension or pronation-supination activity and overuse is obtained (e.g., twisting a screwdriver, lifting heavy luggage with the palm down). Tightly gripping and carrying a heavy briefcase is a very common cause. Raking leaves, baseball, golfing, gardening, and bowling can also cause lateral epicondylitis.

Physical Examination

- Point tenderness typically occurs over the ECRB origin at the lateral epicondyle (see Fig. 2-24B).
- The tenderness may be more generalized over the common extensor wad insertion at the lateral epicondyle (just distal and anterior to the lateral epicondyle).
- The pain is often exacerbated by wrist extension against resistance with the forearm pronated (palm down).
- Elbow extension may be mildly limited.
- The *Mill test* may be positive. With this test, pain occurs over the lateral epicondyle when the wrist and fingers are completely flexed (Fig. 2-26).
- With the *Maudsley test*, the patient may feel pain on resisted extension of the middle finger at the metacarpophalangeal joint when the elbow is fully extended (Fig. 2-27).
- Evaluation should note possible sensory paresthesias in the superficial radial nerve distribution to rule out *radial tunnel syndrome*. **Radial tunnel syndrome**

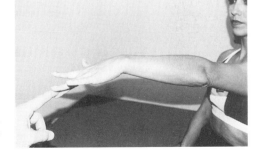

Figure 2–27 Maudsley test for lateral epicondylitis. Pain on resisted extension of the middle finger at the metacarpophalangeal joint when the elbow is fully extended.

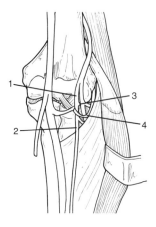

Figure 2–28 Radial tunnel syndrome. Four anatomic elements are potentially compressive: (1) fibrous bands overlying the radial head and capsule, (2) fibrous origin of the extensor carpi radialis brevis, (3) radial recurrent arterial fan, and (4) arcade of Frohse. (Adapted from Moss S, Switzer H: Radial tunnel syndrome: A spectrum of clinical presentations. J Hand Surg [Am] 8:415, 1983.)

(Fig. 2-28) is the most common cause of refractory lateral pain and coexists with lateral epicondylitis in 10% of patients.

- The *cervical nerve roots* should be examined to rule out cervical radiculopathy.
- Other conditions that should be considered include bursitis of the bursa below the conjoined tendon, chronic irritation of the radiohumeral joint or capsule, radiocapitellar chondromalacia or arthritis, radial neck fracture, Panner's disease, little leaguer's elbow, and osteochondritis dissecans of the elbow.

Differential Diagnosis of Lateral Elbow Pain

	Type, Site of Pain	Provocative Test	Neurologic Findings
Lateral epicondylitis	Well localized point tenderness over lateral epicondyle; pain increases with use	Resisted wrist extension, resisted forearm pronation, chair-lift test	None
Intra-articular pathology	Generalized elbow pain	Axial compression test	None
Cervical radiculopathy	Diffuse lateral arm pain, neck pain and/or stiffness	Limited neck ROM, Spurling test positive	Abnormal reflex, sensory, or motor examination results; abnormal EMG/NCS
Radial tunnel syndrome	Vague, diffuse forearm ache; pain more distal than in lateral epicondylitis; pain present at rest	Resisted long-finger extension, resisted forearm supination, positive differential lidocaine injection	Paresthesias in the first dorsal web space of the hand (5%-10%); abnormal EMG/NCS (10%)

EMG, electromyography; NCS, nerve conduction study.
From Warhold LG, Osterman AL, Shirven T: Lateral epicondylitis: How to test it and prevent recurrence. J Musculoskel Med 10(10):243, 1993.

Nonoperative Treatment

Activity Modification

- In nonathletes, **elimination of the activities that are painful** is key to improvement (e.g., repetitive valve opening).
- Treatments such as ice and NSAIDs may lessen the inflammation, but continued repetition of the aggravating motion will prolong any recovery.
- Often, repetitive pronation-supination motions and lifting heavy weights at work can be modified or eliminated. Activity modifications such as avoidance of grasping in pronation (Fig. 2-29) and substituting controlled supination lifting with both arms instead may relieve the symptoms (Fig. 2-30).
- Lifting should be done with the palms *up* (supination) whenever possible, and *both* upper extremities should be used in a manner that reduces forcible elbow extension, supination, and wrist extension.

Correction of Mechanics

- If a late or poor backhand causes pain, **correction of the mechanics of the stroke** is warranted.
- Avoidance of ball impact that lacks forward body weight transference is stressed.
- If typing with unsupported arms exacerbates the pain, placing the elbows on stacked towels for support will help.

Nonsteroidal Anti-inflammatory Drugs

- If not contraindicated, we use cyclooxygenase-2 (COX-2) inhibitors such as celecoxib (Celebrex) or over-the-counter drugs such as ibuprofen (Advil).

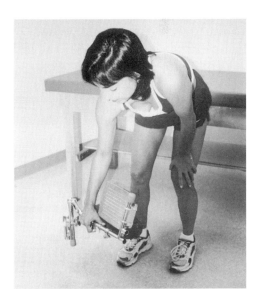

Figure 2–29 Modify activity by avoiding grasping heavy objects in pronation (i.e., incorrectly).

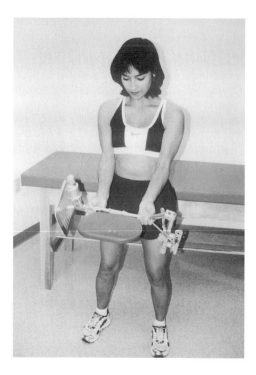

Figure 2–30 Lifting in supination (palm up) with both upper extremities. This is the correct way for patients with lateral epicondylitis of the extensor wad to avoid pain.

Icing
- Ten to 15 minutes of "wet" ice (i.e., a washcloth containing ice that is first soaked in water), four to six times a day.

Stretching
- ROM exercises emphasizing end-range and passive stretching (elbow in full extension and the wrist in flexion with slight ulnar deviation) (Figs. 2-31 and 2-32).

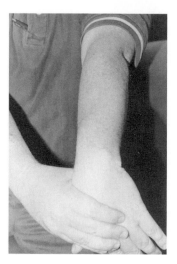

Figure 2–31 Wrist extensor stretch for lateral epicondylitis. With the elbow in extension and the wrist in flexion and slight ulnar deviation, the patient performs five or six stretches while holding for 30 seconds. Repeat two or three times a day.

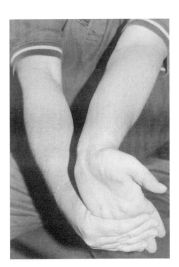

Figure 2–32 Wrist flexor wad stretching for medial epicondylitis. With the elbow in extension and the wrist in extension and slight radial deviation, the patient performs five or six stretches while holding for 30 seconds. Repeat two or three times a day.

Counterforce Bracing (Tennis Elbow Bracing)

- Bracing is used only during actual play or aggravating activity.
- The tension of the band is adjusted to comfort *while the muscles are relaxed* so that maximal contraction of the finger and wrist extensors is inhibited by the band (Fig. 2-33).
- The band is placed two fingerbreadths distal to the painful area of the lateral epicondyle.
- Some authors also recommend 6 to 8 weeks' use of a **wrist splint** positioned in 45 degrees of dorsiflexion.
- Tennis players may reduce racquet string tension, change the size of the grip (usually to a larger grip), and change to a better dampening racquet. For grip size, Nirschl recommended measuring the length from the proximal palmar crease to the tip of the ring finger with a ruler (Fig. 2-34). If the distance is 4½ inches, the grip should be a 4½.

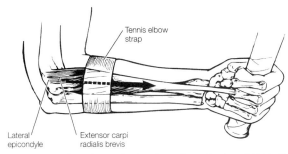

Tennis elbow strap

Lateral epicondyle

Extensor carpi radialis brevis

Figure 2–33 Lateral counterforce brace for the elbow (lateral epicondylitis). Place the brace two fingerbreadths distal to the lateral epicondyle (snug). This attempts to work as a counterforce brace that places some stress on the brace itself rather than causing proximal insertional pain at the lateral epicondyle.

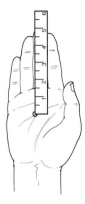

Figure 2–34   Nirschl technique for proper handle size measured from the proximal palmar crease to the tip of the ring finger. Place the measuring rule between the ring and the long fingers for proper ruler placement on the palmar crease. The measurement obtained is the proper handle size—that is, if this distance is 4½ inches, the proper handle size is 4½ inches.

Cortisone Injection
- We have had excellent results with injection of cortisone for tennis elbow.
- We recommend injecting no more often than every 3 months and no more than three injections a year to avoid possible tendon rupture.

TECHNIQUE
- Use 2 ml of lidocaine in a 25-gauge, 1-inch needle centered at the point of maximal tenderness at the ECRB origin; do not enter the tendon.
- The needle is left in place, and then the syringe is changed and 0.5 ml of betamethasone (Celestone) is injected. This is preferred rather than skin infiltration with cortisone to avoid skin and subcutaneous tissue atrophy from the steroid.

Range-of-Motion Exercises (see Figs. 2-31 and 2-32)
- Exercises emphasize end-range and passive stretching (elbow in full extension and wrist in flexion with slight ulnar deviation).
- Soft tissue mobilization is performed perpendicular to the tissue involved.
- Phonophoresis or iontophoresis may be helpful.

Strengthening Exercises (Last Phase)
- A gentle strengthening program should be used for grip strength and wrist extensor, wrist flexor, biceps, triceps, and rotator cuff strengthening.
- *However, the acute inflammatory phase must have resolved first, with 2 weeks of no pain during activities of daily living before initiation of graduated strengthening exercises*.
- Development of symptoms (i.e., pain) modifies the exercise progression, with a lower level of intensity and more icing if pain recurs.
- The exercise program includes
  - Active motion and submaximal isometrics
  - Isotonic eccentric hand exercises with graduated weights not to exceed 5 pounds
  - Wrist curls
    Sit with the hand over the knee. With the palm up (supination), bend the wrist 10 times while holding a 1- to 2-pound weight. Increase to two sets of 10 daily; then increase the weight by 1 pound up to 5 to 6 pounds. Repeat with the palm down (pronation), but progress to only 4 pounds.
  - Forearm strengthening

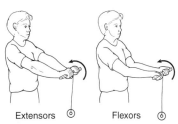

Figure 2–35 Wrist flexors and extensors. The patient rolls up a string with a weight tied on the end. The weight may be progressively increased. Flexors are worked with the palms up, extensors with the palms down.

Extensors   Flexors

Hold the arm out in front of the body, palm down. The patient clenches the fingers, bends the wrist up (extension), and holds it tight for 10 seconds. Next, with the other hand, the patient attempts to push the hand down. Hold for 10 seconds, 5 repetitions; slowly increase to 20 repetitions two to three times a day.

Weight on the end of a rope (Fig. 2-35) can be used to strengthen the wrist flexors and extensors. The patient rolls up a string with a weight tied on the end. The weight can be progressively increased. Flexors are worked with the palms up, extensors with the palm down.

Elbow flexion and extension exercises (Figs. 2-36 and 2-37).

Squeeze a racquetball repetitively for forearm and hand strength.

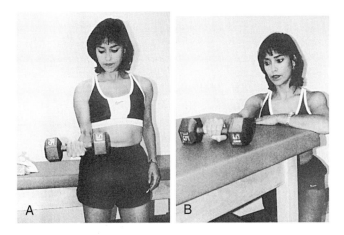

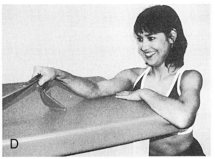

Figure 2–36 **A**, Wrist flexion—resistive training. **B**, Wrist extension—resistive training. **C**, Elbow flexion—Thera-Band training. **D**, Elbow extension—Thera-Band training.

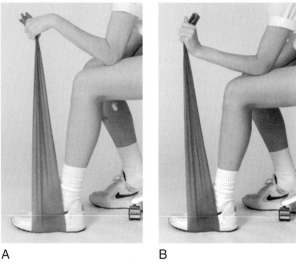

A   B

Figure 2–37   Elbow Thera-Band strengthening exercises.

REHABILITATION PROTOCOL	***Evaluation-Based Rehabilitation of Medial and Lateral Epicondylitis*** Galloway, DeMaio, and Mangine

Rationale: Patients begin a rehabilitation protocol based on their symptoms and objective physical findings. The *initial phase* of each protocol is directed toward restoring ROM at the wrist and elbow. *Phase 2* involves strength training and a structured return to activity. First, obtain relief of acute pain and then increase forearm extensor power, flexibility, and endurance.

When	Protocol 1 (Severe Symptoms)	Protocol 2 (Mild/Moderate Symptoms)	Protocol 3 (Symptoms Resolved)
	• Pain at rest • Point tenderness • Pain with minimally resisted wrist extension • Swelling • Grip strength difference (GSD) >50% • >5 degrees motion loss at wrist or elbow	• Pain with activity only • Minimal point tenderness • Minimal pain with resisted wrist flexion-extension • GSD <50% • No motion loss	• No pain with daily activity • No referred pain • Full ROM • GSD <10%

REHABILITATION PROTOCOL: *Evaluation-Based Rehabilitation of Medial and Lateral Epicondylitis*   *Continued*

Evaluation	• Duration of symptoms • Referred pain • Grip strength measurement • Elbow palpation • Motion measurement • History of injury or inciting activity • Differential diagnosis	• Duration of symptoms • Referred pain • Grip strength measurement • Elbow palpation • Motion measurement • History of injury or inciting activity • Differential diagnosis	• Review initial injury or inciting activity • Identify requirements for returning to desired activity • Identify remaining functional deficits
Treatment	**Phase 1 (Reduce Inflammation)** • Rest • Passive ROM • Cold therapy • Medications **Phase 2 (Rehabilitation)** • Limit activity • Cold therapy • Stretching (static) • Strengthening (isometric) • Ultrasound • HVGS • Proceed to protocol 2 when tolerating above • Surgical indications	**Phase 1 (Reduce Inflammation)** • Rest • Passive ROM • Cold therapy • Medications **Phase 2 (Rehabilitation)** • Limit activity • Flexibility • Strengthening • Transverse friction massage • Cold therapy • HVGS • Ultrasound • Proceed to protocol 3	• Preactivity flexibility • Strengthening • Isokinetics • Isotonic • Modalities • Whirlpool • Ice after activity • Technique modification • Equipment modification • Counterforce bracing • Friction massage • Gradual return to activity
Goals	• Resolution of pain at rest • Tolerate stretching/strengthening with minimal discomfort • Improve ROM • Maintain cardiovascular conditioning	• No pain with daily activity • No pain with stretching/(PREs) • Full ROM • Prepare for functional rehabilitation • Maintain cardiovascular conditioning	• Pain-free return to activity • Prevent recurrence—maintenance program of stretching

- Progress strength, flexibility, and endurance in a *graduated* fashion with slow-velocity exercises involving the application of gradually increasing resistance. A "no pain, no gain" philosophy is incorrect here.

Galloway, DeMaio, and Mangine divide their approach to patients with epicondylitis (medial or lateral) into three stages: The *initial phase* is directed toward reducing inflammation and preparing the patient for phase 2. The *second phase* emphasizes return of strength and endurance. Specific inciting factors are identified and modified. *Phase 3* involves functional rehabilitation designed to return the patient to the desired activity level. This protocol is also based on the severity of the initial symptoms and objective findings at initiation of treatment.

Surgical Treatment

Surgical treatment of tennis elbow is not considered unless the patient has had recalcitrant symptoms for more than 1 year despite the nonoperative treatment previously discussed. Various operations have been described for tennis elbow pain. Many authors have recommended excision of torn, scarred ECRB origin, removal of granulation tissue, and cortical drilling (down to subchondral bone) for stimulation of neovascularization. The elbow capsule is not violated unless intra-articular pathology exists. We prefer to treat these patients arthroscopically whenever possible. Arthroscopic release of the ECRB tendon and decortication of the lateral epicondyle are analogous to the open procedure. Arthroscopic treatment of lateral epicondylitis offers several potential advantages over open procedures, and its success rate is comparable. The lesion is addressed directly, and the common extensor origin is preserved. Arthroscopy also allows intra-articular examination for other disorders. In addition, it permits a shorter postoperative rehabilitation period and earlier return to work or sports.

Postoperatively, we encourage our patients to begin active ROM within the first 24 to 48 hours. The patient is usually seen for follow-up within the first 72 hours. At this time, the patient is encouraged to begin extension and flexion exercises. After the swelling subsides, generally 2 to 3 weeks after surgery, the patient can rapidly regain full ROM and begin strengthening exercises. Return to throwing sports is allowed when the patient has regained full strength.

REHABILITATION PROTOCOL | *After Lateral Epicondylitis Surgery*
Baker and Baker

DAYS 1-7
- Position the extremity in a sling for comfort.
- Control edema and inflammation: apply ice for 20 minutes two or three times a day.
- Gentle hand, wrist, and elbow ROM exercises. Exercises should be done in a pain-free range.
- Active shoulder ROM (glenohumeral joint), lower trapezius setting.

REHABILITATION PROTOCOL: *After Lateral Epicondylitis Surgery*   *Continued*

WEEKS 2-4

- Remove the sling.
- Advance ROM passive motion. Passive motion should be continued and combined with active-assisted motion within the patient's pain tolerance.
- Gentle strengthening exercises with active motion and submaximal isometrics.
- Edema and inflammation control: continue ice application for 20 minutes two or three times a day.
- Shoulder strengthening: manual D1 and D2 proprioceptive neuromuscular facilitation to the glenohumeral joint with the patient supine. Scapular strengthening with manual resistance and continued lower trapezius setting.

WEEKS 5-7

- Advance strengthening as tolerated to include weights or rubber tubing.
- ROM with continued emphasis on end-range and passive overpressure.
- Edema and inflammation control with ice application for 20 minutes after activity.
- Modified activities in preparation for beginning functional training.
- Gentle massage along and against fiber orientation.
- Counterforce bracing.

WEEKS 8-12

- Continue counterforce bracing if needed.
- Begin task-specific functional training.
- Return to sport or activities.

Medial Epicondylitis (Golfer's Elbow)

Medial epicondylitis (often called golfer's elbow) is far less frequent than lateral epicondylitis, but it also requires a detailed examination because of the proximity to other medial structures that may mimic medial epicondylitis. Exclusion of other causes of medial elbow pain is important for appropriate treatment.

Medial epicondylitis is defined as a pathologic condition that involves the pronator teres and flexor carpi radialis origins at the medial epicondyle. However, abnormal changes in the flexor carpi ulnaris and palmaris longus origins at the elbow may also be present.

Repetitive trauma resulting in microtears is a causative factor. An overuse syndrome affecting the medial common flexor origin develops in throwing athletes who place repetitive valgus stress on the elbow with repetitive pull of the flexor forearm musculature. Medial epicondylitis is an example of medial tension overload of the elbow. Tennis, racquetball, squash, and throwing often produce this condition. The serve and forearm strokes are the most likely to bring on pain.

Examination

Medial epicondylitis is diagnosed clinically by pain and tenderness to palpation localized to the medial epicondyle with wrist flexion and pronation against resistance (Fig. 2-38). Medial pain is often elicited after making a tight fist, and grip strength is usually decreased.

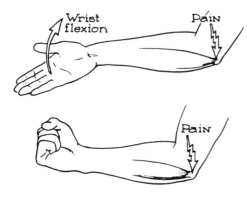

Figure 2–38 Medial epicondylitis may be diagnosed clinically by pain localized to the medial epicondyle during wrist flexion and pronation against resistance. Pain is often elicited after making a tight fist, and grip strength is usually diminished on the affected side. (From Morrey BF: The Elbow and Its Disorders. Philadelphia, WB Saunders, 1985.)

It is *extremely important* to differentiate medial epicondylitis from UCL rupture and instability. In the latter, valgus stress testing reveals UCL pain and opening (instability) of the elbow joint (Fig. 2-39). Concomitant ulnar neuropathy at the elbow may be present with either of these conditions.

Differential Diagnosis

UCL Rupture in Throwers
- Valgus stress testing of the elbow identifies injury to the UCL with opening of the joint on examination.
- A valgus stress is applied to the arm with the elbow slightly flexed and the forearm supinated (see Fig. 2-39B). Opening of the joint is indicative of UCL rupture and instability.

Ulnar Neuropathy
- Tinel's sign is positive at the elbow over the ulnar nerve in the cubital tunnel (elbow) with chronic neuropathy.

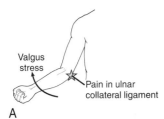

A

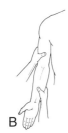

B

Figure 2–39 A, Medial joint pain elicited by placing a valgus stretch on the elbow identifies injury to the ulnar collateral ligament. **B,** To test for valgus instability, the patient's elbow is supinated and flexed 20 to 25 degrees to release the olecranon. The examiner stabilizes the humerus by grasping above the condyles with one hand. The other hand applies valgus stress to the elbow with an abduction force to the distal end of the ulna. (Adapted from Morrey BF: The Elbow and Its Disorders. Philadelphia, WB Saunders, 1985; and Nirschl RP, Kraushaar BS: Assessment and treatment guidelines for elbow injuries. Physician Sports Med 24[5]:230, 1996.)

- Concomitant compression neuropathy symptoms are frequently present and consist of numbness and tingling of the ulnar two (fourth and fifth) fingers.
- Ulnar neuropathy in throwers is seldom isolated and is often found concomitantly with UCL injury or medial epicondylitis because of traction on the nerve in the unstable elbow.
- Other causes of medial elbow pain to be considered are osteochondritis dissecans of the elbow and osteoarthritis.

Nonoperative Treatment

- Nonoperative treatment of medial epicondylitis is similar to that for lateral epicondylitis and begins with modifying or stopping activities that produce tension overload, the underlying etiology of medial epicondylitis, and correction of both training errors (overuse) and throwing mechanics potentially causing the tension overload.
- NSAIDs and icing are used for control of edema and inflammation.
- Braces are available that provide counterforce bracing to the medial flexor wad, but we have enjoyed little success with such braces.
- Stretching and ROM exercises are the same as those described for lateral epicondylitis.
- After the acute pain and inflammation subside, strengthening exercises of the elbow, forearm, wrist, and rotator cuff are begun, with a focus on strengthening of the wrist flexors (see the lateral epicondylitis rehabilitation protocol).
- For persistent symptoms, cortisone injection (0.5 ml betamethasone) into the area of maximal tenderness may be useful, but it should be given no more frequently than every 3 months with no more than three injections per year (see the section on injection technique for lateral epicondylitis). The needle must stay anterior to the medial epicondyle to avoid the ulnar nerve, which lies posterior to the injection site. *If the patient has radiating pain down into the forearm or fingers (accidental nerve injection), do not inject.*
- Surgical intervention may be indicated for symptoms that persist longer than 1 year.

A patient is advanced to high-level functional activities when elbow ROM is normal and pain free and strength is within 10% of the uninvolved extremity. It is imperative to monitor these criteria closely to avoid the tendency of lateral and medial epicondylitis to become chronic.

REHABILITATION PROTOCOL — *Lateral or Medial Epicondylitis*
Wilk and Andrews

PHASE 1—ACUTE PHASE

- Goals
  - Decrease inflammation/pain
  - Promote tissue healing
  - Retard muscle atrophy
- Cryotherapy
- Whirlpool

Continued

REHABILITATION PROTOCOL: *Lateral or Medial Epicondylitis* *Continued*

PHASE 1—ACUTE PHASE—cont'd

- Stretching to increase flexibility
  - Wrist extension-flexion
  - Elbow extension-flexion
  - Forearm supination-pronation
- HVGS
- Phonophoresis
- Friction massage
- Iontophoresis (with an anti-inflammatory such as dexamethasone)
- Avoid painful movements (such as gripping)

PHASE 2—SUBACUTE PHASE

- Goals
  - Improve flexibility
  - Increase muscular strength and endurance
  - Increase functional activities and return to function
- Emphasize concentric-eccentric strengthening
- Concentrate on involved muscle group or groups
- Wrist extension-flexion
- Forearm pronation-supination
- Elbow flexion-extension
- Initiate shoulder strengthening (if deficiencies are noted)
- Continue flexibility exercises
- Use a counterforce brace
- Continue the use of cryotherapy after exercise or function
- Initiate gradual return to stressful activities
- Gradually reinitiate previously painful movements

PHASE 3—CHRONIC PHASE

- Goals
  - Improve muscular strength and endurance
  - Maintain/enhance flexibility
  - Gradually return to high-level sport activities
- Continue strengthening exercises (emphasize eccentric-concentric strengthening)
- Continue to emphasize deficiencies in shoulder and elbow strength
- Continue flexibility exercises
- Gradually diminish use of the counterforce brace
- Use cryotherapy as needed
- Initiate gradual return to sport activity
- Equipment modifications (grip size, string tension, playing surface)
- Emphasize a maintenance program

Summary of Elbow Rehabilitation Principles for Epicondylitis

The guidelines for rehabilitation are centered on tissue-healing limitations and the constraints of pain and activity. The strengthening phase of rehabilitation begins with active motion and submaximal isometrics. When these activities are tolerated for 1.5 to 2 weeks without complications, the patient is progressed with PREs.

We recommend a low load with lower repetitions two times a day initially and then progression to moderate intensity with higher repetitions three times a day.

ROM is very important during the entire rehabilitation process; however, increased emphasis should be placed on ROM during the first 4 weeks to prevent fibrosis of the healing tissues. The therapist must also take into consideration the factor of irritation, which if ignored, will lead to further fibrosis as a result of inflammation.

The differences in the rehabilitation protocols for medial and lateral epicondylitis are, of course, due to the anatomy. However, this protocol can guide the clinician in developing a specific program to meet the patient's needs. One thing remains constant: we must limit harmful forces that can cause further degeneration of the involved tissue during the nonoperative or postoperative rehabilitation period. A factor that should always be considered in a patient undergoing postoperative rehabilitation is the realization that the patient's condition was unresponsive to conservative treatment. Therefore, timelines and progression should always be case specific. If these guidelines are followed with core general principles, patients should return to modification-free activities.

▌ Distal Biceps Repair

- Proximal biceps rupture (long head) at the shoulder is often treated nonoperatively. However, **distal** biceps rupture at the elbow is almost always treated operatively to restore active elbow flexion and supination strength.
- Distal biceps tendon rupture is much less common than proximal biceps rupture (96% of tears are proximal long-head, 1% are proximal short-head, and 3% distal biceps rupture).
- This injury typically occurs in men between the fourth and sixth decades of life (a mean age of 46).
- Predisposing degenerative changes in the biceps tendon at the insertion site are thought to be a predisposing factor for tendon rupture distally.
- Symptoms at the time of injury involve an audible popping sound, intense pain, and noticeable deformity in the biceps.
- The intense pain may give way to a dull ache over a period of several hours.
- The typical history involves a single eccentric contraction of the biceps while attempting to lift a heavy object or load.
- Common physical findings include swelling and tenderness at the antecubital fossa and weakness of supination and elbow flexion.
- Morrey et al. (1985) found a mean loss of 40% of supination strength and a variable loss of flexion strength averaging 30% in patients treated nonoperatively.
- With nonoperative treatment the distal portion of the biceps will scar to the brachialis muscle so that the normal contour does not return. Fatigue is a common complaint in patients treated nonoperatively.
- Boyd and Anderson's two-incision technique usually allows return of nearly full flexion-extension and pronation-supination.
- Operatively treated patients generally regain 100% of strength in their dominant arms and about 90% of strength in their nondominant arms (Baker et al. 1985)
- Objectively and subjectively, patients with distal biceps rupture treated operatively have better results than nonoperatively treated patients do.

REHABILITATION PROTOCOL *Distal Biceps Repair*

PHASE I (WEEK 1)

- Posterior splint at 90 degrees of elbow flexion
- Wrist and hand-gripping exercises

PHASE II (WEEKS 2-6)

- Elbow ROM brace
  - Week 2 at 45-100 degrees
  - Week 4 at 20-115 degrees
  - Week 6 at 15-130 degrees
- Shoulder exercises (rotator cuff)
- Scapular strengthening
- Wrist extensors/flexors
- Gripping exercises
- Week 5-6, isometric triceps exercise

PHASE III (WEEKS 6-10)

- Elbow ROM brace
  - Week 8 at 0-145 degrees
- Week 8 begin
  - Isotonic triceps
  - Isotonic wrist extensors/flexors
  - Shoulder isotonic

PHASE IV (WEEKS 10-16)

- Biceps isometrics at week 12
- Continue flexibility exercises
- ROM/stretching exercises
- Week 10-12, upper body exercises

PHASE V (WEEKS 16-26)

- Biceps isotonic exercises (light) at week 16
- Plyometrics

PHASE VI (WEEK 26 AND BEYOND)

- Return to activities (sport specific)

Isolated Fracture of the Radial Head

Mason's classification of radial head fractures is the most widely accepted and useful for determining treatment (Fig. 2-40; Table 2-1). Rehabilitation is also based on this classification.

REHABILITATION PRINCIPLES

- *Nondisplaced type I* fractures require little or no immobilization.
- Active and passive ROM can begin immediately after injury to promote full ROM.

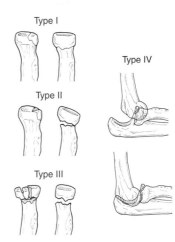

Type I

Type IV

Type II

Type III

Figure 2–40 Mason's classification of radial head fractures.

- Conditioning in the form of elbow flexion and extension, supination and pronation isometrics, and wrist and shoulder isotonics can be implemented immediately after injury (usually within the first week).
- Stress (e.g., heavy lifting) on the radial head is minimized.
- Three to 6 weeks of active elbow flexion and extension can be used, along with wrist isotonics.
- *Type II* and *III* fractures usually require open reduction and internal fixation (ORIF). Frequently, immobilization is required for a very brief time, followed by active and passive ROM exercises.
- *Type IV* comminuted fractures frequently require stabilization of the elbow joint and excision of fragments and generally cause some functional limitation.

Full ROM rarely returns after type IV injuries, and chronic elbow pain often persists.

TABLE 2–1	Mason's Classification of Radial Head Fractures	
Type	**Description**	**Treatment**
I	Nondisplaced fracture Often missed on radiographs Positive posterior fat pad sign	Minimal immobilization and early motion
II	Marginal radial head fracture with displacement, depression, or angulation	ORIF, early motion
III	Comminuted fracture of the entire radial head	ORIF, early motion if possible
IV	Concomitant dislocation of the elbow or other associated injuries	Radial head resection Check distal wrist joint (Essex-Lopresti injury) Guarded prognosis for return to sports

ORIF, open reduction and internal fixation.

REHABILITATION PROTOCOL
After Radial Head Fracture
Type I Fracture or Type II or III Fracture Stabilized with ORIF

PHASE 1—IMMEDIATE MOTION PHASE

Goals

- Decrease pain and inflammation.
- Regain full wrist and elbow ROM.
- Retard muscular atrophy.

Week 1

- Begin elbow active ROM and active-assisted ROM; minimal accepted ROM (15-105 degrees) by 2 weeks.
- Begin putty/gripping exercises.
- Begin isometric strengthening exercises (elbow and wrist).
- Begin isotonic strengthening exercises for the wrist.

PHASE 2—INTERMEDIATE PHASE

Goals

- Maintain full elbow ROM.
- Progress elbow-strengthening exercises.
- Gradually increase functional demands.

Week 3

- Initiate shoulder-strengthening exercises; concentrate on rotator cuff.
- Continue ROM exercises for the elbow (full flexion-extension).
- Initiate light-resistance elbow flexion-extension (1 pound).
- Initiate active-assisted ROM and passive ROM supination-pronation to tolerance.

Week 6

- Continue active-assisted ROM and passive ROM supination-pronation to full range.
- Progress shoulder program.
- Progress elbow-strengthening exercises.

PHASE 3—ADVANCED STRENGTHENING PHASE

Goals

- Maintain full elbow ROM.
- Increase strength, power, and endurance.
- Gradually initiate sporting activities.

Week 7

- Continue active-assisted ROM and passive ROM to full supination-pronation.
- Initiate eccentric elbow flexion-extension.
- Initiate plyometric exercise program.
- Continue isotonic program for the forearm, wrist, and shoulder.
- Continue until 12 weeks.

Elbow Arthroplasty

Indications for elbow arthroplasty include
- Pain, instability, and bilateral ankylosis, such as in patients with advanced stage 3 or 4 rheumatoid arthrosis that is unresponsive to medical management
- Failed interpositional or anatomic arthroplasty
- Failed prosthetic arthroplasty
- Arthrodesis in a poor functional position
- After en bloc resection for tumor
- Degenerative arthrosis after failed débridement and loose body excision
- Rheumatoid arthrosis in which synovectomy and radial head excision have failed

Contraindications to elbow arthroplasty include
- Active infection
- Absent flexors or flail elbow from motor paralysis
- Noncompliant patient with respect to activity limitations
- Inadequate posterior skin quality
- Inadequate bone stock or ligamentous instability with resurfacing implants
- Neurotrophic joint

Elbow prostheses are classified as **semiconstrained** (loose or sloppy hinge), **nonconstrained** (minimally constrained), or **fully constrained**. Fully constrained prostheses are no longer used because of their unacceptable failure rate.

REHABILITATION PROTOCOL | *After Total Elbow Replacement*

3 DAYS

- Remove the bulky dressing and replace with a light compressive dressing.
- Begin active ROM exercises for the elbow and forearm six times a day for 10 to 15 minutes. *Active ROM exercises should be performed with the elbow close to the body to avoid excessive stretch of the reconstructed elbow collateral ligaments.*
- Fit an elbow extension splint to be worn between exercise sessions and at night.

WEEK 2

- Passive ROM exercises of the elbow may be initiated.
- Functional electrical stimulation may be initiated to stimulate the biceps or triceps, or both.

WEEK 6

- Discontinue the elbow extension splint during the day if elbow stability is adequate.
- ROM exercises may now be performed with the elbow away from the body.

WEEK 8

- Discontinue the elbow extension splint at night.
- Initiate gradual, gentle strengthening exercises for the hand and forearm.
- Light resistance exercises may be begun for the elbow.
- Perform therapy within the patient's comfort level.

From Cannon NM: Diagnosis and Treatment Manual for Physicians and Therapists, 3rd ed. Indianapolis, The Hand Rehabilitation Center of Indiana, PC, 1991.

Olecranon Bursitis

Olecranon bursitis, or inflammation (or infection) of the subcutaneous bursa overlying the posterior olecranon process, may be acute (traumatic) or chronic, aseptic or septic. Because the bursa is not developed until after the age of 7 years, this condition is rare in children. The mechanism of injury may be a direct blow (fall on the playing surface) or chronic repeated trauma with gradual fluid accumulation. Infection can result from hematogenous seeding (*Staphylococcus aureus*) or direct inoculation (cut or injection).

Physical examination usually reveals posterior elbow swelling and tenderness with a palpable, often large bursa. In septic bursitis, the area is often warm and erythematous. Although there is no intra-articular involvement, extreme flexion may be limited.

Treatment of aseptic bursitis includes a compression dressing, icing, and a soft elbow pad to avoid constant irritation. We use a Hayes universal elbow pad manufactured by Hely and Weber (1-800-221-5465). These measures should allow gradual resorption of the fluid. If motion of the elbow is severely affected, the bursa is aspirated and the aspirate sent for Gram stain and culture studies. Septic bursitis requires incision and drainage, open wound management, and antibiotic therapy based on culture results. Gentle active ROM can be initiated, but excessive ROM should be avoided until the wound is stable.

Post-traumatic Elbow Stiffness

Michael L. Lee, MD • Melvin P. Rosenwasser, MD

Evaluation and Management

Stiffness of the elbow can result from congenital deformities, paralytic deformities, degenerative arthrosis, burns, or infections, but by far the most common is post-traumatic.

The "normal" arc of motion of the elbow, as defined by the American Academy of Orthopaedic Surgeons, is 0 degrees extension to 146 degrees flexion and 71 degrees pronation to 84 degrees supination. Morrey and coworkers (1981) determined that the ROM required for activities of daily living, or "functional ROM," is 30 to 130 degrees of extension-flexion and 50 to 50 degrees of pronation-supination. Terminal flexion is more important for activities of daily living than terminal extension is.

Classification

Post-traumatic elbow stiffness has been divided by Morrey (1993) into extrinsic (extra-articular), intrinsic (intra-articular), and mixed causes.

Extrinsic causes include everything about the elbow except the articular surface itself, from the skin down to the capsule and collateral ligaments. Skin contractures or subcutaneous scarring from incisions or burns can limit elbow motion. Direct elbow capsular injury, injury to the brachialis, or injury to the triceps causes

Classification of Post-traumatic Elbow Stiffness

EXTRINSIC (EXTRA-ARTICULAR) CAUSES OF ELBOW STIFFNESS

- Skin, subcutaneous tissue
- Capsule (posterior or anterior)
- Collateral ligament contracture
- Myostatic contracture (posterior or anterior)
- Heterotopic ossification

INTRINSIC (INTRA-ARTICULAR) CAUSES OF ELBOW STIFFNESS

- Articular deformity
- Articular adhesions
- Impinging osteophytes
  Olecranon
  Coronoid
- Impinging fibrosis
  Olecranon fossa
  Coronoid fossa
- Loose bodies
- Mixed causes

hematoma resulting in scarring in a contracted position with limitation of motion. Collateral ligament injury with subsequent healing in the contracted position can alter the normal axis of motion, thereby further inhibiting the arc of motion.

In addition, acute pain induces both voluntary and involuntary guarding of the elbow against motion—thus promoting contracture of the elbow capsule and brachialis muscle—and is thought to be the mechanism behind elbow stiffness after minor trauma to the elbow with minimal soft tissue injury. Entrapment neuropathies, most commonly of the ulnar nerve but also reported in the radial and median nerves, can cause pain resulting in guarding against motion.

Intrinsic causes can result from articular incongruity, loss of articular cartilage, hypertrophic callus on the articular surface, intra-articular adhesions, fibrosis within the normal fossa (coronoid or olecranon), or hypertrophic impinging osteophytes.

Evaluation of the Stiff Elbow

History

The two most important answers to be gleaned from the history are

1. The perceived deficits in motion
2. Whether the elbow is painful

Deficits in pronation-supination imply radiocapitellar pathology, and deficits in flexion-extension imply ulnohumeral pathology. Unless there is severe heterotopic ossification or complete ankylosis, either pronation-supination or flexion-extension will predominate in the patient's complaints. Deficits in extension less than 30 degrees or deficits of less than 100 degrees total arc of motion are within the functional ROM, and surgical correction is unlikely to be of benefit.

Normally, post-traumatic elbow stiffness is not painful. Pain implies arthrosis, impingement, entrapment neuropathy, or, less frequently, instability.

Physical Examination

Physical examination begins with inspection of the skin to note scars and areas of fibrosis for preoperative planning of the surgical approach. The nature of skin loss, fibrosis, or adherence and its contribution to stiffness should be evaluated to determine the need for a flap. ROM—passive, active, and active-assisted—should be carefully documented. The endpoint of restricted motion should be noted, with a *soft endpoint* implying soft tissue constraint and a *hard endpoint* implying bony impingement. Unfortunately, this distinction is not usually obvious. The strength and control of major muscle groups about the elbow should be assessed to determine whether the patient would be able to cooperate with the vigorous physical therapy program that will be necessary, whether treated operatively or nonoperatively. Neurovascular examination should focus on the ulnar and median nerves, which may show clinical or subclinical signs and symptoms of entrapment in scar or bony callus.

Radiographic Evaluation

Radiographic evaluation serves three purposes:
1. To evaluate the degree of degenerative changes
2. To rule out impinging hardware
3. To rule out heterotopic ossification

In most patients, anteroposterior elbow, lateral elbow, and radiocapitellar oblique views will suffice. For severe deformity or for bridging heterotopic ossification, an axial computed tomography (CT) scan or lateral tomograms may be necessary to evaluate the joint. Magnetic resonance imaging does not provide more information than CT does, but it may be useful in assessing MCL and lateral collateral ligament (LCL) integrity. It should be noted that focal articular cartilage loss can be difficult to appreciate with any preoperative imaging modality and may become apparent only at surgery.

Treatment

Nonoperative Treatment

Management of elbow stiffness begins with prevention via early motion and treatments related to achieving early motion, including stable internal fixation of fractures. Conditions creating inflammation in or around the elbow should be corrected. Anti-inflammatory medications are helpful in decreasing swelling. Heat before exercise, icing afterward, and physical therapy modalities such as iontophoresis, ultrasound, massage, and electrostimulation can help increase motion. Muscle weakness or imbalance should be corrected with strengthening exercises.

After elbow trauma, whether treated surgically or not, it is crucial to recognize when the patient's elbow motion is not progressing and to initiate more aggressive treatment. **Acute Treatment**. The first-line treatment of elbow stiffness is gradual, patient-controlled, physical therapy–directed stretching exercises. If motion still does not progress, splinting becomes the next step.

Dynamic hinged elbow splints with spring or rubber-band tension are useful to assist with deficits in elbow flexion. Dynamic splints are often poorly tolerated by patients because they impart continuous stretching that may cause cocontraction and spasm of antagonistic muscles, thus leaving the patient with no reprieve other than removing the splint.

Adjustable static (turnbuckle) splints are better tolerated for resistant flexion or extension deficits. If deficits are present in both directions, an adjustable turnbuckle orthosis can be used in alternating directions.

Finally, static splints that exceed the maximum passive extension or flexion capacity by 20 degrees can be made for nighttime use.

Functional electrical stimulation has met with limited success and cannot be recommended at this time. Continuous passive motion machines also have a limited role in established contractures.

Chronic Treatment. Once the elbow becomes nonpainful, yet a motion deficit exists despite splinting (generally after 6 months), further conservative treatment is unlikely to be of benefit.

Closed manipulation under anesthesia, previously thought to be of benefit, is believed to worsen elbow stiffness by inducing new inflammation and tearing of the soft tissue capsule and brachialis muscle, thus causing more hematoma and additional fibrosis. Forceful leveraging can also cause articular cartilage that has been encased in adhesions to delaminate.

Operative Treatment

If conservative measures fail and the patient has reasonable expectations regarding the anticipated results and can cooperate with the arduous postoperative rehabilitation, operative management can be considered.

The degree of degenerative changes within the elbow joint determines the surgical intervention for post-traumatic elbow stiffness. For patients with **no or minimal degenerative changes**, soft tissue releases with or without distraction are indicated. Patients with **moderate degenerative changes** can be treated with limited bony arthroplasty: débridement arthroplasty or Outerbridge-Kashiwagi ulnohumeral arthroplasty. Younger patients with severe degenerative changes can be treated with distraction fascial arthroplasty. For older patients (>60 years), low-demand elbows, or those whose stiffness has failed to be relieved by soft tissue or limited bony procedures, total elbow arthroplasty may be the only option.

For patients with minimal or no degenerative changes, soft tissue releases combined with removal of bony impingement can be helpful.

Surgical Indications. A patient who perceives significant functional deficits from the stiffness and is both cooperative and motivated enough to participate in the extensive physical therapy program is a candidate for operative release. In most cases, surgery offers improvement with flexion contractures greater than 30 degrees and maximum flexion less than 100 degrees. There are no absolute patient age limits for operative release, although young children may be unable to participate in physical therapy and the elderly may have confounding medical problems.

Timing. When the early phase of soft tissue healing has resolved, which can be as early as 3 months after injury, patients can be considered for soft tissue release.

Approaches. In selecting the approach to the elbow, the existing scars and the condition of the skin about the elbow must be considered, along with the direction of motion restriction.

If both flexion and extension are limited, access to both the front and the back of the ulnohumeral joint can be achieved through either a lateral (Kocher) approach or a medial approach. It is helpful to approach the elbow on the side with significant bony impingement. The medial approach is favored if the ulnar nerve requires exploration or release. Both approaches may also be used concurrently.

If there is adequate flexion and only extension is limited (flexion contracture), an anterior approach will allow access to release the anterior capsule, brachialis muscle, and rarely, the biceps tendon. The olecranon fossa is not visualized with this approach, so one must be certain that there are no posterior impediments.

If flexion is limited and extension is good (extension contracture), often a result of postsurgical casting in extension or impinging olecranon fixation, a direct posterior approach can be used to provide access to the triceps muscle, posterior capsule, and olecranon fossa.

If pronation-supination motion is limited, the extended lateral (Kocher) approach allows good visualization of the radiocapitellar joint, in addition to both the anterior and posterior ulnohumeral joints.

Release. After arthrotomy of the elbow joint, the release must be tailored to the offending structures. If the brachialis muscle is tight, it should be released or recessed off the humerus. If the triceps or the biceps is tight, tenolysis or more proximal mobilization of the muscle should be carried out, with tenotomy or Z-lengthening being reserved for more severe cases. If the anterior or posterior capsule is contracted, a capsulotomy or capsulectomy should be performed. Bridging or impinging heterotopic ossification should be excised. Within the joint, impinging marginal osteophytes or hypertrophic callus should be removed. The coronoid and olecranon fossa must be débrided of fibrofatty tissue, which can serve as a block to motion. If either collateral ligament is contracted, it may be released and Z-lengthened. Morrey (1993) believes that if the collateral ligaments are released, a distraction device should be applied to stabilize the elbow during soft tissue healing.

If the radial head is blocking pronation-supination or flexion, the radial head should be excised at the head-neck junction, with care taken to preserve the annular ligament.

For medial approaches, the ulnar nerve must be identified and protected. The stiffer the elbow joint, the more necessary it becomes to transpose the ulnar nerve to allow for nerve gliding and prevent traction injury. It is usually transposed subcutaneously, but if the subcutaneous tissue bed is scarred, submuscular transposition is more appropriate. The wound is closed in layers over suction drains to lessen the hematoma.

Stiff Elbow with Moderate Articular Degenerative Changes. For stiff elbows with moderate degenerative changes, limited bony arthroplasties are necessary in addition to soft tissue releases to help restore motion; débridement arthroplasty or an Outerbridge-Kashiwagi ulnohumeral arthroplasty may be operative options. For symptomatic (painful) arthrosis, radial head excision, olecranon ostectomy, osteophyte excision, olecranon-coronoid fossa débridement, and capsular release through a lateral incision may increase motion and diminish pain. One must be careful not to sacrifice the collateral ligaments, which will result in instability.

Débridement Arthroplasty. Débridement arthroplasty has been described as a treatment of advanced primary osteoarthrosis of the elbow, but it may be considered for post-traumatic stiffness with osteoarthrosis.

The elbow is approached through a posterolateral skin incision as allowed by existing scars. The distal end of the humerus is approached between the triceps and brachioradialis. The radial collateral ligament is Z-lengthened. The joint is opened with flexion and varus. The olecranon and olecranon fossa are débrided of osteophytes. The coronoid and radial head and their corresponding fossa are likewise débrided. They did not recommend resection of the radial head. The radial collateral ligament is repaired and the wound closed over drains. Continuous passive motion is initiated immediately after surgery.

Outerbridge-Kashiwagi Ulnohumeral Arthroplasty. Kashiwagi uses a technique of débridement arthroplasty that allows exploration and débridement of the anterior and posterior compartments with less extensive soft tissue dissection.

The elbow is approached through a small posterior midline incision. The triceps muscle is split, and the posterior capsule is opened. The tip of the olecranon is excised. The olecranon fossa is first fenestrated with a dental burr and then opened up to 1 cm in diameter to allow removal of anterior compartment loose bodies and débridement of the coronoid and radial head. Morrey (1992) modified this procedure and recommended elevation of the triceps (rather than splitting the triceps) and the use of a trephine to open the olecranon fossa.

Advanced Articular Degenerative Changes. Operative options for younger patients with elbow stiffness and severe degenerative changes, which unfortunately make up the largest group of patients with post-traumatic elbow stiffness, are quite limited because of the high demands placed on the elbow. Fascial arthroplasty and total elbow arthroplasty are the two operative options. Because there is no single good position for the elbow, arthrodesis is not an option. Resection arthroplasty usually results in intolerable instability or weakness, or both.

For older patients, total elbow arthroplasty becomes a more attractive option. Total elbow arthroplasty can also be a salvage procedure for patients who have undergone previous unsuccessful soft tissue or limited bony débridement arthroplasty.

Distraction Fascial Arthroplasty. According to Morrey (1992), there are three indications for interpositional arthroplasty:
1. Loss of more than half the articular surface
2. Significant adhesions that avulse more than half the articular surface
3. Malunion causing significant incongruity of the articular surface

An extensile-type posterior approach to the elbow is made through existing scars. Any restrictive capsule, ligaments, and muscles are released to obtain elbow motion. The radial head and any impinging bone are excised, which may afford additional motion. The humeral condyles and olecranon joint surfaces are then recontoured ("anatomic arthroplasty") to provide a smooth surface for rotation. A cutis graft or fascia lata graft (currently most common) may be used as the interpositional material. The graft is stretched over the distal humerus and proximal ulna and securely sutured in place, often through bone tunnels.

To protect and give some degree of stability to the elbow, an external distraction device that allows motion is applied. The distraction device is carefully centered about the projected center of elbow rotation in the distal humerus. The landmarks for the center are the anteroinferior aspect of the medial epicondyle and the center of the capitellum. The distraction device is then attached to the humerus and ulna, and the joint is distracted approximately 3 to 5 mm. Any deficient collateral ligaments should be reconstructed.

Total Elbow Arthroplasty. In general, total elbow arthroplasty for post-traumatic arthrosis has not been able to give the same satisfactory results as arthroplasty performed for rheumatoid arthritis. Total elbow arthroplasty should probably be reserved for patients older than 60 years with low-demand elbows. Nonconstrained implants are not recommended because post-traumatic elbows often lack the ligamentous stability necessary for their success. Semiconstrained total elbow arthroplasty has shown moderate success but may not be durable.

The elbow is approached posteriorly or posteromedially as allowed by existing scars. The ulnar nerve is identified medially and mobilized to allow for anterior transposition. The Bryan-Morrey exposure begins with medial elevation of the triceps muscle and tendon in continuity with a periosteal sleeve off the ulna to allow for elbow subluxation. The anterior and posterior capsules are excised or released. The distal humerus and proximal ulna are prepared with bone cuts specific to the implant, with care taken to preserve the medial and lateral humeral columns. The implant is cemented, adequate hemostasis is achieved, and the wound is closed over drains. Motion begins when the wound is sealed.

Heterotopic Ossification

A thorough discussion of heterotopic ossification (HO) about the elbow is beyond the scope of this review. Direct trauma in the form of intramuscular bleeding and displaced fracture fragments is the most common cause of HO about the elbow. Other risk factors include neural axis trauma (thought to be due to some humoral mediator or systemic cascade), thermal injury ("usually related to the degree, but not necessarily the site of burn"), and forceful passive manipulation of stiff joints.

There appears to be a direct correlation between the frequency of HO and the magnitude of the injury. The incidence of HO in the elbow ranges from 1.6% to 56% and generally increases with fracture severity and with fracture-dislocations.

Clinically, patients have swelling, hyperemia, and diminished motion between 1 and 4 months after injury. The differential diagnosis includes infection, thrombophlebitis, and reflex sympathetic dystrophy. In patients with spinal cord injuries, HO is found distal to the level of the lesion and thus occurs most commonly in the lower extremities. When the upper extremity is involved, it is usually on the side of spasticity, most commonly in the flexor muscles or posterolateral aspect of the elbow. HO is diffuse and does not necessarily follow anatomic structures or planes.

HO can be detected radiographically within the first 4 to 6 weeks. It is important to differentiate periarticular calcifications, indicative of MCL or LCL injury, from true HO. Technetium bone scan turns positive before plain films do. Sensitivity increases with the triple-phase bone scan. CT may help define the internal architecture of the HO to assess its maturity and can be helpful in determining the anatomic location of the HO.

Upper extremity HO has been classified by Hastings and Graham into three types:
Class I—radiographic HO without functional limitation
Class II—subtotal limitation
    Class IIA—limitation in the flexion-extension plane
    Class IIB—limitation in the pronation-supination axis
    Class IIC—limitation in both planes of motion
Class III—complete bony ankylosis

Treatment

HO can be inhibited pharmacologically. Diphosphonates inhibit the crystallization of hydroxyapatite, thus diminishing mineralization of the osteoid. NSAIDs, particularly indomethacin, are thought to decrease HO by interrupting the synthesis of prostaglandin E_2 and also by inhibiting differentiation of precursor cells into active osteoblasts; these drugs should be initiated in the early postoperative or postinjury period. External beam radiation is advocated for use about the hip to prevent HO and after excision of HO (700 to 800 rad in a single dose) within 48 to 72 hours after resection to prevent recurrence.

Obviously, not all patients require surgical intervention. There is evidence that HO may resorb, especially in children and those with neurologic recovery. For increasing limitation of motion and functional impairment unresponsive to physical therapy, surgery can be considered. The timing of surgery is critical. The HO should be metabolically quiescent at the time of surgery, based on the physical appearance of the limb (decreased swelling and erythema) and mature appearance on radiographs. The possibility of progressive soft tissue contracture if surgery is delayed must be balanced against the increased risk for recurrence if excised too early.

Summary

Post-traumatic elbow stiffness can be classified into that resulting from intrinsic causes, extrinsic causes, or a combination of the two. Prevention with modalities aimed at early motion is crucial to the management of stiffness. Treatment of post-traumatic elbow stiffness begins with supervised physical therapy, often combined with splinting. Patients with less than functional motion—30 to 130 degrees of extension-flexion or 50 to 50 degrees of pronation-supination—and who are willing to cooperate with the aggressive, prolonged physical therapy are candidates for operative management.

For patients with no or mild degenerative changes, soft tissue releases are appropriate. The direction of motion limitation will dictate the operative approach and the capsuloligamentous structures to be released. Continuous passive motion postoperatively seems to be of benefit. Results show consistent improvement in the motion arc.

For patients with moderate degenerative changes, limited bony arthroplasty (débridement arthroplasty or Outerbridge-Kashiwagi ulnohumeral arthroplasty) has high satisfaction rates and produces reliable improvement in the motion arc.

For patients with advanced degenerative changes, distraction fascial arthroplasty can be performed in younger patients or total elbow arthroplasty in older patients, although the results are acceptable but not excellent. Fascial arthroplasty outcomes are often unpredictable, and total elbow arthroplasty results have a high rate of loosening (up to 20%), complications (up to 25%), and revisions (up to 18%), but they seem to be improving with refinement in prosthesis design and implantation techniques.

Bibliography

Baker BE, Bierwagen D: Rupture of the biceps brachii: Operative versus non-operative treatment. J Bone Joint Surg Am 67:414, 1985.

Dillman CJ, Fleisig GS, Andrews JR, Escamilla RF: Kinetics of baseball pitching with implications about injury mechanisms. Am J Sports Med 23:233, 1995.

Forster MC, Clark DI, Lunn PG: Elbow osteoarthritis: Prognostic indicators in ulnohumeral debridement—the Outerbridge-Kashiwagi procedure. J Shoulder Elbow Surg 10:557, 2001.

Galloway M, De Maio M, Mangine R: Rehabilitation techniques in the treatment of medial and lateral epicondylitis. Orthopedics 15:1089, 1992.

Gelinas JJ, Faber KJ, Patterson SD, King GJ: The effectiveness of turnbuckle splinting for elbow contractures. J Bone Joint Surg Br 82:74, 2000.

Hastings H 2nd, Graham TJ: The classification and treatment of heterotopic ossification about the elbow and forearm. Hand Clin 10:417, 1994.

Hyman J, Breazeale NM, Altcheck DW: Valgus instability of the elbow in athletes. Clin Sports Med 20:25, 2001.

Mason ML: Some observations on fractures of the head of the radius with a review of one hundred cases. Br J Surg 42:123, 1954.

Morrey BF: Primary degenerative arthritis of the elbow: Treatment by ulnohumeral arthroplasty. J Bone Joint Surg Br 74:409, 1992.

Morrey BF: Post-traumatic stiffness: Distraction arthroplasty. In Morrey BF (ed): The Elbow and Its Disorders, 2nd ed. Philadelphia, WB Saunders, 1993, p 491.

Morrey BF: Biomechanics of the elbow and forearm. Orthop Sports Med 17:840, 1994.

Morrey BF, Askew LJ, An KN: Rupture of the distal tendon of the biceps brachii: A biomechanical study. J Bone Joint Surg Am 67:418, 1985.

Morrey BF, Askew LJ, An KN, Chao EY: A biomechanical study of normal functional elbow motion. J Bone Joint Surg Am 63:872, 1981.

Nirschl, RP, Chumbley EM, O'Connor FG: Evaluation of overuse elbow injuries. Am Fam Physician 61:691, 2000.

Peters T, Baker CL: Lateral epicondylitis. Rev Clin Sports Med 20:549, 2001.

Slocum DB: Classification of elbow injuries from baseball pitching. Tex Med 64:48, 1968.

Tullos HS, Bennett J, Shepard D: Adult elbow dislocations: Mechanisms of instability. Instr Course Lect 35:69, 1986.

Wilk KE: Stretch-shortening drills for the upper extremities: Theory and clinical application. J Orthop Sports Phys Ther 17:225, 1993.

3 Shoulder Injuries

BRIAN S. COHEN, MD • ANTHONY A. ROMEO, MD • BERNARD R. BACH Jr., MD

Physical Findings in Common Conditions of the Shoulder and Upper Arm

IMPINGEMENT SYNDROME

- Hawkins impingement test abnormal
- Neer impingement sign often present
- Supraspinatus isolation testing often painful
- Painful arc of abduction often present
- Subacromial bursa tender (variable)

ROTATOR CUFF TEAR

- Supraspinatus resistance painful and usually weak (supraspinatus isolation test positive)
- Hawkins impingement test abnormal
- Neer impingement sign often present
- Painful arc of abduction present
- Supraspinatus atrophy present (more severe cases)
- Infraspinatus resistance painful and possibly weak (more severe cases)
- Loss of active motion, particularly abduction (variable)
- Drop-arm sign present (only in more severe cases)
- Loss of active external rotation (massive tears)
- After injection into the subacromial space (lidocaine test), pain often improves but weakness of rotator cuff tear remains (versus rotator cuff tendinitis)

ANTERIOR INSTABILITY (RECURRENT SUBLUXATION OR DISLOCATION)

- Apprehension in response to the apprehension test (positive)
- Reduction of apprehension in response to the relocation test
- Increased anterior laxity to passive testing (drawer test, load-and-shift test)
- Signs of axillary nerve injury (occasionally) (deltoid weakness and numbness over the lateral aspect of the shoulder)
- Signs of musculocutaneous nerve injury (rarely) (biceps weakness and numbness over the lateral aspect of the forearm)

POSTERIOR INSTABILITY (RECURRENT SUBLUXATION OR DISLOCATION)

- Increased posterior laxity to passive testing (posterior drawer test, load-and-shift test)
- Mildly abnormal sulcus test (variable)
- Symptoms reproduced by the jerk test or circumduction test (variable)
- Voluntary dislocation or subluxation possible (occasionally)

Physical Findings in Common Conditions of the Shoulder and Upper Arm   *Continued*

MULTIDIRECTIONAL INSTABILITY

- Abnormal sulcus sign
- Increased anterior or posterior laxity, or both, to passive testing (drawer test, load-and-shift test)
- Additional signs of anterior-posterior instability depending on the predominant direction of symptomatic episodes
- Ability to voluntarily dislocate (occasionally)
- Often generalized ligamentous laxity noted (thumb to wrist, elbow hyperextension)

ACROMIOCLAVICULAR JOINT INJURY

- Tenderness of the acromioclavicular (AC) joint
- Localized swelling in the AC joint
- Usually a direct blow to the point of the shoulder (e.g., a fall or football hit)
- Increase in prominence of the distal clavicle (variable, depending on the severity of injury)
- Tenderness of the coracoclavicular ligaments (more severe injuries)
- Pain with cross-chest adduction (see Fig. 3-41)
- Rarely, distal clavicle displaced posteriorly (type IV injuries)
- The O'Brien test produces pain on top of the shoulder (variable)

BICEPS TENDINITIS

- Biceps tendon tender
- Speed test painful
- Yergason test painful (occasionally)
- Biceps instability test abnormal (occasionally, if the biceps tendon unstable)
- Look for signs of concomitant rotator cuff pathology (variable) if the biceps (a secondary humeral head depressor) is "trying to help" a weakened rotator cuff depress the humeral head

SUPRASCAPULAR NERVE COMPRESSION OR INJURY

- Supraspinatus and infraspinatus weakness and atrophy (if compression before innervation of the supraspinatus)
- Infraspinatus weakness and atrophy alone (if compression at the spinoglenoid notch)

RHEUMATOID ARTHRITIS

- Local warmth and swelling
- Muscle atrophy often present
- Signs of rheumatoid involvement at other joints

THORACIC OUTLET SYNDROME

- Symptoms reproduced by the Roos test, Wright maneuver, Adson test, or hyperabduction test (variable)
- Diminution in pulse with the Adson test, Wright maneuver, Halsted test, or hyperabduction test (variable)

ADHESIVE CAPSULITIS (FROZEN SHOULDER)

- Generalized decrease in both active (patient lifts arm) *and* passive (examiner lifts arm) range of motion (ROM), including forward flexion, abduction, internal rotation, and external rotation

Continued

Physical Findings in Common Conditions of the Shoulder and Upper Arm   *Continued*

ADHESIVE CAPSULITIS (FROZEN SHOULDER)—cont'd

- Pain elicited by passive ROM or any passive manipulation that stresses the limits of the patient's reduced motion
- Generalized weakness or atrophy (variable)

STINGER SYNDROME (BURNERS)

- Tenderness over the brachial plexus
- Weakness in muscles innervated by the involved portion of the plexus (deltoid most commonly involved, elbow flexors second most commonly involved)

REFERRED PAIN FROM CERVICAL RADICULOPATHY

- Motor, sensory, or reflex changes noted (radicular)
- Spurling test of neck positive (variable)
- Symptoms of findings distal to the elbow (e.g., hand numbness in the C6 distribution)
- Provocative tests of the shoulder normal

WEIGHTLIFTERS OSTEOLYSIS OF THE ACROMIOCLAVICULAR JOINT

- Point tenderness at the AC joint
- History of repetitive weightlifting
- Irregularity, narrowing of the AC joint noted on radiographs
- Usually no trauma history
- Positive cross-chest adduction sign

Modified from Reider B: The Orthopaedic Physical Examination. Philadelphia, WB Saunders, 1999.

The Disabled Throwing Shoulder: Glenohumeral Internal Rotation Deficit (GIRD) and the Spectrum of Pathology

- Burkhart, Morgan, and Kibler (2003) have proposed a novel concept of a disabled throwing shoulder that rejects much of the "conventional wisdom" regarding microinstability as the cause of the disabled throwing shoulder.
- Review of their three-part series (*Arthroscopy: The Journal of Arthroscopic and Related Surgery*, Vol. 19, No. 4, April 2003, pp. 404-420; No. 5, May-June 2003, pp. 531-539; and Vol. 19, No. 6, July-August 2003, pp. 641-661) is highly recommended for in-depth coverage of this topic.
- Burkhart defines "**dead arm**" in a thrower as any pathologic shoulder condition in which the thrower is unable to throw with preinjury velocity and control because of the combination of pain and subjective unease in the shoulder.
- A throwing athlete usually relates this discomfort to the late cocking or early acceleration phase of the throwing sequence when the arm begins to move forward. At this point the thrower feels a sharp, sudden pain, the arm "goes dead," and the athlete is unable to throw the ball with the usual velocity.
- The story of the dead arm is the "story of the disabled throwing shoulder." Burkhart asserts that the SLAP (superior labrum from anterior to posterior) lesion is the cause of the dead arm.

The Disabled Throwing Shoulder: GIRD and the Spectrum of Pathology   Continued

GLENOHUMERAL INTERNAL ROTATION DEFICIT (GIRD)

- Burkhart believes that the most important pathologic process that occurs in throwers is a "loss of internal rotation of the abducted shoulder."
- Glenohumeral internal rotation deficit (GIRD) is defined as the loss (in degrees) of glenohumeral (GH) internal rotation (in abduction) in comparison to the patient's nonthrowing shoulder.
- By convention, GH rotation is measured with the patient supine, the shoulder abducted 90 degrees in the plane of the body, and the scapula stabilized against the examination table by downward pressure applied by the examiner to the anterior aspect of the shoulder (Fig. 3-1). Internal and external rotation are measured with a goniometer to the point of GH rotation where the scapula just begins to move on the posterior chest wall.
- In symptomatic throwers' shoulders, the loss of internal rotation in abduction (GIRD) far exceeds the external rotation gains.
- **Acquired loss of internal rotation is caused by posteroinferior capsular contracture.** This contracture is the essential lesion that secondarily results in increased external rotation. It can occur with or without anterior capsular stretching, which may develop as a tertiary problem.
- As a result, GIRD should be addressed from a rehabilitation standpoint by focused posterior inferior capsular stretches (Fig. 3-2) to minimize GIRD and prevent secondary intra-articular problems, in particular, posterior type 2 SLAP lesions.
- In these authors' experience, approximately 90% of all throwers with symptomatic GIRD (greater than 25 degrees) will respond positively to a compliant posteroinferior capsular stretching program (above) and reduce GIRD to an acceptable level.
- An acceptable level of GIRD is defined as (1) less than 20 degrees of internal rotation deficit or (2) less than 10% of the total rotation seen in the nonthrowing shoulder.

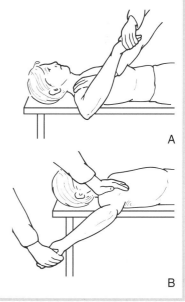

Figure 3–1 **A**, Internal rotation is measured with the patient's shoulder in 90 degrees of flexion while the examiner stabilizes the scapula. The endpoint of internal rotation is taken as the point at which the scapula begins to rotate posteriorly. **B**, External rotation is also measured while stabilizing the scapula. Note that the neutral position (0 degrees) is that in which the forearm is perpendicular to the patient's body (12-o'clock position in a supine patient). (Adapted from Burkhart SS, Morgan CD, Kibler WB: The disabled throwing shoulder: Spectrum of pathology. Part 1: Pathoanatomy and biomechanics. Arthroscopy 19:404-420, 2003.)

A

B

Continued

The Disabled Throwing Shoulder: GIRD and the Spectrum of Pathology   *Continued*

GLENOHUMERAL INTERNAL ROTATION DEFICIT—cont'd

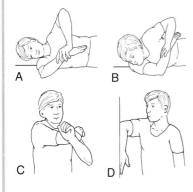

Figure 3–2   Focused posterior inferior capsular stretches. **A**, In the sleeper stretch, the patient is lying on the side with the scapula stabilized against a wall and the shoulder flexed 90 degrees. Passive internal rotation of the arm is applied to the dominant wrist by the nondominant arm. **B**, The roll-over sleeper stretch is the same as the sleeper stretch except that the shoulder is flexed only 50 to 60 degrees and the patient rolls forward 30 to 40 degrees from vertical side lying. **C**, The cross-arm stretch has the patient standing with the shoulder flexed 90 degrees and passive adduction applied to the dominant elbow by the nondominant arm. This traditional posterior stretch primarily stretches the posterior musculature to a greater degree than the posterior inferior capsule. It is imperative that the other stretches in this sequence be done as well. **D**, In the doorway stretch, the shoulder is abducted 90 degrees with the elbow on the edge of an open doorway. The patient leans forward and inferior to apply inferior capsular stretch to the shoulder. (Adapted from Burkhart SS, Morgan CD, Kibler WB: The disabled throwing shoulder: Spectrum of pathology. Part 1: Pathoanatomy and biomechanics. Arthroscopy 19:404-420, 2003.)

- This goal can usually be accomplished over a period of 2 weeks with the use of "sleeper" stretches (Fig. 3-2A).
- Conversely, 10% of throwers do not respond to this stretching regimen. These patients tend to be the older elite pitchers who have been throwing for years (from Little League to major league). These nonresponders tend to be on the severe end of the GIRD spectrum and have long-standing symptoms usually associated with intra-articular pathology (type 2 posterior SLAP lesions).
- Symptomatic nonresponders to stretch may be treated by arthroscopic selective posteroinferior capsulotomy, which in most cases is performed concomitantly with SLAP lesion repair.
- With a selective posteroinferior capsulotomy (Fig. 3-3), one can expect an immediate 65-degree increase in GH internal rotation.
- Verna in 1991 was the first to recognize the relationship of GIRD and shoulder dysfunction in throwing athletes. He monitored 39 professional pitchers in a single season. These pitchers were identified at spring training to have 25 degrees or less of total internal rotation (GIRD, 35 degrees or greater in each of these pitchers), and shoulder problems requiring the pitchers to stop pitching developed in 60% of this group during the study period.
- In a series of 124 pitchers with arthroscopically proven, symptomatic type 2 SLAP lesions (Morgan et al., 1998), all had preoperative severe GIRD in their throwing shoulders. The average GIRD was 53 degrees with a range of 25 to 80 degrees. This is remarkable when compared with an average GIRD of 13 degrees before the season and 16 degrees after the season in asymptomatic professional baseball pitchers (P. Donley, personal communication, November 2000).

The Disabled Throwing Shoulder: GIRD and the Spectrum of Pathology Continued

Figure 3-3 Selective posteroinferior capsulotomy. The capsular contracture is located in the posteroinferior quadrant of the capsule in the zone of the posterior band of the inferior glenohumeral ligament (PIGHL) complex. The capsulotomy is made ¼ inch away from the labrum from the 9- or 3-o'clock position to the 6-o'clock position. (Adapted from Burkhart SS, Morgan CD, Kibler WB: The disabled throwing shoulder: Spectrum of pathology. Part 1: Pathoanatomy and biomechanics. Arthroscopy 19: 404-420, 2003.)

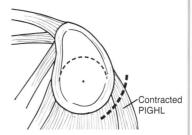

Contracted PIGHL

BIOMECHANICAL BASIS OF THE TETHERED THROWER'S SHOULDER

- Burkhart proposes two mechanisms by which a tight posteroinferior capsule allows hyper–external rotation of the humerus (classically seen in throwers).
- First the tethering effect of a shortened posterior capsule shifts the GH contact point. posterosuperiorly, which allows the greater tuberosity to clear the glenoid rim through a greater arc of motion before internal impingement occurs (Fig. 3-4A and B).
- Second, this shift in the GH contact point minimizes the cam effect of the proximal end of the humerus on the anteroinferior capsule to allow greater external rotation as a result of the redundancy in the capsule.
- An explanation of Burkhart's reciprocal cable model and cam effect in explaining the pathophysiology of this entity is elegant but beyond the scope of this text. This article is strongly recommended reading.
- **Internal impingement** (Fig. 3-5) is defined as intra-articular impingement that occurs in **each and every** shoulder in the abducted, externally rotated position. In this 90 degree–90 degree position, the undersurface of the posterosuperior rotator cuff contacts the posterosuperior glenoid labrum and becomes pinched between the labrum and the greater tuberosity (Walch et al., 1992).

PEEL-BACK MECHANISM IN THROWERS

- Burkhart reports that throwers classically exhibit posterior SLAP lesions or combined anteroposterior SLAP lesions on arthroscopy because of the "peel-back phenomenon."
- **Peel-back** occurs with the arm in the cocked position of abduction and external rotation. It is due to the effect of the biceps tendon as its vector shifts to a more posterior position in the late cocking phase of throwing. At arthroscopy, after removal of the arm from traction and bringing it into abduction and external rotation, the biceps assumes a more posterior and vertical position (Fig. 3-6). This same dynamic angle change during throwing produces a twist at the base of the biceps that transmits a torsional force to the posterior labrum. This "peels back" the posterior superior labrum and biceps (a "thrower's SLAP").
- Successful SLAP repair in throwers requires suture anchors with a simple suture loop (or loops) around the labrum to resist these rotational forces of the peel-back mechanism. Morgan et al. (1998) reported a 97% success rate with suture anchors laced through the labrum versus 71% to 88% with absorbable translabral tacks.

Continued

The Disabled Throwing Shoulder: GIRD and the Spectrum of Pathology Continued

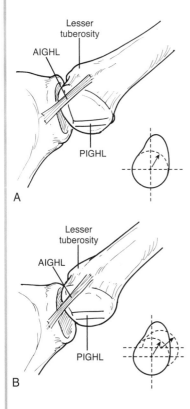

A

B

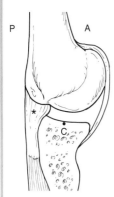

Figure 3–4 **A**, With abduction and external rotation, the two cables obliquely cross the shoulder as reciprocal and equal tension develops. The center of rotation remains approximately at the glenoid bare spot, and the greater tuberosity of the humerus has a well-defined circular arc (*dotted line*) before it contacts the posterior glenoid (internal impingement position). AIGHL, anterior band of the inferior glenohumeral ligament. **B**, When the posterior cable shortens (contracted posterior band), the glenohumeral contact point shifts posterosuperiorly and the allowable arc of external rotation (before the greater tuberosity contacts the posterior glenoid) increases significantly (*dotted lines*). PIGHL, posterior band of the inferior glenohumeral ligament. (Adapted from Burkhart SS, Morgan CD, Kibler WB: The disabled throwing shoulder: Spectrum of pathology. Part 1: Pathoanatomy and biomechanics. Arthroscopy 19: 404-420, 2003.)

Figure 3–5 In abduction and external rotation of the shoulder, the greater tuberosity abuts against the posterosuperior glenoid, and the rotator cuff is entrapped between the two bones (*asterisk*). This has been dubbed internal impingement. A, anterior; C, glenohumeral center of rotation; P, posterior. (Adapted from Burkhart SS, Morgan CD, Kibler WB: The disabled throwing shoulder: Spectrum of pathology. Part 1: Pathoanatomy and biomechanics. Arthroscopy 19:404-420, 2003.)

The Disabled Throwing Shoulder: GIRD and the Spectrum of Pathology *Continued*

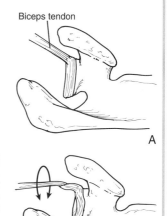

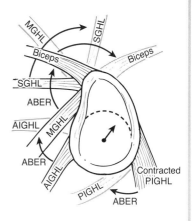

Figure 3–6 **A**, Superior view of the biceps and labral complex of a left shoulder in a resting position. **B**, Superior view of the biceps and labral complex of a left shoulder in the abducted, externally rotated position to show the peel-back mechanism as the biceps vector shifts posteriorly. (Adapted from Burkhart SS, Morgan CD, Kibler WB: The disabled throwing shoulder: Spectrum of pathology. Part 1: Pathoanatomy and biomechanics. Arthroscopy 19:404-420, 2003.)

THE PATHOLOGIC CASCADE FOR THROWERS

- An acquired posteroinferior capsular contracture is believed to be the first and essential abnormality that initiates a pathologic cascade that climaxes in the late cocking phase of throwing.
- At that point, the shift in the GH contact point (Fig. 3-7) causes maximum shear stress on the posterosuperior labrum at exactly the time when the peel-back force and total force are both at their maximum.

Figure 3–7 This diagram shows the shift in position that occurs in the major tendon and capsuloligamentous structures of the glenohumeral joint between the resting position (*solid lines*) and the abducted, externally rotated position (*dotted lines*). In abduction and external rotation, the bowstrung posterior band of the inferior glenohumeral ligament (PIGHL) is beneath the humeral head, thus causing a shift in the glenohumeral rotation point, and the biceps vector shifts posteriorly as the peel-back forces are maximized. ABER, abduction and external rotation; AIGHL, anterior band of the inferior glenohumeral ligament; MGHL, middle glenohumeral ligament; SGHL, superior glenohumeral ligament. (Adapted from Burkhart SS, Morgan CD, Kibler WB: The disabled throwing shoulder: Spectrum of pathology. Part 1: Pathoanatomy and biomechanics. Arthroscopy 19:404-420, 2003.)

Continued

The Disabled Throwing Shoulder: GIRD and the Spectrum of Pathology   *Continued*

THE PATHOLOGIC CASCADE FOR THROWERS—cont'd

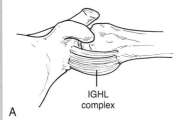

IGHL
complex

A

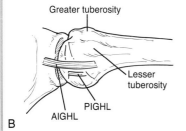

Greater tuberosity

Lesser
tuberosity

PIGHL

AIGHL

B

Figure 3–8 **A,** The hammock of the inferior glenohumeral ligament (IGHL) complex. **B,** The IGHL complex can be mechanically modeled by representing its two dominant structures, the anterior (AIGHL) and posterior (PIGHL) bands, as interdependent cables (reciprocal cable model). (Adapted from Burkhart SS, Morgan CD, Kibler WB: The disabled throwing shoulder: Spectrum of pathology. Part 1: Pathoanatomy and biomechanics. Arthroscopy 19:404-420, 2003.)

- In the presence of a shortened posterior band of the inferior GH ligament complex, the inferior axillary pouch structures are unbalanced and will not allow the normal cradling or hammock effect as described by O'Brien et al. (1990) (Fig. 3-8).
  This hammock effect usually allows the shoulder to wind and unwind in abduction around a relatively fixed central GH rotation point located in the lower half of the glenoid face (the bare spot) (Fig. 3-9).
- As the shoulder attempts to wind up into the cocked position, the contracted posterior band will not allow the head to fully externally rotate around the normal glenoid rotational point, which is acting as a rein or tether that draws the humeral head posterosuperiorly to a new rotation point on the glenoid.
- As the shoulder abducts and excessively externally rotates around this new pathologic posterosuperior rotation point, shear forces at the biceps anchor and the posterosuperior labral attachment increase. These structures began to fail from their attachments via the peel-back mechanism, and posterior type 2 SLAP lesions are produced.
- The anterior capsular structures that were appropriately tensioned before the shift occurred now become lax in the new rotation axis for any given amount of true GH external rotation because of the reduction in the cam effect (Fig. 3-10).
- Excessive external rotation caused by GIRD also causes increase shear and torsional stress in the posterosuperior rotator cuff. This is manifested as undersurface fiber failure as reported by Jobe and Morgan et al.
- Burkhart disagrees with previous reports suggesting that anterior instability is the primary cause of the dead arm syndrome. Burkhart believes that pseudolaxity (caused by a reduction of the cam effect and a break in the labral ring) has been incorrectly identified in the past as anteroinferior instability. Disruption of the labral attachment on one side of the glenoid allows channeling of laxity to the opposite side of the ring (circle concept, Fig. 3-11).
- The ultimate culprit in this theory is a tight posteroinferior capsule. If this is prevented from developing, the authors believe that a dead arm can be prevented.

The Disabled Throwing Shoulder: GIRD and the Spectrum of Pathology   *Continued*

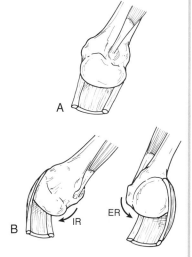

Figure 3–9   The normal hammock effect of the anterior and posterior bands of the inferior glenohumeral ligament complex described by O'Brien et al. permits (**A**) a balanced axillary pouch to direct internal rotation (IR) and external rotation (ER) of the humeral head in abduction (**B**) around a relatively fixed central glenoid rotation point. (Adapted from Burkhart SS, Morgan CD, Kibler WB: The disabled throwing shoulder: Spectrum of pathology. Part 1: Pathoanatomy and biomechanics. Arthroscopy 19:404-420, 2003.)

Figure 3–10   **A**, With the arm in a position of abduction and eternal rotation, the humeral head and the proximal humeral calcar produce a significant cam effect of the anteroinferior capsule in which the capsule is tensioned by virtue of the space-occupying effect. A, anterior; P, posterior. **B**, With a posterosuperior shift of the glenohumeral contact point, the space-occupying effect of the proximal end of the humerus on the anteroinferior capsule is reduced (reduction of the cam effect). This creates a relative redundancy in the anteroinferior capsule that has probably been misinterpreted in the past as microinstability. **C**, A superimposed neutral position (*dotted line*) shows the magnitude of the capsular redundancy that occurs as a result of the shift in the glenohumeral contact point. (Adapted from Burkhart SS, Morgan CD, Kibler WB: The disabled throwing shoulder: Spectrum of pathology. Part 1: Pathoanatomy and biomechanics. Arthroscopy 19:404-420, 2003.)

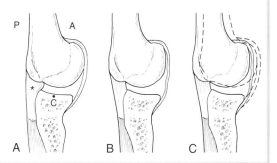

Continued

The Disabled Throwing Shoulder: GIRD and the Spectrum of Pathology   Continued

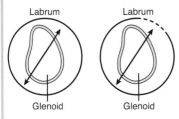

Labrum   Labrum

Glenoid   Glenoid

Figure 3–11   Circle concept of pseudolaxity. With a break in the labral ring, there is a channeling effect of apparent laxity to the opposite side of the ring where there is no disruption. Repair of the labral disruption eliminates the pseudolaxity. Pseudolaxity from a break in the labral ring is augmented by the reduction of the cam effect that occurs when the glenohumeral contact point shifts posterosuperiorly. (Adapted from Burkhart SS, Morgan CD, Kibler WB: The disabled throwing shoulder: Spectrum of pathology. Part 1: Pathoanatomy and biomechanics. Arthroscopy 19:404-420, 2003.)

CULPRITS IN THE DEVELOPMENT OF DEAD ARM

1. A tight posteroinferior capsule causing GIRD and a posterosuperior shift in the GH rotation point, with a resultant increase in the shear stress applied to the posterosuperior glenoid labrum (Fig. 3-12).
2. Peel-back forces in late cocking, which add to the already increased labral shear stress and give rise to the SLAP lesion (Fig. 3-13).
3. Hyper–external rotation of the humerus relative to the scapula caused by the shift in the GH rotation point, which increases the clearance of the greater tuberosity over the glenoid and reduces the humeral head cam effect on the anterior capsule.
4. Scapular protraction.
5. The hyper–external rotation (a) causes a hypertwist phenomenon (Fig. 3-14), which over time can result in a fatigue failure of the posterosuperior rotator cuff fibers from tensile, torsional, and shear overload. This overshadows any damage caused by direct abrasion of the cuff against the posterosuperior glenoid (internal impingement). (b) Torsional overload of the interior GH ligament causing elongation of the anterior stabilizing structures. It should be emphasized that fatigue failure of this inferior GH ligament occurs mainly in veteran elite pitchers and that anterior instability as a part of dead arm syndrome is very unusual, especially in younger athletes.

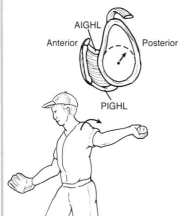

AIGHL

Anterior   Posterior

PIGHL

Figure 3–12   In abduction and external rotation (late cocking), the posterior band of the inferior glenohumeral ligament (PIGHL) is bowstrung beneath the humeral head, which causes a posterosuperior shift in the glenohumeral rotation point. Also in late cocking, the biceps vector shifts posteriorly and twists at its base, thereby maximizing peel-back forces. As a result of the tight posteroinferior capsule, this pitcher shows classic derangements of pitching mechanics: hyper–external rotation, hyper–horizontal abduction (out of the scapular plane), dropped elbow, and premature trunk rotation. (Adapted from Burkhart SS, Morgan CD, Kibler WB: The disabled throwing shoulder: Spectrum of pathology. Part 1: Pathoanatomy and biomechanics. Arthroscopy 19:404-420, 2003.)

The Disabled Throwing Shoulder: GIRD and the Spectrum of Pathology   *Continued*

CULPRITS IN THE DEVELOPMENT OF DEAD ARM—cont'd

Figure 3–13 Three subtypes of type 2 SLAP lesions, designated by anatomic location: **A**, anterior; **B**, posterior; and **C**, combined anteroposterior. (Adapted from Burkhart SS, Morgan CD, Kibler WB: The disabled throwing shoulder: Spectrum of pathology. Part 1: Pathoanatomy and biomechanics. Arthroscopy 19:404-420, 2003.)

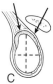

A   B   C

6. Burkhart believes that microinstability is *not* the cause of dead arm syndrome and that "pseudolaxity" from SLAP lesions coupled with a reduction in the cam effect (as a result of the posterosuperior shift of the GH contact point) has been misinterpreted as microinstability.
7. Furthermore, internal impingement is a normal phenomenon that is not usually pathologic in the throwing shoulder.
8. For a thrower with a dead arm and a SLAP lesion, repair of the SLAP lesion combined with an ongoing stretching program of the posteroinferior capsule is usually curative and returns the thrower to the preinjury level of competition in 87% of cases (Morgan et al., 1998).
9. For successful SLAP repair, the surgeon must arthroscopically confirm elimination of the peel-back sign and the drive-through sign.
10. For "stretch nonresponders," the surgeon may need to consider performing an arthroscopic release of the posteroinferior capsule. If there is greater than 130 degrees of external rotation with the scapula stabilized, electrothermal shrinkage versus arthroscopic capsular plication of the anterior band of the inferior GH ligament.
11. The sick scapula syndrome (an extreme form of scapular dyskinesis) can be the cause of a dead arm. Extreme protraction with anterior tilting of the scapula gives the impression that it is inferiorly displaced. This syndrome generally responds to focused rehabilitation of the shoulder.

PREVENTION AND REHABILITATION OF THE DISABLED SHOULDER

Prevention

- Focused posterior and inferior capsular stretches are performed in an attempt to prevent GIRD and its sequelae

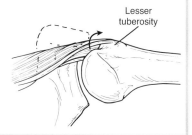

Lesser tuberosity

Figure 3–14 Torsional overload with repetitive hypertwisting of the rotator cuff occurs on the articular surface of the rotator cuff, the most common location of cuff failure in a thrower. (Adapted from Burkhart SS, Morgan CD, Kibler WB: The disabled throwing shoulder: Spectrum of pathology. Part 1: Pathoanatomy and biomechanics. Arthroscopy 19:404-420, 2003.)

Continued

REHABILITATION PROTOCOL	*Following Slap Repair (Burkhart, Morgan, Kibler)*

Immediately Postoperatively

- Operated arm at side in a sling with a small pillow
- Passive external rotation of the shoulder with the arm at the side (not in abduction)
- Flexion and extension of the elbow are emphasized immediately
- In patients requiring a posteroinferior capsulotomy, posteroinferior capsular stretches (sleeper stretches, see Fig. 3-2) on are started the first postoperative day
- Discontinue the sling after 3 weeks

Week 3

- Discontinue the sling
- Passive shoulder elevation is initiated
- Progressive passive motion as tolerated is permitted in all planes
- Sleeper stretches are begun in patients who did not require a posteroinferior capsulotomy

Weeks 6 to16

- Continues stretching and flexibility exercises
- Continue passive posteroinferior capsular stretching
- External rotation stretching in abduction
- Rotator cuff strengthening exercises
- Scapular stabilization exercises
- Deltoid strengthening
- At 8 weeks some biceps strengthening

4 Months Postoperatively

- Interval throwing program on a level surface
- Emphasis on posteroinferior capsular stretching

6 Months Postoperatively

- Pitcher okay to throw full speed

7 Months Postoperatively

- Pitcher throws full velocity from the mound
  All throwers must continue a posteroinferior capsular stretching program indefinitely to avoid the pathologic cascade.

Background

The **primary goal** of the shoulder complex is to position the hand in space for activities of daily living. Secondarily, during overhead athletic activities such as throwing and serving, the shoulder functions as the "funnel" through which the forces from the larger, stronger muscles of the legs and trunk are passed to the muscles of the arm, forearm, and hand, which have finer motor skills. The ability to execute these actions successfully comes from the inherent mobility and functional stability of the GH joint.

"Unrestricted" motion occurs at the GH joint as a result of its osseous configuration (Fig. 3-15). A large humeral head articulating with a small glenoid socket allows extremes of motion at the expense of the stability that is seen in other joints. Similarly, the scapula is very mobile on the thoracic wall, which enables it to follow the humerus and position the glenoid appropriately while avoiding humeral

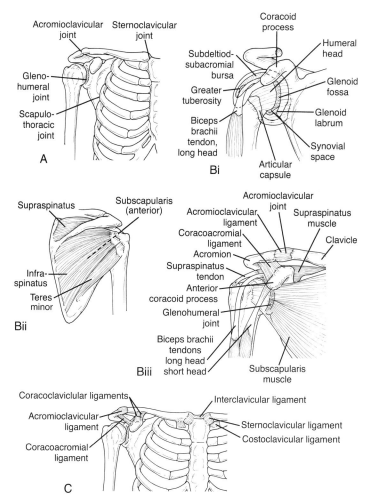

Figure 3–15 **A**, Shoulder joint osteology. **B**, Shoulder musculature. The shallow glenohumeral joint (**Bi**, *anterior view*) derives some stability from the surrounding tendons and musculature, most significantly the rotator cuff (**Bii**, *posterior view*), which consists of the supraspinatus, infraspinatus, teres minor, and subscapularis tendons. The acromioclavicular (AC) articulation (**Biii**, *anterior view*) is surrounded by the AC and coracoclavicular (CC) ligaments. **C**, The AC ligament gives anterior-posterior and medial-lateral stability to the AC joint, and the CC ligaments provide vertical stability. The sternoclavicular joint has little bony stability but strong ligaments—primarily the costoclavicular, sternoclavicular, and interclavicular—that contribute to joint stability. (**B**, From Sartoris DJ: Diagnosing shoulder pain: What's the best imaging approach? Physician Sports Med 20[9]:150, 1992; **C**, from Hutchinson MR, Ahuja GS: Diagnosing and treating clavicle fractures. Physician Sports Med 24[3]:26-35, 1996.)

impingement on the acromion. Osseous stability of the GH joint is enhanced by the fibrocartilaginous labrum, which functions to enlarge and deepen the socket while increasing the conformity of the articulating surfaces. However, the majority of the stability at the shoulder is determined by the soft tissue structures that cross it. The ligaments and capsule form the static stabilizers and function to limit translation and rotation of the humeral head on the glenoid. The **superior GH ligament** has been shown to be an important inferior stabilizer. The **middle GH ligament** imparts stability against anterior translation with the arm in external rotation and abduction less than 90 degrees. The **inferior GH ligament** is the most important anterior stabilizer with the shoulder in 90 degrees of abduction and external rotation, which represents the most unstable position of the shoulder (Fig. 3-16).

The muscles make up the dynamic stabilizers of the GH joint and impart stability in a variety of ways. During muscle contraction, they provide increased capsuloligamentous stiffness, which increases joint stability. They act as dynamic ligaments when their passive elements are put on stretch (Hill, 1951). Most importantly, they make up the components of force couples that control the position of the humerus and scapula, thereby helping to appropriately direct the forces crossing the GH joint.

Proper scapular motion and stability are critical for normal shoulder function. The scapular forms a stable base from which all shoulder motion occurs, and correct positioning is necessary for efficient and powerful GH joint movement. Abnormal scapular alignment and movement, or **scapulothoracic dyskinesis**, can result in clinical findings consistent with instability or impingement syndrome (or with both). Strengthening of the scapular stabilizers is an important component of the rehabilitation protocol after all shoulder injuries and is essential for complete functional recovery of the shoulder complex.

In most patients, rehabilitation after a shoulder injury should initially focus on pain control and regaining coordinated motion throughout all components of the

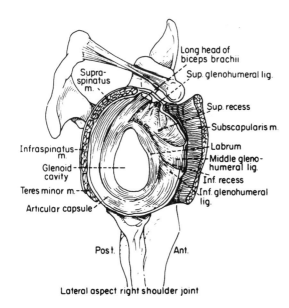

Figure 3–16 Glenohumeral (GH) ligaments and the rotator cuff stabilizers of the GH joint. (From Rockwood CA Jr, Matsen FA III: The Shoulder, 2nd ed. Philadelphia, WB Saunders, 1988, p 255.)

shoulder complex. Once motion is regained, attention is shifted to strengthening and re-educating the muscles around the shoulder to perform their normal tasks. To reproduce the precision with which the shoulder complex functions, the muscles need to be re-educated through "learned motor patterns." These patterns position the shoulder complex in "predetermined" ways and activate the muscles in precise synchronization to maximize recovery of function. Associated conditioning of the lower extremities and trunk muscles is extremely important because more than 50% of the kinetic energy during throwing and serving is generated from the legs and trunk muscles. Therefore, rehabilitation of all components of the kinetic chain is required before successful return to competitive or strenuous overhead athletic activities.

General Principles of Shoulder Rehabilitation

The most important factor that determines the success or failure of a particular shoulder rehabilitation protocol is establishing the correct diagnosis.

Motion, strength, and **stability** are the three components of shoulder function that can be disrupted by an acute or chronic injury. All three can be treated effectively with therapeutic rehabilitation.

Obvious findings of gross instability, massive muscle tears, or severe loss of motion are easily diagnosed, but not necessarily easily treated. Subtle findings, such as increased humeral translation because of loss of GH joint internal rotation, superior humeral head migration as a result of rotator cuff weakness, or abnormal scapular positioning secondary to weakness of the trapezius or serratus anterior muscles, are more difficult to diagnose and just as difficult to treat. For successful rehabilitation, recognition and treatment of the pathology are as important as understanding its impact on normal shoulder function. The goal of rehabilitation, regardless of the pathology, is always functional recovery.

In general, shoulder rehabilitation after an injury or surgery should begin with early active motion to help restore normal shoulder mechanics. The benefits of early joint mobilization have been well documented in other areas of the body. For example, accelerated rehabilitation programs for the knee after anterior cruciate ligament reconstruction have resulted in earlier restoration of motion, strength, and function without compromising stability. Strict immobilization has been shown to be responsible for the development of "functional" instability in the shoulder secondary to rotator cuff inhibition, muscular atrophy, and poor neuromuscular control. A lack of active motion within the shoulder complex compromises the normal kinematic relationship between the GH and scapulothoracic joints and can lead to rotator cuff abnormalities or impingement syndrome. Concerns about early active motion in patients with shoulder pathology are the fear of aggravating an already painful condition and the risk of compromising a surgical repair. The timing of motion and strengthening exercises needs to be well documented by the treating physician and clearly outlined for the patient and physical therapist.

One therapeutic modality that is making advances in shoulder rehabilitation because it puts less stress on tissues is **aquatic physical therapy** (see Chapter 7, Special Topics). The benefit of aquatic rehabilitation is related to the buoyancy effect that water provides for the upper extremity, with the weight of the arm decreased to as little as one eighth its original weight at 90 degrees of abduction or forward flexion.

The apparent decrease in weight of the arm or the shoulder puts less stress on the repaired or inflamed tissues during active exercises. This allows early restoration of active movement in a protected environment and thus early return of normal motor patterns.

Intake Evaluation

Before therapy on the shoulder is initiated, a general intake evaluation is performed. The intake survey begins with a thorough evaluation of all the components of the shoulder complex, as well as all parts of the "kinematic" chain.

The examination starts with a general assessment of the patient's active and passive motion.

The examiner should look for GIRD in the thrower's shoulder (see p. 177). Movement of both scapulae along the thoracic wall should be monitored from behind the patient. Scapular motion should be both smooth and symmetrical. Evidence of scapular winging or asymmetrical movements should alert the examiner to a potential nerve injury or, more often, weakness of the muscles that stabilize the scapula. As discussed earlier, abnormal scapular motion can cause symptoms consistent with anterior instability or impingement.

Analysis of the AC joint for areas of tenderness, as well as degrees of motion, is also important because this small joint can be the source of extremely painful pathology.

The evaluation of the shoulder complex is completed with a thorough examination of the GH joint for ROM, stability, and muscle strength. Once the shoulder complex has been thoroughly evaluated, other areas that function during overhead activities need to be evaluated.

Examination of the patient's hips and knees is performed, with close attention to hip flexion and rotation. ROM and strength of the lumbar spine should be well documented. It is not uncommon to see loss of motion in the hips, knees, or lower part of the back contributing to abnormal shoulder mechanics in a throwing athlete. Evidence of kyphosis or scoliosis of the thoracic spine should be recorded because both of these conditions have been associated with alteration of spine motion during throwing, as well as disruption of normal scapular rhythm.

Differential Diagnosis of Shoulder Pain

Rotator cuff or biceps tendon

    Strain

    Tendinitis

    Tear

GH instability

    Anterior

    Posterior

    Multidirectional

Continued

GH instability with secondary impingement
Primary impingement of the cuff or biceps tendon
Calcific tendinitis
AC joint pathology
  Arthritis
  Separation
  Weightlifter's osteolysis
GH arthritis
  Rheumatoid arthritis
  Septic arthritis
  Inflammatory arthritis
  Neuropathic (Charcot) arthritis
  Crystalline arthritis (gout, pseudogout)
  Hemophilic arthritis
  Osteochondromatosis
Thoracic outlet syndrome (TOS)
Cervical spine/root/brachial plexus injury with referred pain
Suprascapular nerve neuropathy
Shoulder dislocation
  Acute
  Chronic (missed)
Sternoclavicular (SC) injury
Adhesive capsulitis (frozen shoulder)
SLAP lesion
Fracture
  Humerus
  Clavicle
  Scapula
Scapular winging
Little leaguer's shoulder
Reflex sympathetic dystrophy
Tumor
  Metastatic
  Primary
  Multiple myeloma
  Soft tissue neoplasm

Continued on following page

Bone disorders

    Osteonecrosis (avascular necrosis)

    Paget's disease

    Osteomalacia

    Hyperparathyroid disease

Infection

Intrathoracic disorders (referred pain)

    Pancoast's tumor

    Diaphragmatic irritation, esophagitis

    Myocardial infarction

Psychogenic disorders

Polymyalgia rheumatica

Neuralgic amyotrophy (Parsonage-Turner syndrome)

Abdominal disorders (referred pain)

    Gastric ulcer

    Gallbladder

    Subphrenic abscess

The Importance of History Taking in Evaluating Shoulder Pain

It is important to determine whether the shoulder pain results from **acute, traumatic** events or from **chronic, repetitive overuse**. For example, AC joint separation can be ruled out in a pitcher who has AC joint pain that has insidiously developed over a period of 2 months with no history of trauma or a direct blow to the shoulder. The anatomic location of the pain should be pinpointed (e.g., rotator cuff insertion, posterior shoulder) rather than settling for "the whole shoulder hurts."

The patient should be questioned about neck pain or neurologic symptoms indicative of **referred shoulder pain** (e.g., C5-6 lesion or suprascapular nerve).

The patient's **chief complaint** is important and often a good differentiator: weakness, stiffness, pain, catching, popping, subluxation, "dead-arm" impingement, loss of motion, crepitance, radiation into the hand.

In our institution we try to determine which category of shoulder pain that the patient falls into. For **referred neck pain** to the shoulder, are the complaints more radicular in nature with an unimpressive shoulder examination? Is the cause of pain a **frozen shoulder** from not using the arm and a block that **equally** restricts both active and passive shoulder motion? Was there an underlying cause (e.g., rotator cuff tear) that made the patient initially stop using the shoulder?

Is the cause an **unstable shoulder** after a previous dislocation or a very ligamentously lax shoulder (torn loose or born loose)? Is the cause of pain a **rotator cuff tear** with pain and significant weakness on overhead activities, or does the pain originate from the spectrum of rotator cuff tendinitis, partial-thickness tearing, bursitis, impingement, and so forth?

Did the patient have trauma to the shoulder with a clavicle fracture or AC joint tenderness or radiographic evidence of weightlifter's osteolysis of the AC joint? A thorough history and physical examination must be performed to avoid sending the patient to the therapist with a prescription of "shoulder pain—evaluate and treat."

Important History in Throwing Athletes with Shoulder Pain

- General information
  - Age
  - Dominant handedness
  - Years of throwing
  - Level of competition
- Medical information
  - Chronic or acute medical problems
  - Review of systems
  - Preexisting or recurrent shoulder problems
  - Other musculoskeletal problems (acute or distant)
- Shoulder complaints
  - Symptoms
    - Pain
    - Weakness, fatigue
    - Instability
    - Stiffness
    - Functional catching
  - Injury pattern
    - Sudden or acute onset
    - Gradual or chronic onset
    - Traumatic fall or blow
    - Recurrent
  - Symptom characteristics
    - Location
    - Character and severity
    - Provocation
    - Duration
    - Paresthesias
    - Phase of throwing
    - Related activities, disability
  - Related symptoms
    - Cervical
    - Peripheral nerve
    - Brachial plexus
    - Entrapment

From Andrews JR, Zarins B, Wilk KE: Injuries in Baseball. Philadelphia, Lippincott-Raven, 1998.

Examination of the Shoulder

Physical Examination of the Throwing Shoulder

SITTING POSITION

- Inspection
- Palpation
  - SC joint, clavicle, AC joint
  - Acromion, coracoid
  - Bicipital groove
  - Scapula
  - Musculature
- ROM
  - Crepitus
  - GH motion (assymetry of throwing versus nonthrowing shoulder)
  - Scapulothoracic motion
- Rotator cuff, scapular muscle testing
  - Isolated muscle testing
  - Supraspinatus testing
- Scapular winging
- Stability testing
  - Anterior-posterior Lachman test
  - Anterior-posterior apprehension test
- Ligamentous laxity (thumb to wrist, "double-jointed" fingers)
  - Inferior sulcus sign
- Impingement signs
- Biceps testing

SUPINE POSITION

- Motion—rule out GIRD and inspect motion in *all* planes
- Anterior instability tests
  - Anterior shoulder drawer test
  - Apprehension test
  - Relocation test
- Posterior instability tests
  - Posterior shoulder drawer test
  - Apprehension test
- Labral testing
  - Clunk test

PRONE POSITION

- Palpation of posterior structures
- Motion re-evaluation
- Stability—anterior apprehension test

NEUROLOGIC AND CERVICAL EXAMINATION

- Rule out referred or neurologic origin of shoulder pain

RADIOGRAPHIC EXAMINATION

From Andrews JR, Zarins B, Wilk KE: Injuries in Baseball. Philadelphia, Lippincott-Raven, 1998.

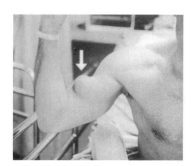

Figure 3–17 Rupture of the long head of the biceps tendon, often referred to as a "Popeye" deformity. (From Reider B: The Orthopaedic Physical Examination. Philadelphia, WB Saunders, 1999.)

DIRECT INSPECTION OF THE SHOULDER

- The presence of atrophy, hypertrophy, scapular winging, asymmetry of the shoulders, swelling, deformity, erythema, or the patient supporting the shoulder with the other arm
- Isolated **atrophy**
  - Supraspinatus and infraspinatus fossa (possible rotator cuff disease, entrapment or injury to the suprascapular nerve, disuse)
  - Deltoid or teres minor muscle atrophy (possible axillary nerve injury)
  - Winging of the scapula (long thoracic nerve injury)
- "Popeye" bulge of the biceps (evidence of a proximal tear of the long head of the biceps) worsened with flexion of the elbow (Fig. 3-17)
- Deformity of the AC joint (grade 2 or 3 AC joint separation)
- Deformity of shoulder (probable dislocation or fracture, or both)
  Palpation of the shoulder begins with palpation of the SC joint and proximal end of the clavicle.
- Prominence, asymmetry, or tenderness to palpation indicates SC dislocation (traumatic), subluxation (traumatic), or arthritis (insidious).
- The **clavicle** is palpated for possible clavicular fracture.
- The **AC** joint is palpated for pain or prominence.
  - A prominence indicates a traumatic grade 2 or 3 AC joint separation.
  - Tenderness, with no prominence (no trauma) may be indicative of weightlifter's osteolysis or arthritis of the AC joint.
- If palpation of the **bicipital groove** identifies tenderness, biceps tendinitis is suggested.
  - Biceps tendinitis often results from the biceps having to "overwork" in its secondary role as a humeral head depressor because of concomitant rotator cuff pathology (biceps tendinitis seldom exists alone, with the exception of a weightlifter performing too many biceps curls). In other words, a weak or torn rotator cuff will recruit the biceps to help with the function that it is struggling to achieve, namely, to depress the humeral head to allow clearance under the arch of the acromion.
  - Absence of the biceps in the groove indicates a rupture of the long head of the biceps.
- Palpation of the **anterior GH joint** and **coracoid** may identify anterior shoulder tenderness, which is a common and very nonspecific finding.

- Tenderness to palpation in the **greater tuberosity** and insertion site of the **rotator cuff insertion** (just distal to the anterolateral border of the acromion) indicates
  - Rotator cuff tendinitis or tear.
  - Primary or secondary impingement.
  - Subacromial bursitis.
- Palpation of the **scapulothoracic muscles** and medial border of the **scapula** checks for
  - Winging of the scapula, indicative of injury to the long thoracic nerve or weakness of the scapulothoracic muscles (possible scapular dyskinesis).
  - Crepitance, which is found with snapping scapula syndrome or tender scapulothoracic bursitis.

RANGE-OF-MOTION TESTING OF THE GLENOHUMERAL AND SCAPULOTHORACIC JOINTS

A **throwing athlete's** shoulder often demonstrates an adaptation of **increased external rotation** of the throwing arm (Fig. 3-18) and **decreased internal rotation** (GIRD—see Fig. 3-1). Testing of the symmetry of active and passive ROM of the shoulder should include

- Internal and external rotation
- Abduction
- Forward flexion (Fig. 3-19)
- Extension

Evaluation of scapulothoracic motion should note subtle scapular winging or lag.

Adhesive capsulitis (frozen shoulder) causes **both restricted active (patient lifts arm) and passive (examiner lifts arm)** shoulder motion, whereas an acute rotator cuff tear results in restricted active motion but nearly normal passive motion.

NEUROLOGIC TESTING

Reflexes, motor strength, sensation, and neck ROM are evaluated. Specific tests are used to rule out thoracic outlet syndrome (TOS) and encroachment on a cervical nerve root.

- The **Adson test** (Fig. 3-20) is used to rule out TOS.
  - The arm of the standing (or seated) patient is abducted 30 degrees at the shoulder and maximally extended.

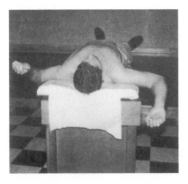

Figure 3–18 Functional adaptation or altered glenohumeral rotational contact point posterosuperiorly (glenohumeral internal rotation deficit [GIRD] hypothesis) (increased external rotation) in a thrower. (From McCluskey GM: Classification and diagnosis of glenohumeral instability in athletes. Sports Med Arthroscopy Rev 8:158-169, 2000.).

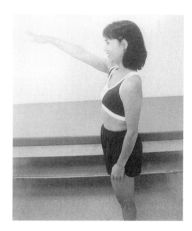

Figure 3–19   Range-of-motion testing: forward flexion.

- The radial pulse is palpated and the examiner grasps the patient's wrist.
- The patient then turns the head toward the symptomatic shoulder and is asked to take a deep breath and hold it.
- The quality of the radial pulse is evaluated in comparison to the pulse taken while the arm is resting at the patient's side.
- Diminution or disappearance of the pulse suggests TOS.
- Some clinicians have patients turn their heads **away** from the side tested in a modified test.
- The **Wright maneuver** is a similar test in which the shoulder is abducted to 90 degrees and fully externally rotated.

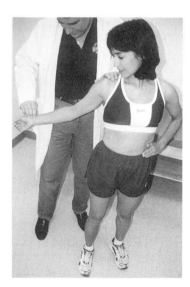

Figure 3–20   Adson test for thoracic outlet syndrome.

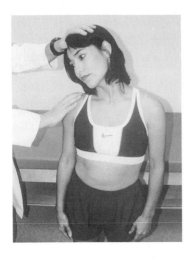

Figure 3–21 Spurling test to detect encroachment on a cervical nerve root.

- The **Roos test** is also used to rule out TOS.
  - The patient abducts the shoulder 90 degrees while flexing the elbow to 90 degrees.
  - The hand is opened and closed 15 times.
  - Numbness, cramping, weakness, or inability to complete the repetitions is suggestive of TOS.
- The **Spurling test** (Fig. 3-21) detects encroachment on a cervical nerve root (cervicular radiculopathy).
  - The neck is extended and rotated toward the involved side before axial compression.
  - The maneuver is designed to exacerbate encroachment on a cervical nerve root by decreasing the dimensions of the neural foramen.
  - Radicular pain (positive result) radiates into the upper extremity in a specific dermatomal distribution (typically radiates below the elbow).
- **Suprascapular nerve compression** is difficult to diagnose. Posterior pain and posterior scapular atrophy (infraspinatus fossa) are often present.
  - Suprascapular notch tenderness is variable. Electromyography studies should be performed to confirm the diagnosis.

BICEPS TESTING

- With the **Speed test,** the examiner resists forward elevation of the athlete's arm with approximately 60 degrees of forward flexion and 45 degrees of abduction and the elbow fully extended and supinated (Fig. 3-22). The test is positive for proximal biceps tendon involvement if the patient complains of pain.
- For the **Yergason test** (Fig. 3-23), the examiner resists the athlete's attempted supination (palm up) from a starting position of elbow flexion of 90 degrees and pronation (palm down). The test is positive when the patient experiences pain about the bicipital groove.
- The **biceps load test** assesses for SLAP lesions of the attachment of the long head of the biceps at the superior glenoid area.
  - With the patient supine on the table, the examiner gently grasps the patient's wrist and elbow.

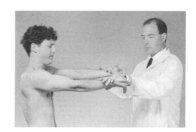

Figure 3–22   Speed test for biceps tendon involvement. (From Reider B: The Orthopaedic Physical Examination. Philadelphia, WB Saunders, 1999.)

- The patient's arm is abducted 90 degrees with the forearm supinated.
- An anterior apprehension test is performed on the relaxed patient.
- When the patient becomes apprehensive during external rotation of the shoulder, the external rotation is stopped.
- The patient is then asked to flex the elbow while the examiner resists the flexion with one hand.
- The examiner asks how the apprehension has changed, if at all. If the apprehension has lessened or the patient feels more comfortable, the test is considered negative for a SLAP lesion.
- If apprehension is unchanged or has become more painful, the test is considered positive for a SLAP lesion.
- The examiner must sit adjacent to the shoulder at the same height as the patient and should face the patient at a right angle.
- This test has a sensitivity of 90.9%, a specificity of 96.9%, a positive predictive value of 83%, and a negative predictive value of 98% according to Kim and colleagues (2001).
- The **SLAP test** is performed with the patient's arm abducted 90 degrees and the hand supinated.
  - The examiner places one hand on the patient's shoulder with the thumb in the 6-o'clock position in the axilla.
  - The examiner's opposite hand exerts a downward force on the patient's hand, thus creating a fulcrum to shift the humeral head superiorly.
  - Crepitation or pain constitutes a positive test.

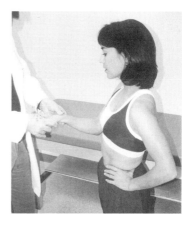

Figure 3–23   Yergason test for biceps pathology.

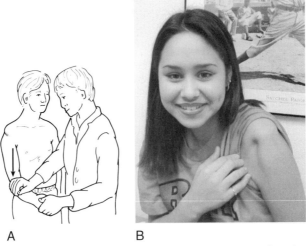

A   B

Figure 3–24 Sulcus sign (see text). **A**, Inferior instability test. Best conducted with the patient standing, this test establishes the sulcus sign, a measure of inferior translation of the humeral head. **B**, Positive sulcus sign of the shoulder. Note the inferior subluxation. (**A**, From Backer M, Warren RF: Recognizing and treating shoulder instability in female athletes. Womens Health Orthop Ed 3[3]: 37-40, 2000.)

GENERALIZED LIGAMENTOUS LAXITY TESTING

- Ligamentous laxity is indicated by the sulcus sign (Fig. 3-24).
  - The patient sits comfortably on the examination table with the arms hanging free down by the side.
  - The examiner stands in front of the patient and applies a traction force along the longitudinal axis of the humerus by pulling it in an inferior direction.
  - Both arms are pulled simultaneously or individually.
  - The distance between the acromion and the humeral head is recorded in centimeters.
  - **A sulcus of 2 cm or larger under the acromion** or an asymmetrical sulcus is positive for inferior subluxation or laxity.
  - The second portion of this test is to have the seated, relaxed patient place the arm in 90 degrees of abduction and resting on the examiner's shoulder. The examiner then applies a caudally directed force to the proximal end of the humerus. Excessive inferior translation with a sulcus defect at the acromion and a feeling of subluxation are considered a positive test.
  - An additional maneuver is to place the patient's arm in maximum external rotation while the longitudinal force is reapplied. The sulcus sign is measured again and compared with the sulcus that is observed when the arm is in the neutral, relaxed position. With external rotation, the anterior capsule and rotator interval are tightened, which should reduce the amount of inferior translation of the head and produce a smaller measurable sulcus sign.

Patients with generalized ligamentous laxity usually demonstrate a positive sulcus sign, elbow hyperextension, finger hyperextension ("double jointed"),

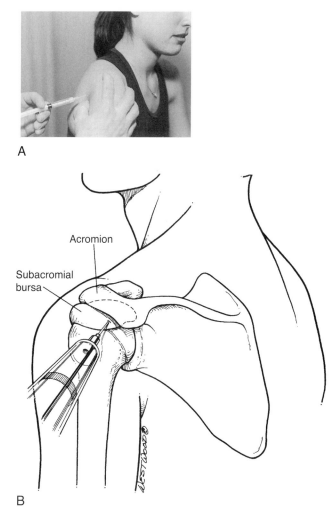

Figure 3–25 **A** and **B**, Injection of the subacromial bursa with 1% lidocaine alleviates pain and allows more accurate testing of the strength of the rotator cuff. (**B**, From Idler RS: Rotator cuff disease: Diagnosing a common cause of shoulder pain. J Musculoskel Med 6[2]:63-69, 1998.)

and a positive thumb-to-forearm test (ability to place the abducted thumb on the ipsilateral forearm). This laxity may at times contribute to multidirectional instability (born loose).

ROTATOR CUFF TESTING

Differentiation between rotator cuff tendinitis, bursitis, and a torn rotator cuff (weakness on motor testing) is often aided by a **lidocaine test** (Fig. 3-25). Injection of lidocaine into the subacromial bursa frequently improves the patient's pain and allows better assessment of true motor strength (now not limited by pain).

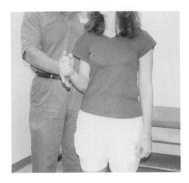

Figure 3–26   External rotation testing of the rotator cuff (infraspinatus portion).

The **infraspinatus** is tested for weakness by resisted external rotation (Fig. 3-26). With the elbows at the side (taking the deltoid out of the examination), the arms are compared for asymmetry of strength.

Internal rotation against resistance tests the **subscapularis** portion of the rotator cuff. The **"lift-off" test** is also used to test the subscapularis. The patient's hand is placed behind the back and lifted away from the body against resistance (Fig. 3-27).

The **supraspinatus** portion of the rotator cuff **is the most commonly torn part of the cuff**. With the arm slightly abducted, forward flexed, and internally rotated, the patient attempts to maintain the arm's position while the examiner pushes downward on the patient's hand (Fig. 3-28). This is called the **supraspinatus isolation test**.

The **"drop-arm" test** may **suggest a very large full-thickness rotator cuff tear**.

- The patient is asked to lower the arm from full elevation to 90 degrees of abduction (with the arm extended straight out to the side).
- Patients with large, full-thickness rotator cuff tears often cannot perform this exercise and are unable to smoothly lower the arm to the side. Instead it "drops," even with repeated attempts.

IMPINGEMENT TESTS

Secondary impingement often results in a "relative narrowing" of the subacromial space that produces inflammation and tenderness at the rotator cuff, which gets "banged on" by the overlying acromial arch in overhead throwing. The painful, weakened rotator cuff is not as able to perform its normal humeral head depressor

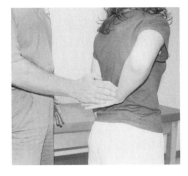

Figure 3–27   "Lift-off" test to evaluate the subscapularis portion of the rotator cuff.

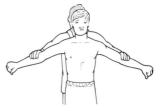

Figure 3–28 The supraspinatus isolation test is performed by resisting the athlete's abduction from the starting position of 90 degrees of abduction and about 30 degrees of forward flexion. The examiner applies a downward force toward the floor and the athlete resists.

role, thus allowing even less subacromial "clearance" during throwing or overhead activities and secondary impingement, and a vicious circle is begun.

In the **Neer impingement test**, the examiner performs forward elevation of the internally rotated humerus. Pain on this test indicates rotator cuff impingement or inflammation, or both (often positive with rotator cuff tendinitis, tears, and primary and secondary subacromial impingement) (Fig. 3-29).

The **Hawkins impingement test** is done with across-the-chest adduction of the internally rotated, forward-flexed arm (Fig. 3-30); pain indicates coracoacromial arch impingement on the rotator cuff. The differential diagnosis is the same as with the Neer test (rotator cuff tendinitis, tear, subacromial impingement).

Assessment of underlying shoulder stability is very important in evaluation of the rotator cuff because rotator cuff signs and symptoms (e.g., tender rotator cuff insertion, tendinitis) are often a secondary manifestation of an underlying problem in shoulder instability.

Internal impingement (see Fig. 3-5) is defined as intra-articular impingement that occurs when the shoulder is in the abducted, externally rotated position. In this 90 degree–90 degree position, the undersurface of the posterosuperior rotator cuff contacts the posterosuperior glenoid labrum and becomes "pinched" between the labrum and the greater tuberosity (Walch et al., 1992).

There is some disagreement between experts on whether this is a relatively innocuous physiologic daily occurrence with all shoulders versus a major pathologic entity with resultant significant consequences in the thrower's shoulder.

ANTERIOR INSTABILITY TESTING

The **anterior drawer test** (Lachman test of the shoulder) is used to determine whether the patient has anterior instability (i.e., anterior glenohumeral joint laxity).

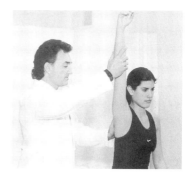

Figure 3–29 Neer impingement test (see text).

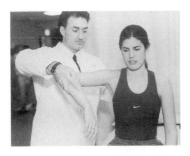

Figure 3–30 Hawkins impingement test (see text).

The humeral head is passively translated anteriorly on the glenoid with the shoulder as shown in Figure 3-31.

The **anterior apprehension test** (**crank test**) (Fig. 3-32) is used to assess (recurrent) anterior instability.

- The patient lies supine on the table with the shoulder at the edge of the table.
- With the arm at 90 degrees of abduction, the elbow is grasped by the examiner with one hand and slowly externally rotated.
- The other hand is placed with fingertips posterior to the humeral head, and a gentle anterior force is applied to the humeral head.
- The test is considered positive for anterior instability if the patient expresses apprehension by verbal communication, facial expression, or reflex contracture of the shoulder muscles.
- The test also can be done at 45 and 135 degrees of abduction. At 45 degrees of abduction, the test stresses the subscapularis and middle GH ligament complex. At more than 90 degrees of abduction, the test stresses the inferior GH ligament complex.

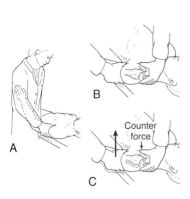

Figure 3–31 Anterior shoulder drawer test. **A,** The examiner stands at the athlete's axilla with the athlete's arm in 80 to 90 degrees of abduction and 10 to 20 degrees of external rotation. The athlete's hand is placed between the examiner's outside arm and flank, thereby freeing both examining hands. The examiner should adduct his arm against the side to hold the patient's hand in place. **B,** Next, the examiner places the hand that is closest to the athlete on the shoulder to be examined with the thumb anteriorly on the coracoid and the finger posteriorly on the scapular spine. This position will allow the examiner to stabilize the scapula and feel the motion of the shoulder translation. With the outside hand (the one holding the athlete's hand in the axilla), the examiner grasps the athlete's upper arm just distal to the deltoid insertion. **C,** The examiner applies an anteriorly directed force similar to that used in performing an anterior drawer test in the knee. A counterforce should be maintained on the scapula and coracoid with the other hand. This technique allows the examiner to feel the degree of anterior translation of the humeral head and compare it with the opposite shoulder. (**A-C,** From Andrews J, Zarins R, Wilk KE: Injuries in Baseball. Philadelphia, Lippincott-Raven, 1998.)

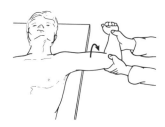

Figure 3–32 Anterior apprehension ("crank") test to evaluate recurrent anterior instability. (From Backer M, Warren RF: Recognizing and treating shoulder instability in female athletes. Womens Health Orthop Ed 3[3]:37-40, 2000.)

The **anterior release test** (Fig. 3-33) evaluates possible anterior instability.
- The patient lies supine on a table with the affected arm over the edge of the table.
- The patient abducts the arm 90 degrees while the examiner applies a posteriorly directed force on the humeral head.
- The posterior force is maintained while the arm is brought into extreme external rotation.
- The humeral head is then released suddenly.
- The test is considered positive when the patient experiences sudden pain or a distinct increase in pain or when symptoms that occurred during athletic or work activities are reproduced.
- This test has a sensitivity of 91.9%, a specificity of 88.9%, a positive predictive value of 87.1%, a negative predictive value of 93%, and an accuracy of 90.2% according to Gross and Distefano (1997).

The **shoulder relocation test** (Fig. 3-34) evaluates the patient for internal impingement, recurrent anterior subluxation, and recurrent anterior inferior instability.
- The test is done with the patient supine on the table and usually after an anterior apprehension test.
- *This test can be used to differentiate between anterior instability and impingement.*
- The supine patient's arm is placed in abduction, external rotation, and hyperextension (the apprehension position), and a posteriorly directed force is applied to the proximal end of the humerus.
- Diminished pain or apprehension with the posteriorly directed force is considered a positive relocation test.
- *If apprehension is eliminated,* the test is more specific for anterior instability.

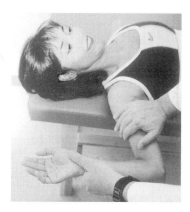

Figure 3–33 Anterior release test (see text).

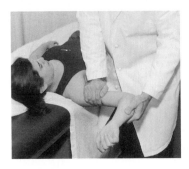

Figure 3–34   Relocation test for anterior instability (see text).

- *If pain is eliminated,* the test is more specific for internal impingement.
- Patients with external impingement generally do not have pain in this position. If they do, the relocation test is negative and does not relieve pain.

The **load-and-shift test** (Fig. 3-35) defines passive anterior and posterior translation of the humeral head on the glenoid in patients with hyperlaxity or instability of the shoulder The test can be done with the patient sitting or supine.

- Sitting position
  - The examiner stands behind the patient and places one hand over the acromion and scapula to stabilize the shoulder while the other hand cups the proximal end of the humerus with the thumb on the posterior joint line and the index finger on the anterior aspect of the shoulder.
  - The humeral head is loaded by pushing it into the glenoid fossa and is moved relative to the glenoid in the anteroposterior direction (shifting).
  - The degree of translation is recorded along with pain, crepitation, and apprehension.
- Supine position
  - With the patient supine and the shoulder over the edge of the table, the arm is abducted 45 degrees in the scapular plane with neutral rotation.
  - While one hand cups the proximal end of the humerus and the other cups the elbow, an axial load is applied to the humerus with the hand grasping the elbow to compress the humeral head into the glenoid fossa (loading).
  - The other hand then shifts the proximal end of the humerus in the anteroposterior direction relative to the glenoid fossa.
  - The degree of translation, crepitation, pain, or apprehension is noted.

POSTERIOR INSTABILITY AND LABRAL TESTING

Posterior instability is evaluated with the **posterior apprehension test** (Fig. 3-36) and the **posterior shoulder drawer test** (Fig. 3-37).

The "**clunk**" test (Fig. 3-38) is used to assess for *labral tears*.

- The examiner places one hand on the humeral head with the fingers posterior while the other hand grasps the athlete's humeral condyles at the elbow to provide a back-and-forth motion between internal and external rotation.
- The athlete's shoulder is brought into overhead abduction past 120 degrees, and the examiner's hand on the humeral head provides an anteriorly directed levering force while rotating the humerus with the other hand.

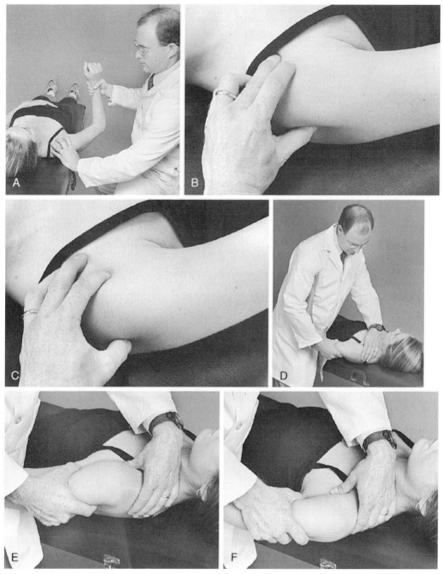

Figure 3–35 Load-and-shift test. **A**, Standard position. **B**, Anterior translation. **C**, Posterior translation. **D**, Alternative technique. **E**, Anterior translation. **F**, Posterior translation. These tests define passive shoulder translation (increased instability or hyperlaxity). (**A-F**, From Reider B: The Orthopaedic Physical Examination. Philadelphia, WB Saunders, 1999.)

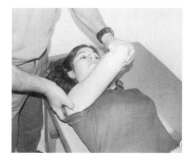

Figure 3–36 Posterior apprehension test. The athlete's shoulder is flexed to at least 90 degrees and internally rotated as the examiner applies a posteriorly directed force on the humerus while increasing the degree of adduction. The examiner should use greater forward flexion to 120 degrees to evaluate for posterior and inferior apprehension.

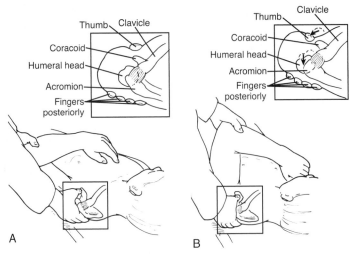

Figure 3–37 Posterior shoulder drawer test. **A**, The examiner uses the hand that is closest to the athlete to grasp the elbow and position the shoulder in about 90 to 120 degrees of abduction and 30 degrees of forward flexion. The examiner's other hand is placed on the athlete's shoulder with the fingers posteriorly on the scapular spine and the thumb on the coracoid (*inset*). **B**, The examiner's thumb on the coracoid is then brought down over the anterior humeral head, and a posteriorly directed force is applied (*inset*) as the shoulder is brought into greater flexion and internal rotation. The amount of posterior translation can be appreciated by the motion of the examiner's thumb and by the feeling of the humeral head moving toward the fingers placed posteriorly on the shoulder. (**A** and **B**, From Andrews JR, Zarins B, Wilk KE: Injuries in Baseball. Philadelphia, Lippincott-Raven, 1998. Artist: D. Nichols.)

- The examiner is attempting to capture any labral tear with the humeral head and make it snap or pop with the circumduction motion of the humeral head.
- The test is positive if a "clunk" or reproducible intra-articular pop is appreciated.

The **labral crank test** (Fig. 3-39) to assess for a superior labral tear can be done with the patient standing or supine.

- The patient's arm is elevated to 160 degrees in the scapular plane.
- An axial load is applied along the humerus while the arm is rotated maximally in internal rotation and external rotation.

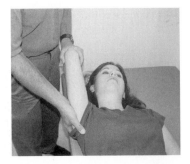

Figure 3–38 "Clunk" test to evaluate glenoid labral tears.

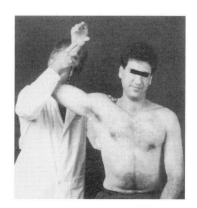

Figure 3–39 Crank test. The examiner abducts the arm to 90 degrees, translating the humeral head anteriorly by posterior force, and palpates and feels for crepitus, or grinding, on the anterior rim of the glenoid. (From Andrews JR, Wilk KE: The Athlete's Shoulder. New York, Churchill Livingstone, 1994.)

- The test is considered positive if pain is elicited during this maneuver (usually in external rotation), with or without a click, or if there is reproduction of symptoms (catching or pain) similar to the those felt by the patient during athletic or work activities.
- This test has a sensitivity of 91% and a specificity of 93% according to Liu and coworkers (1996).

The **O'Brien test** (Fig. 3-40) (active compression test), used to evaluate superior labral tears, SLAP lesions, AC joint pathology, and intra-articular biceps pathology, is done with the patient standing.

- The patient forward-flexes the arm 90 degrees with the elbow in complete extension and then adducts the arm 10 to 15 degrees medial to the sagittal plane of the body.
- The arm is placed in maximal internal rotation so that the thumb is down.
- The examiner stands behind the patient and applies a downward force to the arm while the patient resists this downward motion.
- The second portion of the test is done with the arm in the same position but the patient fully supinates the forearm with the palm facing the ceiling. The same maneuver is repeated.
- The test is considered positive if pain is elicited during the first step and reduced or eliminated with the second step of this maneuver.
- A click or pop is sometimes heard.
- The test is also considered positive for AC joint pathology when the pain is localized to the top of the shoulder.
- This test is more commonly positive with the palm toward the ceiling.

ACROMIOCLAVICULAR JOINT TESTING

Passive cross-chest adduction (Fig. 3-41) may reproduce AC joint pain if AC joint injury, arthritis, or weightlifter's osteolysis is present.

The **O'Brien test** was originally conceived as a test for the AC joint, but it may indicate tears of the glenoid labrum as well.

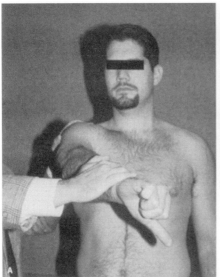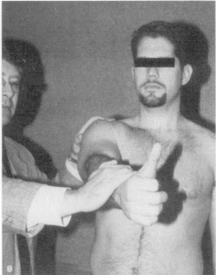

Figure 3–40   The O'Brien test (active compression test) is used to evaluate superior labral tears, superior labrum from anterior to posterior (SLAP) lesions, acromioclavicular joint pathology, and intra-articular biceps pathology. **A**, The patient forward-flexes the arm to 90 degrees with the elbow extended and adducted 15 degrees medial to the midline of the body and with the thumb pointed down. The examiner applies a downward force on the arm that the patient resists. **B**, Next, the test is performed with the arm in the same position, but the patient fully supinates the arm with the palm facing the ceiling. The same maneuver is repeated. The test is positive for a superior labral injury if pain is elicited in the first step and reduced or eliminated in the second step of this maneuver. (**A** and **B**, From Cannon WD, DeHaven KE: Evaluation and diagnosis of shoulder problems in the throwing athletes. Sports Med Arthrosc Rev 8:168, 2000.)

General Shoulder Rehabilitation Goals

MOTION

Once the intake evaluation is completed, the therapist should be more comfortable anticipating the patient's response to the therapeutic regimen. The key to recovery is motion. The main deterrent to motion is pain, which is also responsible for a high

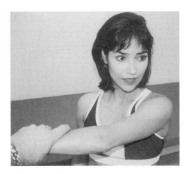

Figure 3–41   Passive cross-chest adduction to test for acromioclavicular joint pathology.

degree of muscle inhibition. Pain can result from injury or surgery. Pain relief can be achieved by a variety of modalities, including rest, avoidance of painful motions, cryotherapy, ultrasound, galvanic stimulation, and medications. Once the discomfort is controlled, motion exercises can be started. **Early motion** should focus on pain-free ranges below 90 degrees of abduction or 90 degrees of forward flexion. For most patients, **the early goal is to achieve 90 degrees of elevation and 45 degrees of external rotation with the arm comfortably at the side**. These positions of the shoulder are consistent with most skilled-length and force-dependent motor patterns. For surgical patients, it is the responsibility of the surgeon to obtain at least 90 degrees of stable elevation in the operating room for the therapist to be able to gain this motion soon after surgery. Exercises that are used to regain motion around the shoulder include active-assisted pulley or wand maneuvers and passive joint mobilization and stretching (Figs. 3-42 and 3-43).

We initially begin ROM exercises with the patient supine, the arm comfortably at the side with a small cushion or towel under the elbow, and the elbow bent. This position reduces the forces crossing the shoulder joint by decreasing the effect of gravity and **shortening the lever arm** of the upper extremity. As the patient begins to recover pain-free motion, the exercises are performed in the seated and standing positions.

MUSCLE STRENGTHENING

The timing at which muscle strengthening enters the rehabilitation regimen is related to the diagnosis and treatment. For instance, patients who have undergone rotator cuff repair should generally avoid active motion and muscle strengthening of the rotator cuff muscles for 6 weeks after surgery to allow the repaired tendon time to heal securely to the bone of the greater tuberosity of the humerus. Strengthening of

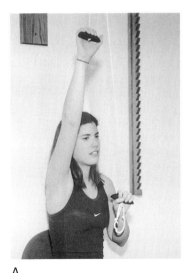
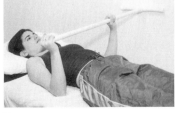

A   B

Figure 3–42   Exercises to regain motion: active-assisted range-of-motion exercises using a pulley system (**A**) and a dowel stick (**B**).

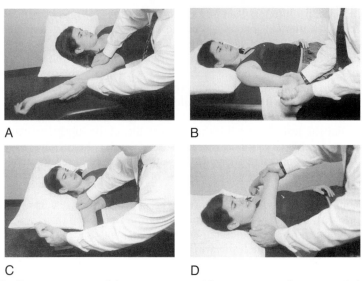

Figure 3–43 Passive joint mobilization. **A**, Forward flexion. **B**, External rotation with the arm at the side. **C**, External rotation with the arm in 90 degrees of abduction. **D**, Cross-body adduction.

the muscles around the shoulder can be accomplished through different exercises. Initially, basic **closed-chain exercises** are the safest strengthening exercises (Fig. 3-44). The advantage of closed-chain exercises is co-contraction of both the agonist and antagonist muscle groups. These exercises closely replicate normal physiologic motor patterns and function to stabilize the shoulder and limit the amount of shear force crossing the joint. A closed-chain exercise is one in which the distal segment is stabilized against a fixed object, which for the shoulder can include a wall, a door, or a table. The goal is to generate resistance through motion of the shoulder and scapula. One example is the "clock" exercise, in which the hand is stabilized against a wall or table, depending on the amount of abduction allowed, and the hand is rotated to different positions of the clock face. This motion effectively stimulates rotator cuff activity. Initially, the maneuvers are done with the shoulder in less than 90 degrees of abduction or flexion. As the tissues heal and motion is recovered, strengthening progresses to greater amounts of abduction and forward flexion.

Strengthening of the scapular stabilizers is very important early in the rehabilitation program. Scapular strengthening begins with closed-chain exercises (Fig. 3-45) and advances to open-chain exercises (Fig. 3-46).

Recovery can be enhanced by using **proprioceptive neuromuscular facilitation (PNF) exercises**. The therapist can apply specific sensory input to facilitate a specific activity or movement pattern. One example is the **D2 flexion-extension pattern for the upper extremity**. During this maneuver, the therapist applies **rhythmic stabilization** at different positions of arm elevation, such as 30 degrees, 60 degrees, 90 degrees, and 120 degrees. This results in improved stability of the GH joint through isometric strengthening of the dynamic stabilizers.

As recovery continues and more motion is regained, more aggressive strengthening can be instituted. **Closed-chain exercises can be advanced to open-chain exercises,**

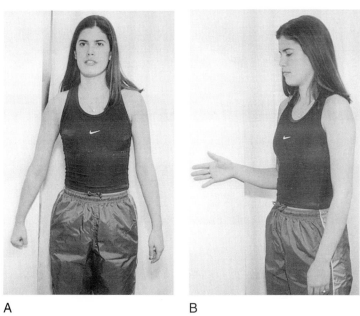

Figure 3–44   Closed-chain shoulder exercises. **A**, Isometric strengthening of the rotator cuff in abduction (pushing out against the wall). **B**, Isometric strengthening of the rotator cuff in external rotation.

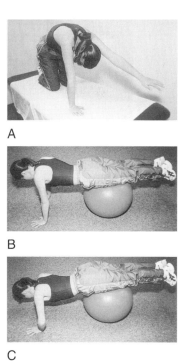

Figure 3–45   Closed-chain strengthening exercises of the scapular stabilizers. **A**, Scapular protraction. **B** and **C**, Scapular retraction.

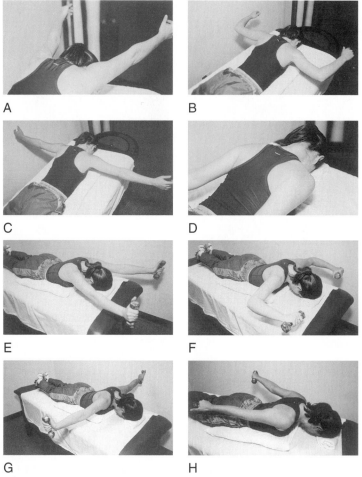

Figure 3–46 Open-chain strengthening exercises of the scapular stabilizers without (**A-D**) and with (**E-H**) lightweight dumbbells.

in which the hand is no longer stabilized against a fixed object. This results in increased shear forces crossing the shoulder joint. Internal and external rotation exercises are one form of open-chain activity and should be done with the shoulder positioned in the scapular plane (Fig. 3-47). **The scapular plane position** is recreated with the arm situated between 30 and 60 degrees anterior to the coronal plane of the thorax, or approximately at the halfway point between directly out to the side (coronal plane) and directly in front (sagittal plane) of the patient. This orientation has been shown to put minimal stress on the joint capsule and orient the shoulder in the position of functional movement. Rotational exercise should begin with the arm comfortably at the patient's side and advanced to 90 degrees based on the patient's healing stage and level of discomfort. The variation in position positively stresses the dynamic stabilizers by altering the stability of the GH joint from

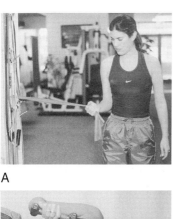

A

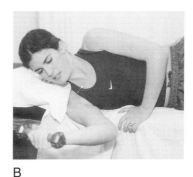

B

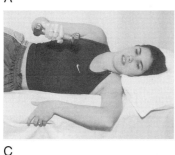

C

Figure 3–47 Open-chain isotonic strengthening of the rotator cuff (internal rotation) using Thera-Band tubing (**A**), lightweight dumbbells (**B**), and external rotation strengthening (**C**).

maximum stability with the arm at the side to minimum stability with the arm at 90 degrees of abduction.

The most functional of the open-chain exercises are **plyometric exercises**. Plyometric activities are **defined by a stretching and shortening cycle of the muscle**. This is a component of all athletic activity. Initially, the muscle is eccentrically stretched and then slowly loaded. The higher level of stress that these exercises place on the tissue requires that they be incorporated into the rehabilitation program only after healing is completed and full motion is attained. Plyometric exercises are successful in helping the muscle recover strength and power. Thera-Band tubing, a medicine ball, or free weights are all acceptable plyometric devices (Fig. 3-48). These exercises require close observation by the therapist to help the patient avoid injury.

It is important that while rehabilitation of the shoulder is being undertaken, the remainder of the musculoskeletal system not be neglected. **Overall conditioning**, including stretching, strengthening, and endurance training of the other components of the kinematic chain should be performed simultaneously with shoulder rehabilitation.

Patient motivation is a critical component of the rehabilitation program. Without self-motivation, any treatment plan is destined to fail. For complete recovery, most rehabilitation protocols require patients to perform some of the exercises on their own at home. This requires not only an understanding of the maneuvers but also the discipline to execute them on a regular basis. **Patient self-motivation** is even more crucial in the present medical environment because of increased attention directed at cost control. Many insurance carriers limit coverage for physical therapy. As a result,

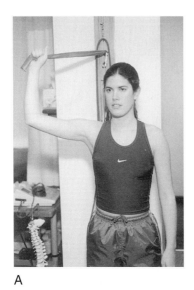

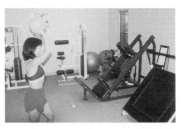

B

A

Figure 3–48 Plyometric shoulder-strengthening exercises using Thera-Band tubing (**A**) and an exercise ball (**B**).

a comprehensive home exercise program should also be outlined early in the rehabilitation process. This allows patients to augment their rehabilitation exercises at home and gives them a feeling of responsibility for their own recovery.

Impingement Syndrome

The term "impingement syndrome" was popularized by Neer in 1972 as a clinical entity in which the rotator cuff was pathologically compressed against the anterior structures of the coracoacromial arch, the anterior third of the acromion, the coracoacromial ligament, and the AC joint (Fig. 3-49).

Irritation of the rotator cuff muscle compromises its function as a depressor of the humeral head during overhead activities (i.e., less clearance of the humeral head under the arch), which further intensifies the impingement process (Fig. 3-50).

A reactive progression of this syndrome is defined by a narrowing of the subacromial outlet by spur formation in the coracoacromial ligament and on the undersurface of the anterior third of the acromion (Fig. 3-51). All these factors result in an increase in pressure on the rotator cuff, which can lead to chronic wearing and subsequent tearing of the rotator cuff tendons. Neer also defined three stages of impingement involving patient age, physical findings, and clinical course.

Patients with subacromial impingement often complain of shoulder pain, weakness, and possible paresthesias in the upper part of the arm. It is very important to rule out other causes of these symptoms, such as cervical spine pathology. When subacromial impingement is suspected, **it is necessary to differentiate primary from secondary impingement**. Correct identification of the cause of the problem is essential for successful treatment.

Progressive Stages of Shoulder Impingement

STAGE 1: EDEMA AND INFLAMMATION

Typical age	Younger than 25 years, but may occur at any age
Clinical course	Reversible lesion
Physical signs	• Tenderness to palpation over the greater tuberosity of the humerus
	• Tenderness along the anterior ridge or acromion
	• Painful arc of abduction between 60 and 120 degrees, increased with resistance at 90 degrees
	• Positive impingement sign
	• Shoulder ROM may be restricted with significant subacromial inflammation

STAGE 2: FIBROSIS AND TENDINITIS

Typical age	25-40 years
Clinical course	Not reversible by modification of activity
Physical signs	Stage 1 signs plus the following:
	• Greater degree of soft tissue crepitus may be felt because of scarring in the subacromial space
	• Catching sensation with lowering of the arm at approximately 100 degrees
	• Limitation of active and passive ROM

STAGE 3: BONE SPURS AND TENDON RUPTURES

Typical age	Older than 40 years
Clinical course	Not reversible
Physical signs	Stages 1 and 2 signs plus the following:
	• Limitation of ROM, more pronounced with active motion
	• Atrophy of the infraspinatus
	• Weakness of shoulder abduction and external rotation
	• Biceps tendon involvement
	• AC joint tenderness

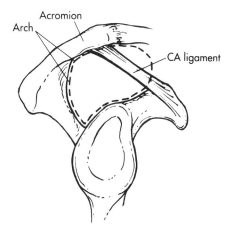

Figure 3–49 The normal coracoacromial (CA) arch. (From Jobe FW [ed]: Operative Techniques in Upper Extremity Sports Injuries. St Louis, CV Mosby, 1996.)

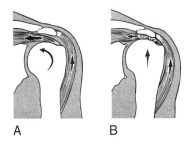

Figure 3–50 The supraspinatus tendon (rotator cuff) helps stabilize the head of the humerus against the upward pull of the deltoid. **A**, Subacromial impingement is prevented by the normal rotator cuff function of humeral head depression. **B**, Deep surface tearing of the supraspinatus tendon (rotator cuff tear) weakens the ability of the cuff to hold the humeral head down (i.e., depress the humeral head to allow clearance under the acromion) and results in impingement of the tendon at the acromion with overhead activities. (**A** and **B**, Redrawn from Matsen FA III, Arntz CT: Subacromial impingement. In Rockwood CA Jr, Matsen FA III [eds]: The Shoulder. Philadelphia, WB Saunders, 1990, p 624.)

PRIMARY IMPINGEMENT

Primary subacromial impingement is the result of an abnormal mechanical relationship between the rotator cuff and the coracoacromial arch. It also includes other "primary" factors that can lead to narrowing of the subacromial outlet (Table 3-1). Patients with primary impingement are usually older than 40 years and complain of anterior shoulder and upper lateral arm pain with an inability to sleep on the affected side. They have complaints of "shoulder weakness" and difficulty performing overhead activities. On physical examination, patients may exhibit loss of motion or weakness of rotator cuff strength secondary to pain. They will usually demonstrate a positive Hawkins sign (see Fig. 3-30) and a positive impingement sign as described by Neer (see Fig. 3-29). An **impingement test** may be performed by injecting 10 mL of 1% lidocaine (Xylocaine) into the subacromial space (see Fig. 3-25). If the Xylocaine alleviates pain and improves rotator cuff function, rotator cuff pathology is suspected as the cause of pain (e.g., rotator cuff tendinitis, rotator cuff tear, impingement).

Patients with primary subacromial impingement may have associated AC joint arthritis, which may contribute to their symptoms and compression of their rotator cuff. These patients may report additional discomfort in the AC joint area with

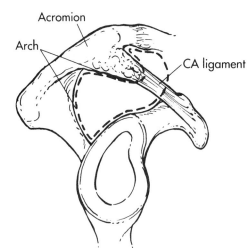

Figure 3–51 Pathologic narrowing of the coracoacromial (CA) arch. (From Jobe FW [ed]: Operative Techniques in Upper Extremity Sports Injuries. St Louis, CV Mosby, 1996.)

TABLE 3–1	Structural Factors That May Increase Subacromial Joint Impingement

Structure	Abnormal Characteristics
Acromioclavicular joint	Congenital anomaly
	Degenerative spur formation
Acromion	Unfused acromion
	Degenerative spurs on the undersurface
	Malunion/nonunion of fracture
Coracoid	Congenital anomaly
	Abnormal shape after surgery or trauma
Rotator cuff	Thickening of tendon from calcific deposits
	Tendon thickening after surgery or trauma
	Upper surface irregularities from partial or complete tears
Humerus	Increased prominence of the greater tuberosity from congenital anomalies or malunion

Modified from Matsen FA III, Arntz CT: Subacromial Impingement. In Rockwood CA Jr, Matsen FA III (eds): The Shoulder. Philadelphia, WB Saunders, 1990.

internal rotation maneuvers, such as scratching their back, or experience pain superiorly with abduction of their shoulder. Findings on physical examination that confirm the diagnosis of AC joint arthritis include "point" tenderness at the AC joint with palpation, worsening of the pain at the AC joint with cross-body adduction (see Fig. 3-41), and resolution of the pain with an injection of lidocaine into the AC joint (Fig. 3-52).

Radiologic evaluation, including axillary and supraspinatus outlet views, may support the diagnosis of primary or "outlet" impingement by demonstrating an os acromiale or a type III acromion (large, hooked acromial spur), respectively (Fig. 3-53).

SECONDARY IMPINGEMENT

Secondary impingement is a clinical phenomenon that reportedly results in a **"relative narrowing" of the subacromial space. It often results from GH or scapulothoracic joint instability**. In patients who have underlying GH instability, the symptoms are

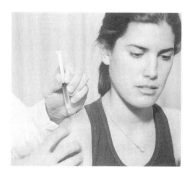

Figure 3–52   Approach for an acromioclavicular joint injection.

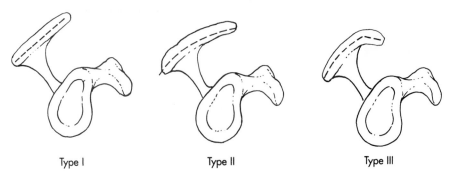

Type I   Type II   Type III

Figure 3–53   Different acromion morphologies. (From Jobe FW [ed]: Operative Techniques in Upper Extremity Sports Injuries. St Louis, CV Mosby, 1996.)

those of rotator cuff dysfunction (caused by an overuse injury of the cuff as a result of the increased work that the muscles are performing to stabilize the shoulder). **Loss of the stabilizing function of the rotator cuff muscles also leads to abnormal superior translation of the humeral head (decreased depression of the humeral head during throwing and less "clearance") and mechanical impingement of the rotator cuff on the coracoacromial arch** (see Fig. 3-50). In patients who have scapular instability, impingement results from **improper positioning of the scapula with regard to the humerus**. The instability leads to insufficient retraction of the scapula, which allows for earlier abutment of the coracoacromial arch on the underlying rotator cuff (Fig. 3-54).

Patients with secondary impingement are usually younger and often participate in overhead sporting activities such as baseball, swimming, volleyball, or tennis. They complain of pain and weakness with overhead motions and may even describe a feeling of the arm going "dead." On physical examination, the examiner should look for possible associated pathology, including GH joint instability with positive apprehension (see Fig. 3-32) and relocation (see Fig. 3-34) tests or abnormal scapular function, such as scapular winging or asymmetrical scapular motion. **Patients with tightening of the posterior capsule have a loss of internal rotation. Posterior capsular tightness leads to obligate translation of the humeral head and rotator cuff in an anterior and superior direction, which contributes to the impingement problem.**

In patients with secondary impingement, treatment of the underlying problem should result in resolution of the "secondary impingement" symptoms. **Often, recognition of the underlying GH joint or scapular instability is missed, and the "secondary impingement" is incorrectly treated as a "primary" (large spur) impingement. Subacromial decompression here worsens the symptoms because the shoulder is rendered even more "unstable."**

TREATMENT

The key to successful treatment of subacromial impingement is defining the underlying cause of the impingement symptoms, whether they are primary or secondary to the pathologic relationship between the coracoacromial arch and the rotator cuff. This factor becomes more critical when conservative management fails and surgical

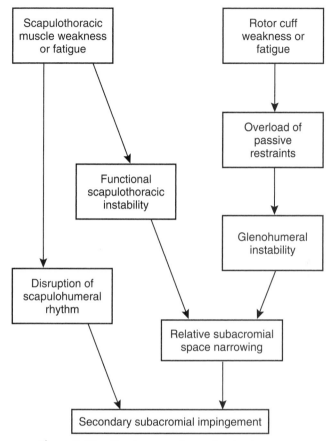

Figure 3–54   Development of secondary impingement.

intervention is indicated because the operative procedures for these two clinical entities may be entirely different.

For primary impingement, surgical treatment involves widening the subacromial outlet by performing subacromial decompression (acromioplasty).

Surgical treatment of secondary impingement is directed toward the *etiology of the symptoms*. For example, if the symptoms of impingement are secondary to anterior GH joint instability, **surgical treatment is anterior stabilization, not acromioplasty**. Performing acromioplasty in this setting may provide short-term benefit, but as the activities related to the onset of the problem resume, the instability symptoms will persist.

Nonoperative Treatment

Nonoperative treatment is very successful and involves a combination of treatment modalities, including anti-inflammatory medications and a well-organized rehabilitation program. In general, the comprehensive rehabilitative protocols for both primary and secondary impingement syndrome are similar and follow the postoperative rehabilitation plan for patients who have undergone subacromial decompression with a normal rotator cuff. The initial goals of the rehabilitative process are to obtain pain relief and regain motion. Along with oral medications, judicious use of subacromial corticosteroid injections may help control the discomfort in the acute stages of the inflammatory process. Other modalities such as cryotherapy and ultrasound are also effective in controlling pain. Improving comfort will allow more successful advances in motion and strengthening. Because the rotator cuff tendon is intact, ROM exercises can be both passive and active. Initially, these exercises are done with the arm below 90 degrees of abduction to avoid impingement of the rotator cuff. As symptoms improve, ROM is increased.

Initially, strengthening exercises start with the arm at the side. The program begins with closed-chain exercises (see Fig. 3-44), and open-chain exercises are initiated after advancing the closed-chain exercises without aggravating shoulder discomfort (see Fig. 3-47). **These exercises help restore the ability of the rotator cuff to dynamically depress and stabilize the humeral head, thereby resulting in a gradual relative increase in the subacromial space**. In patients with secondary impingement, strengthening is started with the arm comfortably at the patient's side to avoid positions that provoke symptoms of instability, such as abduction combined with external rotation. As the dynamic stabilizers respond to the strengthening program, exercises can be added in higher planes of abduction. In general, **strengthening of the deltoid muscle is not emphasized early in the rehabilitation program to avoid a disproportionate increase in the upward force on the humerus**.

Scapular stabilizing exercises are important for patients with primary or secondary impingement (see Figs. 3-45 and 3-46). The scapula forms the base from which the rotator cuff muscles originate. Reciprocal motion is required between the GH and scapulothoracic joint articulations for proper cuff function and correct positioning of the coracoacromial arch.

Abnormal scapular movement or dyskinesia can be treated with a scapular taping program as part of the exercise regimen (Fig. 3-55). Scapular taping can improve the biomechanics of the scapulohumeral and scapulothoracic joints and thus help relieve the patient's symptoms.

Historically, nonoperative treatment was considered unsuccessful if no improvement occurred after a year of proper conservative management. **Today, nonoperative treatment should be considered unsuccessful if the patient shows no improvement after 3 months of a comprehensive and coordinated medical and rehabilitative program**. Furthermore, **after 6 months of appropriate conservative treatment, most patients have achieved maximal improvement from the nonoperative treatment program**. Failed conservative management or a plateau in recovery at an undesirable level of function is an indication for surgical intervention.

Operative Treatment

The success of operative treatment is determined by the choice of an appropriate operative procedure and the technical skill of the surgeon. **For primary impingement**, the current **procedure of choice** is arthroscopic subacromial decompression, although comparable long-term results can be obtained with a traditional open acromioplasty.

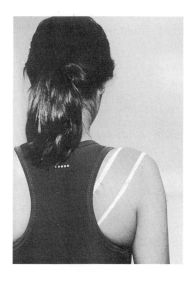

Figure 3–55 Example of scapular taping.

Rehabilitation after surgery focuses on pain control, improved ROM, and muscle strengthening.

When GH joint instability is the reason for secondary impingement, surgical treatment is a stabilization procedure. In our practice we see numerous patients whose impingement was secondary (caused by underlying GH joint instability), but they were incorrectly treated by subacromial decompression, which only worsens the underlying instability.

The most commonly performed procedure is open stabilization with either repair of a torn or avulsed labrum or a capsular shift procedure (capsulorrhaphy), depending on the etiology. With advances in arthroscopic instrumentation, fixation devices, and electrothermal technology, many surgeons are now performing arthroscopic stabilization procedures. Potential advantages of arthroscopic procedures include decreased operative time, less operative morbidity, less loss of motion, and quicker recovery. Currently, the **literature reflects a higher failure rate after arthroscopic stabilization than after open stabilization**. Arthroscopic procedures require advanced arthroscopic skills, complete recognition of the pathoanatomy, challenging fixation techniques, and appropriate diagnosis-related rehabilitation programs. The rehabilitation principles after an arthroscopic stabilization procedure that includes labral repair or suture capsulorrhaphy are similar to those after open stabilization. The biology of healing tissue is the same whether the procedure is done by open means or arthroscopically, unless the tissue has been treated with thermal energy. **Electrothermal arthroscopic capsulorrhaphy, or "shrinking" the shoulder capsule, requires a protective period of approximately 3 weeks after the treatment**. If the rehabilitation program is advanced too early, before the healing response has been adequately initiated, there is a high risk that the capsule will be "stretched" and the procedure will not correct the capsular laxity. The rehabilitation protocol after an open or arthroscopic Bankart repair for anterior shoulder instability is fundamentally the same, except for the 3-week delay for patients who have been treated by electrothermal capsulorrhaphy.

REHABILITATION PROTOCOL	*Conservative (Nonoperative) Treatment of Shoulder Impingement* Wilk and Andrews

Impingement is a chronic inflammatory process produced as the rotator cuff muscles (supraspinatus, infraspinatus, teres major, and subscapularis) and the subdeltoid bursa are "pinched" against the coracoacromial ligament and the anterior acromion when the arm is raised above 80 degrees. The supraspinatus-infraspinatus portion of the rotator cuff is the most common area of impingement. This syndrome is commonly seen in throwing, racquet, and swimming athletes, but it can occur in anyone who uses the arm repetitively in a position greater than 90 degrees of elevation.

PHASE 1: MAXIMAL PROTECTION—ACUTE PHASE

Goals

- Relieve pain and swelling
- Decrease inflammation
- Retard muscle atrophy
- Maintain/increase flexibility

Active Rest

- Eliminate any activity that causes an increase in symptoms (e.g., throwing)

Range of Motion

- Pendulum exercises
- Active-assisted ROM-limited symptom-free available range
  - Rope and pulley
    - Flexion
  - L-bar
    - Flexion
    - Neutral external rotation

Joint Mobilizations

- Grades 1 and 2
- Inferior and posterior glides in the scapular plane

Modalities

- Cryotherapy
- Transcutaneous electrical stimulation (TENS), high-voltage galvanic stimulation (HVGS)

Strengthening Exercises

- Isometrics-submaximal
  - External rotation
  - Internal rotation
  - Biceps
  - Deltoid (anterior, middle, posterior)

Patient Education and Activity Modification

- Regarding activity, pathology, and avoidance of overhead activity, reaching, and lifting activity

Conservative (Nonoperative) Treatment of Shoulder Impingement   *Continued*

PHASE 2: MOTION PHASE—SUBACUTE PHASE

Criteria for Progression to Phase 2

- Decreased pain and/or symptoms
- Increased ROM
- Painful arc in abduction only
- Improved muscular function

Goals

- Re-establish nonpainful ROM
- Normalize athrokinematics of the shoulder complex
- Retard muscular atrophy without exacerbation of pain.

Range of Motion

- Rope and pulley
  - Flexion
  - Abduction (symptom-free motion only)
- L-bar
  - Flexion
  - Abduction (symptom-free motion)
  - External rotation in 45 degrees of abduction; progress to 90 degrees of abduction
  - Internal rotation in 45 degrees of abduction; progress to 90 degrees of abduction
- Initiate anterior and posterior capsular stretching (Fig. 3-56).

Joint Mobilization

- Grades 2, 3, and 4
- Inferior, anterior, and posterior glides
- Combined glides as required

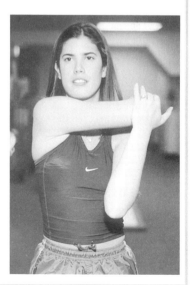

Figure 3–56   Stretching of the posterior capsule.

Continued

Conservative (Nonoperative) Treatment of Shoulder Impingement Continued

PHASE 2: MOTION PHASE—SUBACUTE PHASE—cont'd

Modalities

- Cryotherapy
- Ultrasound/phonophoresis

Strengthening Exercises

- Continue isometrics exercises
- Initiate scapulothoracic strengthening exercises (see the scapulothoracic section)
- Initiate neuromuscular control exercises

PHASE 3: INTERMEDIATE STRENGTHENING PHASE

Criteria for Progression to Phase 3

- Decrease in pain and symptoms
- Normal active-assisted ROM
- Improved muscular strength

Goals

- Normalize ROM
- Symptom-free normal activities
- Improve muscular performance

Range of Motion

- Aggressive L-bar active-assisted ROM in all planes
- Continue self-assisted capsular stretching (anterior-posterior)

Strengthening Exercises

- Initiate isotonic dumbbell program
  - Side-lying neutral
    - Internal rotation
    - External rotation
  - Prone
    - Extension
    - Horizontal abduction
  - Standing
    - Flexion to 90 degrees
    - Supraspinatus
- Initiate serratus exercises
  - Wall push-ups
- Initiate tubing progression in slight abduction for internal and external rotation strengthening
- Initiate arm ergometer for endurance

PHASE 4: DYNAMIC ADVANCED STRENGTHENING PHASE

Criteria for Progression to Phase 4

- Full, nonpainful ROM
- No pain or tenderness
- 70% of contralateral strength

Conservative (Nonoperative) Treatment of Shoulder Impingement   *Continued*

PHASE 4: DYNAMIC ADVANCED STRENGTHENING PHASE—cont'd

Goals

- Increase strength and endurance
- Increase power
- Increase neuromuscular control

Isokinetic Testing

- Modified neutral internal and external rotation
- Abduction-adduction

Initiate "Thrower's Ten" Exercise Program (see Thrower's Ten section)

Isokinetics

- Velocity spectrum, 180-300 degrees/sec
- Progress from modified neutral to 90/90 position as tolerated

Initiate Plyometric Exercises (Late in this Phase)

PHASE 5: RETURN-TO-ACTIVITY PHASE

Criteria for Progression to Phase 5

- Full, nonpainful ROM
- No pain or tenderness
- Isokinetic test that fulfills the criteria
- Satisfactory clinical examination

Goal

- Unrestricted symptom-free activity

Isokinetic Test

- 90/90 internal and external rotation, 180 degrees/sec, 300 degrees/sec
- Abduction-adduction, 180 degrees/sec, 300 degrees/sec

Initiate Interval Throwing Program

- Throwing
- Tennis
- Golf

MAINTENANCE EXERCISE PROGRAM

Flexibility Exercises

- L-bar
  - Flexion
  - External rotation
  - Self-assisted capsular stretches

Isotonic Exercises

- Supraspinatus
- Prone extension
- Prone horizontal abduction

Continued

Conservative (Nonoperative) Treatment of Shoulder Impingement   *Continued*

MAINTENANCE EXERCISE PROGRAM—cont'd

Thera-Band Tubing Exercises

- Internal and external rotation
- Neutral or 90/90 position
- D2 proprioceptive neuromuscular facilitation (PNF) pattern

Serratus Push-ups

Interval Throwing Phase II for Pitchers

| REHABILITATION PROTOCOL | *After Arthroscopic Subacromial Decompression—Intact Rotator Cuff (Distal Clavicle Resection)* Bach, Cohen, and Romeo |

PHASE 1: WEEKS 0-4

Restrictions

- ROM
  - 140 degrees of forward flexion
  - 40 degrees of external rotation
  - 60 degrees of abduction
- ROM exercises begin with the arm comfortably at the patient's side, progress to 45 degrees of abduction and eventually 90 degrees. Abduction is advanced slowly, depending on patient comfort level
- No abduction or rotation until 6 weeks after surgery—this combination re-creates the impingement maneuver
- No resisted motions until 4 weeks postoperatively
- (No cross-body adduction until 8 weeks postoperatively if distal clavicle resection is performed)

Immobilization

- Early motion is important
- Sling immobilization for comfort only during the first 2 weeks
- Sling should be discontinued by 2 weeks after surgery
- Patients can use the sling at night for comfort

Pain Control

- Reduction of pain and discomfort is essential for recovery
  - Medications
    - Narcotics—10 days to 2 weeks after surgery
    - Nonsteroidal anti-inflammatory drugs (NSAIDs)—for patients with persistent discomfort after surgery
  - Therapeutic modalities
    - Ice, ultrasound, HVGS
    - Moist heat before therapy; ice at end of session

After Arthroscopic Subacromial Decompression— Intact Rotator Cuff (Distal Clavicle Resection)   *Continued*

PHASE 1: WEEKS 0-4—cont'd

Motion: Shoulder

- Goals
  - 140 degrees of forward flexion
  - 40 degrees of external rotation
  - 60 degrees of abduction
- Exercises
  - Begin with Codman pendulum exercises to promote early motion
  - Passive ROM exercises (see Fig. 3-43)
  - Stretching of the anterior, posterior, and inferior capsule with the opposite arm (see Fig. 3-56)
  - Active-assisted ROM exercises (see Fig. 3-42)
    - Shoulder flexion
    - Shoulder extension
    - Internal and external rotation
  - Progress to active ROM exercises as comfort improves

Motion: Elbow

- Passive—progress to active
  - 0-130 degrees
  - Pronation and supination as tolerated

Muscle Strengthening

- Grip strengthening with racquetball, putty, Nerf ball

PHASE 2: WEEKS 4-8

Criteria for Progression to Phase 2

- Minimal pain and tenderness
- Nearly complete motion
- Good "shoulder strength" ⁴/₅ motor

Restrictions

- Progress ROM goals to
  - 160 degrees of forward flexion
  - 45 degrees of internal rotation (vertebral level L1)

Immobilization

- None

Pain Control

- NSAIDs—for patients with persistent discomfort
- Therapeutic modalities
  - Ice, ultrasound, HVGS
  - Moist heat before therapy; ice at end of session
- Subacromial injection: lidocaine/steroid—for patients with acute inflammatory symptoms that do not respond to NSAIDs

Continued

After Arthroscopic Subacromial Decompression— Intact Rotator Cuff (Distal Clavicle Resection) Continued

PHASE 2: WEEKS 4-8—cont'd

Motion

- Goals
  - 160 degrees of forward flexion
  - 60 degrees of external rotation
  - 80 degrees of abduction
  - 45 degrees of internal rotation (vertebral level L1)
- Exercises
  - Increasing active ROM in all directions
  - Focus on prolonged, gentle passive stretching at end ranges to increase shoulder flexibility
  - Use joint mobilization for capsular restrictions, especially the posterior capsule (see Fig. 3-56)

Muscle Strengthening

- Rotator cuff strengthening (only three times per week to avoid rotator cuff tendinitis)
  - Begin with closed-chain isometric strengthening (see Fig. 3-44)
    - Internal rotation
    - External rotation
    - Abduction
  - Progress to open-chain strengthening with Thera-Bands (see Fig. 3-46)
    - Exercises performed with the elbow flexed to 90 degrees
    - Starting position is with the shoulder in the neutral position of forward flexion, abduction, and external rotation (arm comfortably at the patient's side)
    - Exercises are performed through an arc of 45 degrees in each of the five planes of motion
    - Six color-coded Thera-Band bands are available; each provides increasing resistance from 1 to 6 pounds, at increments of 1 pound
    - Progression to the next band occurs usually at 2- to 3-week intervals. Patients are instructed to not progress to the next band if there is any discomfort at the present level
    - Thera-Band exercises permit both **concentric and eccentric strengthening** of the shoulder muscles and are a form of isotonic exercise (characterized by variable speed and fixed resistance)
      - Internal rotation
      - External rotation
      - Abduction
      - Forward flexion
      - Extension
    - Progress to light isotonic dumbbell exercises (see Fig. 3-47B)
      - Internal rotation
      - External rotation
      - Abduction
      - Forward flexion
      - Extension

After Arthroscopic Subacromial Decompression— Intact Rotator Cuff (Distal Clavicle Resection) *Continued*

PHASE 2: WEEKS 4-8—cont'd

- Scapular stabilizer strengthening
  - Closed-chain strengthening exercises (see Fig. 3-45)
    - Scapular retraction (rhomboideus, middle trapezius)
    - Scapular protraction (serratus anterior)
    - Scapular depression (latissimus dorsi, trapezius, serratus anterior)
  - Progress to open-chain scapular stabilizer strengthening (see Fig. 3-46)

Note: Do not perform more than 15 repetitions for each set or more than three sets of repetitions. If this regimen is easy for the patient, increase the resistance, not the repetitions. Upper body strengthening with excessive repetitions is counterproductive.

PHASE 3: WEEKS 8-12

Criteria for Progression to Phase 3

- Full painless ROM
- Minimal or no pain
- Strength at least 50% of contralateral shoulder
- "Stable" shoulder on clinical examination—no impingement signs

Goals

- Improve shoulder strength, power, and endurance
- Improve neuromuscular control and shoulder proprioception
- Prepare for gradual return to functional activities

Motion

- Achieve motion equal to that of contralateral side
- Use both active and passive ROM exercises to maintain motion

Muscle Strengthening

- Advance strengthening of rotator cuff and scapular stabilizers as tolerated
- 8-15 repetitions for each exercise, for three sets
- Continue strengthening only three times per week to avoid rotator cuff tendinitis from overtraining

Functional Strengthening

- Plyometric exercises (see Fig. 3-48)

For Patients with Concomitant Distal Clavicle Resections

- Now begin cross-body adduction exercises
  - First passive; advance to active motion when AC joint pain is minimal

PHASE 4: WEEKS 12-16

Criteria for Progression to Phase 4

- Full, painless ROM
- No pain or tenderness
- Shoulder strength that fulfills established criteria
- Satisfactory clinical examination

Continued

After Arthroscopic Subacromial Decompression— Intact Rotator Cuff (Distal Clavicle Resection) Continued

PHASE 4: WEEKS 12-16—cont'd

Goals

- Progressive return to unrestricted activities
- Advancement of shoulder strength and motion with a home exercise program that is taught throughout rehabilitation

Progressive, Systematic Interval Program for Returning to Sports

- Throwing athletes (see pp. 271 to 276)
- Tennis players (see p. 276)
- Golfers (see p. 281)
- Institute "Thrower's Ten" program (p. 238) for overhead athletes

   Maximum improvement is expected by 4-6 months after acromioplasty and 6-12 months after acromioplasty combined with distal clavicle resection.

Warning Signals

- Loss of motion—especially internal rotation
- Lack of strength progression—especially abduction
- Continued pain—especially at night

Treatment of Above "Problems"

- These patients may need to move back to earlier routines
- May require increased utilization of pain control modalities as outlined earlier
- If no improvement, patients may require repeat surgical treatment as outlined
  - It is important to determine that the appropriate surgical procedure was performed initially
  - Issues of possible secondary gain must be evaluated

Rotator Cuff Tendinitis in Overhead Athletes

During overhead sports, the rotator cuff is continually being challenged to keep the humeral head centered in the glenoid and prevent pathologic displacement as a result of the extreme forces acting on the shoulder. Because of this highly stressed environment, the joint capsule and rotator cuff can demonstrate a secondary inflammatory response. Prolonged rotator cuff tendinitis can result in decreased muscular efficiency and loss of dynamic stability, with a final pathway of functional instability and progressive tissue failure. **Posterior capsular tightness, which is manifested as a loss of internal rotation, is often present in overhead throwers and may lead to anterior-superior humeral head translation, thus further contributing to irritation of the rotator cuff.**

   The biomechanics of throwing has been closely analyzed. As a result, it serves as an appropriate model to examine the motions and arm positions of overhead athletic activities. The **throwing motion** and its related biomechanics are divided into **six stages**: wind-up, early cocking, late cocking, acceleration, deceleration, and follow-through (Fig. 3-57).

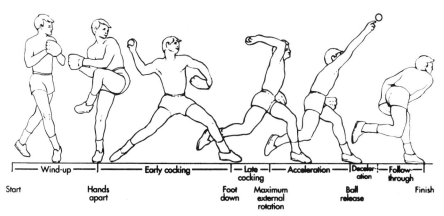

Figure 3–57 Six phases of throwing. (From Jobe FW [ed]: Operative Techniques in Upper Extremity Sports Injuries. St Louis, CV Mosby, 1996.)

THE SIX PHASES OF THROWING

- **Wind-up:** Serves as the preparatory phase. Includes body rotation and ends when the ball leaves the nondominant hand.
- **Early cocking:** As the ball is released from the glove hand, the shoulder abducts and externally rotates. The body starts moving forward, thereby generating momentum. Early cocking terminates as the forward foot contacts the ground.
- **Late cocking:** As the body rapidly moves forward, the dominant shoulder achieves maximal abduction and external rotation. Significant torque and force are placed on the shoulder restraints at this extreme ROM.
- **Acceleration:** Begins with further forward body motion and internal rotation of the humerus leading to internal rotation of the throwing arm. Acceleration ends with ball release.
- **Deceleration:** Begins after ball release and constitutes 30% of the time required to dissipate the excess kinetic energy of the throwing motion.
- **Follow-through:** Completes the remaining 70% of the time required to dissipate the excess kinetic energy. All major muscle groups must eccentrically contract to accomplish this result. Follow-through ends when all motion is complete.

Patients with rotator cuff tendinitis are a diagnostic challenge to the physician. A considerable amount of information can be obtained from the history (see the section "The Importance of History-Taking in Evaluating Shoulder Pain"). It is important to identify the specific throwing phase associated with the onset of symptoms.

- Localization of pain is important, as well as documenting any recent change in the athlete's training routine. This includes both the general conditioning program and the throwing regimen.
- **On physical examination, one needs to examine for shoulder instability, GIRD, posterior capsular tightness, impingement, and rotator cuff pathology.**
- Findings on physical examination that are indicative of rotator cuff tendinitis include rotator cuff tenderness and possibly weakness with resisted external rotation or abduction in the scapular plane.

- Pain with resistance is known as the "tendon sign" and at a minimum represents inflammation of the cuff tendons. Resolution of the symptoms and recovery of strength after injection of lidocaine in the subacromial space strongly suggest cuff tendinitis rather than a cuff tear. A cuff tear would still have weakness despite numbing of the painful cuff because of the structural defect or "hole" involving one or more of the four tendons.

Rotator cuff tendinitis can lead to a secondary type impingement and also make a primary impingement syndrome more symptomatic. Rehabilitation focuses on resolution of the inflammation, recovery of motion, and careful strengthening of the rotator cuff muscles and the scapular stabilizers.

Rehabilitation programs for pitchers, position players, tennis players, and golfers are included in the section on interval throwing. **These programs should be implemented for all patients returning to their sport after a period of inactivity.** For sport-specific rehabilitation programs to be successful, the entire body must be re-educated in stepwise fashion to perform the various activities related to the sport. This encourages a smooth transition for the athlete back to sport. These protocols are appropriate for all patients recovering from a shoulder injury, regardless of their treatment. The diagnosis and treatment will dictate when patients can begin sport-specific exercises and at what level they enter the rehabilitation program. The important factor is that the treatment team begin these exercises after the patient has recovered the appropriate motion and strength in the shoulder by following the more traditional physical therapy programs as outlined in this chapter. The team has to advance the patient appropriately. If discomfort develops as a result of "too much" being done, the athlete should take a few days' rest. Additional treatment may be required to decrease inflammation, and return to the previous exercise level may be needed until symptoms have resolved. The details outlined in these protocols are intended to help the athlete and trainer move along a progressive course to achieve full recovery and return to competition. Objective data that can be acquired before resumption of throwing are outlined in Table 3-2.

TABLE 3–2	Isokinetic Criteria for Return to Throwing*	
Bilateral compression	ER	98% to 105%
Bilateral compression	IR	105% to 115%
Bilateral compression	ABD	98% to 103%
Bilateral compression	ADD	110% to 125%
Unilateral ratio	ER/IR	66% to 70%
Unilateral ratio	ABD/ADD	78% to 85%
Peak torque–body weight ratio	ER	18% to 22%
Peak torque–body weight ratio	IR	28% to 32%
Peak torque–body weight ratio	ABD	24% to 30%
Peak torque–body weight ratio	ADD	32% to 38%

*All data represent 180% test speed.
ABD, abduction; ADD, adduction; ER, external rotation; IR, internal rotation.
Modified from Wilk KE, Andrews JK, Arrigo CA: The abductor and adductor strength characteristics of professional baseball pitchers. Am J Sports Med 23:307, 1995.

Common Causes of Injuries to the Pitching Arm*

Even with excellent conditioning, good gradual warm-up, adequate rest, and proper throwing mechanics, the upper extremity of a thrower experiences great stress.

The causes of pitching arm injuries may be divided into four categories: **conditioning problems, fatigue, overuse** (or **overload**), and **mechanical faults**.

CONDITIONING PROBLEMS

Not being properly conditioned
- Lack of total body fitness
- Lack of arm strengthening via a structured progressive pre-season throwing program

Lack of development of good arm strength and stamina over a long period (months to years)
- Need for an off-season throwing program
- Need for a supervised and structured pre-season and in-season throwing program

Improper strengthening and/or weight training program causing
- Restricted ROM in the shoulder and/or trunk
- Imbalance of antagonistic muscle strength
- Shortening or bulking-up of muscle fibers involved in the throwing mechanism

Overstretching the shoulder joint causing too much laxity

Lack of a proper warm-up and stretching program before pitching

Experimenting with new pitches at full velocity, full distance, or throwing too hard for too long early in the season

Pitching in games before being properly conditioned and prepared for competitive situations

FATIGUE, OVERUSE, AND/OR OVERLOAD FACTORS

Throwing too many pitches during one outing

Throwing when tired or fatigued or with tight muscle fibers

Not getting adequate rest and recovery time between pitching turns

Lack of an active in-season maintenance program of running, stretching, light strengthening work, and a controlled throwing program

Playing or practicing at other positions between pitching turns

General body or specific muscle fatigue from strength work that is too fatiguing or strenuous between pitching turns

MECHANICAL FAULTS

Usually negatively affect control and velocity and cause added stress on the throwing arm

*For an outstanding review of pitching faults and their correction, we recommend *Injuries in Baseball* by Wilk, Andrews, and Zarins.

From Wilk KE, Andrews JR, Zarins B: Injuries in Baseball. Philadelphia, Lippincott-Raven, 1998.

Prevention of Arm Injuries in Throwers

Coaches and trainers can help prevent arm injuries in throwers by
- Making sure pitchers are properly conditioned (total body) before throwing full velocity or pitching competitively.
- Making sure pitchers have and use a proper stretching and warm-up and cool-down program before throwing a baseball.
- Developing a year-round throwing program to maintain arm strength and stamina, flexibility, and normal ROM. We recommend a 2- to 3-week rest period at the end of a long season, followed by a limited and modified off-season throwing program.
- Teaching and supervising a proper weight and resistance program. Coaches or medical personnel should be responsible for this program. Many pitchers restrict their flexibility and ROM by improper use of weights. Other pitchers have actually weakened themselves by overstretching the shoulder joint and causing too much laxity.
- Having the pitcher throw at reduced velocity and shorter distances when learning new mechanical techniques or new pitches.
- Making certain that a pitcher pitches with proper throwing mechanics. Although each pitcher throws somewhat within his own style, through the critical phase of throwing (from hand-break through the deceleration phase), most successful injury-free pitchers use very similar, time-proven techniques.
- Limiting the amount of throwing that the pitcher does during drills and practices if the pitcher plays another defensive position. The defensive positions that would cause the least amount of stress on the arm are first base and the outfield.
- Making certain that the pitcher dresses properly for warmth during cold temperatures or for prevention of early heat exhaustion during very hot weather. Also, be aware of proper intake of fluids to prevent early dehydration and muscle fatigue.
- Finally, even though light weight, full ROM conditioning and strength work are recommended, the best method to build throwing arm strength and stamina is to throw a baseball and throw it biomechanically correctly.

From Wilk KE, Andrews JR, Zarins B: Injuries in Baseball. Philadelphia, Lippincott-Raven, 1998.

THE THROWER'S REHABILITATION REGIMEN

- Self-stretching techniques for pathologic changes in "tightness" of the capsule (see Fig. 3-58)
- Off-season adherence to rotator cuff, scapulothoracic, and shoulder girdle strengthening with the "**Thrower's Ten**" program (Fig. 3-59)
- Excellent conditioning of the "entire" athlete
- Warm-up and cool-down period with practice and games
- Avoidance of "overuse"—i.e., avoidance of throwing while fatigued
- Use of the throwing program described by Wilk and coworkers (1997)

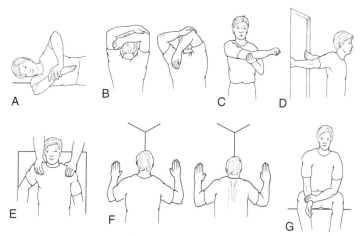

Figure 3–58   Self-stretching of the shoulder. (**A**, From Burkhart SS, Morgan CD, Kibler WB: The disabled throwing shoulder: Spectrum of pathology. Part 1: Pathoanatomy and biomechanics. Arthroscopy 19:404-420, 2003. **B-G**, from Wilk KE, Andrews JR: The Athlete's Shoulder. New York, Churchill Livingstone, 1994.)

A, Sleeper stretch. In the sleeper stretch, the patient is side-lying with the scapula stabilized against a wall, the shoulder flexed 90 degrees, and the elbow flexed 90 degrees. Passive internal rotation of the arm is applied to the dominant wrist by the nondominant arm.

B, Inferior capsular stretch. Hold the involved arm overhead with the elbow bent and the arm straight ahead. Using the uninvolved arm, stretch the arm farther overhead. When a stretching sensation is felt, hold for 5 seconds and repeat.

C, Posterior capsular stretch. With the uninvolved arm, grasp the elbow of the involved arm. Pull the involved arm across the chest to stretch the back of the involved shoulder. Hold at the endpoint for 5 seconds and repeat. This stretch is very important in throwers because of a tight posterior capsule.

D, Anterior capsular stretch. Standing in a doorway, the patient holds onto the door frame with the elbow straight and the shoulder abducted to 90 degrees and externally rotated. Walk through the doorway until a stretch is felt at the front of the shoulder. Hold for 5 seconds and repeat. **Avoid this stretch in patients with generalized ligamentous laxity or multidirectional instability**.

E, Pectoralis minor stretch. Lie on the back while pushing the shoulders toward the ceiling with a partner giving resistance. Relax and have the partner stretch the shoulder down. Hold the stretch for 5 seconds.

F, Pectoralis major corner stretch. Stand facing a corner. Position one arm on each side of the corner with the arms approximately 90 degrees away from the side and the forearms resting on the wall. Lean forward into the corner until a stretch is felt on the front of the shoulders. Hold __ seconds. Repeat __ times.

G, Biceps stretch. Sit with the elbow extended and resting on the leg. With the uninvolved arm pushing on the forearm, straighten the elbow and hold the stretch for 5 seconds.

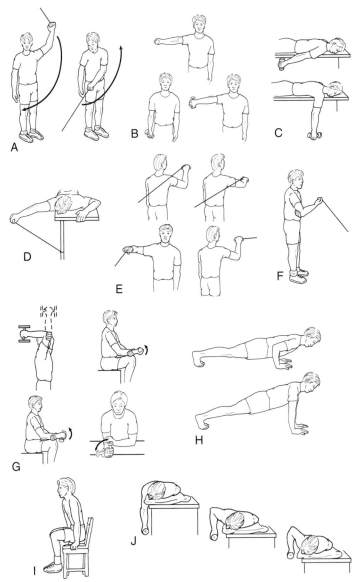

Figure 3–59   A-J, **"Thrower's Ten" program**. The "Thrower's Ten" program is designed to exercise the major muscles necessary for throwing. The program's goal is to be an organized and concise exercise program. In addition, all exercises included are specific to the thrower and are designed to improve strength, power, and endurance of the shoulder complex musculature. (From Andrews JR, Wilk KE: The Athlete's Shoulder. New York, Churchill Livingstone, 1994.)

A, Diagonal pattern D2 extension. Grip the tubing handle overhead and out to the side with the hand of the involved arm. Pull the tubing down and across the body to the opposite side of the leg. During the motion, lead with the thumb. Perform __ sets of __ repetitions __ times daily.

Diagonal pattern D2 flexion. Grip the tubing handle in the hand of the involved arm, beginning with the arm 45 degrees out from the side and the palm facing backward. After turning the palm forward, flex the elbow and bring the arm up and over the uninvolved shoulder. Turn the palm down and reverse to take the arm to the starting position. The exercise should be performed in a controlled manner. Perform __ sets of __ repetitions __ times daily.

Figure 3–59, cont'd

B, Dumbbell exercises for deltoid and supraspinatus deltoid strengthening. Stand with the arm at the side, the elbow straight, and the palm against the side. Raise the arm to the side, palm down, until the arm reaches 90 degrees. Perform __ sets of __ repetitions __ times daily.

Supraspinatus strengthening. Stand with the elbow straight and the thumb up. Raise the arm to shoulder level at a 30-degree angle in front of the body. Do not go above shoulder height. Hold for 2 seconds and lower slowly. Perform __ sets of __ repetitions __ times daily.

C, Prone shoulder abduction for the rhomboids: diagonal pattern D2 flexion. With the involved hand, grip the tubing handle across the body and against the thigh of the opposite leg. Starting with the palm down, rotate the palm up. Flex the elbow and bring the arm up and over the involved shoulder with the palm facing inward. Turn the palm down and reverse to take the arm to the starting position. The exercise should be performed in a controlled manner. Perform __ sets of __ repetitions __ times daily.

D, Prone shoulder extension for the latissimus dorsi. Lie on the table, face down, with the involved arm hanging straight to the floor and the palm facing down. Raise the arm straight back as far as possible. Hold for 2 seconds and lower slowly. Perform __ sets of __ repetitions __ times daily.

E, Internal rotation at 90 degrees abduction. Stand with the shoulder abducted to 90 degrees and externally rotated 90 degrees and the elbow bent to 90 degrees. Keep the shoulder abducted and rotate the shoulder forward while keeping the elbow at 90 degrees. Return the tubing and the hand to the starting position slowly and in a controlled manner.

Left, Slow-speed sets: perform __ sets of __ repetitions __ times daily.

Right, Fast-speed sets: perform __ sets of __ repetitions __ times daily.

External rotation at 90 degrees abduction. Stand with the shoulder abducted to 90 degrees and the elbow flexed to 90 degrees. Grip the tubing handle while the other hand is fixed straight ahead. Keep the shoulder abducted and rotate the shoulder back while keeping the elbow at 90 degrees. Return the tubing and the hand to the starting position slowly and in a controlled manner.

Left, Slow-speed sets: perform __ sets of __ repetitions __ times daily.

Right, Fast-speed sets: perform __ sets of __ repetitions __ times daily.

F, Biceps strengthening with tubing. Stand with one end of the tubing securely in the involved hand and the opposite end under the foot of the involved side while controlling tension. Assist with the opposite hand so that the arm is flexed through the full range of motion. Return to the starting position with a slow 5 count. Repeat three to five sets of 10 repetitions.

G, Dumbbell exercises for the triceps and wrist extensors-flexors. Triceps curls: Raise the involved arm overhead. Provide support at the elbow with the uninvolved hand. Straighten the arm overhead. Hold for 2 seconds and lower slowly. Perform __ sets of __ repetitions __ times daily.

Wrist flexion. Support the forearm on a table with the hand off the edge, the palm facing upward. Hold a weight or hammer in the involved hand and lower it as far as possible; then curl it up as high as possible. Hold for a 2 count. Perform __ sets of __ repetitions __ times daily.

Wrist extension. Support the forearm on a table with the hand off the edge, the palm facing downward. Hold a weight or hammer in the involved hand and lower it as far as possible; then curl it up as high as possible. Hold for a 2 count. Perform __ sets of __ repetitions __ times daily.

Forearm pronation. Support the forearm on a table with the wrist in neutral position. Hold a weight or hammer in a normal hammering position and roll the wrist to bring the hammer into pronation as far as possible. Hold for a 2 count. Raise to the starting position. Perform __ sets of __ repetitions __ times daily.

Forearm supination. Support the forearm on a table with the wrist in neutral position. Hold a weight or hammer in a normal hammering position and roll the wrist to bring the hammer into full supination. Hold for a 2 count. Raise back to the starting position. Perform __ sets of __ repetitions __ times daily.

H, Serratus anterior strengthening. Start with a push-up into the wall. Gradually progress to the tabletop and eventually to the floor as tolerable. Perform __ sets of __ repetitions __ times daily.

I, Press-ups. Sit on a chair or a table and place both hands firmly on the sides of the chair or table, the palm down and fingers pointed outward. The hands should be placed as far apart as the width of the shoulders. Slowly push downward through the hands to elevate the body. Hold the elevated position for 2 seconds. Repeat. Perform __ sets of __ repetitions __ times daily.

J, Rowing. Lie on the stomach with the involved arm hanging over the side of a table, the dumbbell in the hand, and the elbow straight. Slowly raise the arm while bending the elbow, and bring the dumbbell as high as possible. Hold at the top for 2 seconds; then lower slowly. Repeat. Perform __ sets of __ repetitions __ times daily.

Rotator Cuff Tears

Rotator cuff tears and subacromial impingement are among the most common causes of shoulder pain and disability. The frequency of rotator cuff tears increases with age, with full-thickness tears uncommon in patients younger than 40 years. The **rotator cuff "complex"** refers to the tendons of **four muscles: subscapularis, supraspinatus, infraspinatus, and teres minor**. These four muscles originate on the scapula, cross the GH joint, and then transition into tendons that insert onto the tuberosities of the proximal end of the humerus. **The rotator cuff has three well-recognized functions: rotation of the humeral head, stabilization of the humeral head in the glenoid socket by compressing the round head into the shallow socket, and the ability to provide "muscular balance" and stabilize the GH joint when other larger muscles crossing the shoulder contract**. Injury to the rotator cuff may occur in progressive stages. Rotator cuff tears can be classified as either acute or chronic, based on their timing, and as partial (articular or bursal side) or complete, based on the depth of the tear. Complete tears can be classified according to the size of the tear in square centimeters as described by Post (1983): **small** (0 to 1 cm^2), **medium** (1 to 3 cm^2), **large** (3 to 5 cm^2), or **massive** (>5 cm^2). All these factors, as well as the patient's demographic and medical background, play a role in determining the treatment plan.

Surgical repair of a torn rotator cuff is done in an effort to decrease pain, increase function, and improve ROM. Postoperative care must strike a precarious balance between restrictions that allow for tissue healing, activities that return ROM, and gradual restoration of muscle function and strength. It is not uncommon to have residual postoperative stiffness and pain despite an excellent operative repair if the postoperative rehabilitation is not correct.

Wilk and Andrews described multiple factors that significantly affect the postoperative rehabilitation program after repair of rotator cuff tears.

Factors Affecting Rehabilitation after Repair of Rotator Cuff Tears

TYPE OF REPAIR

- Open
- Mini-open
- Arthroscopic

SIZE OF TEAR

- Absolute size
- Number of tendons involved

PATIENT'S TISSUE QUALITY

- Good, fair, poor

LOCATION OF TEAR

- Superior tear
- Superoposterior
- Superoanterior

Factors Affecting Rehabilitation after Repair of Rotator Cuff Tears   *Continued*

SURGICAL APPROACH

ONSET OF TISSUE FAILURE

- Acute or gradual onset
- Timing of repair

PATIENT VARIABLES

- Age
- Dominant or nondominant arm
- Preinjury level
- Desired level of function (work and sports)
- Work situation
- Patient compliance with therapy regimen

REHABILITATION SITUATION

- Supervised or unsupervised

PHYSICIAN'S PHILOSOPHIC APPROACH

From Wilk KE, Crockett HC, Andrews JR: Rehabilitation after rotator cuff surgery. Tech Shoulder Elbow Surg 1:128, 2000.

TYPE OF REPAIR

Patients who have undergone detachment or release of the deltoid muscle from the acromion or clavicle (e.g., **traditional open rotator cuff repair**) may not perform active muscle contractions of the deltoid for 6 to 8 weeks to prevent avulsion of the deltoid.

Arthroscopic repair of the cuff actually has a slightly *slower* rate of rehabilitation progression because of weaker fixation of the repair than with the open procedure. A **mini-open** procedure, involving a vertical split with orientation of the deltoid fibers, allows mild, earlier deltoid muscular contractions. Regardless of the surgical approach performed, the underlying biology of healing tendons must be respected in all patients.

SIZE OF THE TEAR

Functional outcome and expectation after rotator cuff surgery are directly related to the size of the tear repaired. Wilk and Andrews (2002) base the rate of rehabilitation on the size and extent of the tear (see "Rehabilitation Protocol").

TISSUE QUALITY

The quality of the tendon, muscular tissue, and bone helps determine the speed of rehabilitation. Thin, fatty, or weak tissue is progressed slower than excellent tissue.

LOCATION OF THE TEAR

Tears that involve posterior cuff structures require a slower progression in external rotation strengthening. **Rehabilitation after subscapularis repair (anterior structure) should limit resisted internal rotation for 4 to 6 weeks**. The amount of passive external rotation motion should also be restricted until early tissue healing has occurred. Most tears are confined to the supraspinatus tendon, the critical site of wear, which often corresponds to the site of subacromial impingement.

PATIENT VARIABLES

Several authors have reported a less successful outcome in older patients, possibly because they typically have larger and more complex tears, which probably affects the outcome.

Several studies have noted no difference in outcome based on arm dominance. Hawkins and Montadi (1991) noted that workers' compensation patients required twice as long to return to work as did their non–workers' compensation cohorts.

Finally, researchers have noted a correlation between preoperative shoulder function and outcome after surgical repair. Generally, patients who had an active lifestyle before surgery return to the same postoperatively.

REHABILITATION SITUATION AND SURGEON'S PHILOSOPHIC APPROACH

We recommend treatment by a skilled shoulder therapist rather than a home therapy program. Some physicians prefer more aggressive progression, whereas others remain very conservative in their approach.

Rehabilitation after rotator cuff surgery emphasizes immediate motion, early dynamic GH joint stability, and gradual restoration of rotator cuff strength. Throughout rehabilitation, overstressing of the healing tissue is to be avoided by striking a balance between regaining shoulder mobility and allowing soft tissue healing.

Basic Rehabilitation Goals after Rotator Cuff Repair

Goal 1	Maintain integrity of the repaired rotator cuff. *Never overstress healing tissue.*
Goal 2	Re-establish full passive ROM as quickly and safely as possible.
Goal 3	Re-establish dynamic humeral head control. *Do not work through a shoulder shrug!*
Goal 4	Improve external rotation muscular strength. *Re-establish muscular balance.*
Goal 5	Initiate resisted shoulder abduction and flexion when muscular balance is restored.
Goal 6	Caution against overaggressive activities (tissue-healing constraints).
Goal 7	Restore functional use of the shoulder, but do so gradually.
Goal 8	Activate rotator cuff muscles through inhibition of pain.

From Wilk KE, Crockett HC, Andrews JR: Rehabilitation after rotator cuff surgery. Tech Shoulder Elbow Surg 1:128, 2000.

ACUTE TEARS

Patients with acute tears of the rotator cuff usually seek treatment from their physician after a traumatic injury. They have complaints of pain and sudden weakness, which may be manifested as an inability to elevate the arm. On physical examination, they have shoulder motion weakness during forward elevation, external rotation, or internal rotation, depending on which cuff muscles are involved. Passive motion is usually intact, depending on the time after injury. If the injury is chronic and the patient has been avoiding using the shoulder because of pain, there may be concomitant adhesive capsulitis (limitation of passive shoulder motion) and weakness of active ROM (underlying rotator cuff tear).

It is important to remember that **the likelihood of an associated rotator cuff tear with a shoulder dislocation increases with age**. In patients older than 40 years, an associated rotator cuff tear is present with shoulder dislocation in more than 30%; in patients older than 60 years, it is present in more than 80%. Therefore, serial examinations of the shoulder are necessary after a dislocation to evaluate the integrity of the rotator cuff. If significant symptoms of pain and weakness persist after 3 weeks, an imaging study of the rotator cuff is required. A torn rotator cuff after a dislocation is a surgical problem, so once the diagnosis is made, surgical repair is indicated.

Treatment

The recommended treatment for active patients with acute tears of the rotator cuff is surgical repair. Advantages of early operative repair include mobility of the rotator cuff, which allows technically easier repairs; good quality of the tendon, which allows a more stable repair; and in patients with cuff tears associated with a dislocation, improved GH joint stability.

CHRONIC TEARS

Chronic rotator cuff tears may be an asymptomatic pathologic condition associated with the normal aging process. A variety of factors, including poor vascularity, a "hostile" environment between the coracoacromial arch and the proximal part of the humerus, decreased use, or gradual deterioration in the tendon, contribute to senescence of the rotator cuff, especially the supraspinatus. Lehman and colleagues (1995) found rotator cuff tears in 30% of cadavers older than 60 years and in only 6% of those younger than 60 years. In a study by Romeo and coworkers (1999), **the average age of their patients treated for a rotator cuff tear was 58 years**. Many patients with chronic rotator cuff tears are older than 50 years, have no history of shoulder trauma, and express vague complaints of intermittent shoulder pain that has become progressively more symptomatic. These patients may also have a history that is indicative of a primary impingement etiology.

Examination

- On physical examination, some evidence of muscular atrophy may be seen in the supraspinatus fossa.
- Depending on the size of the tear, there may also be atrophy in the infraspinatus fossa.

- Passive motion is usually maintained, but it may be associated with subacromial crepitance.
- Smooth active motion is diminished, and symptoms are reproduced when the arm is lowered from an overhead position.
- Muscle weakness is related to the size of the tear and the muscles involved.
- Subacromial injection of lidocaine may help differentiate weakness caused by associated painful inflammation from that caused by a cuff tendon tear.
- Provocative maneuvers, including the Neer impingement sign (see Fig. 3-29) and the Hawkins sign (see Fig. 3-30), may be positive but are nonspecific because they may be positive with other conditions such as rotator cuff tendinitis, bursitis, or partial-thickness rotator cuff tears.
- It is important that other potential causes be investigated. Patients with cervical radiculopathy at the C5-6 level can have an insidious onset of shoulder pain, rotator cuff weakness, and muscular atrophy in the supraspinatus and infraspinatus fossa.

Imaging

Imaging studies may be helpful in confirming the diagnosis of a chronic rotator cuff tear and may help determine the potential success of operative treatment.

- A "trauma shoulder series" may show some proximal (superior) humeral migration, which is indicative of a large chronic rotator cuff tear/insufficiency.
- Plain radiographs can also show degenerative conditions or bone collapse consistent with a cuff tear arthropathy in which both the cuff deficiency and the arthritis contribute to the patient's symptoms.
- A magnetic resonance imaging (MRI) examination of the shoulder may help demonstrate a rotator cuff tear, its size, and the degree of retraction. MRI can also help assess the rotator cuff musculature. Evidence of fatty or fibrous infiltration of the rotator cuff muscles is consistent with a long-standing cuff tear and is a poor prognostic indicator for successful return of cuff function.
- MRI with intra-articular injection of contrast (gadolinium) is performed in younger patients in whom labral pathology or concomitant instability is suspected.

Treatment

Treatment of most patients with a chronic tear of the rotator cuff follows a conservative rehabilitation program. Operative intervention in this patient population is indicated for patients who are unresponsive to conservative management or demonstrate acute tearing of a chronic injury. The primary goal of surgical management of rotator cuff tears is to obtain pain relief. Additional goals, which are easier to achieve with acute rotator cuff tears than with chronic rotator cuff tears, include improved ROM, improved strength, and return of function.

REHABILITATION PROTOCOL	*For Patients with Chronic Rotator Cuff Tears Treated Conservatively (Nonoperatively)* Bach, Cohen, and Romeo

PHASE 1: WEEKS 0-4

Restrictions

- Avoid provocative maneuvers or exercises that cause discomfort
  - Includes both offending ROM exercises and strengthening exercises
- Patients may have an underlying subacromial bursitis; therefore, ROM exercises and muscle strengthening exercises should begin with the arm in less than 90 degrees of abduction
- **Avoid** abduction-rotation—re-creates the impingement maneuver
- **Avoid** "empty-can" exercises

Immobilization

- Brief sling immobilization for comfort only

Pain Control

- Reduction of pain and discomfort is essential for recovery
- Medications
  - NSAIDs—Consider cyclooxygenase-2 (COX-2) inhibitors (e.g., celecoxib [Celebrex])
  - Subacromial injection of corticosteroid and local anesthetic; judicious use for patients with acute inflammatory symptoms of a concomitant bursitis; limit of three injections
- Therapeutic modalities
  - Ice, ultrasound, HVGS
  - Moist heat before therapy; ice at end of session

Shoulder Motion

Goals

- Internal and external rotation equal to that on the contralateral side, with the arm positioned in less than 90 degrees of abduction

Exercises

- Begin with Codman pendulum exercises to gain early motion
- Passive ROM exercises (see Fig. 3-43)
  - Shoulder flexion
  - Shoulder extension
  - Internal and external rotation
  - Capsular stretching for the anterior, posterior, and inferior capsule by using the opposite arm (see Fig. 3-56)
- **Avoid** assisted-motion exercises (see Fig. 3-42)
  - Shoulder flexion
  - Shoulder extension
  - Internal and external rotation
- Progress to active ROM exercises
  - "Wall walking" (Fig. 3-60)

Elbow Motion

- Passive to active motion; progress as tolerated
  - 0-130 degrees
  - Pronation to supination as tolerated

Continued

For Patients with Chronic Rotator Cuff Tears Treated Conservatively (Nonoperatively) Continued

PHASE 1: WEEKS 0-4—cont'd

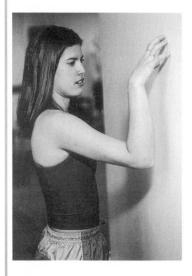

Figure 3–60 Demonstration of active range of motion of the shoulder, "wall walking."

Muscle Strengthening

- Grip strengthening (putty, Nerf ball, racquetball)
- Use of the arm for activities of daily living **below shoulder level**

PHASE 2: WEEKS 4-8

Criteria for Progression to Phase 2

- Minimal pain and tenderness
- Improvement of passive ROM
- Return of functional ROM

Goals

- Improve shoulder complex strength, power, and endurance

Restrictions

- Avoid provocative maneuvers or exercises that cause discomfort for the patient
- Includes both ROM exercises and strengthening exercises

Immobilization

- None

Pain Control

- Reduction of pain and discomfort is essential for recovery
- Medications
  - NSAIDs—Consider NSAIDs such as a COX-2 inhibitor (e.g., Celebrex).
  - Subacromial injection of corticosteroid and local anesthetic; judicious use in patients with acute inflammatory symptoms of a concomitant bursitis; limit of three injections

For Patients with Chronic Rotator Cuff Tears Treated Conservatively
(Nonoperatively)   *Continued*

PHASE 2: WEEKS 4-8—cont'd

- Therapeutic modalities
  - Ice, ultrasound, HVGS
  - Moist heat before therapy; ice at end of session

Motion

Goal

- Equal to contralateral shoulder in all planes of motion

Exercises

- Passive ROM
- Capsular stretching
- Active-assisted motion exercises
- Active ROM exercises

Muscle Strengthening

- Three times per week, 8-12 repetitions, for three sets
- Strengthening of the remaining muscles of the rotator cuff
- Begin with closed-chain isometric strengthening (see Fig. 3-44)
  - Internal rotation
  - External rotation
  - Abduction
- Progress to open-chain strengthening with Thera-Bands (see Fig. 3-47)
  - Exercises performed with the elbow flexed to 90 degrees
  - Starting position is with the shoulder in the neutral position of 0 degrees of forward flexion, abduction, and external rotation
  - Exercises are done through an arc of 45 degrees in each of the five clinical planes of motion
  - Six color-coded bands are available; each provides increasing resistance from 1 to 6 pounds at increments of 1 pound
  - Progression to the next band occurs usually at 2- to 3-week intervals. Patients are instructed to not progress to the next band if there is any discomfort at the present level
  - Thera-Band exercises permit concentric and eccentric strengthening of the shoulder muscles and are a form of isotonic exercises (characterized by variable speed and fixed resistance)
    - Internal rotation
    - External rotation
    - Abduction
    - Forward flexion
    - Extension
- Progress to light isotonic dumbbell exercises (see Fig. 3-47B)
  - Internal rotation
  - External rotation
  - Abduction
  - Forward flexion
  - Extension
- Strengthening of the deltoid (Fig. 3-61)

Continued

For Patients with Chronic Rotator Cuff Tears Treated Conservatively (Nonoperatively) Continued

PHASE 2: WEEKS 4-8—cont'd

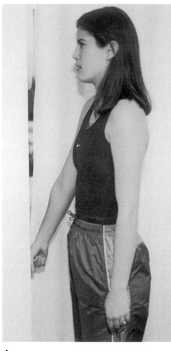

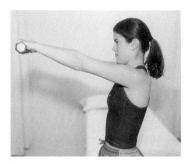

B

A

Figure 3–61 Strengthening of the anterior deltoid. **A**, Closed-chain isometric. **B**, Open-chain isotonic.

- Strengthening of scapular stabilizers
  - Closed-chain strengthening exercises (see Fig. 3-45)
    - Scapular retraction (rhomboideus, middle trapezius)
    - Scapular protraction (serratus anterior)
    - Scapular depression (latissimus dorsi, trapezius, serratus anterior)
    - Shoulder shrugs (upper trapezius)
  - Progress to open-chain scapular stabilizer strengthening (see Fig. 3-46)

PHASE 3: WEEKS 8-12

Criteria for Progression to Phase 3

- Full painless ROM
- No pain or tenderness with strengthening exercises

Goals

- Improve neuromuscular control and shoulder proprioception
- Prepare for gradual return to functional activities
- Establish a home exercise maintenance program that is performed at least three times per week for both stretching and strengthening

For Patients with Chronic Rotator Cuff Tears Treated Conservatively
(Nonoperatively)   *Continued*

PHASE 3: WEEKS 8-12—cont'd

Functional Strengthening

- Plyometric exercises (see Fig. 3-48)

Progressive, Systematic Interval Program for Returning to Sports

- Throwing athletes—see pages 271 and 274
- Tennis players—see page 276
- Golfers—see page 281

Maximal improvement is expected by 4-6 months.

Warning Signals

- Loss of motion—especially internal rotation
- Lack of strength progression—especially abduction, forward elevation
- Continued pain—especially at night

Treatment of Warning Signals

- These patients may need to move back to earlier routines
- May require increased utilization of pain control modalities as outlined earlier
- May require surgical intervention

REHABILITATION PROTOCOL *After Surgical Repair of the Rotator Cuff*
Bach, Cohen, and Romeo

PHASE 1: WEEKS 0-6

Restrictions

- No active ROM exercises
- Initiation of active ROM exercises based on size of tear
  - **Small tears** (0-1 cm)—no active ROM before 4 weeks
  - **Medium tears** (1-3 cm)—no active ROM before 6 weeks
  - **Large tears** (3-5 cm)—no active ROM before 8 weeks
  - **Massive tears** (>5 cm ROM)—no active ROM before 12 weeks
- Delay active-assisted ROM exercises for similar periods based on size of the tear
- Passive ROM only
  - 140 degrees of forward flexion
  - 40 degrees of external rotation
  - 60-80 degrees of abduction without rotation
- No strengthening/resisted motions of the shoulder until 12 weeks after surgery
  - For tears with high healing potential (small tears, acute, patients younger than 50 years, nonsmoker), isometric strengthening progressing to Thera-Band exercises may begin at 8 weeks. Strengthening exercises before 12 weeks should be performed with the arm at less than 45 degrees of abduction

Continued

After Surgical Repair of the Rotator Cuff   *Continued*

PHASE 1: WEEKS 0-6—cont'd

Immobilization

- The type of immobilization depends on the amount of abduction required to repair rotator cuff tendons with little or no tension
- Use of sling—if tension on the repair is minimal or none with the arm at the side
  - Small tears—1-3 weeks
  - Medium tears—3-6 weeks
  - Large and massive tears—6-8 weeks
- Abduction orthosis—if tension on the repair is minimal or none with the arm in 20-40 degrees of abduction
  - Small tears—6 weeks
  - Medium tears—6 weeks
  - Large and massive tears—8 weeks

Pain Control

- Patients treated by arthroscopic rotator cuff repair experience less postoperative pain than do those treated by mini-open or open repair (but more tenuous repair)
- Medications
  - Narcotic—for 7-10 days after surgery
  - NSAIDs—for patients with persistent discomfort after surgery. Consider COX-2 inhibitor formulas
- Therapeutic modalities
  - Ice, ultrasound, HVGS
  - Moist heat before therapy; ice at end of session

Shoulder Motion

- Passive only
  - 140 degrees of forward flexion
  - 40 degrees of external rotation
  - 60-80 degrees of abduction
- For patients immobilized in an abduction pillow, avoid adduction (i.e., bringing the arm toward the midline)
- Exercises should begin "above" the level of abduction in the abduction pillow
  - Begin Codman pendulum exercises to promote early motion
  - Passive ROM exercises only (see Fig. 3-43)

Elbow Motion

- Passive—progress to active motion
  - 0-130 degrees
  - Pronation and supination as tolerated

Muscle Strengthening

- Grip strengthening only in this phase

PHASE 2: WEEKS 6-12

Criteria for Progression to Phase 2

- At least 6 weeks of recovery has elapsed
- Painless passive ROM to
  - 140 degrees of forward flexion
  - 40 degrees of external rotation
  - 60-80 degrees of abduction

After Surgical Repair of the Rotator Cuff   *Continued*

PHASE 2: WEEKS 6-12—cont'd

Restrictions

- No strengthening/resisted motions of the shoulder until 12 weeks after surgery
- During phase 2, no active ROM exercises for patients with massive tears

Immobilization

- Discontinuation of the sling or abduction orthosis
- Use for comfort only

Pain Control

- NSAIDs for patients with persistent discomfort after surgery
- Therapeutic modalities
  - Ice, ultrasound, HVGS
  - Moist heat before therapy; ice at end of session

Shoulder Motion

Goals

- 140 degrees of forward flexion—progress to 160 degrees
- 40 degrees of external rotation—progress to 60 degrees
- 60-80 degrees of abduction—progress to 90 degrees

Exercises

- Continue with passive ROM exercises to achieve above goals (see Fig. 3-43)
- Begin active-assisted ROM exercises for the above goals (see Fig. 3-42)
- Progress to active ROM exercises as tolerated after full motion achieved with active-assisted exercises
- Light passive stretching at end ROM

Muscle Strengthening

- Begin rotator cuff and scapular stabilizer strengthening for small tears with excellent healing potential—as outlined below in phase 3
- Continue with grip strengthening

PHASE 3: MONTHS 4-6

Criteria for Progression to Phase 3

- Painless active ROM
- No shoulder pain or tenderness
- Satisfactory clinical examination

Goals

- Improve shoulder strength, power, and endurance
- Improve neuromuscular control and shoulder proprioception
- Prepare for gradual return to functional activities
- Establish a home exercise maintenance program that is performed at least three times per week for strengthening
- Stretching exercises should be performed daily

Continued

After Surgical Repair of the Rotator Cuff   *Continued*

PHASE 3: MONTHS 4-6—cont'd

Motion

- Achieve motion equal to that on the contralateral side
- Use passive, active-assisted, **and active** ROM exercises
- Passive capsular stretching at end ROM, especially cross-body (horizontal) adduction and internal rotation to stretch the posterior capsule

Muscle Strengthening

- Strengthening of the rotator cuff
  - Begin with closed-chain isometric strengthening (see Fig. 3-44)
    - Internal rotation
    - External rotation
    - Abduction
    - Forward flexion
    - Extension
  - Progress to open-chain strengthening with Thera-Bands (see Fig. 3-47)
    - Exercises performed with the elbow flexed to 90 degrees
    - Starting position is with the shoulder in the neutral position of 0 degrees of forward flexion, abduction, and external rotation. The arm should be comfortable at the patient's side
    - Exercises are performed through an arc of 45 degrees in each of the five planes of motion
    - Six color-coded bands are available; each provides increasing resistance from 1 to 6 pounds at increments of 1 pound
    - Progression to the next band occurs usually at 2- to 3-week intervals. Patients are instructed to not progress to the next band if there is any discomfort at the present level
    - Thera-Band exercises permit concentric and eccentric strengthening of the shoulder muscles and are a form of isotonic exercises (characterized by variable speed and fixed resistance)
      - Internal rotation
      - External rotation
      - Abduction
      - Forward flexion
      - Extension
  - Progress to light isotonic dumbbell exercises (see Fig. 3-47B)
    - Internal rotation
    - External rotation
    - Abduction
    - Forward flexion
    - Extension
- Strengthening of the deltoid—especially the anterior deltoid (see Fig. 3-61)
- Strengthening of scapular stabilizers
  - Closed-chain strengthening exercises (Fig. 3-62; see also Fig. 3-45)
    - Scapular retraction (rhomboideus, middle trapezius)
    - Scapular protraction (serratus anterior)
    - Scapular depression (latissimus dorsi, trapezius, serratus anterior)
    - Shoulder shrugs (trapezius, levator scapulae)
  - Progress to open-chain scapular stabilizer strengthening (see Fig. 3-46)

After Surgical Repair of the Rotator Cuff   Continued

PHASE 3: MONTHS 4-6—cont'd

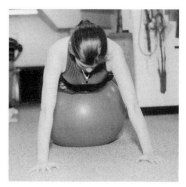

A

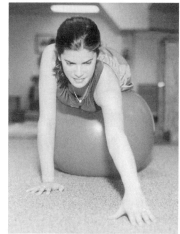

B

Figure 3–62 Additional closed-chain scapular stabilizer strengthening. **A**, Start. **B**, Finish (the right arm is the focus of rehabilitation).

Goals

- Three times per week
- Begin with 10 repetitions for one set, advance to 8-12 repetitions for three sets
- Functional strengthening (begins after 70% of strength recovered):
  - Plyometric exercises (see Fig. 3-48)
- Progressive, systematic interval program for returning to sports
  - Throwing athletes—see pages 271 and 274
  - Tennis players—see page 276
  - Golfers—see page 281

Maximal Improvement

- Small tears—4-6 months
- Medium tears—6-8 months
- Large and massive tears—8-12 months
  Patients will continue to show improvement in strength and function for at least 12 months.

Warning Signals

- Loss of motion—especially internal rotation
- Lack of strength progression—especially abduction
- Continued pain—especially at night

Treatment

- These patients may need to move back to earlier routines
- May require increased utilization of pain control modalities as outlined earlier
- May require repeat surgical intervention

Continued

> *After Surgical Repair of the Rotator Cuff*   *Continued*
>
> **PHASE 3: MONTHS 4-6—cont'd**
> - Indications for repeat surgical intervention
>   - Inability to establish more than 90 degrees forward elevation by 3 months
>   - Steady progress interrupted by a traumatic event and/or painful pop during the healing phase with a lasting loss of previously gained active motion
>   - Radiographic evidence of loosened intra-articular implants (e.g., corkscrews) after an injury in the postoperative rehabilitation period. The patient has a loss of active motion and/or crepitance of the joint as well

ROTATOR CUFF TEARS IN OVERHEAD ATHLETES

Overhead athletes are at an increased risk for rotator cuff injuries because of the repetitive, high-velocity (7000 degrees/sec), mechanical stress placed on their shoulders. **Athletes who have an underlying degree of instability may experience compression of the cuff as well as the posterior-superior glenoid labrum along the upper third of the posterior glenoid.** This condition, known as *internal impingement,* **is believed by some authors to be a contributing factor to the development of articular-sided partial-thickness tears and full-thickness tears in overhead athletes.**

Successful treatment of this patient population depends on recognition of the underlying instability.

Burkhart et al. (2003) believe that GIRD (glenohumeral internal rotation deficit) caused by posteroinferior capsular contracture is the most pathologic process involved in throwers' shoulder injuries.

Advocates of this theory work hard to stretch this capsular contracture to obtain symmetry with the unaffected shoulder to stop the pathologic cascade described in the first section of this chapter.

Burkhart found rotator cuff tears in 31% of throwers with arthroscopically confirmed SLAP lesions. In posterior type 2 SLAP lesions, the humerus is thought to sublux posterosuperiorly because of the break in the labral ring, which repetitively produces high tensile force in the posterosuperior cuff. This force may ultimately contribute to tearing of the rotator cuff.

In addition, the hypertwist phenomenon caused by hyper–external rotation of the shoulder can lead to torsional and shear overload with fatigue failure of cuff fibers in the same area of the posterosuperior rotator cuff.

The diagnosis requires a comprehensive history focusing on the timing and quality of the pain and a complete physical examination that includes provocative maneuvers to test for instability.

- Radiologic evaluation with an arthrogram-enhanced MRI (gadolinium) may identify partial-thickness tears.
- In this population, patients with partial-thickness tears **rarely require operative repair** because of resolution of symptoms after proper shoulder rehabilitation and/or an operative stabilization procedure.

- Overhead athletes in whom a full-thickness rotator cuff tear is diagnosed in the setting of anterior instability should be treated aggressively with surgical repair of the rotator cuff and a stabilization procedure. This recommendation is at odds with historical recommendations in older patients to treat the rotator cuff tear and then evaluate the need for additional treatment of the instability.
- Maximal athletic performance requires an intact rotator cuff and a stable shoulder.
- Aggressive débridement of partial-thickness tears is discouraged because of the risk for thinning of the tendons and propagation to a full-thickness tear.

Rehabilitation for patients with partial tears treated nonoperatively is similar to the program on page 245. Patients treated by operative stabilization procedures follow the postoperative routine on page 296, and patients who have an associated cuff repair follow the rehabilitation on page 259. Once the repair has completely healed in an overhead athlete and full ROM and a significant amount of strength have been recovered, the athlete can advance to the sport-specific rehabilitation program (see section on interval throwing).

Rehabilitation after Arthroscopically Assisted Mini-open Repair of the Rotator Cuff

We use three different rehabilitation programs based on the *size of the tear* and the *condition of the repaired tissues* (Table 3-3). The three programs differ mainly in their rates of rehabilitation progression:

- The **type 1 program** is used for small tears in younger patients with good to excellent tissues. This program is much more progressive than type 2 or 3.
- The **type 2 program** is used for medium to large tears in active individuals with good tissues.
- The **type 3 program** is used for patients with large to massive tears with a tenuous repair and fair to poor tissue quality.

TABLE 3–3	Criteria for Rehabilitation after Mini–Open Repair of the Rotator Cuff	
Size of Tear	**Guidelines**	**Rehabilitation Program**
Small (≤1 cm)	Sling 7-10 days Restore full ROM within 4-6 wk	Type 1
Medium to large (2-4 cm)	Sling 2-3 wk Restore ROM within 8-10 wk	Type 2
Large to massive (≥5 cm)	Abduction pillow 1-2 wk Sling 2-3 wk Restore full ROM within 10-14 wk	Type 3

Important General Points for Rehabilitation after Rotator Cuff Repair*

- Re-establishing early passive ROM is considered paramount.
- On postoperative day 1, the patient's arm is *passively* moved through a ROM (flexion in the scapular plane and internal and external rotation in the scapular plane at 45 degrees of abduction).
- Allow active-assisted external and internal rotation with an L-bar (Breg Corp., Vista, CA) in the scapular plane (Fig. 3-63). The patient moves the arm to tolerance but no farther and gently progresses ROM over subsequent days.
- Active-assisted arm elevation with the L-bar in the scapular plane is allowed at 7 to 10 days. The therapist must provide assistance or support as the patient lowers the arm from 80 to 30 degrees of elevation or the patient will have pain secondary to an inability to control the arm while lowering it.
- As motion progresses, exercises are done with the arm abducted to 75 degrees during external and internal rotation active-assisted ROM stretching.
- The patient is then progressed to 90 degrees of abduction for these ROM exercises.
- Finally, the arm is placed at the side (0 degrees of abduction) during external and internal rotation.

Goals for obtaining full passive motion of the shoulder after rotator cuff repair:

Type 1—3 to 4 weeks
Type 2—4 to 6 weeks
Type 3—6 to 8 weeks

- **Restoration of *active* motion is much slower because of healing constraints, pain inhibition, and weakness of the rotator cuff.**
- Motions such as excessive shoulder extension, adduction behind the back, and horizontal adduction are **prohibited** for at least 6 to 8 weeks.
- Cryotherapy is used four to eight times a day for the first 7 to 10 days to suppress inflammation, decrease muscle spasm, and enhance analgesia.

---

*From Wilk KE, Meister K, Andrews JR: Current concepts in the rehabilitation of the overhead throwing athlete. Am J Sports Med 30:136, 2002.

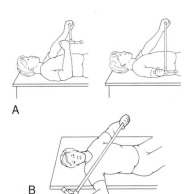

A

B

Figure 3–63 Active-assisted range-of-motion exercises, external rotation. (**A** and **B**, From Andrews JR, Wilk KE: The Athlete's Shoulder. New York, Churchill Livingstone, 1994.)

A, Lie on the back with the involved arm against the body and the elbow at 90 degrees. Grip the T-bar handle in the hand of the involved arm, and with the uninvolved arm, push the involved shoulder into external rotation. Hold for 5 seconds. Return to the starting position and repeat.

B, Lie on the back with the involved arm 45 degrees from the body and the elbow at 90 degrees. Grip the T-bar in the hand of the involved arm and keep the elbow in the flexed position. Using the opposite arm, push the involved arm into external rotation. Hold for 5 seconds. Return to the starting position and repeat.

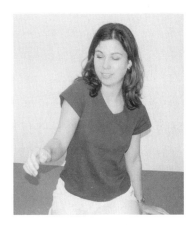

Figure 3–64 "Shrug" sign. Note the superior displacement of the humerus and compensatory scapular muscle activity.

- Active **submaximal, pain-free multiangle isometrics** are used for the internal and external rotators, abductors, flexors, and elbow flexor muscle groups.
- **Rhythmic stabilization exercises** (in the supine position) are begun at 10 to 14 days postoperatively (type 2 protocol) to restore dynamic stabilization of the GH joint through co-contractions of the surrounding musculature. These exercises are designed to prevent and treat the **"shrug" sign** (Fig. 3-64).
- These exercises are done in the **"balanced position,"** defined as 100-110 degrees of elevation and 10 degrees of horizontal abduction (Fig. 3-65).
- In this position, the therapist provides an **extremely low** (3-4 pounds of force) isometric force to resist flexion and extension and horizontal abduction and adduction.

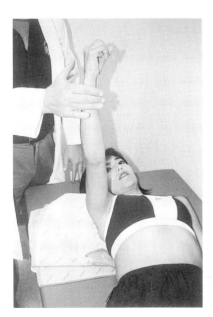

Figure 3–65 Rhythmic stabilization exercise drills. The patient's arm is placed in the balanced position and reciprocal static isometric contractions are done to resist shoulder flexion and horizontal abduction and adduction.

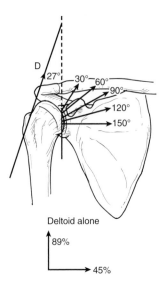

Deltoid alone

89%

45%

Figure 3–66   Deltoid muscle resultant vectors. With the arm at the side, the line of the deltoid muscle insertion into the humerus is 27 degrees. Thus, the resultant vector is superior migration of the humeral head. At 90 to 100 degrees of arm elevation, the deltoid muscle generates a compressive force into the glenoid. (From Andrews JR, Zarins B, Wilk KE: Injuries in Baseball. Philadelphia, Lippincott-Raven, 1997.)

- The "**balanced position**" (100 to 110 degrees of elevation) is used so that the deltoid muscle generates a more horizontal (and thus compressive) force (Fig. 3-66). This exercise at 100 to 125 degrees activates the rotator cuff with assistance from the deltoid to **avoid superior migration** of the humeral head.
- The "**shrug sign**" occurs if a **strong deltoid muscle overpowers the weakened rotator cuff and causes the humeral head to migrate superiorly** (see Fig. 3-50). This is related to lack of humeral head control. At initiation of arm elevation to 25 to 30 degrees, the entire shoulder elevates or "shrugs." Dynamic stabilization drills should alleviate this problem.
- As GH joint control is regained and re-established, the drills can be done at lower flexion angles (30, 60, 90 degrees). The progression is (1) supine (scapula support) to (2) side-lying (Fig. 3-67), and then (3) seated.
- Rhythmic stabilization drills (low 3- to 4-pound force) are done for the internal and external rotators in the plane of the scapula (start at 7 to 10 days) (Fig. 3-68).
- At 3 weeks, isotonic tubing is used for the external and internal rotator muscles with the arm at the side (see Fig. 3-47). As strength improves, side-lying external rotator strengthening is begun. External rotation strength is emphasized.
- **Emphasis is on external rotation strength** because this strength is critical in re-establishing functional use of the arm.

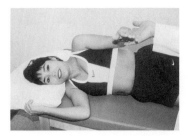

Figure 3–67   Rhythmic stabilization drills to re-establish dynamic glenohumeral joint stability.

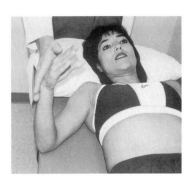

Figure 3–68 Rhythmic stabilization drills to resist external and internal rotation of the glenohumeral joint.

- The patient is not allowed to progressively exercise through a shrug sign (deleterious to the repair). Emphasis should be on re-establishing dynamic stabilization.
- **Once external rotation strength is achieved, active abduction and flexion are allowed.**
- At 8 weeks, light isotonic strengthening and flexibility exercises are begun, with low weight and high repetition for muscle endurance and strength.
- At 3 months, the patient can progress to the fundamental shoulder exercise program.
- Tennis players
  - Ground strokes are allowed at 5 to 6 months.
  - Serving is allowed when pain free (10 to 12 months).
  - Interval training tables are on pages 271 to 282.
- Golfers
  - Golf swing is begun at 16 weeks.
  - Gradual return to play is allowed at 6 to 7 months.
- Internal training programs for overhead athletes should be used after periods of prolonged inactivity or after the surgically repaired athlete has healed and is cleared to play. These programs encourage gradual resumption of activity rather than immediate full-velocity throwing, which may produce an injury (see the section on interval throwing).
  - Patients with **arthroscopic repairs** are generally progressed **2 to 3 weeks slower** than those with arthroscopically-assisted mini-open procedures because the fixation is not as strong.

REHABILITATION PROTOCOL	*After Type 1 Rotator Cuff Surgical Repair (Arthroscopically Assisted Mini-Open Repair for Small to Medium Tears [<1 cm])* Wilk, Crockett, and Andrews

CANDIDATES FOR TYPE 1 PROTOCOL

- **Young patient**
- **Excellent tissue quality**
- **Small tear (<1 cm)**

Continued

After Type 1 Rotator Cuff Surgical Repair (Arthroscopically Assisted Mini-Open Repair for Small to Medium Tears [<1 cm])   *Continued*

PHASE 1: IMMEDIATE POSTSURGICAL PHASE (DAYS 1-10)

Goals

- Maintain integrity of repair
- Gradually increase passive ROM
- Diminish pain and inflammation
- Prevent muscular inhibition

Days 1-6

- Sling
- Pendulum exercises
- Active-assisted ROM exercise (L-bar)
  - External and internal rotation in the scapular plane
- Passive ROM
  - Flexion to tolerance
  - External and internal rotation in the scapular plane
- Elbow/hand gripping and ROM exercises
- Submaximal pain-free isometrics
  - Flexion
  - Abduction
  - External rotation
  - Internal rotation
  - Elbow flexors
- Cryotherapy for pain and inflammation (ice 15-20 minutes every hour)
- Sleeping (in sling)

Days 7-10

- Discontinue sling at days 7-10
- Pendulum exercises (e.g., flexion, circles)
- Progress passive ROM to tolerance
  - Flexion to at least 115 degrees
  - External rotation in the scapular plane to 45-55 degrees
  - Internal rotation in the scapular plane to 45-55 degrees
- Active-assisted ROM exercises (L-bar)
  - External and internal rotation in the scapular plane
  - Flexion to tolerance (therapist provides assistance by supporting the arm)
- Continue elbow/hand ROM and gripping exercises
- Continue isometrics
  - Flexion with bent elbow
  - Extension with bent elbow
  - Abduction with bent elbow
  - External and internal rotation with the arm in the scapular plane
  - Elbow flexion
  - May initiate external and internal rotation tubing exercises at 0 degrees abduction if the patient exhibits the necessary active ROM
- Continue the use of ice for pain control (use ice at least 6-7 times daily)
- Sleeping (continue sleeping in a sling until the physician instructs [usually day 7])

After Type 1 Rotator Cuff Surgical Repair (Arthroscopically Assisted Mini-Open Repair for Small to Medium Tears [<1 cm]) Continued

PHASE 1: IMMEDIATE POSTSURGICAL PHASE (DAYS 1-10)—cont'd

Precautions

- No lifting of objects
- No excessive shoulder motion behind the back
- No excessive stretching or sudden movements
- No supporting of body weight by the hands
- Keep the incision clean and dry

PHASE 2: PROTECTION PHASE (DAY 11-WEEK 5)

Goals

- Allow healing of soft tissue
- Do not overstress healing tissue
- Gradually restore passive ROM (weeks 2-3)
- Re-establish dynamic shoulder stability
- Decrease pain and inflammation

Days 11-14

- Passive ROM to tolerance
  - Flexion at 0-145/160 degrees
  - External rotation at 90 degrees abduction: at least 75-80 degrees
  - Internal rotation at 90 degrees abduction: at least 55-60 degrees
- Active-assisted ROM to tolerance
  - Flexion
  - External and internal rotation in the scapular plane
  - External and internal rotation at 90 degrees abduction
- Dynamic stabilization drills (i.e., rhythmic stabilization drills [see Fig. 3-68])
  - External and internal rotation in the scapular plane
  - Flexion-extension at 100 degrees flexion
- Continue isotonic external and internal rotation with tubing
- Initiate prone rowing, elbow flexion
- Initiate active exercise (flexion-abduction)
- Continue use of cryotherapy

Weeks 3-4

- Patient should exhibit full passive ROM and be nearing full active ROM
- Continue all exercises listed above
- Initiate scapular muscular strengthening program
- Initiate side-lying external rotation strengthening (light dumbbell)
- Initiate isotonic elbow flexion
- Continue use of ice as needed
- May use pool for light ROM exercises

Week 5

- Patient should exhibit full active ROM
- Continue active-assisted ROM and stretching exercises

Continued

After Type 1 Rotator Cuff Surgical Repair (Arthroscopically Assisted Mini-Open Repair for Small to Medium Tears [<1 cm])   *Continued*

PHASE 2: PROTECTION PHASE (DAY 11-WEEK 5)—cont'd

- Progress isotonic strengthening exercise program
  - External rotation with tubing
    - Side-lying internal rotation
    - Prone rowing
    - Prone horizontal abduction
    - Shoulder flexion (scapular plane)
    - Shoulder abduction
    - Biceps curls

Precautions

- No lifting of heavy objects
- No supporting of body weight by hands and arms
- No sudden jerking motions

PHASE 3: INTERMEDIATE PHASE (WEEKS 6-11)

Goals

- Gradual restoration of shoulder strength and power
- Gradual return to functional activities
- Continue stretching and passive ROM (as needed to maintain full ROM)
- Continue dynamic stabilization drills
- Progress isotonic strengthening program
  - External and internal rotation with tubing
  - Side-lying external rotation
  - Lateral raises
  - Full can in the scapular plane
  - Prone rowing
  - Prone horizontal abduction
  - Prone extension
  - Elbow flexion
  - Elbow extension
- If the physician permits, the patient may initiate *light* functional activities

Weeks 8-10

- Continue all exercises listed above
- Progress to fundamental shoulder exercises
- Initiate interval golf program (slow rate of progression)

PHASE 4: ADVANCED STRENGTHENING PHASE (WEEKS 12-19)

Goals

- Maintain full nonpainful active ROM
- Enhance functional use of the upper extremity
- Improve muscular strength and power
- Gradual return to functional activities

After Type 1 Rotator Cuff Surgical Repair (Arthroscopically Assisted Mini-Open Repair for Small to Medium Tears [<1 cm]) Continued

PHASE 4: ADVANCED STRENGTHENING PHASE (WEEKS 12-19)—cont'd

Week 12

- Continue ROM exercises and stretching to maintain full ROM
- Self-assisted capsular stretches
- Progress shoulder strengthening exercises to fundamental shoulder exercises
- Initiate swimming or tennis program (if appropriate)

Week 15

- Continue all exercises listed above
- Progress golf program to playing golf (if appropriate)

PHASE 5: RETURN-TO-ACTIVITY PHASE (WEEKS 20-26)

Goals

- Gradual return to strenuous work activities
- Gradual return to recreational sport activities

Week 20

- Continue fundamental shoulder exercise program (at least four times per week)
- Continue stretching if motion is tight
- Continue progression to sport participation

REHABILITATION PROTOCOL

After Type 2 Rotator Cuff Surgical Repair (Arthroscopically Assisted Mini-open Repair for Medium to Large Tears [>1 cm, <5 cm])
Wilk, Crockett, and Andrews

CANDIDATES FOR TYPE 2 REHABILITATION

- Medium to large tear
- Active patient
- Good tissue quality

PHASE 1: IMMEDIATE POSTSURGICAL PHASE (DAYS 1-10)

Goals

- Maintain integrity of the repair
- Gradually increase passive ROM
- Diminish pain and inflammation
- Prevent muscular inhibition

Days 1-6

- Sling or abduction brace (physician's decision)
- Pendulum stretches
- Active-assisted ROM exercises (L-bar)
  - External and internal rotation in the scapular plane

Continued

After Type 2 Rotator Cuff Surgical Repair (Arthroscopically Assisted Mini-Open Repair for Medium to Large Tears [>1 cm, <5 cm])   *Continued*

PHASE 1: IMMEDIATE POSTSURGICAL PHASE (DAYS 1-10)—cont'd

- Passive ROM
  - Flexion to tolerance
  - External and internal rotation in the scapular plane
- Elbow/hand gripping and ROM exercises
- Submaximal pain-free isometrics
  - Flexion
  - Abduction
  - External rotation
  - Internal rotation
  - Elbow flexors
- Cryotherapy for pain and inflammation (ice 15-20 minutes every hour)
- Sleeping in a sling or brace

Days 7-10

- Discontinue brace at days 10-14
- Pendulum exercises (e.g., flexion, circles)
- Progress passive ROM to tolerance
  - Flexion to at least 105 degrees
  - External rotation in the scapular plane to 35-45 degrees
  - Internal rotation in the scapular plane to 35-45 degrees
- Active-assisted ROM exercises (L-bar)
  - External and internal rotation in the scapular plane
  - Flexion to tolerance (therapist provides assistance by supporting the arm)
- Continue elbow/hand ROM and gripping exercises
- Continue isometrics
  - Flexion with bent elbow
  - Extension with bent elbow
  - Abduction with bent elbow
  - External and internal rotation with arm in the scapular plane
  - Elbow flexion
- Continue use of ice for pain control (at least 6-7 times daily)
- Sleeping (in a brace until physician instructs)

Precautions

- No lifting of objects
- No excessive shoulder extension
- No excessive stretching or sudden movements
- No supporting of body weight by hands
- Keep incision clean and dry

PHASE 2: PROTECTION PHASE (DAY 11-WEEK 6)

Goals

- Allow healing of soft tissue
- Do not overstress healing tissue
- Gradually restore full passive ROM (weeks 4-5)
- Re-establish dynamic shoulder stability
- Decrease pain and inflammation

After Type 2 Rotator Cuff Surgical Repair (Arthroscopically Assisted Mini-Open Repair for Medium to Large Tears [>1 cm, <5 cm])   *Continued*

PHASE 2: PROTECTION PHASE (DAY 11-WEEK 6)—cont'd

Days 11-14

- Discontinue use of sling or brace
- Passive ROM to tolerance
  - Flexion at 0-125/145 degrees
  - External rotation at 90 degrees abduction: at least 45 degrees
  - Internal rotation at 90 degrees abduction: at least 45 degrees
- Active-assisted ROM to tolerance
  - Flexion
  - External and internal rotation in the scapular plane
  - External and internal rotation at 90 degrees abduction
- Dynamic stabilization drills (i.e., rhythmic stabilization drills [see Fig. 3-68])
  - External and internal rotation in the scapular plane
  - Flexion-extension at 100 degrees flexion
- Continue all isometric contractions
- Continue use of cryotherapy as needed
- Continue all precautions

Weeks 3-4

- Patient should exhibit full passive ROM
- Continue all exercises listed above
- Initiate gentle external and internal rotation strengthening with exercise tubing at 0 degrees of abduction
- Initiate manual resistance external rotation supine in the scapular plane
- Initiate prone rowing to neutral arm position
- Initiate isotonic elbow flexion
- Continue use of ice as needed
- May use heat before ROM exercises
- May use pool for light ROM exercises

Weeks 5-6

- May use heat before exercises
- Continue active-assisted ROM and stretching exercises
- Initiate active ROM exercises
  - Shoulder flexion in the scapular plane
  - Shoulder abduction
- Progress isotonic strengthening exercise program
  - External rotation with tubing
  - Side-lying internal rotation
  - Prone rowing
  - Prone horizontal abduction
  - Biceps curls

Precautions

- No heavy lifting of objects
- No excessive behind-the-back movements
- No supporting of body weight by hands and arms
- No sudden jerking motions

Continued

After Type 2 Rotator Cuff Surgical Repair (Arthroscopically Assisted Mini-Open Repair for Medium to Large Tears [>1 cm, <5 cm])   *Continued*

PHASE 3: INTERMEDIATE PHASE (WEEKS 7-14)

Goals

- Full active ROM (weeks 8-10)
- Full passive ROM
- Dynamic shoulder stability
- Gradual restoration of shoulder strength and power
- Gradual return of functional activities

Week 7

- Continue stretching and passive ROM (as needed to maintain full ROM)
- Continue dynamic stabilization drills
- Progress strengthening program
  - External and internal rotation with tubing
  - Side-lying external rotation
  - Lateral raises*
  - Full can in the scapular plane*
  - Prone rowing
  - Prone horizontal abduction
  - Prone extension
  - Elbow flexion
  - Elbow extension

Week 8

- Continue all exercises listed above
- If physician permits, may initiate *light* functional activities

Week 14

- Continue all exercises listed above
- Progress to fundamental shoulder exercises

PHASE 4: ADVANCED STRENGTHENING PHASE (WEEKS 15-22)

Goals

- Maintain full nonpainful ROM
- Enhance functional use of the upper extremity
- Improve muscular strength and power
- Gradual return to functional activities

Week 15

- Continue ROM and stretching to maintain full ROM
- Self-assisted capsular stretches
- Progress shoulder strengthening exercises to fundamental shoulder exercises
- Initiate interval golf program (if appropriate)

Week 20

- Continue all exercises listed above
- Progress golf program to playing golf (if appropriate)
- Initiate interval tennis program (if appropriate)
- May initiate swimming

After Type 2 Rotator Cuff Surgical Repair (Arthroscopically Assisted Mini-Open Repair for Medium to Large Tears [>1 cm, <5 cm])   *Continued*

PHASE 5: RETURN-TO-ACTIVITY PHASE (WEEKS 23-30)

Goals

- Gradual return to strenuous work activities
- Gradual return to recreational sport activities

Week 23

- Continue fundamental shoulder exercises program (at least four times per week)
- Continue stretching if motion is tight
- Continue progression to sport participation

*Patient must be able to elevate the arm without shoulder or scapular hiking before initiating isotonics; if unable, continue GH joint exercises.

REHABILITATION PROTOCOL

After Type 3 Rotator Cuff Surgical Repair (Arthroscopically Assisted Mini-Open Repair for Large to Massive Tears [>5 cm])
Wilk, Crockett, and Andrews

CANDIDATES FOR TYPE 3 REHABILITATION

- Large to massive tear
- Poor tissue quality
- Tenuous repair

PHASE 1: IMMEDIATE POSTSURGICAL PHASE (DAYS 1-10)

Goals

- Maintain integrity of the repair
- Gradually increase passive ROM
- Diminish pain and inflammation
- Prevent muscular inhibition

Days 1-6

- Sling or slight abduction brace (physician's decision)
- Pendulum exercises
- Active-assisted ROM exercise (L-bar)
  - External and internal rotation in the scapular plane
- Passive ROM
  - Flexion to tolerance
  - External and internal rotation in the scapular plane (gentle ROM)
- Elbow/hand gripping and ROM exercises
- Submaximal gentle isometrics
  - Flexion
  - Abduction
  - External rotation
  - Internal rotation
  - Elbow flexors

Continued

After Type 3 Rotator Cuff Surgical Repair (Arthroscopically Assisted Mini-Open Repair for Large to Massive Tears [>5 cm])   *Continued*

PHASE 1: IMMEDIATE POSTSURGICAL PHASE (DAYS 1-10)—cont'd

- Cryotherapy for pain and inflammation (ice 15-20 minutes every hour)
- Sleeping (in a sling or brace)

Days 7-10

- Continue use of a brace or sling
- Pendulum exercises (e.g., flexion, circles)
- Progress passive ROM and gripping exercises
  - Flexion to at least 90 degrees
  - External rotation in the scapular plane to 35 degrees
  - Internal rotation in the scapular plane to 35 degrees
- Continue elbow/hand ROM and gripping exercises
- Continue submaximal isometrics
  - Flexion with bent elbow
  - Extension with bent elbow
  - Abduction with bent elbow
  - External and internal rotation with the arm in the scapular plane
  - Elbow flexion
- Continue use of ice for pain control (at least 6-7 times daily)
- Sleeping (in a brace until physician instructs)

Precautions

- Maintain arm in brace; remove only for exercise
- No lifting of objects
- No excessive shoulder extension
- No excessive or aggressive stretching or sudden movements
- No supporting of body weight by hands
- Keep incision clean and dry

PHASE 2: PROTECTION PHASE (DAY 11-WEEK 6)

Goals

- Allow healing of soft tissue
- Do not overstress healing tissue
- Gradually restore full passive ROM (weeks 4-5)
- Re-establish dynamic shoulder stability
- Decrease pain and inflammation

Days 11-14

- Continue use of brace
- Passive ROM to tolerance
  - Flexion at 0 to approximately 125 degrees
  - External rotation at 90 degrees abduction: at least 45 degrees
  - Internal rotation at 90 degrees abduction: at least 45 degrees
- Active-assisted ROM to tolerance
  - External and internal rotation in the scapular plane
  - Flexion-extension at 100 degrees flexion
- Continue all isometric contractions
- Continue use of cryotherapy as needed
- Continue all precautions

After Type 3 Rotator Cuff Surgical Repair (Arthroscopically Assisted Mini-Open Repair for Large to Massive Tears [>5 cm])   Continued

PHASE 2: PROTECTION PHASE (DAY 11-WEEK 6)—cont'd

Weeks 3-4

- Initiate active-assisted ROM flexion in the supine position (therapist supports the arm during motion)
- Continue all exercises listed above
- Initiate external and internal rotation strengthening with exercise tubing at 0 degrees of abduction
- Progress passive ROM until approximately full ROM at weeks 4-5
- Initiate prone rowing to neutral arm position
- Initiate isotonic elbow flexion
- Continue use of ice as needed
- May use heat before ROM exercises
- May use pool for light ROM exercises
- Continue use of brace during sleeping until end of week 4
- Discontinue use of brace at end of week 4

Weeks 5-6

- May use heat before exercises
- Continue active-assisted ROM and stretching exercises
- Initiate active ROM exercises
  - Shoulder flexion in the scapular plane
  - Shoulder abduction
- Progress isotonic strengthening exercise program
  - External rotation with tubing
  - Side-lying internal rotation
  - Prone rowing
  - Prone horizontal abduction
  - Biceps curls

Precautions

- No lifting
- No excessive behind-the-back movements
- No supporting of body weight by hands and arms
- No sudden jerking motions

PHASE 3: INTERMEDIATE PHASE (WEEKS 7-14)

Goals

- Full active ROM (weeks 10-12)
- Maintain full passive ROM
- Dynamic shoulder stability
- Gradual restoration of shoulder strength and power
- Gradual return to functional activities

Week 7

- Continue stretching and passive ROM (as needed to maintain full ROM)
- Continue dynamic stabilization drills

Continued

After Type 3 Rotator Cuff Surgical Repair (Arthroscopically Assisted Mini-Open Repair for Large to Massive Tears [>5 cm])   Continued

PHASE 3: INTERMEDIATE PHASE (WEEKS 7-14)—cont'd

- Progress strengthening program
  - External and internal rotation with tubing
  - Side-lying external rotation
  - Lateral raises* (active ROM only)
  - Full can in the scapular plane* (active ROM only)
  - Prone rowing
  - Prone horizontal abduction
  - Elbow flexion
  - Elbow extension

Week 10

- Continue all exercises listed above
- If physician permits, may initiate *light* functional activities

Week 14

- Continue all exercises listed above
- Progress to fundamental shoulder exercises

PHASE 4: ADVANCED STRENGTHENING PHASE (WEEKS 15-22)

Goals

- Maintain full nonpainful ROM
- Enhance functional uses of the upper extremity
- Improve muscular strength and power
- Gradual return to functional activities

Week 15

- Continue ROM and stretching to maintain full ROM
- Self-assisted capsular stretches
- Progress shoulder strengthening exercises to fundamental shoulder exercises

Week 20

- Continue all exercises listed above
- Continue to perform ROM stretching if motion is not complete

PHASE 5: RETURN-TO-ACTIVITY PHASE (WEEKS 23-30)

Goals

- Gradual return to strenuous work activities
- Gradual return to recreational sport activities

Week 23

- Continue fundamental shoulder exercise program (at least four times per week)
- Continue stretching if motion is tight

Week 26

- May initiate interval sport program (e.g., golf)

*The patient must be able to elevate the arm without shoulder or scapular hiking before initiating isotonics; if unable, continue GH joint exercises.

REHABILITATION PROTOCOL	*Interval Throwing Program for Pitchers* Wilk

STEP 1

Toss the ball (no wind-up) against a wall on alternate days. Start with 25-30 throws, build up to 70 throws, and gradually increase the throwing distance.

Number of Throws	Distance (ft)
20	20 (warm-up phase)
25-40	30-40
10	20 (cool-down phase)

STEP 2

Toss the ball (playing catch with an easy wind-up) on alternate days.

Number of Throws	Distance (ft)
10	20 (warm-up)
10	30-40
30-40	50
10	20-30 (cool-down)

STEP 3

Continue increasing the throwing distance while still tossing the ball with an easy wind-up.

Number of Throws	Distance (ft)
10	20 (warm-up)
10	30-40
30-40	50-60
10	30 (cool-down)

STEP 4

Increase throwing distance to a maximum of 60 feet. Continue tossing the ball with an occasional throw at no more than half speed.

Number of Throws	Distance (ft)
10	30 (warm-up)
10	40-45
30-40	60-70
10	30 (cool-down)

STEP 5

During this step, gradually increase the distance to 150 feet maximum.

Phase 5-1

Number of Throws	Distance (ft)
10	40 (warm-up)
10	50-60
15-20	70-80
10	50-60
10	40 (cool-down)

Continued

Interval Throwing Program for Pitchers *Continued*

STEP 5—cont'd

Phase 5-2

Number of Throws	Distance (ft)
10	40 (warm-up)
10	50-60
20-30	80-90
20	50-60
10	40 (cool-down)

Phase 5-3

Number of Throws	Distance (ft)
10	40 (warm-up)
10	60
15-20	100-110
20	60
10	40 (cool-down)

Phase 5-4

Number of Throws	Distance (ft)
10	40 (warm-up)
10	60
15-20	120-150
20	60
10	40 (cool-down)

STEP 6

Progress to throwing off the mound at half to three-fourths speed. Try to use proper body mechanics, especially when throwing off the mound.
- Stay on top of the ball.
- Keep the elbow up.
- Throw over the top.
- Follow through with the arm and trunk.
- Use the legs to push.

Phase 6-1

Number of Throws	Distance (ft)
10	60 (warm-up)
10	120-150 (lobbing)
30	45 (off the mound)
10	60 (off the mound)
10	40 (cool-down)

Phase 6-2

Number of Throws	Distance (ft)
10	50 (warm-up)
10	120-150 (lobbing)
20	45 (off the mound)
20	60 (off the mound)
10	40 (cool-down)

Interval Throwing Program for Pitchers   *Continued*

STEP 6—cont'd

Phase 6-3

Number of Throws	Distance (ft)
10	50 (warm-up)
10	60
10	120-150 (lobbing)
10	45 (off the mound)
30	60 (off the mound)
10	40 (cool-down)

Phase 6-4

Number of Throws	Distance (ft)
10	50 (warm-up)
10	120-150 (lobbing)
10	45 (off the mound)
40-50	60 (off the mound)
10	40 (cool-down)

At this time, if the pitcher has successfully completed phase 6-4 without pain or discomfort and is throwing approximately three-fourths speed, the pitching coach and trainer may allow the pitcher to proceed to step 7: "up/down bullpens." Up/down bullpens is used to simulate a game. The pitcher rests between a series of pitches to reproduce the rest period between innings.

STEP 7

• Up/down bullpens (half to three-fourths speed)

Day 1

Number of Throws	Distance (ft)
10 warm-up throws	120-150 (lobbing)
10 warm-up throws	60 (off the mound)
40 pitches	60 (off the mound)
Rest 10 min	
20 pitches	60 (off the mound)

Day 2

• Off

Day 3

Number of Throws	Distance (ft)
10 warm-up throws	120-150 (lobbing)
10 warm-up throws	60 (off the mound)
30 pitches	60 (off the mound)
Rest 10 min	
20 pitches	60 (off the mound)
Rest 10 min	
10 warm-up throws	60 (off the mound)
20 pitches	60 (off the mound)

Continued

Interval Throwing Program for Pitchers   Continued

STEP 7—cont'd

Day 4

• Off

Day 5

Number of Throws	Distance (ft)
10 warm-up throws	120-150 (lobbing)
10 warm-up throws	60 (off the mound)
30 pitches	60 (off the mound)
Rest 8 min	
20 pitches	60 (off the mound)
Rest 8 min	
20 warm-up throws	60 (off the mound)
Rest 8 min	
20 pitches	60 (off the mound)

At this point the pitcher is ready to begin a normal routine, from throwing batting practice to pitching in the bullpen. This program can and should be adjusted as needed by the trainer or physical therapist. Each step may take more or less time than listed, and the program should be monitored by the trainer, physical therapist, and physician. The pitcher should remember that it is necessary to work hard but not overdo it.

REHABILITATION PROTOCOL

Interval Throwing Program for Catchers, Infielders, and Outfielders
Wilk

Note: Perform each step three times. All throws should have an arc or "hump."
The maximum distance thrown by infielders and catchers is 120 feet. The maximum distance thrown by outfielders is 200 feet.

STEP 1

Toss the ball with no wind-up. Stand with your feet shoulder-width apart and face the player to whom you are throwing. Concentrate on rotating and staying on top of the ball.

Number of Throws	Distance (ft)
5	20 (warm-up)
10	30
5	20 (cool-down)

STEP 2

Stand sideways to the person to whom you are throwing. Feet are shoulder-width apart. Close up and pivot onto your back foot as you throw.

Number of Throws	Distance (ft)
5	30 (warm-up)
5	40
10	50
5	30 (cool-down)

Interval Throwing Program for Catchers, Infielders, and Outfielders   *Continued*

STEP 3

Repeat the position in step 2. Step toward the target with your front leg and follow through with your back leg.

Number of Throws	Distance (ft)
5	50 (warm-up)
5	60
10	70
5	50 (cool-down)

STEP 4

Assume the pitcher's stance. Lift and stride with your lead leg. Follow through with your back leg.

Number of Throws	Distance (ft)
5	60 (warm-up)
5	70
10	80
5	60 (cool-down)

STEP 5

Outfielders: Lead with your glove-side foot forward. Take one step, crow-hop, and throw the ball.

Infielders: Lead with your glove-side foot forward. Take a shuffle step and throw the ball. Throw the last five throws in a straight line.

Number of Throws	Distance (ft)
5	70 (warm-up)
5	90
10	100
5	80 (cool-down)

STEP 6

Use the throwing technique presented in step 5. Assume your playing position. Infielders and catchers do not throw farther than 120 feet. Outfielders do not throw farther than 150 feet (mid-outfield).

Number of Throws	Infielders' and Catchers' Distance (ft)	Outfielders' Distance (ft)
5	80 (warm-up)	80 (warm-up)
5	80-90	90-100
5	90-100	110-125
5	110-120	130-150
5	80 (cool-down)	80 (cool-down)

STEP 7

Infielders, catchers, and outfielders all may assume their playing positions.

Number of Throws	Infielders' and Catchers' Distance (ft)	Outfielders' Distance (ft)
5	80 (warm-up)	80-90 (warm-up)
5	80-90	110-130
5	90-100	150-175

Continued

Interval Throwing Program for Catchers, Infielders, and Outfielders   Continued

STEP 7—cont'd

Number of Throws	Infielders' and Catchers' Distance (ft)	Outfielders' Distance (ft)
5	110-120	180-200
5	80 (cool-down)	90 (cool-down)

STEP 8

Repeat step 7. Use a fungo bat to hit to the infielders and outfielders while in their normal playing positions.

REHABILITATION PROTOCOL	*Interval Program for Tennis Players* Wilk

This tennis protocol is designed to be performed every other day. Each session should begin with the warm-up exercises as outlined below. Continue with your strengthening, flexibility, and conditioning exercises on days that you are not following the tennis protocol.

WARM-UP

Lower Extremity

* Jog four laps around the tennis court
* Stretches
  * Gastrocnemius
  * Achilles tendon
  * Hamstring
  * Quadriceps

Upper Extremity

* Shoulder stretches
  * Posterior cuff
  * Inferior capsule
  * Rhomboids
    * Forearm/wrist stretches
    * Wrist flexors
    * Wrist extensors

Trunk

* Side bends
* Extension
* Rotation

Forehand Ground Strokes

Hit toward the fence on the opposite side of the court. Do not worry about getting the ball in the court.

   During all of the strokes listed above, remember the following key steps:

* Bend your knees
* Turn your body

Interval Program for Tennis Players   *Continued*

WARM-UP—cont'd

- Step toward the ball
- Hit the ball when it is out in front of you

Avoid hitting with an open stance because this places undue stress on your shoulder. It is especially more stressful during the forehand stroke if you have had anterior instability or impingement problems. It is also true during the backhand if you have had problems of posterior instability.

On the very first day of these sport-specific drills, start with bouncing the ball and hitting it. Try to bounce the ball yourself and hit it at waist level. This will allow for consistency in the following:

- How the ball comes to you
- Approximating your timing between hits
- Hitting toward a target to ensure follow-through and full extension
- Using the proper mechanics, thereby placing less stress on the anterior aspect of the shoulder

WEEK 1

Day 1

- 25 forehand strokes
- 25 backhand strokes

Day 2

If there are no problems after the first-day workout, increase the number of forehand and backhand strokes.
- 50 forehand strokes
- 50 backhand strokes

Day 3

- 50 forehand strokes (waist level)
- 50 backhand strokes (waist level)
- 25 high forehand strokes
- 25 high backhand strokes

WEEK 2

Progress to having the ball tossed to you in a timely manner so that you have enough time to recover from your deliberate follow-through (i.e., wait until the ball bounces on the other side of the court before tossing another ball). Always aim the ball at a target or at a spot on the court.

If you are working on basic ground strokes, have someone bounce the ball to you consistently at waist height.

If you are working on high forehands, have the ball bounced to you at shoulder height or higher.

Day 1

- 25 high forehand strokes
- 50 waist-high forehand strokes
- 50 waist-high backhand strokes
- 25 high backhand strokes

Continued

Interval Program for Tennis Players   *Continued*

WEEK 2—cont'd

Day 2

- 25 high forehand strokes
- 50 waist-high forehand strokes
- 50 waist-high backhand strokes
- 25 high backhand strokes

Day 3

Alternate hitting the ball cross-court and down the line with waist-high and high forehand and backhand strokes
- 25 high forehand strokes
- 50 waist-high forehand strokes
- 50 waist-high backhand strokes
- 25 high backhand strokes

WEEK 3

Continue the three-times-per-week schedule. Add regular and high forehand and backhand volleys. At this point you may begin having someone hit tennis balls to you from a basket of balls. This will allow you to get the feel of the ball as it comes off another tennis racket. Your partner should wait until the ball that you hit has bounced on the other side of the court before hitting another ball to you. This will give you time to emphasize your follow-through and not hurry to return for the next shot. As always, emphasis is placed on proper body mechanics.

Day 1

- 25 high forehand strokes
- 50 waist-high forehand strokes
- 50 waist-high backhand strokes
- 25 high backhand strokes
- 25 low backhand and forehand volleys
- 25 high backhand and forehand volleys

Day 2

Same as day 1, week 3

Day 3

Same as day 2, week 3 with emphasis on direction (i.e., down the line and cross-court). Remember, good body mechanics is still a must:
- Keep your knees bent
- Hit the ball on the rise
- Hit the ball in front of you
- Turn your body
- Do not hit the ball with an open stance
- Stay on the balls of your feet

WEEK 4

Day 1

Continue having your partner hit tennis balls to you from out of a basket. Alternate hitting forehand and backhand strokes with lateral movement along the baseline. Again, emphasis is on good mechanics as described previously.

Interval Program for Tennis Players   *Continued*

WEEK 4—cont'd

Alternate hitting the ball down the line and cross-court. This drill should be done with a full basket of tennis balls (100-150 tennis balls).

Follow this drill with high and low volleys using half a basket of tennis balls (50-75 balls). This drill is also performed with lateral movement and returning to the middle of the court after the ball is hit.

Your partner should continue allowing enough time for you to return to the middle of the court before hitting the next ball so that you avoid rushing your stroke and using faulty mechanics.

Day 2

Same drills as day 1, week 4

Day 3

Same drills as day 2, week 4

WEEK 5
Day 1

Find a partner able to hit consistent ground strokes (able to hit the ball to the same area consistently, e.g., to your forehand with the ball bouncing about waist high).

Begin hitting ground strokes with the partner alternating hitting the ball to your backhand and to your forehand. Rally for about 15 minutes; then add volleys with your partner hitting to you from the baseline. Alternate between backhand and forehand volleys and high and low volleys. Continue volleying another 15 minutes. You will have rallied for a total of 30 to 40 minutes.

At the end of the session, practice a few serves while standing along the baseline. First, warm up by shadowing for 1 to 3 minutes. Hold the tennis racquet loosely and swing across your body in a figure 8. Do not swing the racquet hard. When you are ready to practice your serves with a ball, be sure to keep your toss out in front of you, get your racquet up and behind you, bend your knees, and hit up on the ball. Forget about how much power you are generating, and forget about hitting the ball between the service lines. Try hitting the ball as though you are hitting it toward the back fence.

Hit approximately 10 serves from each side of the court. Remember, this is the first time you are serving, so do not try to hit at 100% of your effort.

Day 2

Same as day 1, week 5, but now increase the number of times you practice your serve. After working on your ground strokes and volleys, return to the baseline and work on your second serve. Hit up on the ball, bend your knees, follow through, and keep the toss in front of you. This time hit 20 balls from each side of the court (i.e., 20 into the deuce court and 20 into the ad court).

Day 3

Same as day 2, week 5, with ground strokes, volleys, and serves. Do not add to the serves. Concentrate on the following:
• Bending your knees
• Preparing the racket
• Using footwork
• Hitting the ball out in front of you

Continued

Interval Program for Tennis Players   *Continued*

WEEK 5—cont'd

- Keeping your eyes on the ball
- Following through
- Getting in position for the next shot
- Keeping the toss in front of you during the serve

The workout should be the same as day 2, but if you emphasize the proper mechanics listed previously, you should feel as though you had a harder workout than on day 2.

WEEK 6

Day 1

After the usual warm-up program, start with specific ground stroke drills, with you hitting the ball down the line and your partner on the other side hitting the ball cross-court. This will force you to move quickly on the court. Emphasize good mechanics as mentioned previously.

Perform this drill for 10 to 15 minutes before reversing the direction of your strokes. Now have your partner hit down the line while you hit cross-court.

Proceed to the next drill with your partner hitting the ball to you. Return balls using a forehand, then a backhand, then a put-away volley. Repeat this sequence for 10 to 15 minutes. End this session by serving 50 balls to the ad court and 50 balls to the deuce court.

Day 2

Same as day 1, week 6, plus returning serves from each side of the court (deuce and ad court). End with practicing serves, 50 to each court.

Day 3

Perform the following sequence: warm-up; cross-court and down-the-line drills; backhand, forehand, and volley drills; return of serves; and practice serves.

WEEK 7

Day 1

Perform the warm-up program. Perform drills as before and practice return of serves. Before practicing serving, work on hitting 10 to 15 overhead shots. Continue emphasizing good mechanics. Add the approach shot to your drills.

Day 2

Same as day 1, week 7, except double the number of overhead shots (25-30 overheads).

Day 3

Perform warm-up exercises and cross-court drills. Add the overhead shot to the backhand, forehand, and volley drill to make it the backhand, forehand, volley, and overhead drill.

If you are a serious tennis player, you will want to work on other strokes or other parts of your game. Feel free to gradually add them to your practice and workout sessions. Just as in other strokes, the proper mechanics should be applied to drop volley, slice, heavy topspin, drop shots, and lobs, offensive and defensive.

Interval Program for Tennis Players Continued

WEEK 8

Day 1

Warm-up and play a simulated one-set match. Be sure to take rest periods after every third game. Remember, you will have to concentrate harder on using good mechanics.

Day 2

Perform another simulated game but with a two-set match.

Day 3

Perform another simulated game, this time a best-of-three-set match.

If all goes well, you may make plans to return to your regular workout and game schedule. You may also practice or play on consecutive days if your condition allows it.

REHABILITATION PROTOCOL *Interval Program for Golfers* Wilk

This sport-specific protocol is designed to be performed every other day. Each session should begin with the warm-up exercises outlined here. Continue the strengthening, flexibility, and conditioning exercises on the days you are not playing or practicing golf. Advance one stage every 2 to 4 weeks, depending on the severity of the shoulder problem, as each stage becomes pain free in execution.

WARM-UP

Lower extremities: Jog or walk briskly around the practice green area three or four times; stretch the hamstrings, quadriceps, and Achilles tendon.

Upper extremities: Stretch the shoulder (posterior cuff, anterior cuff, rhomboid) and wrist flexors and extensors.

Trunk: Do side bends, extension, and rotation stretching exercises.

Stage 1
Putt	50	3 times/wk
Medium long	0	0 times/wk
Long	0	0 times/wk

Stage 2
Putt	50	3 times/wk
Medium long	20	2 times/wk
Long	0	0 times/wk

Stage 3
Putt	50	3 times/wk
Medium long	40	3 times/wk
Long	0	0 times/wk

Not more than one third best distance

Stage 4
Putt	50	3 times/wk
Medium long	50	3 times/wk
Long	10	2 times/wk

Up to half best distance

Continued

Interval Program for Golfers   *Continued*

WARM-UP—cont'd

Stage 5

Putt	50	3 times/wk
Medium long	50	3 times/wk
Long	10	3 times/wk

Stage 6

Putt	50	3 times/wk
Medium long	50	3 times/wk
Long	20	3 times/wk

Play a round of golf in lieu of one practice session per week

---

Rehabilitation after Débridement of Irreparable or Massive Rotator Cuff Tears

The rehabilitation program for patients with **"irreparable"** massive rotator cuff tears after undergoing arthroscopic subacromial decompression and rotator cuff débridement focuses on **four critical treatment areas:**

- Gradual **attainment of motion** through passive and active-assisted stretching techniques. Full motion should be obtained by 3 to 4 weeks after surgery.
- Gradual restoration of shoulder **strength**, beginning with the rotator cuff and scapulothoracic muscles (Fig. 3-69) and then progressing to the deltoid muscles.
- Re-establishment of "balance of muscular forces" at the GH joint to allow arm elevation.
- **The key to restoring active shoulder elevation in these patients is strengthening of the *posterior rotator cuff muscles.***
- Burkhart (2001) reported that weakness of the posterior rotator cuff otherwise "uncouples" the force couple and leads to anterior-superior translation of the humeral head with active arm elevation.
- Restoration of dynamic stability to the GH joint through proprioceptive and neuromuscular training drills.
  - Internal and external rotation rhythmic stabilization drills are done at various degrees of nonpainful arm elevation (see Fig. 3-68).

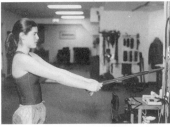   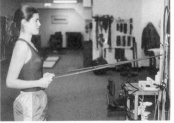

A   B

Figure 3–69   Open-chain scapular strengthening with Thera-Band tubing. **A,** Start. **B,** Finish.

- External rotation is strengthened with light isotonic and isometric exercises.
- Patients should continue their preinjury exercise programs three times a week or more. The fundamental shoulder exercise program is continued.

Shoulder Instability

The GH joint is inherently lax or loose because of its osseous configuration. It exhibits the greatest amount of motion found in any joint in the body. The shoulder sacrifices stability for mobility and, as a result, is the most common joint dislocated, with over 90% of dislocations occurring anteriorly. "Shoulder instability" is an all-encompassing term that includes the entire range of disorders, such as dislocation, subluxation, and "pathologic" laxity. To understand the terminology related to shoulder instability, the various terms commonly associated with this condition must be defined. **Translation** is movement of the humerus with respect to the glenoid articular surface. **Laxity** is the amount of translation that occurs. Some laxity is expected in normal shoulders. In fact, more than a centimeter of posterior laxity is common, especially in athletes. Consequently, **instability must be defined as unwanted translations of the GH joint experienced by the patient**. The ability of the examiner to translate the humerus greater than 1 cm or onto the rim of the glenoid does not represent instability. However, if that maneuver reproduces the symptoms, which the patient may describe as "**slipping**," "**giving way**," or "**painful**," this is supportive evidence of GH joint instability. Finally, a **shoulder dislocation** is defined as complete loss of the articulation between the humeral head and the glenoid socket. **Subluxation** refers to partial loss of GH joint articulation to the extent that symptoms are produced.

The stability of the GH joint is dependent on its static and dynamic stabilizers. The **static stabilizers**, such as the glenoid labrum and articular congruity, can be affected only by surgical means, not rehabilitation. However, the **dynamic stabilizers**, which primarily consist of the rotator cuff and coordination between scapular movement and humeral movement, can be dramatically influenced by a proper rehabilitation program. **Strengthening of the musculature around the shoulder is the foundation of all rehabilitation programs for shoulder instability**.

We have already focused on the diagnosis and treatment of overhead athletes who have underlying micro-instability that may predispose them to secondary impingement, internal impingement, rotator cuff tendinitis, rotator cuff tears, or any combination of these conditions. This section focuses on the diagnosis and treatment of patients with symptomatic anterior, posterior, and multidirectional instability.

Classification of Shoulder Instability

FREQUENCY

Acute
Recurrent
Fixed (chronic)

Continued

Classification of Shoulder Instability   *Continued*

CAUSE

Traumatic event (macrotrauma)
Atraumatic event (voluntary, involuntary)
Microtrauma
Congenital
Neuromuscular condition (Erb's palsy, cerebral palsy, seizures)

DIRECTION

Anterior
Posterior
Inferior
Multidirectional

DEGREE

Dislocation
Subluxation
Microtrauma (transient)

From Warren RF, Craig EV, Altcheck DW: The Unstable Shoulder. Philadelphia, Lippincott-Raven, 1999.

Directional Classification

ANTERIOR SHOULDER INSTABILITY

Traumatic, acute dislocation (subcoracoid, subglenoid, subclavicular, intrathoracic)
Traumatic, acute subluxation
Recurrent anterior instability
- Chronic recurrent anterior dislocation
- Chronic recurrent anterior subluxation
Fixed (locked) anterior dislocation

POSTERIOR SHOULDER INSTABILITY

Traumatic, acute dislocation (subacromial, subglenoid, subspinous)
Traumatic, acute subluxation
Recurrent posterior instability
- Recurrent posterior dislocation
- Recurrent posterior subluxation
Voluntary (atraumatic) subluxation-dislocation
- Positional type
- Muscular type
Chronic (locked) dislocation (size of a reversed Hill-Sachs lesion)
- <25% of the articular surface
- 25% to 40% of the articular surface
- <40% of the articular surface

Directional Classification   *Continued*

MULTIDIRECTIONAL SHOULDER INSTABILITY

Type I	Global instability: atraumatic multidirectional instability
Type II	Anterior-inferior instability: acute macrotraumatic episode in the setting of underlying hyperlaxity
Type III	Posterior-inferior instability: repetitive microtraumatic episodes in the setting of underlying hyperlaxity
Type IV	Anterior-posterior instability

From Warren RF, Craig EV, Altcheck DW: The Unstable Shoulder. Philadelphia, Lippincott-Raven, 1999.

ANTERIOR SHOULDER INSTABILITY

Anterior shoulder instability is the most common type of GH joint instability and can be caused by a traumatic dislocation or repetitive microtrauma that results in symptomatic episodes of subluxation. More than 90% of shoulder dislocations occur anteriorly, **usually with the arm in abduction and external rotation.** This represents the "weakest position of the GH joint biomechanically" and is the "**classic position" for anterior instability**.

The **diagnosis of traumatic anterior dislocation** is usually straightforward when one takes a detailed history, including the position of the arm at the time of injury and the mechanism of injury, and performs a detailed physical examination. The mechanism of injury generally involves indirect levering of the humeral head anteriorly with the shoulder positioned in a combination of abduction and external rotation. Less commonly, the dislocation can be caused by a direct blow to the posterior of the shoulder with the force directed anteriorly.

Physical Examination

- The affected shoulder is usually held in slight abduction and external rotation, with the forearm cradled by the unaffected arm.
- There may be a palpable fullness in the anterior aspect of the shoulder.
- Internal rotation and adduction may be limited.
- Evaluation for neurologic injuries is critical before any relocation maneuver is performed. **The axillary nerve is most commonly injured with an anterior dislocation.** This risk increases with patient age, duration of dislocation, and the severity of trauma that caused the dislocation.
- Critical in the evaluation process is a complete radiographic "trauma shoulder series" to rule out a concomitant fracture.
- Initial treatment includes a reduction procedure and some form of analgesic control, with radiographs taken after reduction to confirm successful relocation and a repeat neurologic examination performed to ensure that no nerve injury or entrapment has occurred during the reduction.

Recurrent anterior instability is the most common problem after a primary anterior dislocation. The most consistent and significant factor influencing recurrence is **age at primary dislocation**, but in reality, it may be a reflection of the activities more common in a younger population than an older population. **Patients younger than 30 years have an average risk of approximately 70% for recurrent dislocation when treated via a nonsurgical rehabilitation program**. Overall, the average recurrence rate is approximately 50% with nonoperative management. Recurrent instability is diagnosed by the history and confirmed by a thorough physical examination in patients demonstrating a positive apprehension sign (see Fig. 3-32) and positive relocation test (see Fig. 3-34). The natural history of recurrent anterior instability is altered if early operative stabilization is performed. In a prospective, randomized study, Kirkley and coworkers (1999) showed a significant difference in the rate of recurrent anterior dislocation in two groups of patients with an average age of 22 years. **One group was treated with a rehabilitation program and had a redislocation rate of 47%, whereas the other group was treated with an arthroscopic stabilization procedure and had a redislocation rate of 15% at an average follow-up of 2 years**.

Nonoperative Treatment

Conservative management of anterior shoulder instability has been associated with a more successful outcome in patients older than 30 years. Younger patients treated conservatively usually require a longer course of immobilization in the hope of achieving a successful outcome. However, it should be recognized that the length of immobilization has been only loosely associated with decreasing the risk for recurrence, and further scientific studies are needed to prove its value. **Because recurrence is the most common complication, the goal of the rehabilitation program is to optimize shoulder stability**. Avoidance of any provocative maneuvers and careful muscle strengthening are important components of the rehabilitation program as outlined in the following protocols.

REHABILITATION PROTOCOL — *Nonoperative Management of Anterior Shoulder Instability*
Bach, Cohen, and Romeo

PHASE 1: WEEKS 0-2

Restrictions

- Avoid provocative positions of the shoulder that risk recurrent instability, including
  - External rotation
  - Abduction
  - Distraction

Immobilization

- Sling immobilization—remove for exercises.
- Duration of immobilization is age dependent
  - <20 years old—3 to 4 weeks
  - 20-30 years old—2 to 3 weeks
  - >30 years old—10 days to 2 weeks
  - >40 years old—3 to 5 days

Nonoperative Management of Anterior Shoulder Instability   *Continued*

PHASE 1: WEEKS 0-2—cont'd

Pain Control

- Reduction of pain and discomfort is essential for recovery
  - Medications
    - ○ Narcotics—for 5-7 days after a traumatic dislocation
    - ○ NSAIDs—to reduce inflammation (e.g., celecoxib [Celebrex])
  - Therapeutic modalities
    - ○ Ice, ultrasound, HVGS
    - ○ Moist heat before therapy; ice at end of session

Motion: Shoulder

- Begins during phase 1 for patients 30 years and older
- Follows the protocol as outlined in phase 2

Motion: Elbow

- Passive—progress to active
  - 0-130 degrees of flexion
  - Pronation and supination as tolerated

Muscle Strengthening

- Scapular stabilizer strengthening begins during phase 1 for patients 30 years and older
  - Follows the protocol as outlined in phase 2
- Grip strengthening

PHASE 2: WEEKS 3-4

Criteria for Progression to Phase 2

- Reduced pain and tenderness
- Adequate immobilization

Restrictions

- Avoid provocative positions of the shoulder that risk recurrent instability
- Shoulder motion
  - 140 degrees of forward flexion
  - 40 degrees of external rotation with the arm at the side
- Avoid extension—**puts additional stress on anterior structures**

Immobilization

- Sling—as per criteria outlined in phase 1

Motion: Shoulder

Goals

- 140 degrees of forward flexion
- 40 degrees of external rotation with the arm at the side

Exercises

- Begin with Codman pendulum exercises to promote early motion.
- Passive ROM exercises (see Fig. 3-43).
- Active-assisted ROM exercises (see Fig. 3-42).
- Active ROM exercises.

Continued

Nonoperative Management of Anterior Shoulder Instability   Continued

PHASE 2: WEEKS 3-4—cont'd

Muscle Strengthening

- Rotator cuff strengthening
  - Begin with closed-chain isometric strengthening with the elbow flexed to 90 degrees and the arm comfortably at the side (see Fig. 3-44)
    - Internal rotation
    - External rotation
    - Forward flexion
- Strengthening of scapular stabilizers
  - Closed-chain strengthening exercises (see Figs. 3-45 and 3-62)
    - Scapular retraction (rhomboideus, middle trapezius)
    - Scapular protraction (serratus anterior)
    - Scapular depression (latissimus dorsi, trapezius, serratus anterior)
    - Shoulder shrugs (trapezius, levator scapulae)

PHASE 3: WEEKS 4-8

Criteria for Progression to Phase 3

- Pain-free motion of 140 degrees of forward flexion and 40 degrees of external rotation with the arm at the side
- Minimal pain or tenderness with strengthening exercises
- Improvement in strength of the rotator cuff and scapular stabilizers

Restrictions

- Avoid positions that exacerbate instability
  - Abduction-external rotation
- Shoulder motion
  - 160 degrees of forward flexion
  - 40 degrees of external rotation with the arm in 30-45 degrees of abduction

Motion: Shoulder

Goals

- 160 degrees of forward flexion
- 40 degrees of external rotation with the arm in 30-45 degrees of abduction

Exercises

- Passive ROM exercises (see Fig. 3-44)
- Active-assisted ROM exercises (see Fig. 3-42)
- Active ROM exercises

Muscle Strengthening

- Rotator cuff strengthening
  - Closed-chain isometric strengthening with the arm in 35-45 degrees of abduction
  - Progress to open-chain strengthening with Thera-Bands (see Fig. 3-47A)
    - Exercises performed with the elbow flexed to 90 degrees
    - Starting position is with the shoulder in the neutral position of 0 degrees of forward flexion, abduction, and external rotation. The arm should be comfortable at the patient's side
    - Exercises are performed through an arc of 45 degrees in each of the five planes of motion

Nonoperative Management of Anterior Shoulder Instability   *Continued*

PHASE 3: WEEKS 4-8—cont'd

- ○ Six color-coded bands are available; each provides increasing resistance from 1 to 6 pounds at increments of 1 pound
- ○ Progression to the next band occurs usually at 2- to 3-week intervals. Patients are instructed to not progress to the next band if there is any discomfort at the present level
- ○ Thera-Band exercises permit concentric and eccentric strengthening of the shoulder muscles and are a form of isotonic exercises (characterized by variable speed and fixed resistance)
  - ▪ Internal rotation
  - ▪ External rotation
  - ▪ Abduction
  - ▪ Forward flexion
- • Progress to light isotonic dumbbell exercises
  - ○ Internal rotation
  - ○ External rotation
  - ○ Abduction
  - ○ Forward flexion
- • Strengthening of scapular stabilizers
  - ○ Continue with closed-chain strengthening exercises (see Figs. 3-45 and 3-62)
  - ○ Advance to open-chain, isotonic strengthening exercises (see Fig. 3-46)
- • Initiate deltoid strengthening in the plane of the scapula to 90 degrees of elevation

PHASE 4: WEEKS 8-12

Criteria for Progression to Phase 4

- • Pain-free motion of 160 degrees of forward flexion and 40 degrees of external rotation with the arm in 30-45 degrees of abduction
- • Minimal pain or tenderness with strengthening exercises
- • Continued improvement in strength of the rotator cuff and scapular stabilizers
- • Satisfactory physical examination

Goals

- • Improve shoulder strength, power, and endurance
- • Improve neuromuscular control and shoulder proprioception
- • Restore full shoulder motion

Restriction

- • Avoid positions that exacerbate instability

Pain Control

- • As outlined in phase 3

Motion: Shoulder

Goals

- • Obtain motion that is at least equal to that on the contralateral side

Exercises

- • Use passive, active-assisted, and active ROM exercises to obtain motion goals

Continued

Nonoperative Management of Anterior Shoulder Instability   *Continued*

PHASE 4: WEEKS 8-12—cont'd

Capsular Stretching

• Especially the posterior capsule (see Fig. 3-56)

Muscle Strengthening

• Continue with strengthening of the rotator cuff, scapular stabilizers, and deltoid
  • 8-12 repetitions for three sets

Upper Extremity Endurance Training

• Incorporated endurance training for the upper extremity
  • Upper body ergometer

Proprioceptive Training

• PNF patterns (Fig. 3-70)

PHASE 5: WEEKS 12-16

Criteria for Progression to Phase 5

• Pain-free ROM
• No evidence of recurrent instability
• Recovery of 70% to 80% of shoulder strength
• Satisfactory physical examination

Goals

• Prepare for gradual return to functional and sporting activities
• Establish a home exercise maintenance program that is performed at least three times per week for both stretching and strengthening

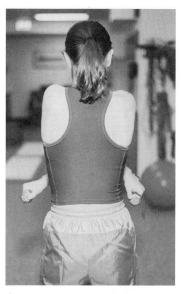

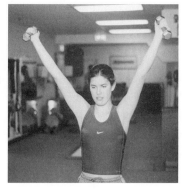

A

B

Figure 3–70 Example of one proprioceptive neuromuscular facilitation pattern. **A**, Start. **B**, Finish.

Nonoperative Management of Anterior Shoulder Instability   *Continued*

PHASE 5: WEEKS 12-16—cont'd

Functional Strengthening

- Plyometric exercises (see Fig. 3-48)

Progressive, Systematic Interval Program for Returning to Sports

- Golfers—see page 281
- Overhead athletes not before **6 months**
  - Throwing athletes—see pages 271 to 276
  - Tennis players—see page 276

Maximum improvement is expected by 6 months.

Warning Signs

- Persistent instability
- Loss of motion
- Lack of strength progression—especially abduction
- Continued pain

Treatment of Complications

- These patients may need to move back to earlier routines
- May require increased utilization of pain control modalities as outlined above
- May require surgical intervention
  - Recurrent instability is defined as three or more instability events within a year or instability that occurs at rest or during sleep. These findings are strong indications for surgical management

---

REHABILITATION PROTOCOL | *Nonoperative Rehabilitation for Anterior Shoulder Instability*
Wilk

The program will vary in length for each individual, depending on several factors:
- Severity of injury
- Acute versus chronic condition
- ROM/strength status
- Performance/activity demands

PHASE 1: ACUTE MOTION PHASE

Goals

- Re-establish nonpainful ROM
- Retard muscular atrophy
- Decrease pain/inflammation

Note: During the early rehabilitation program, caution must be applied in placing the anterior capsule under stress (i.e., avoid abduction, external rotation) until dynamic joint stability is restored.

Continued

Nonoperative Rehabilitation for Anterior Shoulder Instability   *Continued*

PHASE 1: ACUTE MOTION PHASE—cont'd

Decrease Pain and Inflammation

- Therapeutic modalities (e.g., ice, electrotherapy)
- NSAIDs
- *Gentle* joint mobilization

Range-of-Motion Exercises

- Pendulums
- Circumduction
- Rope and pulley
  - Flexion
  - Abduction to 90 degrees; progress to full ROM
- L-bar
  - Flexion
  - Abduction
  - Internal rotation with the arm in the scapular plane
  - External rotation with the arm in the scapular plane (*progress arm to 90 degrees of abduction as tolerated*)
- Posterior capsular stretching
- Upper extremity ergometer

Shoulder hyperextension is contraindicated.

Strengthening Exercises

- Isometrics
  - Flexion
  - Abduction
  - Extension
  - Internal rotation (multiple angles)
  - External rotation (scapular plane)
- Weight shifts (closed-chain exercises)

PHASE 2: INTERMEDIATE PHASE

Criteria for Progression to Phase 2

- Full ROM
- Minimal pain or tenderness
- "Good" manual muscle test (MMT) of internal rotation, external rotation, flexion, and abduction

Goals

- Regain and improve muscular strength
- Normalize arthrokinematics
- Improve neuromuscular control of shoulder complex

Initiate Isotonic Strengthening

- Flexion
- Abduction to 90 degrees
- Internal rotation
- Side-lying external rotation to 45 degrees
- Shoulder shrugs
- Extension
- Horizontal adduction

Nonoperative Rehabilitation for Anterior Shoulder Instability   *Continued*

PHASE 2: INTERMEDIATE PHASE—cont'd

- Supraspinatus
- Biceps
- Push-ups

Initiate Eccentric (Surgical Tubing) Exercises at 0 Degrees Abduction

- Internal rotation
- External rotation

Normalize Arthrokinematics of the Shoulder Complex

- Continue joint mobilization
- Patient education on mechanics and modification of activity/sport

Improve Neuromuscular Control of the Shoulder Complex

- Initiation of PNF (see Fig. 3-70)
- Rhythmic stabilization drills (see Figs. 3-67 and 3-68)

Continue Use of Modalities (As Needed)

- Ice, electrotherapy modalities

PHASE 3: ADVANCED STRENGTHENING PHASE

Criteria for Progression to Phase 3

- Full nonpainful ROM
- No palpable tenderness
- Continued progression of resistive exercises

Goals

- Improve strength, power, and endurance
- Improve neuromuscular control
- Prepare patient/athlete for activity

Continue Use of Modalities (as Needed)

Continue Posterior Capsular Stretches

Continue Isotonic Strengthening (Progressive Resistance Exercises)

Continue Eccentric Strengthening

Emphasize PNF

Initiate Isokinetics

- Flexion-extension
- Abduction-adduction
- Internal-external rotation
- Horizontal abduction/adduction

Initiate Plyometric Training

- Surgical tubing
- Wall push-ups
- Medicine ball
- Boxes

Continued

Nonoperative Rehabilitation for Anterior Shoulder Instability   *Continued*

PHASE 3: ADVANCED STRENGTHENING PHASE—cont'd

Initiate Military Press

Precaution—avoid excessive stress on the anterior capsule.

PHASE 4: RETURN-TO-ACTIVITY PHASE

Criteria for Progression to Phase 4

- Full ROM
- No pain or palpable tenderness
- Satisfactory isokinetic test
- Satisfactory clinical examination

Goals

- Maintain optimal level of strength, power, and endurance
- Progressively increase activity level to prepare the patient for full functional return to activity/sport

Continue All Exercises as in Phase 3

Continue Posterior Capsular Stretches

Initiate Interval Program

Continue Modalities (as Needed)

Follow-up

- Isokinetic test
- Progress interval program
- Maintenance of exercise program

Operative Treatment

Operative stabilization is indicated in patients with irreducible dislocations, displaced tuberosity fractures, or glenoid rim fractures involving 25% or more of the anterior-inferior glenoid rim. **Patients who experience three or more instability events in a year (recurrent) or instability during rest or sleep are also appropriate candidates for surgical management.** A **relative indication** for surgical intervention is a younger patient, especially an **athlete who desires continued participation in sports** or work activities. **In this population, early surgical intervention will reduce the statistically high risk for recurrent instability and allow return to sports**. The problem with conservative treatment in this patient group is that it is less likely to alter the natural history of the shoulder instability. The athlete may have fewer or no episodes of instability with a conservative treatment program during the "off-season." However, with the return of the next season, if the instability becomes symptomatic, the athlete will risk losing two seasons, which essentially ends competitive participation, especially for a high-level athlete.

The **traditional open Bankart repair** is the **standard of care** for open stabilization procedures, with a **recurrence rate of less than 5%**. Recurrence after arthroscopic stabilization procedures has been highly variable, with early reports suggesting recurrence rates anywhere from 0% to 45%. The higher failure rates are probably the result of poor surgical technique and an accelerated rehabilitation program that ignored the normal biology of tissue repair, which is the same for both operative procedures. **Recent literature has shown a recurrence rate of 8% to 17% after arthroscopic Bankart repairs**, which is related to better surgical technique and more traditional postoperative rehabilitation. Advantages of arthroscopic stabilization procedures include cosmetic incisions, less postoperative pain, and earlier recovery of external rotation.

The operative technique chosen depends on which technique the surgeon is most comfortable with. Like arthroscopic rotator cuff repairs, arthroscopic stabilization procedures are technically more challenging and require a clear understanding of the pathoanatomy. Rehabilitation after stabilization procedures is detailed on page 296. The rehabilitation program is essentially the same for open and arthroscopic techniques because the biology of healing tissue is the same, and the consideration of subscapularis tendon healing is contained within the time frame of healing for the GH capsulolabral complex.

Complications after Shoulder Stabilization Surgery

Numerous complications may develop after shoulder stabilization surgery for instability and may include
- Limitation of motion
- Recurrent instability
- Inability to return to the preinjury level of play in the sport
- Development of osteoarthritis

The most common complication after shoulder stabilization surgery is loss of motion (especially external rotation).

For these reasons, the goals of rehabilitation after shoulder stabilization are
1. Maintenance of integrity of the surgically corrected stability
2. Gradual restoration of full functional ROM
3. Enhancement of dynamic stability (of muscles surrounding the shoulder)
4. Return to full unrestricted activity and sport

Factors Affecting Rehabilitation after Shoulder Stabilization Procedures

TYPE OF SURGICAL PROCEDURE

Exposure
  Open
  Arthroscopic
Type of procedure
  Bankart
  Capsular shift, etc.

METHOD OF FIXATION

Suture anchors
Bioabsorbable sutures

Continued

Factors Affecting Rehabilitation after Shoulder Stabilization Procedures   *Continued*

TYPE OF INSTABILITY

Anterior
Posterior
Multidirectional

TISSUE STATUS OF PATIENT

Normal
Hyperelasticity
Hypoelasticity

PATIENT'S RESPONSE TO SURGERY

DYNAMIC STABILIZERS STATUS

Muscle development
Muscle strength
Dynamic stability
Proprioceptive abilities

PATIENT'S PREINJURY ACTIVITY STATUS

Athletic versus nonathletic
Overhead thrower versus sedentary
Postoperative goals

PHYSICIAN'S PHILOSOPHIC APPROACH

REHABILITATION PROTOCOL	*After an Anterior Surgical Stabilization Procedure*
	Bach, Cohen, and Romeo

PHASE 1: WEEKS 0-4

Restrictions

- Shoulder motion
  - 140 degrees of forward flexion
  - 40 degrees of external rotation
    - Initially with the arm at the side
    - After 10 days, can progress to 40 degrees of external rotation with the arm in increasing amounts of abduction, up to 45 degrees
- Active ROM only—no passive ROM or manipulation by the therapist
  - Patients after an open stabilization procedure with a take-down of the subscapularis insertion are restricted from active internal rotation for 4 weeks
- Avoid provocative maneuvers that re-create position of instability (e.g., abduction-external rotation)

Immobilization

- Sling immobilization
  - 4-week duration—during day and **especially at night**

After an Anterior Surgical Stabilization Procedure   Continued

PHASE 1: WEEKS 0-4—cont'd

Pain Control

- Reduction of pain and discomfort is essential for recovery
  - Medications
    - ○ Narcotics—for 7-10 days after surgery
    - ○ NSAIDs—for patients with persistent discomfort after surgery
  - Therapeutic modalities
    - ○ Ice, ultrasound, HVGS
    - ○ Moist heat before therapy; ice at end of session

Motion: Shoulder

- Goals: **Active ROM exercises only**
  - 140 degrees of forward flexion
  - 40 degrees of external rotation with the arm at the side
  - After 10 days, can progress to external rotation with the arm abducted up to 45 degrees
  - **No active internal rotation for patients after an open stabilization procedure with removal and subsequent repair of the subscapularis insertion**
- Exercises
  - Begin with Codman pendulum exercises to promote early motion
  - Active ROM exercises
    - ○ Passive internal rotation to the stomach for patients restricted from active internal rotation

Motion: Elbow

- Passive—progress to active
  - 0-130 degrees of flexion
  - Pronation and supination as tolerated

Muscle Strengthening

- Rotator cuff strengthening—within the limits of the active ROM exercises
  - Closed-chain isometric strengthening with the elbow flexed to 90 degrees and the arm at the side (see Fig. 3-44B)
    - ○ Internal rotation
      - ■ No internal rotation strengthening before 6 weeks after open stabilization with removal and subsequent repair of the subscapularis insertion
    - ○ External rotation
    - ○ Abduction
    - ○ Forward flexion
  - Grip strengthening

PHASE 2: WEEKS 4-8

Criteria for Progression to Phase 2

- Minimal pain and discomfort with active ROM and closed-chain strengthening exercises
- No sensation or findings of instability with above exercises

Continued

After an Anterior Surgical Stabilization Procedure   *Continued*

PHASE 2: WEEKS 4-8—cont'd

Restrictions

- Shoulder motion: active ROM only
  - 160 degrees of forward flexion
  - 60 degrees of external rotation
  - 70 degrees of abduction
- **Avoid provocative maneuvers that re-create the position of instability**
  - *Abduction-external rotation*
- *Note*: For overhead athletes, the restrictions are less. Although there is a higher risk for recurrent instability, the need for full motion to perform overhead sports requires that most athletes regain motion to within 10 degrees of normal for the affected shoulder by 6-8 weeks after surgery

Immobilization

- Sling—discontinue

Pain Control

- Medications
  - NSAIDs—for patients with persistent discomfort
- Therapeutic modalities
  - Ice, ultrasound, HVGS
  - Moist heat before therapy; ice at end of session

Motion: Shoulder

- Goals
  - 160 degrees of forward flexion
  - 50 degrees of external rotation
  - 70 degrees of abduction
- Exercises
  - Active ROM exercises
- *Note:* For overhead athletes, the motion goals should be within 10 degrees of normal for the affected shoulder

Muscle Strengthening

- Rotator cuff strengthening—within the limits of active ROM exercises
  - Closed-chain isometric strengthening with the elbow flexed to 90 degrees and the arm at the side (see Fig. 3-44B)
    - Internal rotation
      - No internal rotation strengthening before 6 weeks after open stabilization with removal and subsequent repair of the subscapularis insertion
    - External rotation
    - Abduction
    - Forward flexion
  - Progress to light open-chain and isotonic strengthening with Thera-Bands (see Fig. 3-47A)
    - Exercises performed with the elbow flexed to 90 degrees
    - Starting position is with the shoulder in the neutral position of 0 degrees of forward flexion, abduction, and external rotation
    - Exercises are performed through an arc of at least 45 degrees in each of the five planes of motion—within the guidelines of allowed motion

After an Anterior Surgical Stabilization Procedure   *Continued*

PHASE 2: WEEKS 4-8—cont'd

- ○ Six color-coded bands are available; each provides increasing resistance from 1 to 6 pounds at increments of 1 pound
- ○ Progression to the next band occurs usually at 2- to 3-week intervals. Patients are instructed to not progress to the next band if there is any discomfort at the present level
- ○ Thera-Band exercises permit concentric and eccentric strengthening of the shoulder muscles and are a form of isotonic exercises (characterized by variable speed and fixed resistance)
- ○ Internal rotation
  - ▪ Hold internal rotation strengthening until 6 weeks for the subscapularis repair group
- ○ External rotation
- ○ Abduction
- ○ Forward flexion
- • Strengthening of scapular stabilizers
  - • Closed-chain strengthening exercises (Fig. 3-71; see also Figs. 3-45 and 3-62)
    - ○ Scapular retraction (rhomboideus, middle trapezius)
    - ○ Scapular protraction (serratus anterior)
    - ○ Scapular depression (latissimus dorsi, trapezius, serratus anterior)
    - ○ Shoulder shrugs (trapezius, levator scapulae)

PHASE 3: WEEKS 8-12

Criteria for Progression to Phase 3

- • Minimal pain or discomfort with active ROM and muscle strengthening exercises
- • Improvement in strengthening of the rotator cuff and scapular stabilizers
- • Satisfactory physical examination

Goals

- • Improve shoulder strength, power, and endurance
- • Improve neuromuscular control and shoulder proprioception
- • Restore full shoulder motion
- • Establish a home exercise maintenance program that is performed at least three times per week for both stretching and strengthening

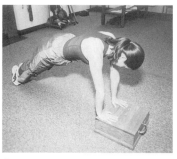 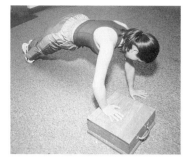

A   B

Figure 3–71   Closed-chain strengthening of the scapular stabilizers. **A**, Start. **B**, Finish.

Continued

After an Anterior Surgical Stabilization Procedure Continued

PHASE 3: WEEKS 8-12—cont'd

Pain Control

- Medications
  - NSAIDs—for patients with persistent discomfort
  - Subacromial injection: corticosteroid/local anesthetic combination
    ○ For patients with findings consistent with secondary impingement
  - GH joint: corticosteroid/local anesthetic combination
    ○ For patients whose clinical findings are consistent with GH joint pathology
- Therapeutic modalities
  - Ice, ultrasound, HVGS
  - Moist heat before therapy; ice at end of session

Motion: Shoulder

Goals

- Obtain motion equal to that on the contralateral side
- Active ROM exercises
- Active-assisted ROM exercises (see Fig. 3-42)
- Passive ROM exercises (see Fig. 3-43)
- Capsular stretching (especially the posterior capsule [see Fig. 3-56])

Muscle Strengthening

- Rotator cuff strengthening—three times per week, 8-12 repetitions for three sets
  - Continue with advancing Thera-Band strengthening
  - Progress to light isotonic dumbbell exercises (see Fig. 3-47B)
- Scapular stabilizer strengthening
  - Continue with closed-chain strengthening
  - Progress to open-chain strengthening (see Figs. 3-46 and 3-47)

Upper Extremity Endurance Training

- Incorporated endurance training for the upper extremity
  - Upper body ergometer

Proprioceptive Training

- PNF patterns (see Fig. 3-70)

Functional Strengthening

- Plyometric exercises (see Fig. 3-48)

Progressive, Systematic Interval Program for Returning to Sports

- Golfers—see page 281
- Overhead athletes not before 6 months
  - Throwing athletes—see pages 271 to 276
  - Tennis players—see page 276

Maximum improvement is expected by 12 months; most patients can return to sports and full-duty work status by 6 months.

After an Anterior Surgical Stabilization Procedure   *Continued*

PHASE 3: WEEKS 8-12—cont'd

Warning Signs

- Persistent instability
- Loss of motion
- Lack of strength progression—especially abduction
- Continued pain

Treatment of Complications

- These patients may need to move back to earlier routines
- May require increased utilization of pain control modalities as outlined above
- May require imaging work-up or repeat surgical intervention

---

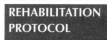

REHABILITATION PROTOCOL

After Open (Bankart) Anterior Capsulolabral Reconstruction
Wilk

PHASE 1: IMMEDIATE POSTOPERATIVE PHASE

Goals

- Protect the surgical procedure
- Minimize the effects of mobilization
- Diminish pain and inflammation

Weeks 0-2

- Sling for comfort (1 week)
- May wear immobilizer for sleep (2 weeks) —physician's decision
- Elbow/hand ROM
- Gripping exercises
- Passive ROM and active-assisted ROM (L-bar)
  - Flexion to tolerance
  - Abduction to tolerance
  - External and internal rotation in the scapular plane
- Submaximal isometrics
- Rhythmic stabilization
- Cryotherapy, modalities as needed

Weeks 3-4

- Gradually progress ROM
  - Flexion to 120-140 degrees
  - External rotation in the scapular plane to 35-45 degrees
  - Internal rotation in the scapular plane to 45-60 degrees
  - Shoulder extension
- Initiate light isotonics for the shoulder musculature
  Tubing for external and internal rotation
  Dumbbell exercises for the deltoid, supraspinatus, biceps, and scapular musculature
  Continue dynamic stabilization exercises, PNF
- Initiate self-assisted capsular stretching

Continued

After Open (Bankart) Anterior Capsulolabral Reconstruction Continued

PHASE 1: IMMEDIATE POSTOPERATIVE PHASE—cont'd

Weeks 5-6

- Progress ROM as tolerated
  - Flexion to 160 degrees (maximum)
  - External and internal rotation at 90 degrees abduction
    - ○ Internal rotation to 75 degrees
    - ○ External rotation to 70-75 degrees
  - Shoulder extension to 30-35 degrees
- Joint mobilization, stretching, etc.
- Continue self-assisted capsular stretching
- Upper body ergometer with the arm at 90 degrees abduction
- Progress all strengthening exercises
  - Continue PNF diagonal patterns (rhythmic stabilization techniques)
  - Continue isotonic strengthening
  - Dynamic stabilization exercises

Weeks 6-7

- Progress ROM to
  - External rotation at 90 degrees abduction: 80-85 degrees
  - External rotation at 90 degrees abduction: 70-75 degrees
  - Flexion: 165-175 degrees

PHASE 2: INTERMEDIATE PHASE

Goals

- Re-establish full ROM
- Normalize arthrokinematics
- Improve muscular strength
- Enhance neuromuscular control

Weeks 8-10

- Progress to full ROM (weeks 7-8)
- Continue all stretching exercises
  - Joint mobilization, capsular stretching, passive and active stretching
- In overhead athletes, progress external rotation past 90 degrees
- In nonoverhead athletes, maintain 90-degree external rotation
- Continue strengthening exercises
  - "Thrower's Ten" program (for overhead athletes)
  - Isotonic strengthening for entire shoulder complex
  - PNF manual technique
  - Neuromuscular control drills
  - Isokinetic strengthening

Weeks 10-14

- Continue all flexibility exercises
- Continue all strengthening exercises
- May initiate *light* plyometric exercises
- May initiate *controlled* swimming, golf swings, etc.
- May initiate *light isotonic machine weight* training (weeks 12-14)

After Open (Bankart) Anterior Capsulolabral Reconstruction   *Continued*

PHASE 3: ADVANCED STRENGTHENING PHASE (MONTHS 4-6)

Criteria for Progression to Phase 3

- Full ROM
- No pain or tenderness
- Satisfactory stability
- Strength 70% to 80% of contralateral side

Goals

- Enhance muscular strength, power, and endurance
- Improve muscular endurance
- Maintain mobility

Weeks 14-20

- Continue all flexibility exercises
  - Self-assisted capsular stretches (anterior, posterior, and inferior)
  - Maintain external rotation flexibility
- Continue isotonic strengthening program
- Emphasize muscular balance (external and internal rotation)
- Continue PNF manual resistance
- May initiate and continue plyometrics
- Initiate interval throwing program (physician's approval necessary) (see pp. 271 to 276)

Weeks 20-24

- Continue all exercises listed above
- Continue and progress all elements of the interval sport program (throwing, etc.)

PHASE 4: RETURN-TO-ACTIVITY PHASE (MONTHS 6-9)

Criteria for Progression to Phase 4

- Full nonpainful ROM
- Satisfactory stability
- Satisfactory strength (isokinetics)
- No pain or tenderness

Goals

- Gradual return to sport activities
- Maintain strength and mobility of shoulder

Exercises

- Continue capsular stretching to maintain mobility
- Continue strengthening program
  - Either "Thrower's Ten" or fundamental shoulder exercise program
- Return to sport participation (unrestricted)

REHABILITATION PROTOCOL

After Arthroscopic Anterior Shoulder Stabilization
Wilk

PHASE 1: IMMEDIATE POSTOPERATIVE PHASE—"RESTRICTIVE MOTION"

Goals

- Protect the anatomic repair
- Prevent negative effects of immobilization
- Promote dynamic stability
- Diminish pain and inflammation

Weeks 0-2

- No active external rotation or extension or abduction
- Sling for 2 weeks
- Sleep in immobilizer for 2-4 weeks
- Elbow/hand ROM
- Hand gripping exercises
- Passive and gentle active-assisted ROM exercises
  - Flexion to 60 degrees
  - Elevation in the scapular plane to 60 degrees
  - External and internal rotation with the arm in 20 degrees of abduction
  - External rotation to 5-10 degrees
  - Internal rotation to 45 degrees
  - Submaximal isometrics for shoulder musculature
  - Cryotherapy, modalities as indicated

Weeks 3-4

- Discontinue sling
- May use immobilizer for sleep (physician's decision)
- Continue gentle ROM exercises (passive and active-assisted ROM)
  - Flexion to 90 degrees
  - Abduction to 75-85 degrees
  - External rotation in the scapular plane to 15-20 degrees
  - Internal rotation in the scapular plane to 55-60 degrees
- *Note:* The rate of progression is based on evaluation of the patient.
- **No active external rotation, extension, or elevation**
- Continue isometrics and rhythmic stabilization (submaximal)
- Continue use of cryotherapy

Weeks 5-6

- Gradually improve ROM
  - Flexion to 135-140 degrees
  - External rotation at 45 degrees abduction: 25-30 degrees
  - External rotation at 45 degrees abduction: 55-60 degrees
- May initiate stretching exercises
- Initiate external and internal rotation (arm at the side) with exercise tubing
- PNF manual resistance

After Arthroscopic Anterior Shoulder Stabilization   Continued

PHASE 2: INTERMEDIATE PHASE—MODERATE PROTECTION PHASE

Goals

- Gradually restore full ROM (week 10)
- Preserve the integrity of the surgical repair
- Restore muscular strength and balance

Weeks 7-9

- Gradually progress ROM
  - Flexion to 160 degrees
  - External rotation at 90 degrees abduction: 70-75 degrees
  - Internal rotation at 90 degrees abduction: 70-75 degrees
- Continue to progress isotonic strengthening program
- Continue PNF strengthening

Weeks 10-14

- May initiate slightly more aggressive strengthening
- Progress isotonic strengthening exercises
- Continue all stretching exercises
- Progress ROM to functional demands (i.e., overhead athlete)

PHASE 3: MINIMAL PROTECTION PHASE

Criteria for Progression to Phase 3

- Full nonpainful ROM
- Satisfactory stability
- Muscular strength (good grade or better)
- No pain or tenderness

Goals

- Establish and maintain full ROM
- Improve muscular strength, power, and endurance
- Gradually initiate functional activities

Weeks 15-18

- Continue all stretching exercises (capsular stretches)
- Continue strengthening exercises
  - "Thrower's Ten" program or fundamental exercises
  - PNF manual resistance
  - Endurance training
  - Initiate light plyometric program
  - Restricted sport activities (light swimming, half golf swings)

Weeks 18-21

- Continue all exercise listed earlier
- Initiate interval sport program (throwing, etc.)

Continued

After Arthroscopic Anterior Shoulder Stabilization   *Continued*

PHASE 4: ADVANCED STRENGTHENING PHASE

Criteria for Progression to Phase 4

- Full nonpainful ROM
- Satisfactory static stability
- Muscular strength 75% to 80% of the contralateral side
- No pain or tenderness

Goals

- Enhance muscular strength, power, and endurance
- Progress functional activities
- Maintain shoulder mobility

Weeks 22-24

- Continue flexibility exercises
- Continue isotonic strengthening program
- PNF manual resistance patterns
- Plyometric strengthening
- Progress interval sport programs

PHASE 5: RETURN-TO-ACTIVITY PHASE (MONTHS 6-9)

Criteria for Progression to Phase 5

- Full functional ROM
- Satisfactory isokinetic test that fulfills criteria
- Satisfactory shoulder stability
- No pain or tenderness

Goals

- Gradual return to sport activities
- Maintain strength, mobility, and stability

Exercises

- Gradually progress sport activities to unrestricted participation
- Continue stretching and strengthening program

POSTERIOR SHOULDER INSTABILITY

Posterior instability is much less common than anterior instability. Posterior dislocations are most frequently caused by a generalized muscle contraction after a **seizure**, which can be related to epilepsy, alcohol abuse, or severe electric shock. Patients with a posterior shoulder dislocation hold the arm in adduction and internal rotation. A fullness may be palpable in the posterior aspect of the shoulder, and **abduction and external rotation may be limited**. A complete radiographic evaluation of the shoulder is required, **especially an axillary lateral view**. If an axillary lateral radiograph cannot be obtained, a computed tomography (CT) scan of the GH joint should be done. **In approximately 80% of patients with posterior dislocation of** the GH joint, the diagnosis is not made by the initial treating physician because of incomplete radiographic evaluation, which is why *all* shoulder injuries must have an axillary lateral view as part of the radiograph series.

Posterior instability in athletes commonly results in subluxation, usually secondary to repetitive microtrauma. For example, posterior instability may develop in an offensive lineman in football because of the forward-flexed and internally rotated shoulder position needed for blocking. On physical examination, patients with posterior instability demonstrate increased posterior translation on posterior drawer testing. Symptoms are reproduced when a posteriorly directed force is placed on the patient's arm in the adducted, forward-flexed position.

Treatment of Traumatic Posterior Dislocation

Treatment of a traumatic posterior dislocation that is successfully reduced usually **begins with immobilization in a brace that maintains the shoulder in external rotation and neutral to slight extension**. Immobilization is continued for 6 weeks, and then a structured rehabilitation program is followed, similar to the one outlined on page 308. Variations may be required, depending on the position of immobilization, positions producing recurrent instability, freedom of full external rotation, and restriction of internal rotation. **The basic premise of treating an unstable shoulder with physical therapy is to strengthen the dynamic stabilizers (muscles and tendons) while the static stabilizers (including the glenoid labrum) heal**.

Indications for surgical stabilization of a posterior shoulder dislocation include
- A displaced lesser tuberosity fracture
- A posterior glenoid rim fracture of more than 25%
- An impaction fracture of the anterior-superior humeral articular surface (reverse Hill-Sachs lesion) of more than 40%
- An irreducible dislocation
- Recurrent posterior dislocations
- An unstable reduction (usually associated with a reverse Hill-Sachs lesion of 20% to 40%)

Patients with unstable reductions may have pathology similar to that after anterior dislocation, namely, avulsion of the capsule and labrum from the posterior glenoid rim. This can be repaired with an open or arthroscopic technique. The rehabilitation protocol after surgical repair of the capsulolabral complex for posterior dislocation is outlined on page 310.

Patients who have symptomatic posterior instability with no history of a traumatic dislocation usually benefit from a rehabilitation program that focuses on strengthening of the dynamic stabilizers. Patients who do not improve after an organized rehabilitation program for 3 to 6 months may require surgical treatment. These patients typically have a lax posterior capsule, which can be treated with an arthroscopic technique (capsular suture plication, electrothermal capsulorrhaphy [shrinkage]), followed by rehabilitation as outlined on page 308, or with an open posterior stabilization procedure followed by rehabilitation as outlined on page 310.

REHABILITATION PROTOCOL	*Nonoperative Rehabilitation for Posterior Shoulder Instability*
	Wilk

This program is designed to return the patient/athlete to activity/sport as quickly and safely as possible. The program will vary in length for each individual, depending on the severity of injury, ROM/strength status, and performance/activity demands.

PHASE 1: ACUTE PHASE

Goals

- Decrease pain and inflammation
- Re-establish nonpainful ROM
- Retard muscle atrophy

Decrease Pain and Inflammation

- Therapeutic modalities (e.g., ice, heat, electrotherapy)
- NSAIDs
- Gentle joint mobilization

Range-of-Motion Exercises

- Pendulum
- Rope and pulley
- L-bar
  - Flexion
  - Abduction
  - Horizontal abduction
  - External rotation

Strength Exercises

- Isometric
  - Flexion
  - Abduction
  - Extension
  - External rotation
- Weight shifts (closed-chain exercises)

Note: Avoid any motion that may place stress on the posterior capsule, such as excessive internal rotation, abduction, or horizontal adduction.

PHASE 2: IMMEDIATE PHASE

Criteria for Progression to Phase 2

- Full ROM
- Minimal pain and tenderness
- "Good" MMT

Goals

- Regain and improve muscular strength
- Normal arthrokinematics
- Improve neuromuscular control of the shoulder complex

Nonoperative Rehabilitation for Posterior Shoulder Instability   *Continued*

PHASE 2: IMMEDIATE PHASE—cont'd

Initiate Isotonic Strengthening

- Flexion
- Abduction to 90 degrees
- External rotation
- Internal rotation (from full external rotation to 0 degrees)
- Supraspinatus
- Extension
- Horizontal abduction (prone)
- Push-ups

Initiate Eccentric (Surgical Tubing) Strengthening

- External rotation (from 0 degrees to full external rotation)
- Internal rotation (from full external rotation to 0 degrees)

Normalize Arthrokinematics of the Shoulder Complex

- Continue joint mobilization
- Patient education on mechanics of activity/sport

Improve Neuromuscular Control of the Shoulder Complex

- Initiate PNF
- Rhythmic stabilization drills

Continue Use of Modalities (As Needed)

- Ice, electrotherapy modalities

PHASE 3: ADVANCED STRENGTHENING PHASE

Criteria for Progression to Phase 3

- Full nonpainful ROM
- No palpable tenderness
- Continued progression of resistive exercises

Goals

- Improve strength, power, and endurance
- Improve neuromuscular control
- Prepare athlete for activity

Continue Use of Modalities (As Needed)

Continue Anterior Capsule Stretch

Continue Isotonic Strengthening

Continue Eccentric Strengthening

Emphasize PNF (D2 Extension)

Initiate Isokinetics

- Flexion-extension
- Abduction-adduction
- Internal and external rotation
- Horizontal abduction-adduction

Continued

Nonoperative Rehabilitation for Posterior Shoulder Instability   *Continued*

PHASE 3: ADVANCED STRENGTHENING PHASE—cont'd

Initiate Plyometric Training

- Surgical tubing
- Medicine ball
- Wall push-ups

Initiate Military Press

PHASE 4: RETURN-TO-ACTIVITY PHASE

Criteria for Progression to Phase 4

- Full ROM
- No pain or tenderness
- Satisfactory clinical examination
- Satisfactory isokinetic test

Goals

- Maintain optimal level of strength, power, and endurance
- Progressively increase activity level to prepare patient/athlete for full functional return to activity/sport

Continue All Exercises as in Phase 3

Initiate and Progress Interval Program

REHABILITATION PROTOCOL   *Posterior Capsular Shift*
Wilk

The goal of this rehabilitation program is to return the patient/athlete to activity/sport as quickly and safely as possible while maintaining a stable shoulder. This program is based on shoulder anatomy, biomechanics, and the healing constraints of the surgical procedure.

The posterior capsular shift procedure is one in which the orthopaedic surgeon makes an incision into the ligamentous capsule of the posterior aspect of the shoulder then pulls the capsule tighter and sutures it together.

PHASE 1: PROTECTION PHASE (WEEKS 0-6)

Precautions

- Postoperative brace in 30-45 degrees abduction, 15 degrees external rotation for 4-6 weeks
- Brace must be worn at all times with the exception of exercise activity and bathing
- No overhead activity
- Must sleep in brace

Goals

- Allow healing of sutured capsule
- Initiate early protected ROM
- Retard muscular atrophy
- Decrease pain and inflammation

Posterior Capsular Shift   *Continued*

PHASE 1: PROTECTION PHASE (WEEKS 0-6)—cont'd

Weeks 0-4

Exercises

- Gripping exercises with putty
- Active elbow flexion-extension and pronation-supination
- Active ROM of cervical spine
- Passive ROM progressing to active-assisted ROM
- Active-assisted ROM
  - External rotation at 30-45 degrees of abduction: 25-30 degrees
  - Flexion to 90 degrees as tolerated
  - Internal rotation at 30-45 degrees of abduction (week 3): 15-25 degrees
- Submaximal shoulder isometrics
  - Flexion
  - Abduction
  - Extension
  - External rotation

Note: In general, all exercises begin with one set of 10 repetitions and should increase by one set of 10 repetitions daily as tolerated to five sets of 10 repetitions.

Cryotherapy: Ice before and after exercises for 20 minutes. Ice up to 20 min/hr to control pain and swelling.

Criteria for Hospital Discharge

- Passive shoulder ROM to 90 degrees flexion and 25 degrees external rotation
- Minimal pain and swelling
- "Good" proximal and distal muscle power

Weeks 4-6

Goals

- Gradual increase in ROM
- Normalize arthrokinemetrics
- Improve strength
- Decrease pain and inflammation

Range-of-Motion Exercises

T-bar active-assisted exercises
- External rotation from 45-90 degrees of shoulder abduction
- Shoulder flexion to tolerance
- Shoulder abduction to 90 degrees
- Internal rotation at 45 degrees of abduction: 35 degrees
- Rope and pulley
  - Shoulder abduction to tolerance
  - Shoulder flexion to 90 degrees
- All exercises should be performed to tolerance
- Take to the point of pain and/or tolerance and hold (5 seconds)
- *Gentle* self-assisted capsular stretches

Continued

Posterior Capsular Shift Continued

PHASE 1: PROTECTION PHASE (WEEKS 0-6)—cont'd

Gentle Joint Mobilization to Re-establish Normal

- Arthrokinetmatics
- Scapulothoracic joint
- GH joint—avoid posterior glides
- SC joint

Strengthening Exercises

- Active abduction to 90 degrees
- Active external rotation from neutral to 90 degrees
- Elbow/wrist progressive resistance exercise program

Conditioning Program For

- Trunk
- Lower extremities
- Cardiovascular endurance

Decrease Pain and Inflammation

- Ice, NSAIDs, modalities

Brace

- Discontinue 4-6 weeks after surgery per physician's direction

PHASE 2: INTERMEDIATE PHASE (WEEKS 6-12)

Goals

- Full, nonpainful ROM at week 8 (except internal rotation)
- Normalize arthrokinematics
- Increase strength
- Improve neuromuscular control

Weeks 6-9

Range-of-Motion Exercises

- T-bar active-assisted exercises
  - External rotation to tolerance
  - Shoulder abduction to tolerance
  - Shoulder flexion to tolerance
  - Rope and pulley: flexion-abduction

Joint Mobilization

- Continue as above

Strengthening Exercises

- Tubing for internal and external rotation at 0 degrees abduction
- Initiate isotonic dumbbell program
  - Shoulder abduction
  - Shoulder flexion
  - Latissimus dorsi
  - Rhomboids

Posterior Capsular Shift   *Continued*

PHASE 2: INTERMEDIATE PHASE (WEEKS 6-12)—cont'd

- Biceps curl
- Triceps kick-out over table
- Shoulder shrugs
- Push-ups into wall (serratus anterior)

Initiate Neuromuscular Control Exercises for Sternoclavicular Joint

Weeks 10-12

- Continue all exercises listed above

Initiate

- Active-assisted internal rotation to the 90/90 position
- Dumbbells for the supraspinatus
- Tubing exercises for the rhomboids, latissimus dorsi, biceps, and triceps
- Progressive push-ups

PHASE 3: DYNAMIC STRENGTHENING PROGRAM (WEEKS 12-18)

Criteria for Progression to Phase 3

- Full, nonpainful ROM
- No pain/tenderness
- Strength 70% of contralateral side

Weeks 13-15

Goals

- Improve strength, power, and endurance
- Improve neuromuscular control

Emphasis of Phase 3

- High-speed/high-energy strengthening exercises
- Eccentric exercises
- Diagonal patterns

Exercises

- Continue internal and external rotation tubing exercises at 0 degrees abduction (arm at side)
- Tubing for rhomboids
- Tubing for latissimus dorsi
- Tubing for biceps and triceps
- Continue dumbbell exercise for supraspinatus and deltoid
- Progressive serratus anterior push-up—anterior flexion
- Continue trunk and lower extremity strengthening and conditioning exercises
- Continue self-assisted capsular stretches

Weeks 16-20

- Continue all exercises as above
- Emphasis on gradual return to recreational activities

Continued

Posterior Capsular Shift   *Continued*

PHASE 4: RETURN-TO-ACTIVITY PHASE (WEEKS 21-28)

Criteria for Progression to Phase 4

- Full ROM
- No pain or tenderness
- Satisfactory clinical examination
- Satisfactory isokinetic test

Goal

- Progressively increase activities to prepare patient for unrestricted functional return

Exercises

- Continue tubing and dumbbell exercises outlined in phase 3
- Continue ROM exercises
- Initiate internal programs between 28 and 32 weeks (if the patient is a recreational athlete)

REHABILITATION PROTOCOL   *After Posterior Shoulder Stabilization*
Bach, Cohen, and Romeo

PHASE 1: WEEKS 0-4

Restrictions

- No shoulder motion

Immobilization

- Use of a gunslinger orthosis for 4 weeks

Pain Control

- Reduction of pain and discomfort is essential for recovery
- Patients treated with an arthroscopic stabilization procedure experience less postoperative pain than do patients treated with an open stabilization procedure
  - Medications
    - Narcotics—for 7-10 days after surgery
    - NSAIDs—for patients with persistent discomfort after surgery
  - Therapeutic modalities
    - Ice, ultrasound, HVGS
    - Moist heat before therapy; ice at end of session

Motion: Shoulder

- None

Motion: Elbow

- Passive—progress to active
  - 0-130 degrees of flexion
  - Pronation and supination as tolerated

After Posterior Shoulder Stabilization   *Continued*

PHASE 1: WEEKS 0-4—cont'd

Muscle Strengthening

- Grip strengthening only

PHASE 2: WEEKS 4-8

Criteria for Progression to Phase 2

- Adequate immobilization

Restrictions

- **Shoulder motion: active ROM only**
  - Forward flexion to 120 degrees
  - Abduction to 45 degrees
  - External rotation as tolerated
  - Internal rotation and adduction to the stomach
- Avoid provocative maneuvers that re-create the position of instability
  - Avoid excessive internal rotation

Immobilization

- Gunslinger—discontinue

Pain Control

- Medications
  - NSAIDs—for patients with persistent discomfort
- Therapeutic modalities
  - Ice, ultrasound, HVGS
  - Moist heat before therapy; ice at end of session

Shoulder Motion: Active Range of Motion Only

Goals

- Forward flexion to 120 degrees
- Abduction to 45 degrees
- External rotation as tolerated
- Internal rotation and adduction to the stomach

Exercises

- Active ROM only

Muscle Strengthening

- Rotator cuff strengthening
- Closed-chain isometric strengthening with the elbow flexed to 90 degrees and the arm at the side (see Fig. 3-44)
  - Forward flexion
  - External rotation
  - Internal rotation
  - Abduction
  - Adduction

Continued

After Posterior Shoulder Stabilization   *Continued*

PHASE 2: WEEKS 4-8—cont'd

- Strengthening of scapular stabilizers
  - Closed-chain strengthening exercises (see Figs. 3-45, 3-62, and 3-71).
  - Scapular retraction (rhomboideus, middle trapezius)
  - Scapular protraction (serratus anterior)
  - Scapular depression (latissimus dorsi, trapezius, serratus anterior)
  - Shoulder shrugs (trapezius, levator scapulae)

PHASE 3: WEEKS 8-12

Criteria for Progression to Phase 3

- Minimal pain and discomfort with active ROM and closed-chain strengthening exercises
- No sensation or findings of instability with above exercises

Restrictions

- Shoulder motion: active and active-assisted motion exercises
  - 160 degrees of forward flexion
  - Full external rotation
  - 70 degrees of abduction
  - Internal rotation and adduction to the stomach

Pain Control

- Medications
  - NSAIDs—for patients with persistent discomfort
- Therapeutic modalities
  - Ice, ultrasound, HVGS
  - Moist heat before therapy; ice at end of session

Motion: Shoulder

Goals

- 160 degrees of forward flexion
- Full external rotation
- 70 degrees of abduction
- Internal rotation and adduction to the stomach

Exercises

- Active ROM exercises
- Active-assisted ROM exercises (see Fig. 3-42)

Muscle Strengthening

- Rotator cuff strengthening—three times per week, 8-12 repetitions for three sets
  - Continue with closed-chain isometric strengthening
  - Progress to open-chain strengthening with Thera-Bands (see Fig. 3-47A)
    - Exercises performed with the elbow flexed to 90 degrees
    - Starting position is with the shoulder in the neutral position of 0 degrees of forward flexion, abduction, and external rotation
    - Exercises are performed through an arc of 45 degrees in each of the five planes of motion

After Posterior Shoulder Stabilization   *Continued*

PHASE 3: WEEKS 8-12—cont'd

- ○ Six color-coded bands are available; each provides increasing resistance from 1 to 6 pounds in increments of 1 pound
- ○ Progression to the next band usually occurs at 2- to 3-week intervals. Patients are instructed to not progress to the next band if there is any discomfort at the present level
- ○ Thera-Band exercises permit concentric and eccentric strengthening of the shoulder muscles and are a form of isotonic exercises (characterized by variable speed and fixed resistance)
  - ▪ Internal rotation
  - ▪ External rotation
  - ▪ Abduction
  - ▪ Forward flexion
- • Progress to light isotonic dumbbell exercises
  - ○ Internal rotation (see Fig. 3-47B)
  - ○ External rotation (see Fig. 3-47C)
  - ○ Abduction
  - ○ Forward flexion
- • Strengthening of scapular stabilizers
  - • Continue with closed-chain strengthening exercises
  - • Advance to open-chain isotonic strengthening exercises (see Figs. 3-46 and 3-69)

PHASE 4: MONTHS 3-6

Criteria for Progression to Phase 4

- • Minimal pain or discomfort with active ROM and muscle strengthening exercises
- • Improvement in strengthening of the rotator cuff and scapular stabilizers
- • Satisfactory physical examination

Goals

- • Improve shoulder strength, power, and endurance
- • Improve neuromuscular control and shoulder proprioception
- • Restore full shoulder motion
- • Establish a home exercise maintenance program that is performed at least three times per week for both stretching and strengthening

Pain Control

- • Medications
  - • NSAIDs—for patients with persistent discomfort
  - • Subacromial injection: corticosteroid/local anesthetic combination for patients with findings consistent with secondary impingement
  - • GH joint: corticosteroid/local anesthetic combination for patients whose clinical findings are consistent with GH joint pathology
- • Therapeutic modalities
  - • Ice, ultrasound, HVGS
  - • Moist heat before therapy; ice at end of session

Continued

After Posterior Shoulder Stabilization Continued

PHASE 4: MONTHS 3-6—cont'd

Motion: Shoulder

Goals

- Obtain motion equal to that on contralateral side
- Active ROM exercises
- Active-assisted ROM exercises (see Fig. 3-42)
- Passive ROM exercises (see Fig. 3-43)
- Capsular stretching (especially posterior capsule [see Fig. 3-56])

Muscle Strengthening

- Rotator cuff and scapular stabilizer strengthening as outlined above
  - Three times per week, 8-12 repetitions for three sets

Upper Extremity Endurance Training

- Incorporate endurance training for the upper extremity
  - Upper body ergometer

Proprioceptive Training

- PNF patterns (see Fig. 3-70)

Functional Strengthening

- Plyometric exercises (see Fig. 3-48)

Progressive, Systematic Interval Program for Returning to Sports

- Golfers—see page 281
- Overhead athletes not before 6 months
  - Throwing athletes—see pages 271 to 276
  - Tennis players—see page 276

Maximum improvement is expected by 12 months.

Warning Signs

- Persistent instability
- Loss of motion
- Lack of strength progression—especially abduction
- Continued pain

Treatment of Complications

- These patients may need to move back to earlier routines
- May require increased utilization of pain control modalities as outlined above
- May require imaging work-up or repeat surgical intervention

MULTIDIRECTIONAL INSTABILITY

Multidirectional shoulder instability is not the result of a traumatic injury but is associated with hyperlaxity of the GH joint capsule in conjunction with rotator cuff weakness. Multidirectional shoulder instability can be simply defined as **symptomatic instability in more than one direction**. Patients may have a history of laxity in other joints, as demonstrated by frequent ankle sprains or recurrent patellar dislocations. Physical examination often finds generalized joint laxity, **but the key to diagnosis is the reproduction of symptoms with unwanted GH joint translation**. Patients demonstrate increased laxity in multiple directions and have a positive sulcus sign or varying degrees of inferior translation of the GH joint.

Treatment

Multidirectional instability is treated conservatively with a rehabilitation program focused on strengthening of the rotator cuff, the scapular stabilizers, and the deltoid muscles. Surgical stabilization is considered if an extensive trial of rehabilitation for at least 6 months fails to relieve symptoms. If conservative treatment fails, an open inferior capsular shift via an anterior approach is recommended. The goal of this procedure is to balance tension on all sides of the GH joint and surgically reduce capsular volume. The postoperative rehabilitation protocol is outlined on this page. Arthroscopic treatment of multidirectional instability is currently evolving. Two techniques for reducing capsular volume with promising results are suture capsular plication and electrothermal capsulorrhaphy (shrinkage). The postoperative rehabilitation protocol is outlined below.

REHABILITATION PROTOCOL — *After Open Inferior Capsular Shift for Multidirectional Instability*
Bach, Cohen, and Romeo

PHASE 1: WEEKS 0-6

Restriction

- Shoulder motion: none for 6 weeks

Immobilization

- Sling or gunslinger orthosis
  - 6 weeks—during day and at night

Pain Control

- Reduction of pain and discomfort is essential for recovery
  - Medications
    - Narcotics—for 7-10 days after surgery
    - NSAIDs—for patients with persistent discomfort after surgery
  - Therapeutic modalities
    - Ice, ultrasound, HVGS
    - Moist heat before therapy; ice at end of session

Motion: Shoulder

- None

Motion: Elbow

- Passive—progress to active
  - 0-130 degrees of flexion
  - Pronation and supination as tolerated

Continued

After Open Inferior Capsular Shift for Multidirectional Instability   *Continued*

PHASE 1: WEEKS 0-6—cont'd

Muscle Strengthening

- Rotator cuff strengthening
  - Closed-chain isometric strengthening with the elbow flexed to 90 degrees and the arm at the side in brace (see Fig. 3-44)
    - External rotation
    - Abduction
    - Forward flexion
- Grip strengthening

PHASE 2: WEEKS 7-12

Criteria for Progression to Phase 2

- Minimal pain or discomfort with ROM and closed-chain strengthening exercises
- No sensation or findings of instability with these maneuvers
- Satisfactory physical examination

Restrictions

- Shoulder motion: active ROM only
  - 140 degrees of forward flexion
  - 40 degrees of external rotation
  - 70 degrees of abduction
  - Internal rotation to the stomach
- Avoid positions that re-create instability

Pain Control

- Medications
  - NSAIDs—for patients with persistent discomfort
- Therapeutic modalities
  - Ice, ultrasound, HVGS
  - Moist heat before therapy; ice at end of session

Motion: Shoulder

- Goals
  - 140 degrees of forward flexion
  - 40 degrees of external rotation
  - 70 degrees of abduction
  - Internal rotation to the stomach
- Exercises
  - Active ROM exercises

Muscle Strengthening

- Rotator cuff strengthening—three times per week, 8-12 repetitions for three sets
  - Continue with closed-chain isometric strengthening
  - Progress to open-chain strengthening with Thera-Bands (see Fig. 3-47A)
    - Exercises performed with the elbow flexed to 90 degrees
    - Starting position is with the shoulder in the neutral position of 0 degrees of forward flexion, abduction, and external rotation
    - Exercises are performed through an arc of 45 degrees in each of the five planes of motion

After Open Inferior Capsular Shift for Multidirectional Instability Continued

PHASE 2: WEEKS 7-12—cont'd

- ○ Six color-coded bands are available; each provides increasing resistance from 1 to 6 pounds in increments of 1 pound
- ○ Progression to the next band occurs usually at 2- to 3-week intervals. Patients are instructed to not progress to the next band if there is any discomfort at the present level
- ○ Thera-Band exercises permit concentric and eccentric strengthening of the shoulder muscles and are a form of isotonic exercises (characterized by variable speed and fixed resistance)
  - ▪ Internal rotation
  - ▪ External rotation
  - ▪ Abduction
  - ▪ Forward flexion
- • Progress to light isotonic dumbbell exercises (see Fig. 3-47B and C)
  - ○ Internal rotation
  - ○ External rotation
  - ○ Abduction
  - ○ Forward flexion
- • Strengthening of scapular stabilizers
  - • Closed-chain strengthening exercises (see Figs. 3-45, 3-62, and 3-71)
    - ○ Scapular retraction (rhomboideus, middle trapezius)
    - ○ Scapular protraction (serratus anterior)
    - ○ Scapular depression (latissimus dorsi, trapezius, serratus anterior)
    - ○ Shoulder shrugs (trapezius, levator scapulae)
  - • Progress to open-chain strengthening (Fig. 3-72; see also Figs. 3-46 and 3-62)

PHASE 3: MONTHS 3-6

Criteria for Progression to Phase 3

- • Minimal pain or discomfort with active ROM and muscle strengthening exercises
- • Improvement in strengthening of the rotator cuff and scapular stabilizers
- • Satisfactory physical examination

Goals

- • Improve shoulder complex strength, power, and endurance
- • Improve neuromuscular control and shoulder proprioception
- • Restore full shoulder motion
- • Establish a home exercise maintenance program that is performed at least three times per week for both stretching and strengthening

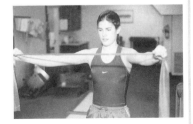

Figure 3–72 Open-chain strengthening of the scapular stabilizers with Thera-Band tubing.

Continued

After Open Inferior Capsular Shift for Multidirectional Instability   *Continued*

PHASE 3: MONTHS 3-6—cont'd

Pain Control

- Medications
  - NSAIDs—for patients with persistent discomfort
  - Subacromial injection: corticosteroid/local anesthetic combination
    - ○ For patients with findings consistent with secondary impingement
  - GH joint: corticosteroid/local anesthetic combination
    - ○ For patients whose clinical findings are consistent with GH joint pathology
- Therapeutic modalities
  - Ice, ultrasound, HVGS
  - Moist heat before therapy; ice at end of session

Motion: Shoulder

- Goals
  - Obtain motion equal to that on the contralateral side
  - Active ROM exercises
  - Active-assisted ROM exercises (see Fig. 3-42)
  - Passive ROM exercises (see Fig. 3-43)
  - Capsular stretching for selective areas of shoulder to "balance" the laxity (do not aim for full ROM)

Muscle Strengthening

- Rotator cuff and scapular stabilizer strengthening as outlined above
  - Three times per week, 8-12 repetitions for three sets
- Deltoid strengthening (Fig. 3-73; see also Fig. 3-61)

Upper Extremity Endurance Training

- Incorporate endurance training for the upper extremity
  - Upper body ergometer

Proprioceptive Training

- PNF patterns (see Fig. 3-70)

Functional Strengthening

- Plyometric exercises (see Fig. 3-48)

Progressive, Systematic Interval Program for Returning to Sports

- Golfers—see page 281
- Overhead athletes not before **6 months**
  - Throwing athletes—see pages 271 to 276
  - Tennis players—see page 276

Maximum improvement is expected by 12 months.

Warning Signs

- Persistent instability after surgery
- Development of instability symptoms from 6 to 12 months suggests failure to re-establish stability of the GH joint
- Loss of motion
- Lack of strength progression—especially abduction
- Continued pain

After Open Inferior Capsular Shift for Multidirectional Instability   Continued

PHASE 3: MONTHS 3-6—cont'd

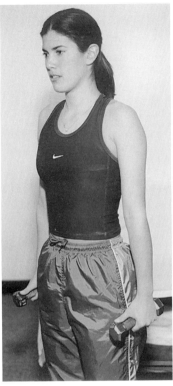

A

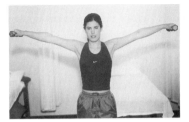

B

Figure 3–73 Isotonic deltoid strengthening with light dumbbells. **A**, Start. **B**, Finish.

Treatment of Complications

- These patients may need to move back to earlier routines
- May require increased utilization of pain control modalities as outlined above
- May require imaging work-up or repeat surgical intervention

---

REHABILITATION PROTOCOL   *After Thermal Capsulorrhaphy for Multidirectional Instability*
Bach, Cohen, and Romeo

PHASE 1: WEEKS 0-6

Restrictions

- Strict shoulder immobilization for 6 weeks
  - Sling or gunslinger orthosis, depending on the degree of instability

Continued

After Thermal Capsulorrhaphy for Multidirectional Instability   *Continued*

PHASE 1: WEEKS 0-6—cont'd

Pain Control

- Reduction of pain and discomfort is essential for recovery
  - Medications
    - Narcotics—for 7-10 days after surgery
    - NSAIDs—for patients with persistent discomfort after surgery
  - Therapeutic modalities
    - Ice, ultrasound, HVGS
    - Moist heat before therapy; ice at end of session

Motion: Shoulder

- None

Motion: Elbow

- Passive—progress to active
- 0-130 degrees of flexion
- Pronation and supination as tolerated

Muscle Strengthening

- Grip strengthening

PHASE 2: WEEKS 6-12

Criteria for Progression to Phase 2

- Adequate immobilization

Restrictions

- Shoulder motion: active ROM only
  - 140 degrees of forward flexion
  - 40 degrees of external rotation with the arm at the side
  - 60 degrees of abduction

Immobilization

- Sling or gunslinger orthosis at night

Pain Control

- Medications
  - NSAIDs—for patients with persistent discomfort
- Therapeutic modalities
  - Ice, ultrasound, HVGS
  - Moist heat before therapy; ice at end of session

Motion: Shoulder

Goals

- 140 degrees of forward flexion
- 40 degrees of external rotation with the arm at the side
- 60 degrees of abduction

Exercises

- Active ROM exercises

After Thermal Capsulorrhaphy for Multidirectional Instability   *Continued*

PHASE 2: WEEKS 6-12—cont'd

Muscle Strengthening

- Rotator cuff strengthening
  - Closed-chain isometric strengthening with the elbow flexed to 90 degrees and the arm at the side (see Fig. 3-44)
    - Internal rotation
    - External rotation
    - Abduction
    - Forward flexion

PHASE 3: MONTHS 3-6

Criteria for Progression to Phase 2

- Minimal pain or discomfort with active ROM and closed-chain strengthening exercises
- No sensation or findings of instability with these maneuvers
- Satisfactory physical examination

Restrictions

- Shoulder motion
  - 160 degrees of forward flexion
  - External rotation as tolerated with the arm at the side
  - 90 degrees of abduction
- Avoid extreme positions that may lead to instability

Pain Control

- Medications
  - NSAIDs—for patients with persistent discomfort
  - Subacromial injection: corticosteroid/local anesthetic combination
    - For patients with findings consistent with secondary impingement
  - GH joint: corticosteroid/local anesthetic combination
    - For patients whose clinical findings are consistent with GH joint pathology
- Therapeutic modalities
  - Ice, ultrasound, HVGS
  - Moist heat before therapy; ice at end of session

Motion: Shoulder

Goals

- 160 degrees of forward flexion
- External rotation as tolerated with the arm at the side
- 90 degrees of abduction
- *Note:* The goal is functional ROM without symptoms of instability, *not* full ROM

Exercises

- Active ROM exercises
- Active-assisted ROM exercises (see Fig. 3-42)
- Passive ROM exercises (see Fig. 3-43)

Continued

After Thermal Capsulorrhaphy for Multidirectional Instability Continued

PHASE 3: MONTHS 3-6—cont'd

Muscle Strengthening

- Rotator cuff strengthening—three times per week, 8-12 repetitions for three sets
  - Continue with closed-chain isometric strengthening
  - Progress to open-chain strengthening with Thera-Bands (see Fig. 3-47A)
    - Exercises performed with the elbow flexed to 90 degrees
    - Starting position is with the shoulder in the neutral position of 0 degrees of forward flexion, abduction, and external rotation
    - Exercises are performed through an arc of 45 degrees in each of the five planes of motion
    - Six color-coded bands are available; each provides increasing resistance from 1 to 6 pounds in increments of 1 pound
    - Progression to the next band occurs usually at 2- to 3-week intervals. Patients are instructed to not progress to the next band if there is any discomfort at the present level
    - Thera-Band exercises permit concentric and eccentric strengthening of the shoulder muscles and are a form of isotonic exercises (characterized by variable speed and fixed resistance)
      - Internal rotation
      - External rotation
      - Abduction
      - Forward flexion
  - Progress to light isotonic dumbbell exercises (see Fig. 3-47B)
    - Internal rotation
    - External rotation
    - Abduction
    - Forward flexion
- Strengthening of scapular stabilizers
  - Closed-chain strengthening exercises (see Figs. 3-45, 3-62, and 3-71)
    - Scapular retraction (rhomboideus, middle trapezius)
    - Scapular protraction (serratus anterior)
    - Scapular depression (latissimus dorsi, trapezius, serratus anterior)
    - Shoulder shrugs (trapezius, levator scapulae)
  - Progress to open-chain strengthening (see Figs. 3-46 and 3-72)
- Deltoid strengthening (see Figs. 3-61 and 3-73)

PHASE 4: MONTHS 6-12

Criteria for Progression to Phase 4

- Minimal pain or discomfort with active ROM and muscle strengthening exercises
- Improvement in strengthening of the rotator cuff and scapular stabilizers
- Satisfactory physical examination

Goals

- Improve shoulder complex strength, power, and endurance
- Improve neuromuscular control and shoulder proprioception
- Restore functional range of shoulder motion
- Establish a home exercise maintenance program that is performed at least three times per week for both stretching and strengthening

After Thermal Capsulorrhaphy for Multidirectional Instability   *Continued*

PHASE 4: MONTHS 6-12—cont'd

Pain Control

- Medications
  - NSAIDs—for patients with persistent discomfort
  - Subacromial injection: corticosteroid/local anesthetic combination
    - For patients with findings consistent with secondary impingement
  - GH joint corticosteroid/local anesthetic combination
    - For patients whose clinical findings are consistent with GH joint pathology
- Therapeutic modalities
  - Ice, ultrasound, HVGS
  - Moist heat before therapy; ice at end of session

Motion: Shoulder

Goals

- Obtain functional ROM without symptoms of instability; usually 10-20 degrees less motion than on opposite side

Exercises

- Active ROM exercises
- Active-assisted ROM exercises (see Fig. 3-42)
- Passive ROM exercises (see Fig. 3-43)
- Capsular stretching
  - Especially posterior capsule (see Fig. 3-56)

Muscle Strengthening

- Rotator cuff, deltoid, and scapular stabilizer strengthening as outlined above
  - Three times per week, 8-12 repetitions for three sets

Upper Extremity Endurance Training

- Incorporate endurance training for the upper extremity
  - Upper body ergometer

Proprioceptive Training

- PNF patterns (see Fig. 3-70)

Functional Strengthening

- Plyometric exercises (see Fig. 3-48)

Progressive, Systematic Interval Program for Returning to Sports

- Throwing athletes—see pages 271 to 276
- Tennis players—see page 276
- Golfers—see page 281

Maximum improvement is expected by 12 months.

Continued

After Thermal Capsulorrhaphy for Multidirectional Instability *Continued*

PHASE 4: MONTHS 6-12—cont'd

Warning Signs

- Persistent instability after surgery
- Development of instability symptoms from 6 to 12 months suggests failure to re-establish stability of the GH joint
- Loss of motion
- Lack of strength progression—especially abduction
- Continued pain

Treatment of Complications

- These patients may need to move back to earlier routines
- May require increased utilization of pain control modalities as outlined above
- May require imaging work-up or repeat surgical intervention

---

REHABILITATION PROTOCOL | *An Accelerated Rehabilitation Program after Anterior Capsular Shift–Acquired Instability in Overhead Athletes*
Wilk

This rehabilitation program's goal is to return the patient/athlete to the activity/sport as quickly and safely as possible while maintaining a stable shoulder. The program is based on muscle physiology, biomechanics, anatomy, and the healing process after surgery for a capsular shift.

The capsular shift procedure is one in which the orthopaedic surgeon makes an incision into the ligamentous capsule of the shoulder, pulls the capsule tighter, and then sutures the capsule together.

The ultimate goal is a functional shoulder and return to the presurgical functional level.

PHASE 1: PROTECTION PHASE (WEEKS 0-6)

Goals

- Allow healing of the sutured capsule
- Begin early protected ROM
- Retard muscular atrophy
- Decrease pain and inflammation

Weeks 0-2

Precautions

- Sleep in an immobilizer for 2 weeks
- No overhead activities for 4-6 weeks
- Wean from the immobilizer and into a sling as soon as possible (the orthopaedist or therapist will tell you when)

An Accelerated Rehabilitation Program after Anterior Capsular Shift–Acquired Instability in Overhead Athletes   Continued

PHASE 1: PROTECTION PHASE (WEEKS 0-6)—cont'd

Exercises

- Gripping exercises
- Elbow flexion-extension and pronation-supination
- Pendulum exercises (nonweighted)
- Rope and pulley active-assisted exercises
  - Shoulder flexion to 90 degrees
  - Shoulder abduction to 60 degrees
- L-bar exercises
  - External rotation to 15-20 degrees with the arm in the scapular plane
  - Shoulder flexion-extension to tolerance
- Active ROM of the cervical spine
- Isometrics
  - Flexion, extension, external and internal rotation, abduction

Criteria for Hospital Discharge

- Shoulder ROM (active-assisted ROM) flexion to 90 degrees, abduction to 45 degrees, external rotation to 40 degrees
- Minimal pain and swelling
- "Good" proximal and distal muscle power

Weeks 2-4

Goals

- Gradual increase in ROM
- Normalize arthrokinematics
- Improve strength
- Decrease pain and inflammation

Range-of-Motion Exercises

- L-bar active-assisted exercises
- External rotation at 45 degrees abduction to 45 degrees
- Internal rotation at 45 degrees abduction to 45 degrees
- Shoulder flexion-extension to tolerance
- Shoulder abduction to tolerance
- Shoulder horizontal abduction-adduction
- Rope and pulley extension-flexion
  - All exercises performed to tolerance
  - Take to point of pain or resistance or both and hold
  - *Gentle* self-assisted capsular stretches

Gentle Joint Mobilization to Re-establish Normal Arthrokinematics to

- Scapulothoracic joint
- GH joint
- SC joint

Strengthening Exercises

- Isometrics
- May initiate tubing for external and internal rotation at 0 degrees of shoulder abduction

Continued

An Accelerated Rehabilitation Program after Anterior Capsular Shift–Acquired Instability in Overhead Athletes   Continued

PHASE 1: PROTECTION PHASE (WEEKS 0-6)—cont'd

Conditioning Program For

- Trunk
- Lower extremities
- Cardiovascular

Decrease Pain and Inflammation

- Ice, NSAIDs, modalities

Weeks 4-5

- Active-assisted ROM flexion to tolerance (approximately 145 degrees)
- Internal and external rotation at 90 degrees abduction to tolerance
- Initiate isotonic (light weight) strengthening
- Gentle joint mobilization (grade III)

Week 6

- Active-assisted ROM; continue all stretching exercises
- Progress external and internal rotation at 90 degrees abduction
- External and internal rotation at 90 degrees abduction: 75 degrees
- Internal and external rotation at 90 degrees abduction: 75 degrees
- Flexion to 165-170 degrees
- Extension to 30 degrees

PHASE 2: INTERMEDIATE PHASE (WEEKS 7-12)

Goals

- Full nonpainful ROM at week 8
- Normalize arthrokinematics
- Increase strength
- Improve neuromuscular control

Weeks 7-9

Range-of-Motion Exercises

- L-bar active-assisted exercises
- Continue all exercises listed above
- Gradually increase ROM to full ROM at week 8
  - External rotation at 90 degrees abduction: 85-90 degrees
  - Internal rotation at 90 degrees abduction: 70-75 degrees
- Continue self-assisted capsular stretches
- Continue joint mobilization

Strengthening Exercises

- Initiate isotonic dumbbell program
  - Side-lying external rotation
  - Side-lying internal rotation
  - Shoulder abduction
  - Supraspinatus
  - Latissimus dorsi
  - Rhomboids
  - Biceps curls

***An Accelerated Rehabilitation Program after Anterior Capsular Shift–Acquired Instability
in Overhead Athletes*** *Continued*

PHASE 2: INTERMEDIATE PHASE (WEEKS 7-12)—cont'd

- Triceps curls
- Shoulder shrugs
- Push-ups into chair (serratus anterior)
- Continue tubing at 0 degrees and at 90 degrees abduction for external and internal rotation

Initiate Neuromuscular Control Exercises for the Scapulothoracic Joint

Weeks 10-12

- Continue all exercises listed above
- Initiate tubing exercises for the rhomboids, latissimus dorsi, biceps, and triceps
- Initiate aggressive stretching and joint mobilization, if needed
- Progressive ROM for an overhead thrower to functional ROM

PHASE 3: DYNAMIC STRENGTHENING PHASE (WEEKS 12-20)

Advanced Strengthening Phase (Weeks13-16)

Criteria for Progression to Phase 3

- Full nonpainful ROM
- No pain or tenderness
- Strength 70% or better in comparison to the contralateral side
- Satisfactory shoulder joint stability

Goals

- Improve strength, power, and endurance
- Improve neuromuscular control
- Maintain shoulder mobility
- Prepare athlete to begin to throw

Emphasis

- High-speed, high-energy strengthening exercises
- Eccentric exercises
- Diagonal patterns
- Functional positions of stretches and strengthening

Exercises

- Continue self-assisted capsular stretches (very important)
- "Thrower's Ten" exercises (p. 238)
  - Tubing exercises in the 90/90 position for internal and external rotation (slow set, fast sets)
  - Isotonics for
    - Rhomboids
    - Latissimus dorsi
    - Biceps
    - Diagonal D2 extension patterns
    - Diagonal D2 flexion patterns
  - Continue dumbbell exercises for the supraspinatus and deltoid
  - Continue serratus anterior strengthening exercises, floor push-ups
  - Continue all isotonic strengthening

Continued

An Accelerated Rehabilitation Program after Anterior Capsular Shift–Acquired Instability in Overhead Athletes   *Continued*

PHASE 3: DYNAMIC STRENGTHENING PHASE (WEEKS 12-20)—cont'd

- Continue trunk–lower extremity strengthening exercises
- Continue neuromuscular exercises
- Initiate plyometric training program

Weeks 17-20

- Initiate interval sport programs
- Continue all exercises
- Progress plyometrics for shoulder
  - External rotation at 90 degrees abduction
  - Internal rotation at 90 degrees abduction
  - D2 extension plyometrics
  - Biceps plyometrics
  - Serratus anterior plyometrics

PHASE 4: THROWING PHASE (WEEKS 20-26)

Criteria for Progression to Phase 4

- Full ROM
- No pain or tenderness
- Isokinetic test that fulfills criteria to throw
- Satisfactory clinical examination

Goals

- Progressively increase activities to prepare the patient for full functional return

Exercise

- Progress interval throwing program
- Continue "Thrower's Ten" exercises
- Continue plyometric five exercises
- Continue all flexibility exercises

Interval Throwing Program

- Interval throwing program phase 2, 22nd week

Return to Sports (Weeks 26-30)

REHABILITATION PROTOCOL	*Regular Rehabilitation after an Anterior Capsular Shift for General Orthopaedic Patients* Wilk

This rehabilitation program's goal is to return the patient/athlete to activity/sport as quickly and safely as possible while maintaining a stable shoulder. The program is based on muscle physiology, biomechanics, anatomy, and the healing process after capsular shift surgery.

Regular Rehabilitation after an Anterior Capsular Shift for General Orthopaedic Patients   Continued

The capsular shift procedure is one in which the orthopaedic surgeon makes an incision into the ligamentous capsule of the shoulder, pulls the capsule tighter, and then sutures the capsule together.

The ultimate goal is a functional shoulder and pain-free return to the patient's presurgical functional level.

Compliance with the rehabilitation program is critical to the patient's ultimate outcome.

Note: This protocol progresses more slowly than that for an overhead athlete because of assumed inadequate capsular structures and relatively poor dynamic stabilizers.

PHASE 1: PROTECTION PHASE (WEEKS 0-6)

Goals

- Allow healing of the sutured capsule
- Begin early protected and restricted ROM
- Retard muscular atrophy and enhance dynamic stability
- Decrease pain and inflammation
  - Brace: patients with bidirectional instability are placed in a sling for 4-6 weeks
  - Patients with multidirectional instability are placed in an abduction brace for 4-6 weeks; **the physician will make the determination**.

Weeks 0-2

Precautions

- Sleep in an immobilizer for 4 weeks
- No overhead activities for 6-8 weeks
- Compliance with the rehabilitation program is critical

Exercises

- Gripping exercises with putty
- Elbow flexion-extension and pronation-supination
- Pendulum exercises (nonweighted)
- Rope and pulley active-assisted exercises
  - Shoulder flexion to 90 degrees
  - Shoulder elevation in the scapular plane to 60 degrees
- L-bar exercises
  - External rotation to 15 degrees with arm abducted at 30 degrees
  - No shoulder abduction or extension
- Active ROM of the cervical spine
- Isometrics
  - Flexion, extension, external and internal rotation, and abduction

Criteria for Hospital Discharge

- Shoulder ROM (active-assisted ROM): flexion to 90 degrees, abduction to 45 degrees, external rotation to 20 degrees
- Minimal pain and swelling
- "Good" proximal and distal muscle power

Continued

Regular Rehabilitation after an Anterior Capsular Shift for General Orthopaedic Patients *Continued*

PHASE 1: PROTECTION PHASE (WEEKS 0-6)—cont'd

Weeks 2-4

Goals

- Gradual increase in ROM
- Normalize arthrokinematics
- Improve strength
- Decrease pain and inflammation

Range-of-Motion Exercises

- L-bar active-assisted exercises, gentle passive ROM exercises
  - External rotation to 25-30 degrees in the scapular plane
  - Internal rotation to 30-35 degrees in the scapular plane
  - Shoulder flexion to 105-115 degrees
  - Shoulder elevation in the scapular plane to 115 degrees
  - Rope and pulley flexion
- All exercises performed to tolerance and therapist/physician motion guidelines
- Take to point of pain or resistance or both and hold
- *Gentle* self-assisted capsular stretches

Gentle Joint Mobilization to Re-establish Normal Arthrokinematics To

- Scapulothoracic joint
- GH joint
- SC joint

Strengthening Exercises

- Isometrics
- Rhythmic stabilization exercises
- May initiate tubing for external and internal rotation at 0 degrees

Conditioning Program For

- Trunk
- Lower extremities
- Cardiovascular

Decrease Pain and Inflammation

- Ice, NSAIDs, modalities

Weeks 4-6

- Continue all exercises listed above
- ROM exercises
  - L-bar active-assisted exercises
    - External rotation at 45 degrees of shoulder abduction: 25-35 degrees
    - Continue all others to tolerance (based on end feel)
- Continue stabilization exercises
  - PNF with rhythmic stabilization, neuromuscular exercises

Regular Rehabilitation after an Anterior Capsular Shift for General Orthopaedic Patients Continued

PHASE 2: INTERMEDIATE PHASE (WEEKS 6-12)

Goals

- Full nonpainful ROM at weeks 10-12
- Normalize arthrokinematics
- Increase strength
- Improve neuromuscular control

Weeks 6-8

Range-of-Motion Exercises

- L-bar active-assisted exercises at 90 degrees abduction
- Continue all exercises listed above
- Gradually increase ROM to full ROM at week 12
- Continue joint mobilization
- May initiate internal and external rotation ROM at 90 degrees of abduction

Strengthening Exercises

- Initiate isotonic dumbbell program
  - Side-lying external rotation
  - Side-lying internal rotation
  - Shoulder abduction
  - Supraspinatus
  - Latissimus dorsi
  - Rhomboids
  - Biceps curls
  - Triceps curls
  - Shoulder shrugs
  - Push-ups into chair (serratus anterior)
- Continue tubing at 0 degrees for external and internal rotation
- Continue stabilization exercises for GH joint

Initiate Neuromuscular Control Exercises for SC Joint

Weeks 8-10

- Continue all exercises listed above; emphasis on neuromuscular control drills, PNF stabilization drills, and scapular strengthening
- Initiate tubing exercises for the rhomboids, latissimus dorsi, biceps, and triceps
- Progress ROM to full ROM
  - External rotation at 90 degrees abduction: 80-85 degrees
  - Internal rotation at 90 degrees abduction: 70-75 degrees
  - Flexion to 165-170 degrees

PHASE 3: DYNAMIC STRENGTHENING PHASE (WEEKS 12-20)—ADVANCED STRENGTHENING PHASE

Note: An aggressive strengthening or stretching program is based on the type of patient. The therapist and/or physician will determine.

Continued

Regular Rehabilitation after an Anterior Capsular Shift for General Orthopaedic Patients Continued

PHASE 3: DYNAMIC STRENGTHENING PHASE (WEEKS 12-20)—ADVANCED STRENGTHENING PHASE—cont'd

Weeks 12-17

Criteria for Progression to Phase 3

- Full nonpainful ROM. The patient must fulfill this criterion before progressing to this phase
- No pain or tenderness
- Strength 70% or better in comparison to the contralateral side

Goals

- Improve strength, power, and endurance
- Improve neuromuscular control
- Prepare an athletic patient for gradual return to sports

Emphasis

- Dynamic stabilization exercises
- Eccentric exercises
- Diagonal patterns, functional movements

Exercises

- Fundamental shoulder exercises
  - Emphasis: neuromuscular control drills, PNF rhythmic stabilization, rotator cuff strengthening, scapular strengthening
- Continue tubing exercises for internal and external rotation at 0 degrees abduction (arm at the side)
- Continue isotonics for
  - Rhomboids
  - Latissimus dorsi
  - Biceps
  - Diagonal D2 extension patterns
  - Diagonal D2 flexion patterns
- Continue dumbbell exercises for the supraspinatus and deltoid
- Continue serratus anterior strengthening exercises, floor push-ups
- Continue trunk and lower extremity strengthening exercises
- Continue neuromuscular exercises
- Continue self-assisted capsular exercises

Weeks 17-20

- Continue all exercises
- Emphasis on gradual return to recreational activities

PHASE 4: RETURN TO ACTIVITY (WEEKS 20-28)

Criteria for Progression to Phase 4

- Full ROM
- No pain or tenderness
- Isokinetic test that fulfills criteria
- Satisfactory clinical examination

Regular Rehabilitation after an Anterior Capsular Shift for General Orthopaedic Patients   Continued

PHASE 4: RETURN TO ACTIVITY (WEEKS 20-28)—cont'd

Goals

• Progressively increase activities to prepare the patient for full functional return

Exercises

• Initiate interval sports programs (if the patient is a recreational athlete)
• Continue tubing exercises as listed in phase 3
• Continue all strengthening exercises
• Continue ROM exercises

Frozen Shoulder (Adhesive Capsulitis)

Codman introduced the term "frozen shoulder" in 1934 to describe patients who had a painful loss of shoulder motion with normal radiographic studies. In 1946, Neviaser named the condition "adhesive capsulitis" based on the arthrographic appearance, which suggested "adhesions" of the capsule of the GH joint limiting overall joint space volume. **Patients with adhesive capsulitis have a painful restriction of *both* active and passive GH joint motion in all planes, or global loss of GH joint motion.**

This condition most commonly occurs in patients 40 to 60 years of age, with a higher incidence in females. The onset of "idiopathic" frozen shoulder has been attributed to extended immobilization, relatively mild trauma (e.g., strain or contusion), and surgical trauma, especially breast or chest wall procedures. Adhesive capsulitis is associated with medical conditions such as diabetes, hyperthyroidism, ischemic heart disease, inflammatory arthritis, and cervical spondylosis. **The most significant association is with insulin-dependent diabetes.** Bilateral disease occurs in approximately 10% of patients, but it can develop in as many as 40% of patients with a history of insulin-dependent diabetes.

Adhesive capsulitis is classically characterized by three stages. The length of each stage is variable, but typically the first stage lasts for 3 to 6 months, the second stage from 3 to 18 months, and the final stage from 3 to 6 months.

The first stage is the "freezing" phase, characterized by the onset of an aching pain in the shoulder. The pain is usually more severe at night and with activities and may be associated with a sense of discomfort that radiates down the arm. Often, a specific traumatic event is difficult for the patient to recall. As symptoms progress, there are fewer arm positions that are comfortable. Most patients will position the arm in adduction and internal rotation. This position represents the "neutral isometric position of relaxed tension for the inflamed glenohumeral capsule, biceps, and rotator cuff." Unfortunately, many of these patients are initially treated by immobilization, which only worsens the "freezing" process.

The second stage is the progressive stiffness or "frozen" phase. Pain at rest usually diminishes during this stage, and the patient is left with a shoulder that has restricted motion in all planes. Activities of daily living become severely restricted. Patients complain about their inability to reach into their back pocket, fasten their bra, comb their hair, or wash their opposite shoulder. When performing these activities, a sharp, acute discomfort can occur as the patient reaches the restraint of the tight capsule. Pain at night is a common complaint and is not easily treated with medications or physical modalities. This stage can last from 3 to 18 months.

The final stage is the resolution or "thawing" phase. This stage is characterized by slow recovery of motion. Aggressive treatment with physical therapy, closed manipulation, or surgical release may accelerate recovery and move the patient from the frozen stage to the thawing phase, as long as ROM activities are practiced daily.

The **diagnosis of adhesive capsulitis** may be suggested by a careful history and physical examination. The history should focus on the onset and duration of symptoms, a description of any antecedent trauma, and any associated medical conditions. The findings on physical examination vary depending on the stage at which the patient is initially seen. **In general, global loss of active *and* passive motion is present; loss of external rotation with the arm at the patient's side is a hallmark of this condition. Loss of *passive* external rotation is the single most important finding on physical examination and helps differentiate the diagnosis from a rotator cuff problem because problems involving the rotator cuff do not generally result in loss of *passive* external rotation.** The diagnosis of a frozen shoulder is confirmed when radiographic studies are normal. Posteriorly dislocated shoulders also lack external rotation and abduction, but an axillary lateral radiograph reveals a dislocated humeral head. The differential diagnoses for shoulder stiffness are listed in Table 3-4. The physician should also be aware of possible underlying disorders that may have caused the adhesive capsulitis (e.g., a painful rotator cuff tear that caused the patient to stop using the arm).

TREATMENT

Even though adhesive capsulitis is believed to be a "self-limited" process, it can be severely disabling for months to years and, as a result, requires aggressive treatment once the diagnosis is made. Initial treatment should include an aggressive physical therapy program to help regain shoulder motion. For patients in the initial painful or freezing phase, pain relief may be obtained with a course of anti-inflammatory medications, the judicious use of corticosteroid injections in the GH joint, or therapeutic modality treatments. Intra-articular corticosteroid injections may help abort the abnormal inflammatory process often associated with this condition. The rehabilitation program for adhesive capsulitis is outlined on page 340. An algorithm for the treatment of shoulder stiffness is shown in Figure 3-74.

Operative intervention is indicated in patients who show no improvement after a 3-month course of aggressive management that includes medications, corticosteroid injection, and physical therapy. In patients who do not have a history of diabetes, our initial intervention is manipulation under anesthesia, followed by outpatient physical therapy. Patients with a history of diabetes in whom conservative management fails and patients who fail to regain shoulder motion after manipulation are treated by arthroscopic surgical release, followed by physical therapy.

TABLE 3-4	Differential Diagnosis of Shoulder Stiffness

Extrinsic Causes

Neurologic

Parkinson's disease
Automatic dystrophy (RSD)
Intradural lesions
Neural compression
  Cervical disk disease
  Neurofibromas
Foraminal stenosis
Neurologic amyotrophy
Hemiplegia
Head trauma

Muscular

Polymyositis

Cardiovascular

Myocardial infarction
Thoracic outlet syndrome
Cerebral hemorrhage

Infections

Chronic bronchitis
Pulmonary tuberculosis

Metabolic

Diabetes mellitus
Thyroid disease
Progressive systemic sclerosis
  (scleroderma)
Paget's disease

Inflammatory

Rheumatologic disorders
Polymyalgia rheumatica

Trauma

Surgery
  Axillary node dissection, sternotomy,
    thoracotomy
Fractures
  Cervical spine, ribs, elbow, hand, etc.

Medications

Isoniazid, phenobarbital

Congenital

Klippel-Feil syndrome
Sprengel's deformity
Glenoid dysplasia
Atresia
Contractures
  Pectoralis major
  Axillary fold

Behavioral

Depression
Hysterical paralysis

Referred Pain

Diaphragmatic irritation

Neoplastic

Pancoast's tumor
Lung carcinoma
Metastatic disease

Intrinsic Causes

Bursitis

Subacromial
Calcific tendinitis
Snapping scapula

Biceps Tendon

Tenosynovitis
Partial or complete tears
SLAP lesions

Rotator Cuff

Impingement syndrome
Partial rotator cuff tears
Complete rotator cuff tears

Trauma

Fractures
  Glenoid
  Proximal humerus
Surgery
  Postoperative shoulder, breast, head,
    neck, chest
Gastrointestinal disorders
  Esophagitis
  Ulcers
  Cholecystitis

Instability—Glenohumeral

Recurrent dislocation, anterior and posterior
Chronic dislocation

Arthritides

Glenohumeral and acromioclavicular
  Osteoarthritis
  Rheumatoid
  Psoriatic
  Infectious
  Neuropathic

Miscellaneous

Avascular necrosis
Hemarthrosis
Osteochondromatosis
Suprascapular nerve palsy

RSD, reflex sympathetic dystrophy; SLAP, superior labrum from anterior to posterior.
From Rockwood CA, Matsen FA: The Shoulder. Philadelphia, WB Saunders, 1990.

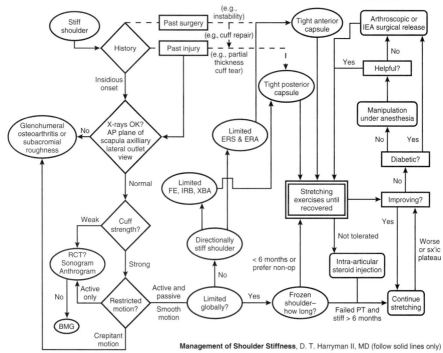

Figure 3–74 Treatment algorithm for patients with a stiff shoulder. AP, anterior-posterior; BMG, below medium grade; ERA, external rotation abduction; ERS, external rotation supine; FE, forward elevation; IRB, internal rotation back; PT, physical therapy; RCT, rotator cuff tissue; sx'ic, symptomatic; XBA, external rotation line on back. (From Rockwood CA Jr, Matsen FA III: The Shoulder, 2nd ed. Philadelphia, WB Saunders, 1988.)

REHABILITATION PROTOCOL	***Frozen Shoulder (Adhesive Capsulitis)*** Bach, Cohen, and Romeo

PHASE 1: WEEKS 0-8

Goals

- Relieve pain
- Restore motion

Restrictions

- None

Immobilization

- None

Pain Control

- Reduction of pain and discomfort is essential for recovery
  - Medications
    - NSAIDs—first-line medications for pain control
    - GH joint injection: corticosteroid/local anesthetic combination

Frozen Shoulder (Adhesive Capsulitis) Continued

PHASE 1: WEEKS 0-8—cont'd

- ○ Oral steroid taper—for patients with refractory or symptomatic frozen shoulder (Pearsall and Speer, 1998)
- ○ Because of potential side effects of oral steroids, patients must be thoroughly questioned about their past medical history
- Therapeutic modalities
  - ○ Ice, ultrasound, HVGS
  - ○ Moist heat before therapy; ice at end of session

Motion: Shoulder

Goals

- Controlled, aggressive ROM exercises
- Focus is on stretching at ROM limits
- No restrictions on range, but therapist and patient have to communicate to avoid injuries

Exercises

- Initially focus on forward flexion and external and internal rotation with the arm at the side and the elbow at 90 degrees
- Active ROM exercises
- Active-assisted ROM exercises (see Fig. 3-42)
- Passive ROM exercises (see Fig. 3-43)
- A home exercise program should be instituted from the beginning
  - Patients should perform their ROM exercises three to five times per day
  - A sustained stretch, of 15-30 seconds, at the end ROM exercises should be part of all ROM routines

PHASE 2: WEEKS 8-16

Criteria for Progression to Phase 2

- Improvement in shoulder discomfort
- Improvement in shoulder motion
- Satisfactory physical examination

Goals

- Improve shoulder motion in all planes
- Improve strength and endurance of the rotator cuff and scapular stabilizers

Pain Control

- Reduction of pain and discomfort is essential for recovery
  - Medications
    - ○ NSAIDs—first-line medications for pain control
    - ○ GH joint injection: corticosteroid/local anesthetic combination
    - ○ Oral steroid taper—for patients with refractory or symptomatic frozen shoulder (Pearsall and Speer, 1998)
    - ○ Because of potential side effects of oral steroids, patients must be thoroughly questioned about their past medical history
  - Therapeutic modalities
    - ○ Ice, ultrasound, HVGS
    - ○ Moist heat before therapy; ice at end of session

Continued

Frozen Shoulder (Adhesive Capsulitis)   *Continued*

PHASE 2: WEEKS 8-16—cont'd

Motion: Shoulder

Goals

- 140 degrees of forward flexion
- 45 degrees of external rotation
- Internal rotation to twelfth thoracic spinous process

Exercises

- Active ROM exercises
- Active-assisted ROM exercises (see Fig. 3-42)
- Passive ROM exercises (see Fig. 3-43)

Muscle Strengthening

- Rotator cuff strengthening—three times per week, 8-12 repetitions for three sets
  - Closed-chain isometric strengthening with the elbow flexed to 90 degrees and the arm at the side (see Fig. 3-44)
    - Internal rotation
    - External rotation
    - Abduction
    - Forward flexion
  - Progress to open-chain strengthening with Thera-Bands (see Fig. 3-47A)
    - Exercises performed with the elbow flexed to 90 degrees
    - Starting position is with the shoulder in the neutral position of 0 degrees of forward flexion, abduction, and external rotation
    - Exercises are performed through an arc of 45 degrees in each of the five planes of motion
    - Six color-coded bands are available; each provides increasing resistance from 1 to 6 pounds in increments of 1 pound
    - Progression to the next band occurs usually at 2- to 3-week intervals. Patients are instructed to not progress to the next band if there is any discomfort at the present level
    - Thera-Band exercises permit concentric and eccentric strengthening of the shoulder muscles and are a form of isotonic exercises (characterized by variable speed and fixed resistance)
      - Internal rotation
      - External rotation
      - Abduction
      - Forward flexion
  - Progress to light isotonic dumbbell exercises
    - Internal rotation (see Fig. 3-47B)
    - External rotation (see Fig. 3-44C)
    - Abduction
    - Forward flexion
- Strengthening of scapular stabilizers
  - Closed-chain strengthening exercises (see Figs. 3-45, 3-62, and 3-71)
    - Scapular retraction (rhomboideus, middle trapezius)
    - Scapular protraction (serratus anterior)
    - Scapular depression (latissimus dorsi, trapezius, serratus anterior)
    - Shoulder shrugs (trapezius, levator scapulae)
  - Progress to open-chain strengthening (see Figs. 3-46 and 3-72)
- Deltoid strengthening (see Figs. 3-46 and 3-73)

Frozen Shoulder (Adhesive Capsulitis)   *Continued*

PHASE 3: MONTHS 4 AND BEYOND

Criteria for Progression to Phase 4

- Significant functional recovery of shoulder motion
  - Successful participation in activities of daily living
- Resolution of painful shoulder
- Satisfactory physical examination

Goals

- Home maintenance exercise program
  - ROM exercises two times a day
  - Rotator cuff strengthening three times a week
  - Scapular stabilizer strengthening three times a week

Maximum improvement is achieved by 6 to 9 months after initiation of the treatment program.

Warning Signs

- Loss of motion
- Continued pain

Treatment of Complications

- These patients may need to move back to earlier routines
- May require increased utilization of pain control modalities as outlined above
- If loss of motion is persistent and pain continues, patients may require surgical intervention
- Manipulation under anesthesia
- Arthroscopic release

Rehabilitation after Shoulder Arthroplasty (Replacement)

Shoulder arthroplasty is one of the few surgical procedures involving the shoulder that require the patient to spend time in the hospital after surgery. As a result, a supervised rehabilitation program to begin mobilization of the reconstructed shoulder joint is started during the hospitalization on the first day after surgery. Rehabilitation after shoulder arthroplasty follows the normal sequence of allowing time for tissue healing, joint mobilization, and finally, muscle strengthening and function.

The ability to begin the rehabilitation process so soon after surgery is the direct result of improvements in the surgical approach to the GH joint. Earlier approaches required release of the deltoid origin to expose the shoulder for prosthetic replacement. This necessitated a more conservative, delayed rehabilitation program to avoid postoperative detachment of the deltoid repair. At present, the only muscle violated during surgical exposure is the subscapularis muscle, and the rehabilitation protocol must be mindful of the time required for the subscapularis tendon to heal. **The amount of external rotation and active internal rotation that the patient can** perform in the first 4 to 6 weeks is limited to motion parameters that can be achieved at the time of surgery. The goal of rehabilitation is to establish a ROM that will allow functional recovery.

Long-term function and rehabilitation progression are affected by the presence or absence of good functional rotator cuff tissue (RCT). Postoperative rehabilitation protocols are often divided into RTC-deficient and RTC-intact groups.

REHABILITATION PROTOCOL | *After Shoulder Arthroplasty*
Bach, Cohen, and Romeo

PHASE 1: WEEKS 0-6

Restrictions

- Shoulder motion
  - Week 1
    - 120 degrees of forward flexion
    - 20 degrees of external rotation with the arm at the side
    - 75 degrees of abduction with 0 degrees of rotation
  - Week 2
    - 140 degrees of forward flexion
    - 40 degrees of external rotation with the arm at the side
    - 75 degrees of abduction with 0 degrees of rotation
  - No active internal rotation
  - No backward extension

Immobilization

- Sling
  - After 7-10 days, sling used for comfort only

Pain Control

- Reduction of pain and discomfort is essential for recovery
  - Medications
    - Narcotics—for 7-10 days after surgery
    - NSAIDs—for patients with persistent discomfort after surgery
  - Therapeutic modalities
    - Ice, ultrasound, HVGS
    - Moist heat before therapy; ice at end of session

Motion: Shoulder

- Goals
  - 140 degrees of forward flexion
  - 40 degrees of external rotation
  - 75 degrees of abduction
- Exercises
  - Begin with Codman pendulum exercises to promote early motion
  - Passive ROM exercises (see Fig. 3-43)
  - Capsular stretching for the anterior, posterior, and inferior capsule by using the opposite arm to assist with motion (see Fig. 3-57)

After Shoulder Arthroplasty   *Continued*

PHASE 1: WEEKS 0-6—cont'd

- Active-assisted motion exercises (see Fig. 3-42)
  - Shoulder flexion
  - Shoulder extension
  - Internal and external rotation
- Progress to active ROM exercises

Motion: Elbow

- Passive—progress to active
- 0-130 degrees
- Pronation and supination as tolerated

Muscle Strengthening

- Grip strengthening only

PHASE 2: WEEKS 6-12

Criteria for Progression to Phase 2

- Minimal pain and tenderness
- Nearly complete motion
- Intact subscapularis without evidence of tendon pain on resisted internal rotation

Restrictions

- Increase ROM goals
  - 160 degrees of forward flexion
  - 60 degrees of external rotation with the arm at the side
  - 90 degrees of abduction with 40 degrees of internal and external rotation

Immobilization

- None

Pain Control

- NSAIDs—for patients with persistent discomfort after surgery
- Therapeutic modalities
  - Ice, ultrasound, HVGS
  - Moist heat before therapy; ice at end of session

Motion: Shoulder

- Goals
  - 160 degrees of forward flexion
  - 60 degrees of external rotation with the arm at the side
  - 90 degrees of abduction with 40 degrees of internal and external rotation
- Exercises
  - Increase active ROM in all directions
  - Focus on passive stretching at end ranges to maintain shoulder flexibility (see Fig. 3-43)
  - Use joint mobilization techniques for capsular restrictions, especially the posterior capsule (see Fig. 3-56)

Continued

After Shoulder Arthroplasty Continued

PHASE 2: WEEKS 6-12—cont'd

Muscle Strengthening

- Rotator cuff strengthening: only three times per week to avoid rotator cuff tendinitis, which will occur with overtraining
  - Begin with closed-chain isometric strengthening (see Fig. 3-44)
    - External rotation
    - Abduction
  - Progress to open-chain strengthening with Thera-Bands (see Fig. 3-47A)
    - Exercises performed with the elbow flexed to 90 degrees
    - Starting position is with the shoulder in the neutral position of 0 degrees of forward flexion, abduction, and external rotation
    - Exercises are performed through an arc of 45 degrees in each of the five planes of motion
    - Six color-coded bands are available; each provides increasing resistance from 1 to 6 pounds in increments of 1 pound
    - Progression to the next band occurs usually at 2- to 3-week intervals. Patients are instructed to not progress to the next band if there is any discomfort at the present level
    - Thera-Band exercises permit concentric and eccentric strengthening of the shoulder muscles and are a form of isotonic exercises (characterized by variable speed and fixed resistance)
      - External rotation
      - Abduction
      - Forward flexion
  - Progress to light isotonic dumbbell exercises
    - External rotation (see Fig. 3-47C)
    - Abduction
    - Forward flexion
- Scapular stabilizer strengthening
  - Closed-chain strengthening exercises (see Figs. 3-45, 3-62, and 3-71)
    - Scapular retraction (rhomboideus, middle trapezius)
    - Scapular protraction (serratus anterior)
    - Scapular depression (latissimus dorsi, trapezius, serratus anterior)
    - Shoulder shrugs (trapezius, levator scapulae)

PHASE 3: MONTHS 3-12

Criteria for Progression to Phase 3

- Full painless ROM
- Satisfactory physical examination

Goals

- Improve shoulder strength, power, and endurance
- Improve neuromuscular control and shoulder proprioception
- Prepare for gradual return to functional activities
- Home maintenance exercise program
  - ROM exercises two times a day
  - Rotator cuff strengthening three times a week
  - Scapular stabilizer strengthening three times a week

After Shoulder Arthroplasty *Continued*

PHASE 3: MONTHS 3-12—cont'd

Motion

- Achieve motion equal to that on the contralateral side
- Use both active and passive ROM exercises to maintain motion

Muscle Strengthening

- Shoulder
  - Begin internal rotation and extension strengthening
    - First closed-chain isometric strengthening and then advance to Thera-Band and lightweight isotonic strengthening
- Scapular stabilizers
  - Progress to open- and closed-chain strengthening (see Figs. 3-46, 3-62, and 3-72)
- Deltoid strengthening (see Figs. 3-61 and 3-73)
- 8-12 repetitions for each exercise for three sets
- Strengthening only three times per week to avoid rotator cuff tendinitis

Functional Strengthening

- Plyometric exercises (see Fig. 3-48)
Maximum improvement is achieved by 12 to 18 months.

Warning Signs

- Loss of motion
- Continued pain

Treatment of Complications

- These patients may need to move back to earlier routines
- May require increased use of pain control modalities as outlined above

---

REHABILITATION PROTOCOL	*After Total Shoulder Arthroplasty (in a Rotator Cuff Tissue–Deficient Group)* Wilk

The goal of the rehabilitation process is to provide greater joint stability to the patient while decreasing pain and improving functional status. The goal of the RTC-deficient group (bone loss, muscle loss) is joint stability and less joint mobility. The key to the success of the rehabilitation after shoulder replacement is compliance with the exercise program.

PHASE 1: IMMEDIATE MOTION PHASE (WEEKS 0-4)

Goals

- Increase passive ROM
- Decrease shoulder pain
- Retard muscular atrophy

Continued

After Total Shoulder Arthroplasty (in a Rotator Cuff Tissue–Deficient Group)   *Continued*

PHASE 1: IMMEDIATE MOTION PHASE (WEEKS 0-4)—cont'd

Exercises

- Continuous passive motion
- Passive ROM
  - Flexion at 0-90 degrees
  - External rotation at 30 degrees abduction: 0-20 degrees
  - Internal rotation at 30 degrees abduction: 0-30 degrees
- Pendulum exercises
- Elbow and wrist ROM
- Gripping exercises
- Isometrics
  - Abductors
  - External and internal rotation
- Ropes and pulley (second week)
- Active-assisted motion exercises (when able)

PHASE 2: ACTIVE MOTION PHASE (WEEKS 5-8)

Goals

- Improve shoulder strength
- Improve ROM
- Decrease pain and inflammation
- Increase functional activities

Exercises

- Active-assisted ROM exercises with the **L**-bar (begin at week 2-3 or when tolerable)
  - Flexion
  - External rotation
  - Internal rotation
- Rope and pulley
  - Flexion
- Pendulum exercises
- Active ROM exercises
  - Seated flexion (short arc at 45-90 degrees)
  - Supine flexion (full available range)
  - Seated abduction at 0-90 degrees
  - Internal and external rotation with exercise tubing (weeks 4-6)
  - Biceps and triceps strengthening exercises with a dumbbell
- Gentle joint mobilization (weeks 6-8)

PHASE 3: STRENGTHENING PHASE (WEEKS 8-12)

Criteria for Progression to Phase 3

- Passive ROM: flexion at 0-120 degrees
  - External rotation at 90 degrees abduction: 30-40 degrees
  - Internal rotation at 90 degrees abduction: 45-55 degrees
- Strength level 4/5 for external and internal rotation and abduction
- *Note:* Some patients will never enter this phase

After Total Shoulder Arthroplasty (in a Rotator Cuff Tissue–Deficient Group)   *Continued*

PHASE 3: STRENGTHENING PHASE (WEEKS 8-12)—cont'd

Goals

- Improve strength of the shoulder musculature
- Improve and gradually increase functional activities

Exercises

- Exercise tubing
  - External rotation
  - Internal rotation
- Dumbbell strengthening
  - Abduction
  - Supraspinatus
  - Flexion
- Stretching exercise
- L-bar stretches
  - Flexion
  - External rotation
  - Internal rotation

▌Biceps Tendon Disorders

IMPORTANT REHABILITATION POINTS

- The long head of the biceps functions as a secondary humeral head depressor and stabilizer.
- In many overhead sports, the biceps aids acceleration and deceleration of the arm.
- Bicipital problems in athletes usually occur in conjunction with other shoulder disorders (rotator cuff pathology, GH joint instability).
- For this reason, a thorough evaluation of the remainder of the shoulder should be performed if a biceps disorder is found (e.g., biceps tendinitis).
- As the long head of the biceps tendon courses from its attachment to the superior glenoid labrum, it exits the GH joint and proceeds through the rotator cuff interval beneath the coracohumeral ligament. It then enters the bicipital groove, where it is restrained by the transverse humeral ligament (Fig. 3-75).
- Synder and colleagues (1990) introduced the term "**SLAP lesion**" to characterize injuries to the superior labrum at the biceps origin. There are four patterns of injury in this classification system (Table 3-5). The SLAP eponym came from the lesions beginning posterior to the biceps anchor and extending anteriorly (superior labrum from anterior to posterior lesion, or **SLAP** lesion).
- See Figure 3-76 for the intraoperative (arthroscopic) appearance of SLAP lesions.
- The most common complaints with SLAP lesions are catching, popping, locking, or grinding of the shoulder. This typically occurs with overhead activities.

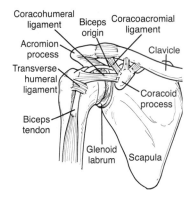

Figure 3-75 Anterior aspect of the right shoulder showing the tendon of the long head of the biceps muscle and its relationships. (From Andrews JR, Zarins B, Wilk KE: Injuries in Baseball. Philadelphia, Lippincott-Raven, 1997, p 112.)

TABLE 3–5	Classification of Superior Labrum from Anterior to Posterior (SLAP) Lesions
Type	**Characteristics**
Type 1 SLAP	Degenerative fraying of the superior labrum but the biceps attachment to the labrum is intact. The biceps anchor is intact (see Fig. 3-76A)
Type 2 SLAP	The biceps anchor has pulled away from the glenoid attachment (see Fig. 3-76B)
Type 3 SLAP	Involves a bucket-handle tear of the superior labrum with an intact biceps anchor (see Fig. 3–76C)
Type 4 SLAP	Similar to a type 3 tears but the tear also extends into the biceps tendon (see Fig. 3-76D). The torn biceps tendon and labrum are displaced into the joint
Complex SLAP	A combination of two or more SLAP types, usually 2 and 3 or 2 and 4

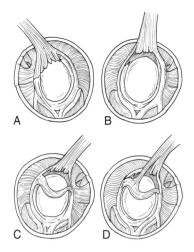

Figure 3–76 SLAP lesions. **A**, Type 1. **B**, Type 2. **C**, Type 3. **D**, Type 4. (**A-D**, From Warren RR, Craig EV, Altchek DW: The Unstable Shoulder. Philadelphia, Lippincott-Raven, 1999.)

- Traction and compression are the most common injuries that lead to SLAP lesions. A sudden pull occurs in many instances, such as grabbing an object in an attempt to avoid a fall.
- Diagnostic examinations for SLAP lesions are reviewed on page 198 (e.g., Speed test, Yergason test).
- Burkhart et al. describe the "peel-back" phenomenon (see "peel-back" text in the section "Peel-Back Mechanism in Throwers").

OPERATIVE TREATMENT—SLAP LESIONS

- Concomitant GH joint pathology must also be treated.
- **Type 1 lesion**—The superior labrum is débrided back to a stable rim with a motorized shaver to prevent subsequent mechanical catching.
- **Type 2 lesion**—The lesion is repaired with suture anchors.
- **Type 3 lesions,** with a bucket-handle tear, are carefully probed to ensure a stable biceps anchor and remaining labrum. The torn fragment is then resected so that a smooth transition zone is left.
- **Type 4 lesions**—Treatment is based on the extent of tearing in the biceps tendon. If the torn segment composes less than 30% of the tendon, the detached labral and biceps tissue can be resected. If more than 30% is involved,
  - *In an older patient* with biceps pain, the labrum is débrided and tenodesis of the biceps is performed.
  - *In a younger patient*, the tendon is preserved (arthroscopic suture repair).

Rehabilitation Considerations

- Type 2 and 4 repairs have a more conservative rehabilitation regimen. A sling is used for 3 weeks with elbow, wrist, and hand exercises.
- Pendulum exercises are begun after 1 week.
- External rotation beyond neutral and extension of the arm behind the body with the elbows extended are **avoided** for at least 4 weeks.
- Protected biceps strengthening is begun, but no stressful biceps activity is allowed for 3 months.

BICEPS RUPTURE (COMPLETE PROXIMAL LONG HEAD TEARS)

- Treatment of complete long head tears is individualized.
- Most patients who are willing to accept the cosmetic deformity ("Popeye" arm) and minimal functional deficit are treated nonoperatively.
- Young, athletic individuals who perform tasks or lifting that requires supination strength may be offered biceps tenodesis and arthroscopic subacromial decompression.

REHABILITATION PROTOCOL   *After Arthrosopic Repair of Type 2 SLAP Lesions*
Wilk

PHASE 1: IMMEDIATE POSTOPERATIVE PHASE—"RESTRICTIVE MOTION" (DAY 1 TO WEEK 6)

Goals

- Protect the anatomic repair
- Prevent negative effects of immobilization
- Promote dynamic stability
- Diminish pain and inflammation

Weeks 0-2

- Sling for 4 weeks
- Sleep in an immobilizer for 4 weeks
- Elbow and hand ROM
- Hand-gripping exercises
- Passive and gentle active-assisted ROM exercise
  - Flexion to 60 degrees (week 2: flexion to 75 degrees)
  - Elevation in the scapular plane to 60 degrees
  - External and internal rotation with the arm in the scapular plane
  - External rotation to 10-15 degrees
  - Internal rotation to 45 degrees
  - *Note:* **No active external rotation or extension or abduction**
- Submaximal isometrics for shoulder musculature
- **NO isolated biceps contractions**
- Cryotherapy, modalities as indicated

Weeks 3-4

- Discontinue use of the sling at 4 weeks
- Sleep in an immobilizer until week 4
- Continue gentle ROM exercises (passive ROM and active-assisted ROM)
  - Flexion to 90 degrees
  - Abduction to 75-85 degrees
  - External rotation in the scapular plane to 25-30 degrees
  - Internal rotation in the scapular plane to 55-60 degrees
  - *Note:* **The rate of progression is based on evaluation of the patient**
- No active external rotation, extension, or elevation
- Initiate rhythmic stabilization drills
- Initiate proprioception training
- Tubing exercises for external and internal rotation at 0 degrees abduction
- Continue isometrics
- Continue use of cryotherapy

Weeks 5-6

- Gradually improve ROM
  - Flexion to 145 degrees
  - External rotation at 45 degrees abduction: 45-50 degrees
  - Internal rotation at 45 degrees abduction: 55-60 degrees
- May initiate stretching exercises
- May initiate light (easy) ROM at 90 degrees abduction
- Continue tubing exercises for external and internal rotation (arm at the side)

After Arthrosopic Repair of Type 2 SLAP Lesions Continued

PHASE 1: IMMEDIATE POSTOPERATIVE PHASE—"RESTRICTIVE MOTION" (DAY 1 TO WEEK 6)—cont'd

- PNF manual resistance
- Initiate active shoulder abduction (without resistance)
- Initiate full can exercise (weight of arm)
- Initiate prone rowing, prone horizontal abduction
- NO biceps strengthening

PHASE 2: INTERMEDIATE PHASE-MODERATE PROTECTION PHASE (WEEKS 7-14)

Goals

- Gradually restore full ROM (week 10)
- Preserve the integrity of the surgical repair
- Restore muscular strength and balance

Weeks 7-9

- Gradually progress ROM
  - Flexion to 180 degrees
  - External rotation at 90 degrees abduction: 90-95 degrees
  - Internal rotation at 90 degrees abduction: 70-75 degrees
- Continue to progress isotonic strengthening program
- Continue PNF strengthening
- Initiate "Thrower's Ten" program

Weeks 10-12

- May initiate slightly more aggressive strengthening
- Progress external rotation to thrower's motion
  - External rotation at 90 degrees abduction: 110-115 in throwers (weeks 10-12)
- Progress isotonic strengthening exercises
- Continue all stretching exercises. **Progress ROM to functional demands (i.e., overhead athlete)**
- Continue all strengthening exercises

PHASE 3: MINIMAL PROTECTION PHASE (WEEKS 14-20)

Criteria for Progression to Phase 3

- Full nonpainful ROM
- Satisfactory stability
- Muscular strength (good grade or better)
- No pain or tenderness

Goals

- Establish and maintain full ROM
- Improve muscular strength, power, and endurance
- Gradually initiate functional activities

Weeks 14-16

- Continue all stretching exercises (capsular stretches)
- Maintain thrower's motion (especially external rotation)

Continued

After Arthrosopic Repair of Type 2 SLAP Lesions *Continued*

PHASE 3: MINIMAL PROTECTION PHASE (WEEKS 14-20)—cont'd

- Continue strengthening exercises
  - "Thrower's Ten" program or fundamental exercises
  - PNF manual resistance
  - Endurance training
  - Initiate light plyometric program
  - Restricted sport activities (light swimming, half golf swings)

Weeks 16-20

- Continue all exercises listed above
- Continue all stretching
- Continue "Thrower's Ten" program
- Continue plyometric program
- Initiate interval sport program (e.g., throwing). **See interval throwing program**

PHASE 4: ADVANCED STRENTHENING PHASE (WEEKS 20-25)

Criteria for Progression to Phase 4

- Full nonpainful ROM
- Satisfactory static stability
- Muscular strength 75% to 80% of contralateral side
- No pain or tenderness

Goals

- Enhanced muscular strength, power, and endurance
- Progress functional activities
- Maintain shoulder mobility

Weeks 20-26

- Continue flexibility exercises
- Continue isotonic strengthening program
- PNF manual resistance patterns
- Plyometric strengthening
- Progress interval sport programs

PHASE 5: RETURN-TO-ACTIVITY PHASE (MONTHS 6-9)

Criteria for Progression to Phase 5

- Full functional ROM
- Muscular performance isokinetic (fulfills criteria)
- Satisfactory shoulder stability
- No pain or tenderness

Goals

- Gradual return to sport activities
- Maintain strength, mobility, and stability

Exercises

- Gradually progress sport activities to unrestrictive participation
- Continue stretching and strengthening program

REHABILITATION PROTOCOL	*After Arthroscopic Débridement of Type 1 or 3 SLAP Lesion and/or Partial Rotator Cuff Débridement (Not a Rotator Cuff Repair)* Wilk

This rehabilitation program's goal is to return the patient/athlete to activity/sport as quickly and safely as possible.

This program is based on muscle physiology, biomechanics, anatomy, and healing response.

PHASE 1: MOTION PHASE (DAYS 1-10)

Goals

- Re-establish nonpainful ROM
- Retard muscular atrophy
- Decrease pain and inflammation

Range of Motion

- Pendulum exercise
- Rope and pulley
- L-bar exercises
  - Flexion-extension
  - Abduction-adduction
  - External and internal rotation (begin at 0 degrees abduction and progress to 45 degrees abduction and then 90 degrees abduction)
- Self-stretches (capsular stretches)

Exercises

- Isometrics. *Note* **No Biceps** isometrics for 5-7 days postoperatively
- May initiate tubing exercises for external and internal rotation at 0 degrees abduction in the late phase (usually 7-10 days postoperatively)

Decrease Pain and Inflammation

- Ice, NSAIDs, modalities

PHASE 2: INTERMEDIATE PHASE (WEEKS 2-4)

Criteria for Progression to Phase 2

- Full ROM
- Minimal pain and tenderness
- "Good" MMT of internal and external rotation and flexion

Goals

- Regain and improve muscular strength
- Normalize arthokinematics
- Improve neuromuscular control of the shoulder complex

Week 2

Exercises

- Initiate isotonic program with dumbbells
  - Shoulder musculature
  - Scapulothoracic

Continued

After Arthroscopic Débridement of Type 1 or 3 SLAP Lesion and/or Partial Rotator Cuff Débridement (Not a Rotator Cuff Repair)   Continued

PHASE 2: INTERMEDIATE PHASE (WEEKS 2-4)—cont'd

- Tubing exercises for external and internal rotation at 0 degrees abduction
- Side-lying external rotation
- Prone rowing external rotation
- PNF manual resistance with dynamic stabilization
- Normalize arthrokinematics of the shoulder complex
  - Joint mobilization
  - Continue stretching of the shoulder (external and internal rotation at 90 degrees abduction)
- Initiate neuromuscular control exercises
- Initiate proprioception training
- Initiate trunk exercises
- Initiate upper extremity endurance exercises

Decrease Pain and Inflammation

- Continue use of modalities, ice, as needed

Week 3

Exercises

- "Thrower's Ten" program
- Emphasis rotator cuff and scapular strengthening
- Dynamic stabilization drills

PHASE 3: DYNAMIC STRENGTHENING PHASE—ADVANCED STRENGTHENING PHASE (WEEKS 5-6)

Criteria for Progression to Phase 3

- Full nonpainful ROM
- No pain or tenderness
- Strength 70% in comparison to the contralateral side

Goals

- Improve strength, power, and endurance
- Improve neuromuscular control
- Prepare athlete to begin to throw, etc.

Exercises

- Continue the "Thrower's Ten" program
- Continue dumbbell strengthening (supraspinatus, deltoid)
- Initiate tubing exercises in the 90/90 position for external and internal rotation (slow/fast sets)
- Exercises for scapulothoracic musculature
- Tubing exercises for biceps
- Initiate plyometrics (two-hand drills progress to one-hand drills)
- Diagonal patterns (PNF)
- Initiate isokinetic strengthening
- Continue endurance exercises: neuromuscular control exercises
- Continue proprioception exercises

After Arthroscopic Débridement of Type 1 or 3 SLAP Lesion and/or Partial Rotator Cuff Débridement (Not a Rotator Cuff Repair) Continued

PHASE 4: RETURN-TO-ACTIVITY PHASE (WEEK 7 AND BEYOND)

Criteria for Progression to Phase 4

- Full ROM
- No pain or tenderness
- Isokinetic test that fulfills criteria to throw
- Satisfactory clinical examination

Goal

- Progressively increase activities to prepare the patient for full functional return

Exercises

- Initiate interval sport program (e.g., throwing, tennis)
- Continue all exercises as in phase 3 (throw and train on same day, lower extremity and ROM on opposite days)
- Progress interval program

Follow-up Visits

- Isokinetic tests
- Clinical examination

REHABILITATION PROTOCOL | *After Proximal Biceps Tendon Repair (Complete Rupture of the Long Head of the Biceps)*
Wilk

- Shoulder brace/immobilizer for 4 weeks
- Pendulums
- Active-assisted ROM of the elbow at 0-145 degrees with gentle ROM into extension
- Shoulder isometrics for 10-14 days
- Shoulder active-assisted ROM with L-bar exercises for external and internal rotation in the scapular plane
- Shoulder passive ROM: flexion, external and internal rotation

4 WEEKS

- Light shoulder progressive resistance exercises

8 WEEKS

- Progress to isotonic program
  - Bench press
  - Shoulder press

REHABILITATION PROTOCOL	*After Distal Biceps Tendon Repair (at the Elbow)* Wilk

IMMOBILIZATION

- Posterior splint, elbow immobilization at 90 degrees for 5-7 days

BRACE

- Elbow placed in a hinged ROM brace at 5-7 days postoperatively; ROM set at 45 degrees to full flexion
- Gradually increase elbow ROM in the brace

RANGE-OF-MOTION PROGRESSION

Week 2	45 degrees to full elbow flexion
Week 3	45 degrees to full flexion
Week 4	30 degrees to full elbow flexion
Week 5	20 degrees to full elbow flexion
Week 6	10 degrees to full elbow flexion; full supination-pronation
Week 8	Full ROM of elbow; full supination-pronation

RANGE-OF-MOTION EXERCISES

Week 2-3	Passive ROM for elbow flexion and supination; active-assisted ROM for elbow extension and pronation
Week 3-4	Initiate active-assisted ROM elbow flexion
Week 4	Active ROM elbow flexion

STRENGTHENING PROGRAM

Week 1	Isometrics for triceps and shoulder muscles
Week 2	Isometrics (submaximal biceps curls)
Week 3-4	Active ROM, no resistance applied
Week 8	Progressive resistance exercise program is initiated for elbow flexion and supination-pronation

- Begin with 1 pound and gradually increase
- Begin shoulder strengthening program
  - Weeks 12-14: May initiate light weight training such as bench press and shoulder press

Interval training programs for return to throwing, tennis, golf after shoulder injury: please see sections for all interval throwing programs.

Acromioclavicular Joint Injury

REHABILITATION RATIONALE

Anatomy

The AC joint is a diarthrodial joint with a fibrocartilaginous intra-articular disk. Two significant ligamentous structures are associated with the joint: the AC ligaments, which provide horizontal stability (Fig. 3-77), and the coracoclavicular ligaments, which are the main suspensory ligaments of the upper extremity and provide vertical stability to the joint.

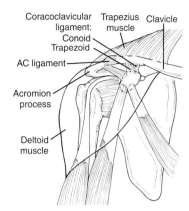

Figure 3–77 An anatomic diagram of a normal acromioclavicular (AC) joint shows the AC and coraco-clavicular (CC) ligaments, which are often injured when an athlete sustains an AC injury. (From Bach BR, Van Fleet TA, Novak PJ: Acromioclavicular injuries: Controversies in treatment. Physician Sports Med 20[12]: 87-95, 1992.)

Recent studies show that only 5 to 8 degrees of motion of the AC joint is possible in any plane.

The most common mechanism of injury to the AC joint is a direct force from a fall on the point of the shoulder (Fig. 3-78).

Rockwood (1990) classifies AC joint injuries into six types (Fig. 3-79).

- Type I
  - Mild sprain of the AC ligament
  - No disruption of the AC or coracoclavicular ligaments
- Type II
  - Disruption of the AC joint
  - AC joint wider because of disruption (<4 mm or 40% difference)
  - Sprained but *intact* coracoclavicular ligaments with coracoclavicular space are essentially the same as the normal shoulder on radiographs
  - A downward force (weight) may disrupt the AC ligament, but *not* the cora-coacromial ligament

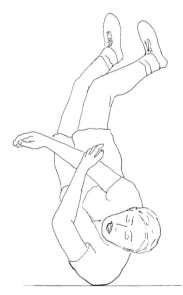

Figure 3–78 The most common mechanism of acromioclavicular joint injury is a direct force that occurs as a result of a fall on the point of the shoulder.

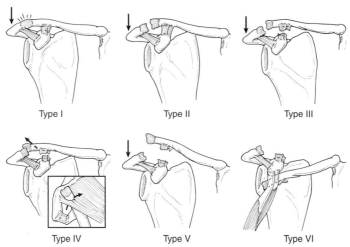

Type I Type II Type III

Type IV Type V Type VI

Figure 3–79 The diagnosis of acromioclavicular (AC) joint injuries includes classification according to the extent of ligament damage. Type I sprains involve partial disruption of the AC ligament and capsule; type II sprains entail a ruptured AC ligament and capsule with incomplete injury to the coracoclavicular (CC) ligament; type III separations exhibit complete tearing of the AC and CC ligaments; type IV injuries involve clavicular displacement posteriorly into or through the trapezius muscles; type V injuries are severe type III injuries with a greater CC interval; and type VI injuries entail displacement of the clavicle inferior to the coracoid process. (From Bach BR, Van Fleet TA, Novak PJ: Acromioclavicular injuries: Controversies in treatment. Physician Sports Med 20[12]:87-95, 1992.)

- Type III
  - Coracoclavicular and AC ligaments disrupted
  - Shoulder complex displaced inferiorly
  - Coracoclavicular interspace 25% to 100% greater than in the normal shoulder, or 4-mm distance (especially with weights applied)
- Type IV
  - The clavicle is displaced posteriorly through fibers of the trapezius
  - The AC and coracoclavicular ligaments are disrupted
  - The deltoid and trapezius muscles are detached from the distal end of the clavicle
- Type V
  - Vertical separation of the clavicle from the scapula is greater than that in a type III injury (100% to 300% more than in the normal shoulder)
- Type VI
  - The clavicle is dislocated inferiorly under the coracoid process

Types I and II injuries are treated conservatively, as are type III injuries in nonactive, nonlaboring patients. Most type IV, V, and VI injuries require open reduction and internal fixation, as do type III injuries in more active individuals.

REHABILITATION PROTOCOL *Acromioclavicular Joint Injuries*
Rockwood and Matsen

TYPE I INJURY

Day 1

- Apply ice to the shoulder for 24-48 hours
- Fit a sling for comfort for up to 7 days
- Perform active ROM of the fingers, wrist, and elbow every 3-4 hours
- Gently maintain normal ROM with rest in a sling as needed
- Begin pendulum exercises on day 2 or 3

Days 7-10

- Symptoms typically subside
- Discontinue sling
- Do not permit any heavy lifting, stress, or contact sports until full painless ROM and no point tenderness over the AC joint (usually at 2 weeks)

TYPE II INJURY

Day 1

- Apply ice for 24-48 hours
- Fit a sling for comfort for 1-2 weeks

Day 7

- Begin gentle ROM exercises of shoulder and allow use of the arm for dressing, eating, and activities of daily living
- Discard the sling at 7-14 days
- Do not permit any heavy lifting, pushing, pulling, or contact sports for at least 6 weeks

TYPE III INJURY

Nonoperative treatment indicated for inactive and nonlaboring patients

Day 1

- Discuss the "bump" remaining on the shoulder: natural history, surgical risks, and recurrence
- Apply ice for 24 hours
- Prescribe mild analgesics for several days
- Place in a sling
- Begin performing activities of daily living at 3-4 days
- Slowly progress to functional ROM with gentle passive ROM exercises at about 7 days
- Patient typically has full ROM at 2-3 weeks with gentle ROM exercises

REHABILITATION PROTOCOL	*After Acromioclavicular Joint Stabilization with Biodegradable Material*
	Wilk

PHASE 1: MOTION PHASE (WEEKS 0-2)

Goals

- Re-establish full nonpainful ROM
- Retard muscular atrophy
- Decrease pain and inflammation

Range-of-Motion Exercises

- T-bar active-assisted ROM exercises
  - Flexion to tolerance
  - External and internal rotation (begin at 0 degrees abduction; progress to 45 degrees abduction and then to 90 degrees abduction)
- Rope and pulley flexion
- Pendulum exercises
- Self-assisted capsular stretches

Note: Restrict horizontal abduction and adduction.

Strengthening Exercises

- Isometrics
- External and internal rotation, abduction, extension exercises for the biceps, triceps

Note: No resisted shoulder flexion is permitted.

- Initiate external and internal rotation with exercise tubing at 0 degrees abduction when pain free.

Decrease Pain and Inflammation

- Ice, NSAIDs, modalities

PHASE 2: INTERMEDIATE PHASE (WEEKS 2-8)

Criteria for Progression to Phase 2

- Full nonpainful ROM
- Minimal pain and tenderness
- Stable AC joint on clinical examination
- Good (grade 4/5) MMT of external and internal rotation and abduction

Goals

- Regain and improve muscular strength
- Normalize arthrokinematics
- Improve neuromuscular control of the shoulder complex

Week 3

Range-of-Motion Exercises

- Continue active-assisted ROM with the T-bar
- Continue self-assisted capsular stretches

After Acromioclavicular Joint Stabilization with Biodegradable Material   *Continued*

PHASE 2: INTERMEDIATE PHASE (WEEKS 2-8)—cont'd

Strengthening Exercises

- Initiate isotonic strengthening (light resistance)
  - Shoulder abduction
  - Shoulder extension
  - Shoulder external and internal rotation
  - Biceps and triceps
  - Scapular musculature
- *Note:* **Restricted shoulder resistance flexion is prohibited.**
- Initiate neuromuscular control exercises (PNF)
- Initiate manual resistance

Pain Control

- Continue use of modalities, ice as needed

Week 6

Range-of-Motion Exercises

- Continue stretching program

Strengthening Exercises

- Continue all strengthening exercises listed above
- Initiate *light* resistance shoulder flexion
- Initiate upper extremity endurance exercises
- Initiate *light* isotonic resistance progression
- **NO** shoulder or bench press or pectoralis deck or pullovers are permitted.
- Rhythmic stabilization exercise for shoulder flexion-extension

PHASE 3: DYNAMIC STRENGTHENING PHASE (WEEKS 8-16)

Criteria for Progression to Phase 3

- Full nonpainful ROM
- No pain or tenderness
- Strength 70% of the contralateral side

Goals

- Improve strength, power, and endurance
- Improve neuromuscular control and dynamic stability of the AC joint
- Prepare the athlete for overhead motion

Strengthening Exercises

- Continue isotonic strengthening exercises
  - Initiate light bench press, shoulder press (progress weight slowly)
  - Continue with resistance exercises for
    - Shoulder abduction
    - Shoulder external and internal rotation
    - Shoulder flexion
    - Latissimus dorsi (rowing, pull-downs)
    - Biceps and triceps

Continued

After Acromioclavicular Joint Stabilization with Biodegradable Material   Continued

PHASE 3: DYNAMIC STRENGTHENING PHASE (WEEKS 8-16)—cont'd

- Initiate tubing PNF patterns
- Initiate external and internal rotation at 90 degrees abduction
- Scapular strengthening (four directions)
  - Emphasis on scapular retractors, elevators
- Neuromuscular control exercises for GH and scapulothoracic joints
  - Rhythmic stabilization
    - Shoulder flexion-extension
    - Shoulder external and internal rotation (90/90)
    - Shoulder abduction-adduction
    - PNF D2 patterns
    - Scapular retraction-protraction
    - Scapular elevation-depression
- Progress to plyometric upper extremity exercises
- Continue stretching to maintain mobility

PHASE 4: RETURN-TO-ACTIVITY PHASE (WEEKS 16 AND BEYOND)

Criteria for Progression to Phase 4

- Full nonpainful ROM
- No pain or tenderness
- Isokinetic test that fulfills criteria (shoulder flexion-extension, abduction-adduction)
- Satisfactory clinical examination

Goal

- Progressively increase activities to prepare patient/athlete for full functional return

Exercises

- Initiate interval sports program
- Continue all exercises listed in phase 3
- Progress resistance exercise levels and stretching

Scapular Dyskinesis

W. Ben Kibler, MD, • John McMullen, MS, ATC

BACKGROUND

The scapula plays many roles in normal shoulder function. It is a stable socket for the normal ball-and-socket kinematics. It retracts and protracts in cocking and follow-through movements, elevates with arm abduction, provides a stable base of origin for the shoulder muscles, and is an important link in the proximal-to-distal activation sequences of the kinetic chains of overhead activity. These roles depend on proper scapular motion and position.

Alterations in scapular motion and position are termed "scapular dyskinesis" and are present in 67% to 100% of shoulder injuries.

Scapular rehabilitation is a key component of shoulder rehabilitation and should be instituted early in shoulder rehabilitation—frequently while the shoulder injury is healing.

The scapular dyskinesis protocol that we use approaches rehabilitation of the scapula from a proximal-to-distal perspective. It uses muscle activation patterns to achieve this objective by facilitation through complementary trunk and hip movement. Lower extremity and trunk activation establishes the normal kinetic chain sequences that yield the desired scapular motion. Once scapular motion is normalized, these kinetic chain movement patterns are the framework for exercises to strengthen the scapular musculature. Closed–kinetic chain (CKC) exercises are begun in the early or acute phase to stimulate co-contractions of the rotator cuff and scapular musculature and promote scapulohumeral control and GH joint stability.

The distal area is an intrinsic load to the scapula, with the magnitude of the load depending on elbow flexion-extension and arm position. Function, rather than time, determines a patient's progress through the stages of the protocol. In this proximal-to-distal perspective, arm motion and strengthening activities are dependent on scapular control. A prerequisite for the addition of arm motion in the scapular program is appropriate, controlled scapular motion. Therefore, the movement pattern of the scapula determines the plane and degree of arm elevation or rotation in an exercise. If scapular compensation occurs with the introduction of a new arm position, new arm motion, or new load on the scapula, the arm position or motion should be changed to ensure that the resulting scapular motion is appropriate. Hip and trunk motion should be used as necessary to facilitate appropriate scapular motion. These facilitating motions may be decreased as scapular control increases.

REHABILITATION PROTOCOL *Scapular Dyskinesis*
Kibler and McMullen

ACUTE PHASE (USUALLY 0-3 WEEKS)

- Initially, avoid painful arm movement and establish scapular motion.
- Begin soft tissue mobilization, electrical modalities, ultrasound, and assisted stretching if muscular inflexibility is limiting motion. The pectoralis minor, levator scapulae, upper trapezius, latissimus dorsi, infraspinatus, and teres minor are frequently inflexible as a result of the injury process.
- Use modalities and active, active-assisted, passive, and PNF stretching techniques for these areas.
- Begin upper extremity weight shifts, wobble board exercises, scapular clock exercises (Fig. 3-80), rhythmic ball stabilization and weight-bearing isometric extension (Fig. 3-81) to promote safe co-contractions.
- Use these CKC exercises in various planes and levels of elevation, but coordinate them with appropriate scapular positioning.
- Initiate scapular motion exercises without arm elevation.
- Use trunk flexion and forward rotation to facilitate scapular protraction and active trunk extension, backward rotation and hip extension to facilitate scapular retraction. These postural changes require that the patient assume a contralateral side foot–forward stance and actively shift body weight forward for protraction and backward for retraction (Fig. 3-82). Patients who are unable to drive the trunk motion with the hips from this stance may actively stride forward and back with each reciprocal motion.

Continued

Scapular Dyskinesis *Continued*

ACUTE PHASE (USUALLY 0-3 WEEKS)—cont'd

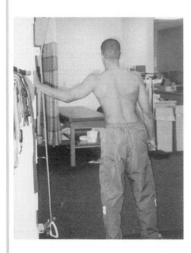

Figure 3–80 Scapular clock exercise. The patient reciprocally moves the scapula in a closed–kinetic chain position.

- Include arm motion with scapular motion exercises because the scapular motion improves to re-establish scapulohumeral coupling patterns. Keep the arm close to the body initially to minimize the intrinsic load.
- Emphasize lower abdominal and hip extensor exercises from the standing position. These muscle groups help stabilize the core and are instrumental in establishing thoracic posture.

Full active scapular motion is often limited by muscular inflexibility and myofascial restrictions. These soft tissue limitations must be alleviated for successful scapular rehabilitation. The pain and restriction in motion associated with these conditions limit progression through rehabilitation and lead to muscular compensation patterns, impingement, and possible GH joint injury.

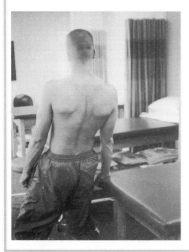

Figure 3–81 Weight-bearing isometric shoulder extension. An axial load with extension muscle activation stimulates thoracic extension and lower trapezius activation.

Scapular Dyskinesis   *Continued*

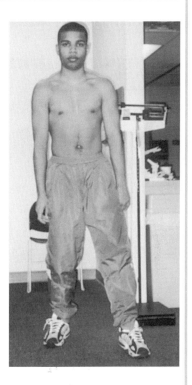

Figure 3–82   Stance for scapular motion exercises.

RECOVERY PHASE (3-8 WEEKS)

Proximal stability and muscular activation are imperative for appropriate scapular motion and strengthening. Strengthening is dependent on motion, and motion is dependent on posture.

- Continue to emphasize lower abdominal and hip extensor exercises along with flexibility exercises for the scapular stabilizers.
- Increase the loads on CKC exercises, such as wall push-ups, table push-ups, and modified prone push-ups.
- Also, increase the level of arm elevation in CKC exercises as scapular control improves.

Position the patient for CKC exercises by placing the hand on a table, wall, or other object and then moving the body relative to the fixed hand to define the plane and degree of elevation. This method ensures appropriate scapular position relative to the position of the arm. If normal scapular positioning cannot be achieved in this manner, the arm position requires adjustment.

- Add arm elevation and rotation patterns to scapular motion exercises, as able (Fig. 3-83). Use diagonal patterns, the scapular plane, and flexion. Progress toward active abduction. If intrinsic loads are too great with the introduction of active elevation, use axially loaded exercises as a transition to open–kinetic chain exercises. In these exercises, the patient applies a moderate load through the upper extremity, as in CKC exercises, but also slides the arm into elevation. Wall slides (Fig. 3-84) and table slides are examples. Incorporate trunk and hip motion with these exercises.

Continued

Scapular Dyskinesis *Continued*

RECOVERY PHASE (3-8 WEEKS)—cont'd

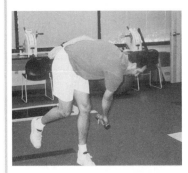

Figure 3–83 Progression of arm motion with scapular motion exercise patterns.

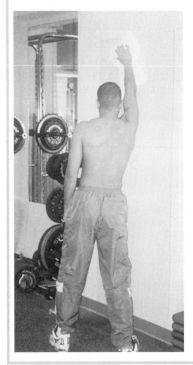

Figure 3–84 Wall slides. While maintaining an axial load, the patient slides the hand in a prescribed pattern.

Scapular Dyskinesis   *Continued*

RECOVERY PHASE (3-8 WEEKS)—cont'd

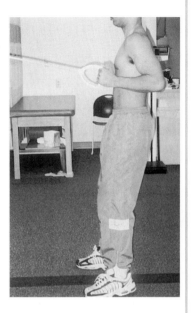

Figure 3–85   Tubing pulls incorporating trunk and hip extension.

- Begin tubing exercises using hip and trunk extension with retraction and hip and trunk flexion with protraction (Fig. 3-85). Use various angles of pull and planes of motion. De-emphasize upward pull until upper trapezius dominance is eliminated.
- As scapulohumeral coupling and control are achieved, dumbbell punches may be introduced. Use complementary strides to incorporate the kinetic chain contribution and reciprocal motions (Fig. 3-86). Vary the height of punches while maintaining scapular control.
- Use lunges with dumbbell reaches to emphasize kinetic chain timing and coordination (Fig. 3-87). Vary the level of arm elevation, amount of external rotation, and degree of elbow flexion in the standing, or return, position to increase the functional demand on the scapular muscles. Vary the direction of the lunge to vary the plane of emphasis for the scapular motion. Avoid scapular compensations such as "winging" or "shrugging." If compensations occur, reduce the load until there is appropriate scapular motion and scapulothoracic congruency with the exercise.

FUNCTIONAL PHASE (6-10 WEEKS)

- When good scapular control and motion have been achieved throughout the range of shoulder elevation, initiate plyometric exercises such as medicine ball toss and catch (Fig. 3-88) and tubing plyometrics.
- Continue to include kinetic chain activation. Move to various planes as scapular control improves.
- Slow, resisted sport skill movements, such as the throwing motion, are good activities to promote kinetic chain stabilization while dynamically loading the scapular muscles.

Continued

Scapular Dyskinesis   *Continued*

FUNCTIONAL PHASE (6-10 WEEKS)—cont'd

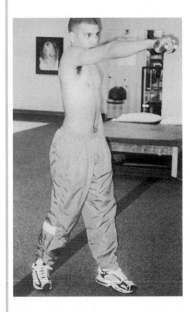

Figure 3–86   Dumbbell punches with a stride.

- Overhead dumbbell presses and punches, in various planes, are advanced exercises requiring good scapular control through a full and loaded GH joint ROM (Fig. 3-89).
- The lunge-and-reach series can be progressed to overhead reaches in the return position.
- Progressively add external resistance to exercises introduced earlier in the program. The volume of work is progressively advanced, as are the difficulty of the exercise and the amount of resistance.
- Challenging lower extremity stability using wobble boards, trampoline, slide boards, and the like also increases the load on the scapular musculature without sacrificing the functional movements.

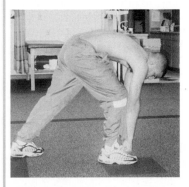

Figure 3–87   Lunge and reach. The return or standing position may be with the hands at the shoulders and the elbows pointing down or may include arm elevation, depending on the stage of recovery.

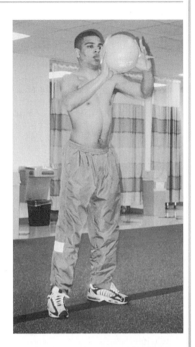

Figure 3–88 Medicine ball plyometric exercise.

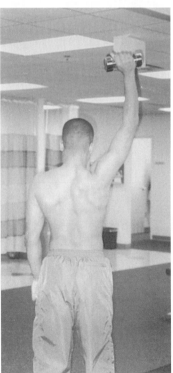

Figure 3–89 Overhead dumbbell press.

Bibliography

Bach BR Jr: Personal communication, November 1999.

Bahr R, Craig EV, Engbresten L: The clinical presentation of shoulder instability including on-the-field management. Clin Sports Med 14:761-776, 1995.

Blom S, Dhalback LO: Nerve injuries in dislocations of the shoulder joint and fractures of the neck of the humerus. Acta Chir Scand 136:461-466, 1970.

Burkhart SS: Arthroscopic treatment of massive rotator cuff tears. Clin Orthop 390:107-118, 2001.

Burkhart SS, Morgan CD: Technical note: The peel-back mechanism. Its role in producing and extending posterior type II SLAP lesions and its effect on SLAP repair rehabilitation. Arthroscopy 14:637-640, 1998.

Burkhart SS, Morgan CD: SLAP lesions in the overhead athlete. Orthop Clin North Am 32:431-441, 2001.

Burkhart SS, Morgan CD, Kibler WB: The disabled throwing shoulder: Spectrum of pathology. Part 1: Pathoanatomy and biomechanics. Arthroscopy 19:404-420, 2003.

Burkhart SS, Morgan CD, Kibler WB: The disabled throwing shoulder: Spectrum of pathology. Part II: Evaluation and treatment of SLAP lesions in throwers. Arthroscopy 19:531-559, 2003.

Burkhart SS, Morgan CD, Kibler WB: The disabled throwing shoulder: Spectrum of pathology. Part III: The SICK scapula, scapular dyskinesis. Arthroscopy 19:641-661, 2003.

Codman EA: The Shoulder: Rupture of the Supraspinatus Tendon and Other Lesions in or about the Subacromial Bursa. Boston, Thomas Todd, 1934.

Cofield RH, Boardman ND, Bengtson KA, et al: Rehabilitation after total shoulder arthroplasty. J Arthroplasty 16:483-486, 2001.

Dines DM, Levinson M: The conservative management of the unstable shoulder including rehabilitation. Clin Sports Med 14:797-816, 1995.

Frieman BG, Albert TJ, Fenlin JM Jr: Rotator cuff disease: A review of diagnosis, pathophysiology, and current trends in treatment. Arch Phys Med Rehabil 75:604-609, 1994.

Gross ML, Distefano MC: Anterior release test: A new test for shoulder instability. Clin Orthop 339:105-108, 1997.

Gusmer PB, Potter HG: Imaging of shoulder instability. Clin Sports Med 14:777-795, 1995.

Halbrecht JL, Tirman P, Atkin D: Internal impingement of the shoulder: Comparison of findings between the throwing and nonthrowing shoulders of college baseball players. Arthroscopy 15:253-258, 1999.

Harryman DT II, Lazarus MD, Rozencwaig R: The stiff shoulder. In Rockwood CA Jr, Matsen FA III (eds): The Shoulder, 2nd ed. Philadelphia, WB Saunders, 1998, pp 1064-1112.

Hawkins RJ, Montadi NG: Clinical evaluation of shoulder instability. Clin J Sports Med 1:59-64, 1991.

Hill AV: The mechanics of voluntary muscle. Lancet 2:947-951, 1951.

Host HH: Scapular taping in the treatment of anterior shoulder impingement. Phys Ther 75:803-811, 1995.

Jobe CM: Posterior superior glenoid impingement: Expanded spectrum. Arthroscopy 11:530-537, 1995.

Kibler WB: Normal shoulder mechanics and function. Instruct Course Lect 46:39-42, 1997.

Kibler WB: Shoulder rehabilitation: Principles and practice. Med Sci Sports Exerc 30:S40-S50, 1998.

Kibler WB: The role of the scapula in athletic shoulder function. Am J Sports Med 2:325-337, 1998.

Kibler WB, Garrett WE Jr: Pathophysiologic alterations in shoulder injury. Instruct Course Lect 46:3-6, 1997.

Kibler WB, Livingston B, Chandler TJ: Current concepts in shoulder rehabilitation. Adv Oper Orthop 3:249-301, 1996.

Kibler WB, Livingston B, Chandler TJ: Shoulder rehabilitation: Clinical application, evaluation, and rehabilitation protocols. Instruct Course Lect 46:43-51, 1997.

Kibler WB, McMullen JB: Accelerated postoperative shoulder rehabilitation. In Norris TR (ed): Orthopaedic Knowledge Update: Shoulder and Elbow 2. Rosemont, IL, American Academy of Orthopaedic Surgeons, 2002, pp 403-409.

Kim SH, Ha KI, Ahn JH, Choi HJ: Biceps local test II: A clinical test for SLAP lesions of the shoulder. Arthroplasty 17:160-164, 2001.

Kim SH, Ha KI, Han KY: Biceps load test: A clinical test for superior labrum anterior and posterior lesions in shoulders with recurrent anterior dislocations. Am J Sports Med 27:300-303, 1999.

Kirkley A, Griffin S, Richards C, et al: Prospective randomized clinical trial comparing effectiveness of immediate arthroscopic stabilization versus immobilization and rehabilitation in first traumatic anterior dislocations of the shoulder. Arthroscopy 15:507-514, 1999.

Lehman C, Cuomo F, Kummer FJ, Zuckerman JD: The incidence of full thickness rotator cuff tears in a large cadaveric population. Bull Hosp Joint Dis 54:30-31, 1995.

Liu SH, Henry MH, Nuccion SL: A prospective evaluation of a new physical examination in predicting glenoid labral tears. Am J Sports Med 24:721-725, 1996.

Matsen FA III, Thomas SC, Rockwood CA Jr, Wirth MA: Glenohumeral instability. In Rockwood CA Jr, Matsen FA III (eds): The Shoulder, 2nd ed. Philadelphia, WB Saunders, 1998, pp 611-754.

McMullen J, Uhl TL: A kinetic chain approach for shoulder rehabilitation. J Athlet Train 35:329-337, 2000.

McQuade KJ, Dawson J, Smidt GL: Scapulothoracic muscle fatigue associated with alterations in scapulohumeral rhythm kinematics during maximum resistive shoulder elevation. J Orthop Sports Phys Ther 28:74-80, 1998.

Morgan CD: The thrower's shoulder. Two perspectives. In McGinty JB, et al (eds): Operative Arthroscopy, 3rd ed. Philadelphia, Lippincott, Williams & Wilkins, 2003, pp 570-584.

Morgan CD, Burkhart SS, Palmeri M, et al: Type II SLAP lesions: Three subtypes and their relationship to superior instability and rotator cuff tears. Arthroscopy 14:553-565, 1998.

Morrey BF, Eiji I, Kai-nan A: Biomechanics of the shoulder. In Rockwood CA Jr, Matsen FA III (ed): The Shoulder, 2nd ed. Philadelphia, WB Saunders, 1998, pp 233-276.

Neer CS II: Anterior acromioplasty for the chronic impingement syndrome in the shoulder. J Bone Joint Surg Am 54:41-50, 1972.

Neviaser RJ, Neviaser TJ: Observations on impingement. Clin Orthop 254:60-63, 1990.

Nichols TR: A biomechanical perspective on spinal mechanisms of coordinated muscular action. Acta Anat 15:1-13, 1994.

O'Brien SJ, Neves MC, Arnoczky SP, et al: The anatomy and histology of the inferior glenohumeral ligament complex of the shoulder. Am J Sports Med 18:449-456, 1990.

Pagnani MJ, Speer KP, Altcheck DW, et al: Arthroscopic fixation of superior labral tears using a biodegradable implant: A preliminary report. Arthroscopy 11:194-198, 1995.

Pearsall AW, Speer KP: Frozen shoulder syndrome: Diagnostic and treatment strategies in the primary care setting. Med Sci Sports Exerc 30:S33-S39, 1998.

Poppen NK, Walker PS: Forces at the glenohumeral joint in abduction. Clin Orthop 135:165-170, 1978.

Post M, Silver R, Singh M: Rotator cuff tear. Clin Orthop 173:78-91, 1983.

Rockwood CA, Matsen FA: The Shoulder. Philadelphia, WB Saunders, 1990.

Romeo AA: Personal communication, October 1999.

Romeo AA, Hang DW, Bach BR Jr, Shott S: Repair of full thickness rotator cuff tears. Gender, age, and other factors affecting outcome. Clin Orthop 367:243-255, 1999.

Samani JE, Marston SB, Buss DD: Arthroscopic stabilization of type II SLAP lesions using an absorbable tack. Arthroscopy 17:19-24, 2001.

Schmitt L, Snyder-Mackler L: Role of scapular stabilizers in etiology and treatment of impingement syndrome. J Orthop Sports Phys Ther 29:31-38, 1999.

Segmüller HE, Hayes MG, Saies AD: Arthroscopic repair of glenolabral injuries with an absorbable fixation device. J Shoulder Elbow Surg 6:383-392, 1997.

Shelbourne KD, Nitz P: Accelerated rehabilitation after anterior cruciate ligament reconstruction. Am J Sports Med 18:192-199, 1990.

Snyder SJ, Karzel RP, Del Pizzo W, et al: SLAP lesions of the shoulder. Arthroscopy 6:274-279, 1990.

Speer KP, Cavanaugh JT, Warren RF: A role for hydrotherapy in shoulder rehabilitation. Am J Sports Med 21:850-853, 1993.

Speer KP, Garret WE Jr: Muscular control of motion and stability about the pectoral girdle. In Matsen FA III, Fu FH, Hawkins RJ (eds): The Shoulder: A Balance of Mobility and Stability. Rosemont, IL, American Academy of Orthopaedic Surgeons, 1993, pp 159-172.

Stollsteimer GT, Savoie FH: Arthroscopic rotator cuff repair: Current indications, limitations, techniques, and results. Instruct Course Lect 47:59-65,1998.

Tauro JC: Arthroscopic rotator cuff repair: Analysis of technique and results at 2 and 3 year follow-up. Arthroscopy 14:45-51, 1998.

Tibone JE, Bradely JP: The treatment of posterior subluxation in athletes. Clin Orthop 29:1124-1137, 1993.

Tyler TF, Nicholas SJ, Roy T, et al: Quantification of posterior capsule tightness and motion loss in patients with shoulder impingement. Am J Sports Med 28:668-674, 2000.

Verna C: Shoulder flexibility to reduce impingement. Paper presented at the Third Annual Meeting of the Professional Baseball Athletic Trainer Society, March 1991, Mesa, AZ.

Walch G, Boileau J, Noel E, et al: Impingement of the deep surface of the supraspinatus tendon on the posterior superior glenoid rim: An arthroscopic study. J Shoulder Elbow Surg 1:238-243, 1992.

Warner JJP, Kann S, Marks P: Arthroscopic repair of combined Bankart and superior labral detachment anterior and posterior lesions: Technique and preliminary results. Arthroscopy 10:383-391, 1994.

Warren RF, Craig EV, Altcheck DW: The Unstable Shoulder. Philadelphia, Lippincott-Raven, 1999.

Wilk KE, Andrews JR, Crockett HC: Rehabilitation after rotator cuff surgery: Techniques in shoulder and elbow. Am J Acad Orthop Surg 5:130-140, 1997.

Wilk KE, Arrigo C: Current concepts in the rehabilitation of the athletic shoulder. J Orthop Sports Phys Ther 18:365-378, 1993.

Wilk KE, Crockett HC, Andrews JR: Rehabilitation after rotator cuff surgery. Tech Shoulder Elbow Surg 1:128-144, 2000.

Wilk KE, Meister K, Andrews JR: Current concepts in the rehabilitation of the overhead throwing athlete. Am J Sports Med 30:136-151, 2002.

Wirth MA, Basamania C, Rockwood CA Jr: Nonoperative management of full-thickness tears of the rotator cuff. Orthop Clin North Am 28:59-66, 1997.

Yamaguchi K, Flatow EL: Management of multidirectional instability. Clin Sports Med 14:885-902, 1995.

Yocum LA, Conway JE: Rotator cuff tear: Clinical assessment and treatment. In Jobe FW (ed): Operative Techniques in Upper Extremity Sports Injuries. St Louis, CV Mosby, 1996, pp 223-245.

Zasler ND: American Association of Orthopaedic Surgeons Annual Meeting: Specialty Society Day, Feb. 7, 1999, Anaheim, CA.

4 | Knee Injuries

MICHAEL D'AMATO, MD •
BERNARD R. BACH, JR., MD

Typical Findings in Common Knee Conditions

MEDIAL KNEE

Medial Meniscal Tear

- Medial (medial meniscus) or lateral (lateral meniscus) joint line pain and tenderness
- Locking is almost pathognomonic for larger tears (locking also seen with loose bodies)
- Joint line pain, clicking or tenderness with twisting, pivoting, deep knee flexion, squatting, or standing from a squatting posture
- Positive clunking or clicking on the McMurray test
- Locked knee (i.e., lack of the ability to completely extend the knee) if a large bucket-handle tear is present
- Apley compression test positive (variable)

Typical Findings in Common Knee Conditions   *Continued*

MEDIAL KNEE—cont'd

Medial Collateral Ligament Injury

- Acute forced valgus mechanism of injury (e.g., clipping injury to the outer aspect of the knee driving the knee medially [inward])
- Medial pain and point tenderness over the medial collateral ligament (MCL)
- Minimal localized effusion (variable) over the MCL (a large associated effusion would suggest a concomitant intra-articular injury such as to the anterior cruciate ligament [ACL] or posterior cruciate ligament [PCL])
- Pain or opening on valgus stress testing at 30 degrees of knee flexion with a type 2 or 3 MCL injury

Pes Anserine Bursitis

- Inflamed bursa below the medial joint line
- Bursa is overlying the insertion point of the sartorius, gracilis, and semitendinosus tendons
- Pain and tenderness located anteromedially 2 to 5 cm *below* the medial joint line
- Most common populations include obese females, athletes, and elderly with concomitant arthritis
- Often the swollen bursa is palpable
- Treatment is intrabursal cortisone injection, ice, and rest from aggravating activities (e.g., stair climbing)

Osteoarthritis

- Insidious or gradual onset
- Morning stiffness and pain
- Joint line narrowing on standing anteroposterior (AP) films
- Angular deformity (variable)
- Effusion (variable)
- Tenderness and pain over affected joint lines (medial and/or lateral)
- Osteophytes (variable)

ANTERIOR KNEE

Patellofemoral Syndrome (Anterior Knee Pain)

- Often bilateral
- Exacerbated by activities that increase patellofemoral joint reaction forces (stair climbing, squats, jumping, running)
- Often underlying biomechanical contributors (see patellofemoral section) such as pes planus, increased Q-angle, positive patellar tilt (tight lateral retinaculum), patella alta
- No mechanical symptoms or findings
- Tender on patellar facet palpation; may have crepitance on compression grind testing of the patella

Osgood-Schlatter Disease

- Active, skeletally immature athlete
- Tender tibial tubercle
- Prominent tibial tubercle

Continued

Typical Findings in Common Knee Conditions *Continued*

ANTERIOR KNEE—cont'd

Jumper's Knee (Patellar Tendinitis)

- Pain at the patellar tendon
- Tender on palpation of the patellar tendon
- History of repetitive jumping, running, or overuse syndrome

Sinding-Larsen–Johansson Syndrome

- Tender at the inferior pole of the patella
- Radiographic changes noted at the inferior pole of the patella (traction apophysitis)
- May have bump palpable at the inferior pole of the patella
- Treatment similar to that for Osgood-Schlatter disease

Acute Patellar Dislocation

- Patient often incorrectly reports "the knee shifted"
- Tender over the medial retinaculum (torn)
- Usually a tense effusion (hemarthrosis)
- Positive patellar apprehension test and increased lateral excursion on lateral glide test
- May have an osteochondral fracture of the patella or a laterally subluxated position of the patella on the sunrise view

Prepatellar Bursitis (Housemaid's Knee)

- Swollen, large bursa noted over the anterior aspect of the knee
- Often a history of repetitive shearing force to the anterior aspect of knee (repetitive kneeling on the knee such as a carpet layer)
- Intra-articular aspiration of the knee joint is negative—no intra-articular effusion; swelling is purely prepatellar

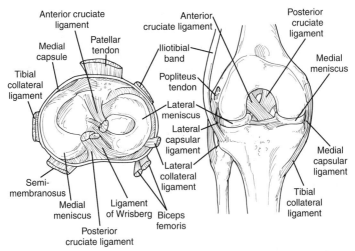

Figure 4–1   Anatomy of the knee. **Left**, Top view showing the plateau of the tibia. **Right**, Front view (with the patella removed).

Typical Findings in Common Knee Conditions   *Continued*

LATERAL KNEE

Iliotibial Band Syndrome

- Lateral knee pain and tenderness over the iliotibial band
- Pain exacerbated by hill climbing, StairMaster, running, or repetitive deep flexion exercises
- Commonly caused by training errors such as hill climbing or too rapid progression of intensity, mileage, or hills (variable)

Lateral Meniscal Tear (See Medial Meniscus)

POSTERIOR KNEE

Baker's (Popliteal) Cyst

- Posterior mass in the back of the knee
- May transilluminate
- High incidence of associated intra-articular pathology (e.g., meniscal tear)

Popliteal Tendinitis

- Posterolateral knee pain in runners
- Positive Garrick test (flex the hip and knee to 90 degrees in a supine patient and internally rotate the leg. The patient is then asked try to keep it there while the examiner applies an external rotation force. This elicits pain at an inflamed popliteus.)
- Treatment is an eccentric quadriceps strengthening program, rest, ice, and nonsteroidal anti-inflammatory drugs (NSAIDs) (e.g., valdecoxib [Bextra], celecoxib [Celebrex])

VARIABLE MANIFESTATION

Anterior Cruciate Ligament Tear (Fig. 4-1)

- Acute injury (hyperextension, valgus clip, etc.)
- Rapid effusion (less than 2 hours after injury) implying hemarthrosis as a result of bleeding from the torn ligament ends
- Inability to continue play
- Subjective instability
- Positive Lachman test, pivot shift test
- Positive anterior drawer sign (less sensitive and specific than the Lachman test)

Osteochondritis Dissecans

- Vague, insidious onset of clicking, popping, locking, mild swelling
- Radiographs (tunnel view) often reveal an osteochondritis dissecans (OCD) lesion
- Magnetic resonance imaging (MRI) useful to some degree for diagnosis and staging

Posterior Cruciate Ligament Tear

- Abnormal posterior drawer test
- PCL mechanism of injury (see Posterior Cruciate Ligament Injuries)
- Effusion (variable)
- Drop-back sign

Continued

Typical Findings in Common Knee Conditions *Continued*

VARIABLE MANIFESTATION—cont'd

Posterolateral Capsuloligamentous Injury

- Acute injury characterized by ecchymosis and swelling on the lateral and posterolateral sides of the knee
- Usually concomitant PCL or ACL injury
- Tearing of a combination of the fibular collateral ligament, popliteus, posterolateral capsule, and possible PCL or ACL
- Look for varus thrust gait during ambulation
- Positive dial test
- Reverse pivot shift
- Posterior drawer, drop-back sign often positive with concomitant PCL injury
- External rotation (Loomer) test positive
- Often other associated ligament(s) injuries

Nontraumatic (Often Chronic) Causes of Knee Pain

Overuse injuries
- Tendinitis
- Bursitis
- Stress fracture

Septic arthritis (EMERGENCY!)
Gonococcal arthritis
Rheumatoid arthritis
Rheumatic fever
Juvenile arthritis
Polymyalgia rheumatica
Crystal-induced disease
- Gout/pseudogout

Charcot joint
OCD
Reflex sympathetic dystrophy (RSD)
Seronegative spondyloarthropathy
- Ankylosing spondylitis
- Reiter's syndrome
- Psoriatic spondylitis
- Inflammatory bowel disease

Collagen vascular disease
- Scleroderma
- Polymyositis
- Polyarteritis nodosa
- Mixed connective tissue disease

Lyme disease
Tuberculosis
Viral synovitis
Fungal infection
Neoplasm (benign or malignant)

Physical Examination

A thorough knee examination begins with a relaxed and comfortable patient. Both knees should be examined simultaneously to allow inspection for asymmetry.

EXAMINATION OF THE ENTIRE EXTREMITY

Before actually examining the knee, the physician should inspect the entire extremity with the knee evident and both shoes and socks off. The patient's gait should be observed at some point during the visit. Sometimes, it is helpful to observe the patient's gait when the patient is not aware of being watched by the examiner (possible secondary gain issues).

With the patient standing, weight-bearing alignment of the knee should be evaluated to document varus, valgus, or normal alignment; any recurvatum deformity or internal or external rotation of the leg (tibial torsion, femoral anteversion); the Q-angle of the patellofemoral joint; and any patella alta, patella baja, or squinting of the patella (Fig. 4-2). Evaluation of the biomechanical alignment of the entire limb includes noting any contributing pes planus deformity that increases the Q-angle at the knee (Fig. 4-3). The skin should be examined for any abnormalities, such as altered appearance (shiny), temperature (hot or cold), sensation (hyperesthetic or hypoesthetic), or sweating that may indicate RSD. Popliteal, dorsalis pedis, and posterior tibial pulses should be documented, as well as function of the sensory and motor (peroneal and tibial) nerves. Examination of the asymptomatic limb is helpful for comparison with the symptomatic side.

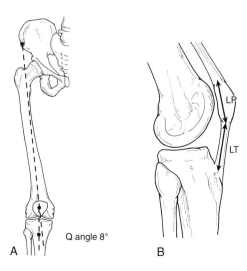

Figure 4–2 **A,** The Q-angle (quadriceps) is an angle formed between lines drawn from the anterior superior iliac spine of the pelvis to the middle of the patella and a line drawn from the middle of the patella to the tibial tubercle. The angle is measured with the knee in full extension. An angle greater than 20 degrees is abnormal and often associated with lateral tracking or instability of the patella. **B,** Insall's technique for measuring patella alta. The length of the patellar tendon (LT) is divided by the length of the patella (LP). A 1.2:1 ratio indicates a normal extensor mechanism. A ratio greater than 1.2:1 indicates patella alta (long patellar tendon). This abnormality is often associated with anterior knee pain, patellar malalignment, and instability. In patella alta, the "high" patella does not properly engage in the trochlear groove. (Adapted from Sebastianelli WJ: Anterior knee pain: Sorting through a complex differential. J Musculoskel Med 10[7]:55-66, 1993.)

Q angle 8°

A

B

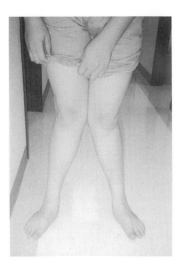

Figure 4–3 Genu valgum (severe) exacerbated by underlying pes planus, which is contributing to an increased Q-angle.

Sometimes, knee pain is referred pain from the hip (anterior thigh pain), and this should be ruled out as a source of pain. In pediatric patients, failure to examine the hip to rule out referred pain to the knee may lead to a missed diagnosis of Legg-Calvé-Perthes disease, slipped capital femoral epiphysis, hip fracture, or septic hip.

Sequential Steps of a Knee Examination

When performing a knee evaluation we usually cover the following important steps:
1. **Visual inspection** for
   a. Effusion
   b. Ecchymosis
   c. Posture of the resting knee (e.g., a locked knee with an inability to completely straighten the knee the last few degrees of extension)
   d. Varus, valgus, or recurvatum deformity when standing
   e. Muscle atrophy
   f. Altered skin temperature, color, appearance (shiny), which might suggest RSD
2. Have the patient perform a straight leg raise (SLR) to demonstrate an **intact extensor mechanism** (i.e., the ability to perform an SLR demonstrates that there is not a complete rupture of the patellar tendon or quadriceps, a displaced patellar fracture, etc.)
3. Perform active and passive **range of motion** (ROM) of the knee and document the ROM
4. **Palpate the anatomic structures** of the knee
   a. MCL and lateral collateral ligament (LCL)
   b. Medial and lateral joint line
   c. Patella, quadriceps, patellar tendon, and tibial tuberosity
   d. Medial retinaculum

Sequential Steps of a Knee Examination   Continued

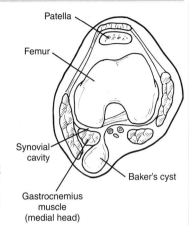

Figure 4–4   Cross section of the knee showing a posterior location for a Baker cyst. (Adapted from Black KP, Skrzynski MC: Arthroscopy in knee diagnosis and surgery: An update. J Musculoskel Med 10[2]79-94, 1993.)

   e. Pes anserine bursa (the attachment site of the semitendinosus, gracilis, and sartorius 1 cm below the medial joint line)
   f. Iliotibial band (laterally) and Gerdy's tubercle (insertion site of the iliotibial band)
   g. Posterior structures (possible Baker's cyst [Fig. 4-4], hamstring and calf muscle insertions, popliteus, plantaris, etc.)
5. **Ligamentous examination**
   a. MCL and LCL (valgus and varus stress testing)
   b. ACL and PCL (Lachman, anterior drawer, posterior drawer, etc.)
   c. Posterolateral corner examination if clinically suspicious
6. **Meniscal examination**
   a. Medial meniscus (McMurray test, Apley compression grind test)
   b. Lateral meniscus (McMurray test, Apley compression grind test)

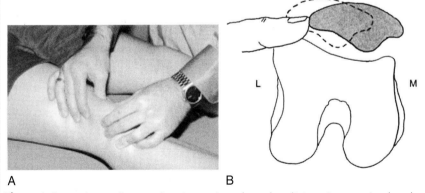

A   B

Figure 4–5   **A**, The patellar apprehension test is performed to elicit anxiety or pain when the examiner laterally displaces or compresses the patella with the thumbs. A positive test indicates underlying patellar instability or subluxation. **B**, Lateral displacement of the patella causing pain or anxiety.

Continued

Sequential Steps of a Knee Examination Continued

---

7. **Patellar examination**
   a. Patellar tracking/maltracking
   b. Q-angle/contributing pes planus
   c. Patellar stability (Fig. 4-5)
   d. Patellar apprehension with lateral glide testing of the patella
   e. Patellar tilt test—tight lateral retinacular structures produce a tilting of the patella toward the lateral trochlear groove and thus a positive patellar tilt test
   f. Patellar glide (lateral and medial)
   g. Vastus medialis obliquus (VMO) atrophy
   h. Patellar crepitance
8. **Hip ROM** to rule out hip pathology referring pain to the knee
9. **Gait**—walking and/or running
10. Generalized ligamentous laxity (positive thumb-to-wrist test)
11. Flexibility of the lower extremity (hamstrings, quadriceps, iliotibial band, etc.)

KNEE LIGAMENT EXAMINATION

Several **stress testing maneuvers** are used for ligamentous and patellar examination (Table 4-1). Valgus stress should be applied to the **medial collateral ligament** and medial capsule with the knee at 0 and 30 degrees of flexion, and the amount of opening of the medial joint line on valgus stressing is recorded (Fig. 4-6). Opening of the medial joint line at 30 degrees of flexion implies a grade II or III MCL tear (see p. 387). Opening at 0 degrees of flexion implies a more severe injury of the MCL with concomitant pathology such as an ACL or PCL injury.

The **lateral collateral ligament** and lateral capsule are stressed by a varus force with the knee in the same positions, and the amount of opening is recorded (Fig. 4-7).

The **posterior cruciate ligament** is checked for a posterior drawer sign with the knee at 90 degrees (Fig. 4-8) and for a positive posterior sag (Fig. 4-9).

A **Lachman test** is used to check the **ACL** with the knee in 30 degrees of flexion (Fig. 4-10A). An **anterior drawer test** (see Fig. 4-10B) can also be done with the knee in 90 degrees of flexion.

The most sensitive test for an ACL tear is a Lachman test with a relaxed patient and relaxed lower extremity.

In very cooperative patients, a **pivot shift test** (see Fig. 4-10C) can be performed, but it is painful and requires significant cooperation. Thus, it should be the last attempted maneuver in the examination because the pain is not tolerated by most patients and may inhibit further examination.

MENISCAL EVALUATION

The most common **meniscal tests** are those described by McMurray and Apley. The **McMurray test** (Fig. 4-11) is done with the knee flexed as far as possible and the foot and tibia either externally rotated (to test the medial meniscus) or internally rotated (to test the lateral meniscus). While the tibia is held in the appropriate position, the knee is brought from the position of acute flexion into extension. The classic finding is a painful pop along the appropriate joint line that is palpable or audible

TABLE 4–1   Ligamentous Testing of the Knee

Test	Purpose	Method	Results
Lachman test	ACL insufficiency	Patient is supine, with the knee in 20 degrees of flexion. Examiner stands on the side of the injured knee and pulls the tibia anteriorly	A "give" reaction or mushy endpoint indicates ACL disruption. Most sensitive ACL test
Anterior drawer test	ACL insufficiency	Patient is supine with the knee flexed to 90 degrees. Examiner attempts to pull the tibia from its anatomic position to a displaced anterior position	Result is positive if the tibia can be anteriorly displaced on the femur
Posterior drawer test	PCL insufficiency	Patient is supine with the knee flexed to 90 degrees. Examiner attempts to posteriorly displace the tibia on the femur by pushing the tibia posteriorly	In PCL insufficiency, there is posterior sagging of the tibia
Varus/valgus stress test	Medial and lateral collateral ligamentous stability; evaluate for possible growth plate injury in a skeletally immature patient	Patient is positioned with the knee first in full extension and then in 30 degrees of flexion. Standing on the side of the injured leg, the examiner applies varus and valgus stress to the knee in both the extended and the 30-degree flexed positions. The degree of joint opening is compared with that in the uninvolved side	Grade I collateral ligament sprains often have tenderness with little or no joint opening. Grade III opening of greater than 15 mm suggests ligament disruption. **Stress radiographs of growth plate injuries show opening or gapping of the affected growth plate**

Continued

TABLE 4–1	Ligamentous Testing of the Knee—cont'd		
Test	Purpose	Method	Results
Pivot shift test	ACL insufficiency (assesses anterior displacement of the lateral tibial plateau on the lateral femoral condyle)	Knee is positioned in 30 degrees of flexion. Examiner places one hand under the heel and the other on the lateral aspect of the proximal end of the tibia and then applies valgus stress. The knee is then brought into extension	In ACL disruption, the lateral tibial plateau is in the anatomic position when the knee is flexed and subluxates anteriorly during extension
Reverse pivot shift test	PCL insufficiency	Knee is positioned in 30 degrees of flexion. Test is done as for the pivot shift test	In PCL and posterolateral insufficiency, the lateral tibial plateau is reduced with the knee in extension and, during flexion, falls posteriorly and rotates with respect to the medial tibial plateau. Straight posterior laxity with isolated PCL injury allows posterior displacement of the tibia on the femur but prevents a reverse pivot shift
Quadriceps active drawer test	Posterior instability	Knees positioned in 90 degrees of flexion. Examiner places posterior pressure on the tibia and then asks the patient to actively fire the quadriceps by trying to slide the heel forward	In posterior laxity, the quadriceps draws the tibia forward

ACL, anterior cruciate ligament; PCL, posterior cruciate ligament.
From Meislin RJ: Managing collateral ligament tears of the knee. J Musculoskel Med 24[3]:90-96, 1996.

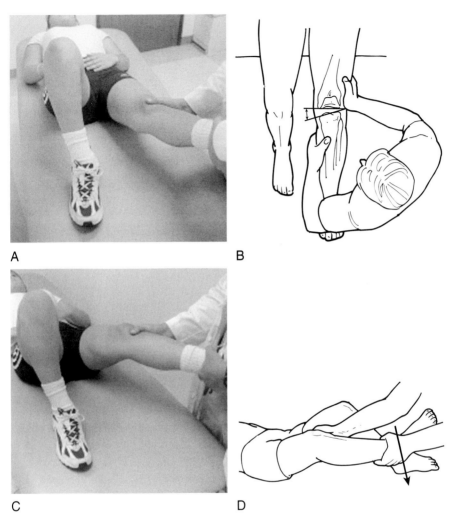

Figure 4–6 Valgus stress testing of the medial collateral ligament (MCL) at 0 degrees of knee flexion (**A** and **B**) and 30 degrees of knee flexion (**C** and **D**). Medial opening at 0 degrees of knee flexion indicates more injury (e.g., anterior cruciate ligament or capsule) than just an isolated MCL tear. (**B**, Adapted from Meislin RJ: Managing collateral ligament tears of the knee. Physician Sports Med 24[3]:90-96, 1996.)

to the examiner. In some knees, significant pain may be elicited over the appropriate joint line without a true popping.

The **Apley compression test** (Fig. 4-12) is done with the patient prone and the knee flexed to 90 degrees. The examiner pushes downward on the sole of the patient's foot toward the examination table to compress the menisci between the tibia and femur. Then, with the tibia in external rotation (for the medial meniscus)

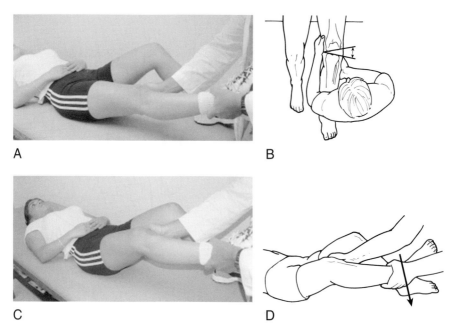

A   B

C   D

Figure 4–7 Lateral collateral ligament testing by applying a varus force to the knee at 0 degrees (**A** and **B**) and 30 degrees (**C** and **D**) of knee flexion. (**B**, Adapted from Meislin RJ: Managing collateral ligament tears of the knee. Physician Sports Med 24[3]:90-96, 1996.)

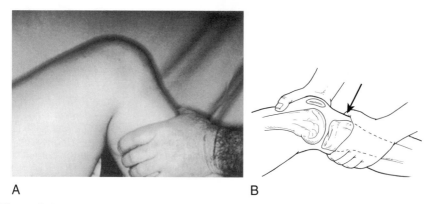

A   B

Figure 4–8 **A,** Posterior drawer test for the posterior cruciate ligament (PCL). The examiner pushes posteriorly on the tibia with the knee relaxed and bent at a 90-degree angle. Increased laxity in comparison to the unaffected limb indicates a probable PCL tear. Compare with the unaffected limb. Laxity is measured by the relationship of the medial tibial plateau to the medial femoral condyle. **B,** The posterior drawer test for PCL injury is performed with the patient supine, the knee flexed 90 degrees, and the quadriceps and hamstring muscles completely relaxed. The examiner holds the tibia in neutral position by sitting on the patient's foot. The examiner gently pushes the proximal end of the tibia posteriorly to assess PCL integrity. Excursion and a soft endpoint, when compared with the opposite side, suggest an injury. (**B,** Adapted from Laprade RF, Wentorf F: Acute knee injuries: On-the-field and sideline evaluation. Physician Sports Med 27[10]:107-111, 1999.)

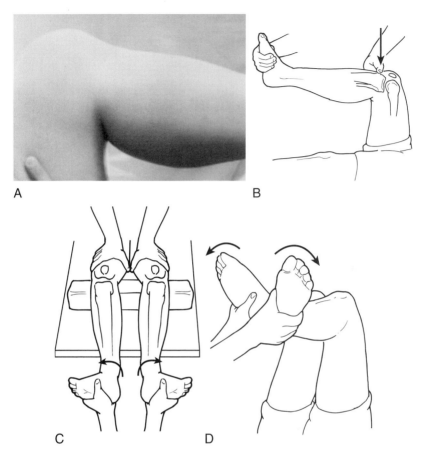

Figure 4–9 **A**, Posterior sag test for the posterior cruciate ligament (PCL). **B**, In the Godfrey test, the tibia sags posteriorly when the hip and knee are flexed at 90 degrees, indicative of PCL damage. Gravity causes the proximal end of the tibia to sag posteriorly, and the normal contour of the bone is lost. **C**, To rule out associated injuries of the posterolateral corner (arcuate complex) and posteromedial corner, the physician evaluates axial rotation. An assistant stabilizes the patient's femurs while the physician externally rotates the tibias. The test is positive if the injured side demonstrates a greater degree of tibial rotation. **D**, In Loomer's variation on the posterolateral drawer test, the patient lies supine. With the patient's hips and knees in 90 degrees of flexion and the knees together, the examiner grasps and maximally externally rotates the patient's feet. Excessive external rotation in one extremity marks a positive test and is easily seen. The examiner will also note mild posterior displacement or sag of the tibia. (**B**, Adapted from Allen AA, Harner CD: When your patient injures the posterior cruciate ligament. J Musculoskel Med 13[2]:44, 1996. Artist: Charles H. Boyter. **C**, Adapted from Meislin RJ: Managing collateral ligament tears of the knee. Physician Sports Med 24[3]:90-96, 1996.)

or internal rotation (for the lateral meniscus), the knee is moved through full ROM while compression is maintained. A positive response is pain over the joint line being tested.

Flexibility of the hamstrings and quadriceps and the Ober test should be documented on the examination as well (see the section on patellofemoral disorders, p. 520).

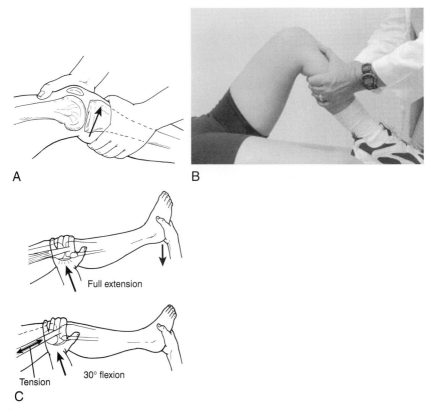

Figure 4–10   **A**, The Lachman test is the most sensitive maneuver for detecting instability of the anterior cruciate ligament (ACL). With the patient's knee in 20 to 30 degrees of flexion, the physician stabilizes the femur with one hand and applies an anteriorly directed force to the proximal end of the tibia with the other hand. Increased anterior translation of the tibia (in comparison to the uninvolved knee) or a soft endpoint indicates ACL disruption. **B**, Anterior drawer test. The patient lies supine with the knee bent at 90 degrees. The examiner places the patient's thigh over the foot to anchor and pulls forward on the relaxed tibia to assess anterior translation and the quality of the endpoint. **C**, For the pivot shift test, internal rotation and valgus forces are applied to the nearly fully extended (straight) knee (*top*). If the ACL is torn, the tibia will sublux slightly anterolaterally. As the knee is then flexed to about 40 degrees (*bottom*), the iliotibial band changes from a knee extensor to a flexor and reduces the subluxated tibia, sometimes with an audible clunk—a positive test for an ACL tear. A positive test should not be repeated because of risk to the meniscus. (**A**, Adapted from Cameron ML, Mizuno Y, Cosgarea AJ: Diagnosing and managing ACL injuries. J Musculoskel Med 17:47-53, 2000. **C**, Adapted from Rey JM: A proposed natural history of symptomatic ACL knee injuries. Clin Sports Med 7:697-709, 1988.)

Aspiration of the Knee

In patients with a tense, painful hemarthrosis, aspiration of the knee provides significant pain relief. Studies have also documented that large effusions (>40 mL of fluid) provide an inhibitory feedback mechanism for the quadriceps and essentially shut down its function. Aspiration of the knee joint is also useful for obtaining synovial

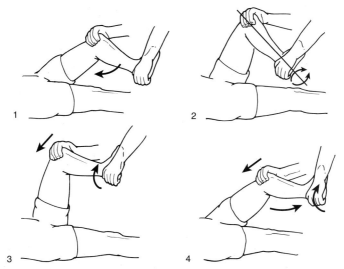

Figure 4–11   McMurray test. Flex the knee maximally. Externally rotate the foot (for the medial meniscus) and passively extend the knee while looking for a click or pain medially. (Adapted from Hunter-Griffin LY [ed]: Athletic Training and Sports Medicine, 2nd ed. Rosemont, IL, American Academy of Orthopaedic Surgeons, 1994.)

fluid to be examined for infection or crystals. Knee aspirate (excluding traumatic hemarthrosis) is sent to the laboratory for

- Cell count and differential cell count (purple-top tube).
- Cultures (Gram stain, aerobic, anaerobic, acid-fast bacilli/fungal).
- Crystals (green-top tube). Gout is negatively birefringent under polarized light, with needle-shaped crystals; pseudogout (chondrocalcinosis) is positively birefringent under polarized light, with a pleomorphic appearance. Some literature suggests that glucose, clot, and viscosity should also be tested.

Fat droplets noted in the knee aspirate after an acute injury indicate a bony injury (fracture) with communication between the marrow cavity and the interior of the joint. Fat droplets in the knee aspirate can typically be seen when the aspirate is squirted into a metal or plastic basin.

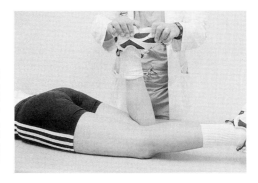

Figure 4–12   Apley compression test (meniscal test). The prone knee is flexed to 90 degrees. The knee is compressed (pushed downward) while alternately externally and internally rotating the foot. Medial pain on external rotation suggests a medial meniscal tear. Lateral pain on internal rotation suggests a probable lateral meniscal tear.

Instillation of 1% lidocaine into the knee during aspiration of blood or fluid may also allow better ligamentous evaluation after the patient's comfort level has improved.

Knee Aspirate

FINDING	NORMAL KNEE	SEPTIC ARTHRITIS	RHEUMATOID ARTHRITIS	DEGENERATIVE JOINT DISEASE
Appearance	Clear	Turbid (cannot read a newspaper through a test tube)	Cloudy	Clear
Cell count/mm^3	200	Usually >50,000*	2000-50,000	2000
Differentiated cell count	Monos	Polys	50/50	Monos
Glucose	Within 60% or more of serum glucose	Very low	Low	Normal

*A count greater than 50,000 white blood cells indicates an infected joint and requires emergency washout (débridement and irrigation) of the joint.

Technique of Knee Aspiration and Cortisone Injection (Brotzman)

- The knee is sterilely prepared with povidone-iodine (Betadine) or alcohol (Fig. 4-13).
- The patient lies flat on the back with the knee straight, relaxed, and well supported.
- A lateral suprapatellar approach is probably safest and easiest.
- Placing a thumb on the medial side of the relaxed patella and pushing the patella laterally identifies the interval for needle insertion (for both 25-gauge and spinal needles). This interval is located between the lateral patellar edge and the lateral femoral condyle. The horizontal needle insertion should be at the superior aspect of the patella to take advantage of the large, fluid-filled suprapatellar pouch that extends superiorly (proximally) from the patella.
- The site is numbed with 5 to 10 mL of 1% lidocaine via a 1.5-inch, 25-gauge needle with sterile technique (see Fig. 4-13 for landmarks).
- After 2 minutes to allow the anesthetic to produce "numbing," an 18- or 20-gauge spinal needle (attached to a 20-mL or larger syringe) is inserted through the "numb" track of the 25-gauge needle with sterile technique.
- As much fluid as possible is aspirated through the spinal needle while maintaining sterility.
- Leaving the spinal needle in place and without contaminating the needle hub, the examiner removes the syringe and attaches a 5-mL syringe containing cortisone to the needle. The cortisone is injected and the needle is removed.

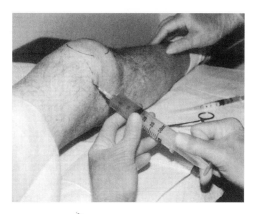

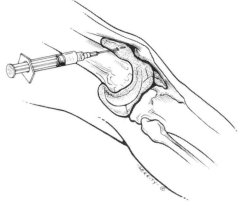

Figure 4–13 Knee injection and aspiration. A lateral approach to a swollen, distended suprapatellar pouch (bursa) is used for knee aspiration. (Adapted from Goss JA, Adams RF: Local injection of corticosteroids in rheumatic diseases. J Musculoskel Med 10[3]:83-92, 1993. Artist: Peg Gerrity.)

- Pressure is maintained on the injection site for 5 minutes after the needle is removed.
- The patient is advised to rest, elevate the limb, and apply ice to the area. Pain medication may be required for 2 or 3 days.

Imaging

Radiographic imaging of the knee should be used to confirm or refute the clinical diagnosis already made from the history and physical examination. In patients with **acute trauma**, **AP**, **lateral**, and **sunrise views** of the knee are usually sufficient to rule out displaced fractures. In older patients or those with **chronic pain, standing AP (weight-bearing), lateral,** and **sunrise views** are appropriate. **Tunnel views** are taken to evaluate possible OCD lesions. Imaging of the contralateral, asymptomatic knee may also help one appreciate differences in joint space width, bone density, physeal fractures, soft tissue swelling, and osteophyte formation.

In all patients older than 30 years, a bilateral weight-bearing AP view should be obtained to look for joint line narrowing indicative of arthritis.

Patients younger than 20 years should have a tunnel view as part of the routine radiographic series to evaluate for otherwise occult OCD lesions.

MRI is not generally needed in the routine evaluation of the knee, but it may be helpful for evaluation of tumors around the knee. When soft tissue masses are identified or bone involvement is seen on radiographs, MRI can help determine their extent. After acute trauma when the knee is too painful or swollen for an accurate examination and immediate diagnosis is necessary, MRI is helpful in distinguishing between a bone bruise, an articular cartilage injury, and a meniscal tear. It is also effective in determining the extent of possible osteomyelitis or avascular necrosis.

The decision to perform MRI, arthroscopy, or both is probably best made by the orthopaedic surgeon rather than the referring primary care physician because MRI may be superfluous if arthroscopy is warranted (e.g., locked knee, hemarthrosis with an ACL tear, symptomatic loose body, septic joint). Several factors should be considered in making this decision. MRI is a noninvasive diagnostic tool. Arthroscopy is invasive, but it is therapeutic as well. It allows treatment of the internal derangement of the knee, in addition to confirming or modifying the clinical diagnosis. MRI is expensive and should be used judiciously. It is not required before every arthroscopic examination. In general, a working diagnosis should be made from the history, physical examination, and plain radiographs before arthroscopic examination, and the findings at arthroscopic examination should confirm this diagnosis.

Computed tomography is helpful for evaluation of complex, intra-articular fractures, such as tibial plateau fractures, and to characterize bone tumors around the knee. It gives no good information on soft tissue structures (ligaments, menisci, etc.)

Arteriograms are helpful when ischemia or claudication may be causing pain around the knee and to rule out vascular injury with acute knee dislocations.

Practitioner Pearls for History and Examination of the Knee

- **Immediate bloody effusion** after acute injury most commonly occurs with intra-articular ligament tears (ACL and PCL, not extra-articular MCL or LCL tears), fractures about the knee, quadriceps rupture, patellar dislocations (torn medial retinaculum), or peripheral meniscal tears (bleeding from the perimeniscal capillary plexus).
- **Locking** of the knee in a slightly flexed position with difficulty working it back into full extension is almost pathognomonic for a meniscal tear (often a bucket-handle tear). A dislocated (or subluxated) patella, an intra-articular loose body, or detached OCD lesions are other probable causes of "locking." True locking is almost always an indication for operative intervention (arthroscopy).
- **Gradual onset of anterior knee pain** in young female athletes (patellofemoral pain) is common. It is typically exacerbated by activities involving deep knee flexion (squatting, kneeling, stairs, running, chair to standing). Knee flexion increases patellofemoral joint reaction forces (PFJRFs) (see the section on patellofemoral disorders, p. 489).
- **Instability or giving way** of the knee is usually indicative of a ligamentous tear (e.g., ACL) or quadriceps atrophy (usually postoperative or after chronic effusion or knee injury causing inhibitory feedback to the quadriceps).
- Pes anserine bursitis, or **Voshell's bursitis**, is a commonly missed cause of **medial** knee pain. Tenderness or inflammation is typically medial, but two to three fingerbreadths below the medial joint line at the pes anserine tendon insertion.

Anterior Cruciate Ligament Injuries

Michael D'Amato, MD • Bernard R. Bach, Jr., MD

BACKGROUND

As our understanding of the biology and biomechanics of knee and graft reconstruction techniques has improved, rehabilitation after ACL injury has also changed. In the 1970s, ACL reconstructions were performed through large arthrotomies via extra-articular reconstruction, and patients were immobilized in casts for long periods after surgery. In the 1980s, arthroscopic techniques led to intra-articular reconstruction and eliminated the need for a large arthrotomy, which allowed the use of "accelerated" rehabilitation protocols that focused on early motion. In the 1990s, the concept of "accelerated" rehabilitation evolved in an effort to return athletes to the playing field quicker than ever. With this emphasis on quick return to sports, issues regarding open– and closed–kinetic chain exercises and graft strain have come to the forefront, as has the role of postoperative and functional bracing. In addition, the value of preoperative rehabilitation to prevent postoperative complications has been recognized.

REHABILITATION RATIONALE

Nonoperative treatment of an ACL-deficient knee may be indicated in older, sedentary people, but in active people, young or old, an ACL-deficient knee has a high incidence of instability that often leads to meniscal tears, articular injury, and subsequent degenerative changes in the knee. Adequate knee function may be maintained in the short term, particularly after hamstring-strengthening programs, but this is unpredictable and function is usually below the preinjury level.

Surgical reconstruction of the ACL can now predictably restore the stability of the knee, and rehabilitation is focused on restoring motion and strength while maintaining knee stability by protecting the healing graft and donor site. Aggressive "accelerated" rehabilitation programs have been made possible through advances in graft material and graft fixation methods and through improved understanding of graft biomechanics and the effects of various exercises and activities on graft strains. Although these protocols may ultimately prove to be safe and appropriate, they must be viewed cautiously until continued research into graft healing further delineates the limits to which rehabilitation after ACL reconstruction can be "accelerated."

Protocols for rehabilitation after ACL reconstruction follow *several basic guiding principles*:

- Achieving full ROM and reduction of inflammation and swelling before surgery to avoid arthrofibrosis
- Early weight-bearing and ROM, with emphasis on obtaining early full extension
- Early initiation of quadriceps and hamstring activity
- Efforts to control swelling and pain to limit muscular inhibition and atrophy
- Appropriate use of open– and closed–kinetic chain exercises while avoiding early open-chain exercises that may shear or tear the weak immature ACL graft (see the section on open– and closed–kinetic chain exercises)
- Comprehensive lower extremity muscle stretching, strengthening, and conditioning
- Neuromuscular and proprioception retraining
- Functional training
- Cardiovascular training
- Stepped progression based on achievement of therapeutic goals

BASIC SCIENCE AND BIOMECHANICS

The ACL is the primary restraint to anterior translation of the tibia and a secondary restraint to tibial rotation and to varus and valgus stress. An intact ACL resists forces up to **2500 N** and strain of about 20% before failing. Older ACLs fail under lower loads than younger ACLs do. The force placed on an intact ACL ranges from about 100 N during passive knee extension to about 400 N with walking and 1700 N with cutting and acceleration-deceleration activities. Loads exceed the ACL's failure capacity only with unusual combinations of loading patterns on the knee.

GRAFT MATERIAL PROPERTIES

The central-third bone–patellar tendon–bone graft has an initial failure strength of up to **2977 N**, and the strength of a quadrupled semitendinosus-gracilis graft complex has been estimated to be as high as **4000 N**. However, strength is greatly reduced after surgical implantation. Current thought is that initial graft strength must exceed that of the normal ACL to maintain sufficient strength because strength is lost during the healing phase and that a stronger graft will allow for safer rehabilitation and return to activity.

GRAFT HEALING

After implantation, ACL grafts undergo sequential phases of avascular necrosis, revascularization, and remodeling. The graft material properties change as the process of *ligamentization* proceeds. Ultimate load to failure in a patellar tendon autograft can drop as low as 11% of the normal ACL, and graft stiffness can fall to as low as 13% of the normal ACL during graft maturation. **Data on human grafts indicate that implanted grafts begin to resemble a native ACL structure as early as 6 months after implantation but that final maturation does not occur until after 1 year.**

GRAFT FIXATION

In the first 6 to 12 weeks of rehabilitation, fixation of the graft rather than the graft itself is the limiting factor for strength in the graft complex. The exercises and activities used in rehabilitation during this time must be carefully chosen so that the ability of the fixation to resist graft slippage is not exceeded.

For **central-third patellar tendon grafts**, interference screw fixation of the bone blocks in the femoral and tibial tunnels has been shown to exceed **500 N** for both metallic and bioabsorbable screws. Graft slippage has not been a problem with this construct.

With **hamstring grafts**, soft tissue fixation and graft slippage vary greatly depending on the fixation (Fig. 4-14). The strongest fixation, with the least amount of graft slippage, is achieved with soft tissue washers, which can provide a construct strength greater than **768 N**. Interference screw fixation has not been as successful, with yield strengths less than 350 N and graft slippage or complete fixation failure with low-level loading.

OPEN- AND CLOSED-KINETIC CHAIN EXERCISE

Considerable debate has occurred in recent years regarding the use of closed–kinetic chain activity versus open–kinetic chain activity after ACL reconstruction (see Glossary for definition of open- and closed-chain exercises). An example of an open–kinetic chain exercise is the use of a leg extension machine (Fig. 4-15). An example of closed–kinetic chain exercise is the use of a leg press machine (Fig. 4-16). **In theory, closed–kinetic chain exercises provide a more significant compression force across the knee while activating co-contraction of the quadriceps and hamstring muscles.** It has been suggested that these two factors help decrease the anterior shear forces in the knee that would otherwise be placed on the maturing ACL graft. Consequently, closed–kinetic chain exercises have been favored over open–kinetic chain exercises during rehabilitation after ACL reconstruction. However, the literature supporting this theory is not definitive. Many common activities cannot be clearly classified as open or closed kinetic chain, which adds to the confusion. Walking, running, stair climbing, and jumping all involve a combination of open– and closed–kinetic chain components.

Jenkins and colleagues (1997) measured side-to-side difference in anterior displacement of the tibia in subjects with unilateral ACL-deficient knees during open–kinetic chain (knee extension) and closed–kinetic chain (leg press) exercises at 30 and 60 degrees of knee flexion and concluded that **open-chain exercises at low flexion angles may produce an increase in anterior shear forces that may cause laxity in the ACL.**

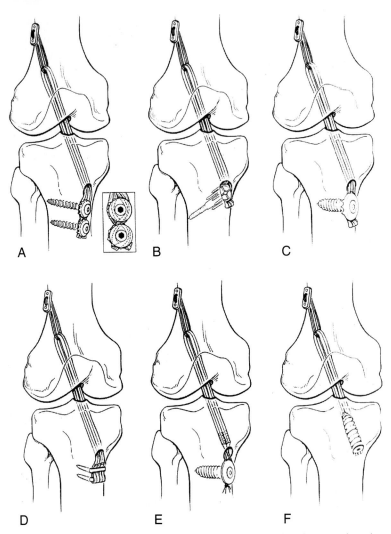

Figure 4–14   A-F, Various tibial fixation methods with a femoral EndoButton for a hamstring anterior cruciate ligament graft. (From Steiner ME, Kowalk DL: Anterior cruciate ligament reconstruction using hamstrings for a two-incision technique. Oper Tech Sports Med 7:172-178, 1999.)

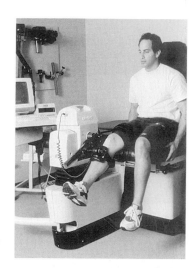

Figure 4–15 Example of an open–kinetic chain exercise (leg extension).

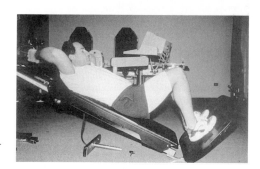

Figure 4–16 Example of a closed–kinetic chain exercise (leg press).

Side-to-Side Differences in Anterior Displacement

	30 Degrees Knee Flexion (mm)	60 Degrees Knee Flexion (mm)
Open kinetic chain (knee extension)	4.7	1.2
Closed kinetic chain (leg press)	1.3	2.1

Three millimeters to 5 mm is abnormal; greater than 5 mm represents arthrometric failure.

Yack and colleagues (1993) also found increased anterior displacement during open–kinetic chain exercise (knee extension) when compared with closed–kinetic chain exercise (parallel squat) through a flexion range of 0 to 64 degrees. Kvist and Gillquist (1999) demonstrated that displacement occurs with even low levels of muscular activity: generation of the first 10% of the peak quadriceps torque produced 80% of the total tibial translation seen with maximal quadriceps torque. Mathematical models have also predicted that shear forces on the ACL are greater with open-chain exercises. Jurist and Otis (1985), Zavetsky and coworkers (1994), and Wilk and Andrews (1993) all noted that changing the position of the resistance pad on isokinetic open–kinetic chain devices could modify anterior shear force and anterior tibial displacement. Wilk and Andrews also found greater anterior tibial displacement at slower isokinetic speed.

Beynnon and associates (1997) used implanted transducers to measure the strain in the intact ACL during various exercises and found no consistent distinction between closed–kinetic chain and open–kinetic chain activities.

Rank Comparison of Peak Anterior Cruciate Ligament Strain Values during Commonly Prescribed Rehabilitation Activities

Rehabilitation Activity	Peak Strain (%)	Number of Subjects
Isometric quadriceps contraction at 15 degrees (30 Nm of extension torque)	4.4	8
Squatting with sport cord	4.0	8
Active flexion-extension of the knee with a 45-N weight boot	3.8	9
Lachman test (150 N of anterior shear load)	3.7	10
Squatting	3.6	8
Active flexion-extension (no weight boot) of the knee	2.8	18
Simultaneous quadriceps and hamstring contraction at 15 degrees	2.8	8
Isometric quadriceps contraction at 30 degrees (30 Nm of extension torque)	2.7	18
Anterior drawer (150 N of anterior shear load)	1.8	10
Stationary bicycling	1.7	8
Isometric hamstring contraction at 15 degrees (to −10 Nm of flexion torque)	0.6	8
Simultaneous quadriceps and hamstring contraction at 30 degrees	0.4	8
Passive flexion-extension of the knee	0.1	10
Isometric quadriceps contraction at 60 degrees (30 Nm of extension torque)	0.0	8
Isometric quadriceps contraction at 90 degrees (30 Nm of extension torque)	0.0	18
Simultaneous quadriceps and hamstring contraction at 60 degrees	0.0	8
Simultaneous quadriceps and hamstring contraction at 90 degrees	0.0	8
Isometric hamstring contraction at 30, 60, and 90 degrees (to −10 Nm of flexion torque)	0.0	8

From Beynnon BD, Fleming BC; Anterior cruciate ligament strain in-vivo: A review of previous work. J Biomech 31:519-525, 1998.

This finding contradicts previous studies and indicates that certain closed-chain activities, such as squatting, may not be as safe as the mathematical force models would predict, particularly at low flexion angles.

A protective effect of the hamstrings has been suggested based on the findings of minimal or absent strain in the ACL with isolated hamstring contraction or when the hamstrings were simultaneously contracted along with the quadriceps. Co-contraction of the quadriceps and hamstrings occurs in closed–kinetic chain exercises, with a progressive decrease in hamstring activity as the flexion angle of the knee increases. Co-contraction does not occur to any significant degree during open–kinetic chain exercise.

Other differences between open– and closed–kinetic chain exercise have been demonstrated. Closed–kinetic chain exercises generate greater activity in the vasti musculature, and open–kinetic chain exercises generate more rectus femoris activity. Open-chain activities generate more isolated muscle activity and thus allow for more specific muscle strengthening. However, with fatigue, any stabilizing effect of these isolated muscles may be lost and can place the ACL at greater risk. Closed-chain exercises, by allowing agonist muscle activity, may not provide focused muscle strengthening, but they may present a safer environment for the ACL in the setting of fatigue.

In summary, closed-chain exercises can be used safely during rehabilitation of the ACL because they appear to generate low anterior shear force and tibial displacement through most of the flexion range, although some evidence now exists that low flexion angles during certain closed–kinetic chain activities may strain the graft as much as open-chain activities and may not be as safe as previously thought. At what level strain becomes detrimental and whether some degree of strain is beneficial during the graft-healing phase are currently unknown. Until these answers are realized, current trends have been to recommend activities that minimize graft strain so that the ACL is placed at the lowest risk for the development of laxity. Open-chain flexion that is dominated by hamstring activity appears to pose little risk to the ACL throughout the entire flexion arc, **but open-chain extension places significant strain on the ACL, as well as the patellofemoral joint, and should be avoided**.

REHABILITATION CONSIDERATIONS AFTER ANTERIOR CRUCIATE LIGAMENT RECONSTRUCTION

Pain and Effusion

Pain and swelling are common after any surgical procedure. Because they cause reflex inhibition of muscle activity and thus postoperative muscle atrophy, it is important to control these problems quickly to facilitate early ROM and strengthening activities. Standard therapeutic modalities to reduce pain and swelling include cryotherapy, compression, and elevation.

Cryotherapy is commonly used to reduce pain, inflammation, and effusion after ACL reconstruction. Cryotherapy acts through local effects and causes vasoconstriction, which reduces fluid extravasation; inhibits afferent nerve conduction, which decreases pain and muscle spasm; and prevents cell death, which limits the release of chemical mediators of pain, inflammation, and edema. Complications such as superficial frostbite and neuropraxia can be prevented by avoiding prolonged placement of the cold source directly on the skin. *Contraindications* to the use of cryotherapy include hypersensitivity to cold, such as Raynaud's phenomenon, lupus erythematosus, periarteritis nodosa, and rheumatoid arthritis.

Motion Loss

Loss of motion is perhaps the most common complication after ACL reconstruction. Loss of extension is more common than loss of flexion **and is poorly tolerated**. Loss of motion can result in anterior knee pain, quadriceps weakness, gait abnormalities, and early articular degenerative changes.

A number of factors can cause or contribute to loss of motion after ACL reconstruction (Shelbourne et al., 1996a):

- Arthrofibrosis, infrapatellar contracture syndrome, patella infra
- Inappropriate ACL graft placement (e.g., tibial tunnel placed too anteriorly) or ACL tensioning
- "Cyclops syndrome"
- Acute surgery on a swollen inflamed knee
- Concomitant MCL repair
- Poorly supervised or poorly designed rehabilitation program
- Prolonged immobilization
- RSD

Prevention is the first and most effective method for treating loss of motion after surgery. Many of the factors leading to loss of knee motion can be prevented with proper surgical timing and technique.

Anterior placement of the tibial tunnel and inadequate notchplasty can both lead to impingement of the graft on the roof of the intercondylar notch with subsequent loss of extension (Fig. 4-17). Anterior femoral tunnel placement may lead to increased graft tension in flexion with subsequent limitation of flexion. Inappropriate tensioning of the graft may overconstrain the knee and also lead to difficulty regaining terminal motion. Inadequate notch preparation and insufficient ACL stump débridement at the tibial plateau may predispose the patient to the formation of a fibroproliferative scar nodule, called a **"cyclops lesion,"** that can impinge anteriorly in the knee and cause pain and limited extension (Fig. 4-18). Symptoms suggestive of a cyclops lesion include loss of extension and a large, painful clunk on attempted terminal extension of the knee.

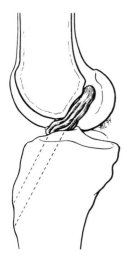

Figure 4–17 Anterior cruciate ligament graft impingement as a result of anterior tibial tunnel placement.

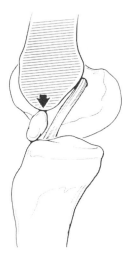

Figure 4–18 "Cyclops lesion." A fibroproliferative scar nodule (cyclops) is causing a popping or clunking on extension of the knee. Cyclops lesions typically occur after inadequate débridement of soft tissue at the interface of the tibial plateau with the tibial tunnel.

ACL reconstruction should be delayed until the acute post-traumatic inflammation and swelling have subsided, full ROM has returned, and the patient has regained strong quadriceps activation.

To meet these goals, preoperative rehabilitation should be started shortly after injury. Modalities to control pain and swelling, such as cryotherapy, elevation, compression, and anti-inflammatory medication, are helpful in eliminating reflex muscular inhibition of the quadriceps. Quadriceps setting, SLR, and closed-chain exercises, accompanied by electrical muscle stimulation and biofeedback, are useful to reactivate the lower extremity musculature, prevent atrophy, and promote strength gain. Proprioception activities can also be started to improve neuromuscular retraining. Activities to increase motion, aided by modalities such as prone hangs, wall slides, and the use of extension boards, are also used in the preoperative period.

There is no one single time frame (such as 3 weeks) for surgical delay to avoid postoperative arthrofibrosis. The condition of the patient's knee rather than any predetermined waiting period determines the appropriate timing for surgery. Less motion loss and faster return of quadriceps strength have been reported when surgery was delayed until motion was restored. **Early ACL reconstruction, before return of motion and "cooling" of the knee, increases the risk for postoperative arthrofibrosis.**

Early passive and active ROM is begun immediately after surgery and may be augmented with the use of a continuous passive motion (CPM) machine. Postoperative immobilization increases the risk that later manipulation will be required to regain motion. Control of pain and swelling, early reactivation of the quadriceps musculature, and early return to weight-bearing all improve the return of motion. Patellar mobilization techniques should be started to prevent patellar tendon shortening or retinacular contracture, both of which can lead to motion loss.

The most important immediate goal is to obtain and maintain full knee extension almost immediately after surgery.

Knee flexion to 90 degrees should be achieved by 7 to 10 days after surgery. Failure to do so should prompt early initiation of countermeasures to prevent a

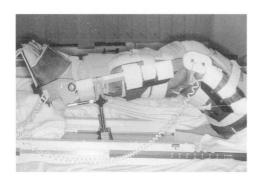

Figure 4–19 Continuous passive motion machine.

chronic problem from occurring. These issues are discussed in detail in the complications/troubleshooting section.

Continuous Passive Motion

The efficacy of CPM after ACL reconstruction is controversial (Fig. 4-19). Historically, its use was advocated to improve cartilage nutrition and limit motion loss during a time when immobilization was common after surgery. With the growing popularity of accelerated rehabilitation and emphasis on early motion and weight-bearing, the benefits of CPM have waned. Few recent studies have demonstrated a significant long-term benefit of CPM. We currently do not believe that the added cost is justified by any short-term benefit and, since 1993, have not routinely recommended the use of CPM. However, there is a role for CPM after manipulation and arthroscopic surgery in patients in whom arthrofibrosis has developed.

Weight-Bearing Status

Theoretical advantages of weight-bearing include improved cartilage nutrition, decreased disuse osteopenia, reduced peripatellar fibrosis, and quicker quadriceps recovery. Tyler and colleagues (1998) showed that immediate weight-bearing reduced muscle inhibition at the knee joint in the early postoperative period, as demonstrated by an increased return of electromyographic (EMG) activity in the VMO within the first 2 weeks after surgery. They also demonstrated a reduction in the development of anterior knee pain in patients who began immediate weight-bearing. No differences in knee laxity, ROM, or functional scores were noted between weight-bearing and non–weight-bearing groups.

One theoretical concern about weight-bearing in the first 4 to 6 weeks after surgery is donor site morbidity in patients in whom a bone–patellar tendon–bone autograft is used. The frequency of proximal tibial fracture, patellar fracture, and patellar tendon rupture in association with weight-bearing is unknown at this time, but it is certainly less than 1%. Though rare, these complications can be difficult to treat and can lead to poor results.

We currently recommend maintaining the knee in a brace locked in full extension during ambulation for the first 4 to 6 weeks after surgery to limit the forces transmitted through the extensor mechanism and to protect the extensor mechanism if the patient slips or falls.

Note: The editors maintain the knee locked in full extension during ambulation for only 2 to 3 weeks.

Muscle Training

Early initiation of muscle training is crucial to prevent muscle atrophy and weakness. *Electrical muscle stimulation* may be helpful to initiate muscle activation in patients who are unable to voluntarily overcome reflex inhibition. *Biofeedback* (such as VMO biofeedback) can be used to enhance the force of muscular contraction. Weight-bearing has also been shown to be beneficial in promoting muscle reactivation. *Muscle balance*, or achieving the appropriate hamstring-to-quadriceps ratio, improves dynamic protection of the ACL. Barratta and colleagues (1988) reported an increased risk of injury with reduced hamstring antagonist activity and demonstrated improved coactivation ratios in response to exercise. *Fatigue* has been shown to significantly affect not only the strength of muscular contraction but also the electromechanical response time and rate of muscular force generation. Because deficits in these critical elements of dynamic knee stabilization reduce the ability to protect the knee during activity, endurance training should be included in the rehabilitation program.

Electrical Muscle Stimulation and Biofeedback

Electrical muscle stimulation (Fig. 4-20) and biofeedback (Fig. 4-21) may be useful as adjuncts to conventional muscle training techniques. Although no convincing evidence has shown that *electrical muscle stimulation* alone is superior to voluntary muscle contraction alone in promoting muscle strength after surgery, it may be of benefit in the early postoperative period when reflex inhibition of the quadriceps as a result of pain and swelling prevents the initiation of voluntary muscle activity. Anderson and Lipscomb (1989) noted a positive effect of electrical muscle stimulation in limiting quadriceps strength loss and patellofemoral crepitus after ACL reconstruction. **The most appropriate use of electrical muscle stimulation seems to be in conjunction with volitional muscle activity in the early postoperative period.**

Biofeedback may be useful for re-education of the muscles. Using EMG monitoring, a visual or auditory signal is provided to the patient when a preset threshold of muscle activity is achieved. The threshold limits can be modified as the patient progresses. Through the use of positive "rewards," biofeedback encourages increased

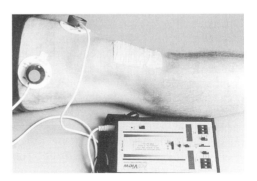

Figure 4–20 Electrical stimulation of the quadriceps.

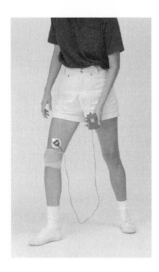

Figure 4–21 Electromyographic biofeedback of the vastus medialis obliquus muscle.

muscular contraction, which is beneficial during strength training. It can also promote the improved timing of muscle activation, which in turn benefits dynamic stabilization of the knee.

Proprioception

The role of the ACL in proprioception of the knee is still under investigation. Altered proprioception has been reported to reduce the effectiveness of the individual to protect the knee and perhaps predispose the ACL to repetitive microtrauma and ultimately failure. Patients with ACL-deficient knees have been shown to have decreased proprioceptive abilities, which in turn has a detrimental effect on the dynamic hamstring stabilization reflex. Differences in proprioception have been demonstrated in asymptomatic and symptomatic patients after ACL injury, and a relationship between proprioception and outcome after ACL reconstruction has been noted. The mechanism by which rehabilitation after ACL reconstruction has a beneficial effect on improving proprioception is not clear. However, improvement has been shown in both ACL-reconstructed and ACL-deficient patients after proprioceptive training programs.

Lephart and coworkers (1992 and 1998) recommended a program designed to affect all three levels of neuromuscular control. *Higher brain center control* is developed through conscious, repetitive positioning activities, which maximizes sensory input to reinforce proper joint stabilization activity. *Unconscious control* is developed by incorporating *distraction techniques* into the exercises, such as the addition of ball throwing or catching while performing the required task (Fig. 4-22).

To improve *brainstem control*, balance and postural maintenance activities are implemented, beginning with visual activities with the eyes open and progressing to exercises with the eyes closed to remove the visual input. The rehabilitation program also includes a progression of activities from stable to unstable surfaces and from bilateral to unilateral stance.

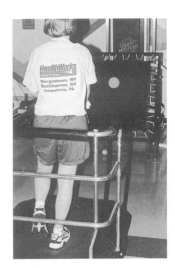

Figure 4–22 Distraction technique involving a mini-tramp, single-leg balance during ball toss to develop unconscious control.

To enhance proprioceptive control at the *spinal level*, activities involving sudden changes in joint position are used. Plyometric activities and rapid movement exercises on changing surfaces improve the reflex dynamic stabilization arc.

Anterior Cruciate Ligament Bracing

The effectiveness of and need for bracing after ACL reconstruction are controversial. Two forms of braces are currently in use, *rehabilitation* (transitional) braces (Fig. 4-23A) and *functional* braces (Fig. 4-23B). Rehabilitation braces are used in the early postoperative period to protect the donor site while ROM, weight-bearing, and muscle activity are initiated. Functional braces are used when the patient returns to strenuous

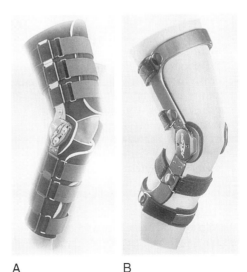

Figure 4–23 **A**, Transitional anterior cruciate ligament (ACL) rehabilitation brace. **B**, Functional knee brace (ACL).

A   B

activity or athletics to provide increased stability to the knee and protect the reconstructed ligament while it matures. **The efficacy of prophylactic functional bracing in preventing reinjury after graft maturation has not been supported in the literature, and such bracing is not recommended.** Beynnon and associates (1997) demonstrated a protective effect of bracing under low-level loading conditions, but this effect was diminished with progressively increasing loads. Bracing has been shown to increase quadriceps atrophy and inhibit the return of quadriceps strength after surgery. These effects appear to resolve once brace use is discontinued.

No long-term benefits of bracing on knee laxity, ROM, or function have been demonstrated.

We currently recommend the use of a drop-lock rehabilitation brace for the first 4 to 6 weeks after surgery. The brace is locked in extension during sleep to prevent potential loss of extension, and for patients with bone–patellar tendon–bone autografts, it is locked in extension during weight-bearing to protect the extensor mechanism. The brace is removed or unlocked several times a day during ROM and non–weight-bearing exercises. We believe that the risk for postoperative patellar fracture or patellar tendon rupture, though rare, outweighs the cost and inconvenience of transitional brace use.

Gender Issues

In recent years, a tremendous increase in women's participation in athletics has made it apparent that **women are at an increased risk for ACL injury**. A number of differences between women and men have been hypothesized as possible causes for this increased susceptibility.

Specific rehabilitation modifications may help compensate for these anatomic, neuromuscular, and flexibility differences and should be incorporated into the standard protocol being used.

The *anatomic differences* (a wider pelvis, increased genu valgum, increased external tibial torsion, and underdeveloped musculature) place a woman's ACL at an inherent mechanical disadvantage, especially during jumping activities when increased rotational forces at landing may overload the ligament.

Among the differences in *neuromuscular characteristics* of men and women is a decreased ability in women to generate muscular force, even when corrections are made for size differences. This limits the ability to resist displacing loads through dynamic stabilization of the knee. Other differences in dynamic knee stabilization that place women at greater risk for ACL injury include slower muscle activation and force generation, as well as recruitment of the quadriceps muscles rather than the hamstrings or gastrocnemius muscles. An inherently lower hamstring-to-quadriceps muscle ratio may further strain the ACL.

Women have greater *laxity* than men do. There may be a hormonal basis for this difference because changes in laxity have been documented during the menstrual cycle. As a result, women have increased hyperextension at the knee, which places the knee in a less favorable position for the hamstrings to generate a protective force. Women also generate less dynamic knee stability than men do in response to muscle contraction. These factors lead to greater anterior tibial displacement in women and may place the ACL at greater risk for injury.

Hewett and colleagues (1996) developed a *prophylactic training program* designed specifically for women in an attempt to reduce their risk for knee injury. They demonstrated a reduction in landing force, increased muscle power, and improved hamstring-to-quadriceps ratio with a 6-week training program. They also found that the program, when done before a sport season, significantly reduced the number of knee injuries in women athletes.

Wilk and colleagues (1999) proposed *eight key factors that should be considered during rehabilitation after reconstruction of the ACL in women* and designed a set of specific exercises to counteract problem areas (see p. 412). Another key to avoiding ACL injuries in female athletes is to train the athlete to land from a jump with both knees slightly flexed. This will help avoid a hyperextension mechanism and reduce the risk for ACL injury.

Gender Issues That May Contribute to Increased Risk for Anterior Cruciate Ligament Injuries in Females

Anatomic Differences	Muscular and Neuromuscular Differences	Laxity and Range of Motion
Wider pelvis	Diminished muscular force	Greater ROM
Increased flexibility	Dependence on the quadriceps muscle for stability	Genu recurvatum
Less well developed thigh musculature	Longer time for development of force	Increased knee laxity
Narrower femoral notch	Longer electromechanical response time	Increased hip rotation
Smaller ACL		
Increased genu valgum		
Increased external tibial torsion		

From Wilk KE, Arrigo C, Andrews JR, Clancy WG: Rehabilitation after anterior cruciate ligament reconstruction in the female athlete. J Athletic Train 34:177-193, 1999.

REHABILITATION PROTOCOL
Jump-Training Program for Prevention of Anterior Cruciate Ligament Injuries in Female Athletes
Hewett

EXERCISE	DURATION OR REPETITIONS BY WEEK	
Phase 1: Technique	**Week 1**	**Week 2**
1. Wall jumps	20 sec	25 sec
2. Tuck jumps*	20 sec	25 sec
3. Broad jump stick (hold) landing	5 reps	10 reps
4. Squat jumps*	10 sec	15 sec
5. Double-legged cone jumps*	30 sec/30 sec	30 sec/30 sec (side-to-side and back-to-front)
6. 180-degree jumps	20 sec	25 sec
7. Bounding in place	20 sec	25 sec

Continued

REHABILITATION PROTOCOL: *Jump-Training Program for Prevention of Anterior Cruciate Ligament Injuries in Female Athletes*   *Continued*

EXERCISE	DURATION OR REPETITIONS BY WEEK	
Phase 2: Fundamentals	**Week 3**	**Week 4**
1. Wall jumps	30 sec	30 sec
2. Tuck jumps*	30 sec	30 sec
3. Jump, jump, jump, vertical jump	5 reps	8 reps
4. Squat jumps*	20 sec	20 sec
5. Bounding for distance	1 run	2 runs
6. Double-legged cone jumps*	30 sec/30 sec	30 sec/30 sec (side to side and back to front)
7. Scissors jump	30 sec	30 sec
8. Hop, hop, stick landing*	5 reps/leg	5 reps/leg
Phase 3: Performance	**Week 5**	**Week 6**
1. Wall jumps	30 sec	30 sec
2. Step, jump up, down, vertical	5 reps	20 reps
3. Mattress jumps	30 sec/30 sec	30 sec/30 sec (side-to-side and back-to-front)
4. Single-legged jumps, distance*	5 reps/leg	5 reps/leg
5. Squat jumps*	25 sec	25 sec
6. Jump into bounding*	3 runs	4 runs
7. Hop, hop, stick landing	5 reps/leg	5 reps/leg

GLOSSARY OF JUMP-TRAINING EXERCISES

- 180-degree jump: two-footed jump. Rotate 180 degrees midair, hold the landing for 2 seconds, and repeat in the reverse direction.
- Bounding for distance: start bounding in place; slowly increase the distance with each step while keeping the knees high.
- Bounding in place: jump from one leg to the other, straight up and down, while progressively increasing rhythm and height.
- Broad jump stick (hold) landing: two-footed jump as far as possible; hold the landing for 5 seconds.
- Cone jump: double-legged jump with the feet together; quickly jump side to side over cones and repeat forward and backward.
- Hop, hop, stick landing: single-legged hop; stick the second landing for 5 seconds, and increase the distance of the hop as technique improves.
- Jump into bounding: two-footed broad jump; land on a single leg, and then progress into bounding for distance.

REHABILITATION PROTOCOL: *Jump-Training Program for Prevention of Anterior Cruciate Ligament Injuries in Female Athletes* *Continued*

GLOSSARY OF JUMP-TRAINING EXERCISES—cont'd

- Jump, jump, jump, vertical jump: three broad jumps with a vertical jump immediately after landing the third broad jump.
- Mattress jump: two-footed jump on a mattress, trampoline, or other easily compressed device; perform side to side and back to front.
- Scissors jump: start in stride position with one foot well in front of other.
- Single-legged jump, distance: single-legged hop for distance; hold the landing (knees bent) for 5 seconds.
- Squat jump: standing jump while raising both arms overhead; land in a squatting position, and touch both hands to the floor.
- Step, jump up, down, vertical: two-footed jump onto a 6- to 8-inch step; jump off the step with two feet, and then make a vertical jump.
- Tuck jump: from a standing position, jump and bring both knees up to the chest as high as possible; repeat quickly
- Wall jump (ankle bounces): with the knees slightly bent and arms raised overhead, bounce up and down off the toes.

STRETCHING AND WEIGHT-TRAINING PROGRAM

Stretches†	Weight-Training Exercises‡	Stretches†	Weight-Training Exercises‡
1. Calf stretch with a bent knee	1. Abdominal curl	6. Iliotibial band/lower back	6. Bench press
2. Calf stretch with a straight knee	2. Back hyperextension	7. Posterior deltoids	7. Latissimus dorsi pull-down
3. Quadriceps	3. Leg press	8. Latissimus dorsi	8. Forearm curl
4. Hamstring	4. Calf raise	9. Pectorals/biceps	9. Warm-down short stretch
5. Hip flexors	5. Pullover		

Note: Before jumping exercises: stretching (15 to 20 minutes), skipping (two laps), side shuffle (two laps).
During training: each jump exercise is followed by a 30-second rest period.
After training: cool-down walk (2 minutes), stretching (5 minutes), weight training (after 15-minute rest).
*These jumps are performed on mats.
†Stretching consists of three sets lasting 30 second each.
‡Weight training consists of one set of each exercise, generally 12 repetitions for upper body exercises and 15 repetitions for the trunk and lower body exercise.
From Hewett TE, Lindenfeld TN, Riccobene JV, Noyes FR: The effect of neuromuscular training on the incidence of knee injury in female athletes. Am J Sports Med 27:699-706, 1999.

Factors That Potentially Increase the Risk for Anterior Cruciate Ligament Injuries in Female Athletes and Measures for Prevention

FACTOR	MEASURE FOR PREVENTION
Females exhibit a wider pelvis and increased genu valgum	Establish dynamic control of valgus moment at the knee joint
Female athletes recruit the quadriceps muscle to stabilize the knee	Retrain the neuromuscular pattern for the female athlete to use the hamstrings
Females generate muscular force more slowly than males do	Train for fast speeds and reaction timing
Jumping athletes lose hip control on landing	Train hip and trunk control
Less developed thigh musculature	Train the hip musculature to assist in stabilization
Genu recurvatum and increased knee laxity	Train the athlete to control knee extension (stability position)
Exhibit less effective dynamic stabilization	Enhance neuromuscular control and protective pattern reflexes
Poorer muscular endurance rates	Train the female athlete to enhance muscular endurance

From Wilk KE, Arrigo C, Andrews JR, Clancy WG: Rehabilitation after anterior cruciate ligament reconstruction in the female athlete. J Athletic Train 34:177-193, 1999.

REHABILITATION PROTOCOL

Eight Specific Exercise Drills Used after Anterior Cruciate Ligament Reconstruction in Women
Wilk, Arrigo, Andrews, and Clancy

HIP MUSCULATURE TO STABILIZE THE KNEE

- Lateral step-overs (regular, fast, very slow)
- Step-overs with ball catches
- Step-overs with rotation
- Lateral step-ups on foam
- Dip walk
- Squats (foam) (Balance Master)
- Front diagonal lunges onto foam

RETRAIN NEUROMUSCULAR PATTERN FOR HAMSTRING CONTROL

- Lateral lunges straight
- Lateral lunges
- Lateral lunges with rotation
- Lateral lunges onto foam
- Lateral lunges with ball catches
- Squats, unstable pattern
- Lateral lunges jumping
- Lateral lunges, unstable pattern
- Coactivation balance through biofeedback
- Slide board
- Fitter (Fitter International, Calgary, Alberta, Canada)

REHABILITATION PROTOCOL: *Eight Specific Exercise Drills Used after Anterior Cruciate Ligament Reconstruction in Women*   *Continued*

CONTROL VALGUS MOMENT

- Front step-downs
- Lateral step-ups with Thera-Band (Hygienic Corporation, Akron, OH)
- Tilt board balance throws

CONTROL HYPEREXTENSION

- Plyometric leg press
- Plyometric leg press with four corners
- Plyometric jumps
  - 1 box
  - 2 boxes
  - 4 boxes
  - 2 boxes rotation
  - 2 boxes with catches
- Bounding drills
- Forward and backward step-over drills

HIGH-SPEED TRAINING, ESPECIALLY HAMSTRINGS

- Isokinetics
- Backward lunging
- Shuttle
- Lateral lunges (fast jumps)
- Resistance tubing for hamstrings
- Backward running

NEUROMUSCULAR REACTION

- Squats on tilt board
- Balance beam with cords
- Dip walk with cords
- Balance throws
- Balance throws with perturbations
- Lateral lunges with perturbations onto tilt board

LESS WELL DEVELOPED THIGH MUSCULATURE

- Knee extensor and flexor strengthening exercises
- Squats
- Leg press
- Wall squats
- Bicycling

POORER MUSCULAR ENDURANCE

- Stair climbing
- Bicycling
- Weight training (low weights, high repetitions)
- Cardiovascular training
- Balance drills for longer durations

From Wilk KE, Arrigo C, Andrews JR, Clancy WG: Rehabilitation after anterior cruciate ligament reconstruction in the female athlete. J Athletic Train 34:177-193, 1999.

OLDER PATIENTS WITH ANTERIOR CRUCIATE LIGAMENT INJURIES

An awareness of the health benefits of improved physical fitness has led to an increase in the activity level of the older population and an increase in ACL injuries. Traditionally, ACL injuries in older patients were treated nonoperatively, but much better outcomes have been demonstrated with surgical treatment.

Patients older than 35 years do benefit from ACL reconstruction and can expect results comparable to those of younger patients; however, the ACL deficiency must be treated early after injury, before chronic degenerative changes occur.

Results of ACL reconstruction in older patients with long-term, chronic ACL deficiency are not as predictable. Rehabilitation protocols developed specifically for the older population have not been studied, and it is unclear whether modifications in the standard programs are needed. *Patients older than 26 years have been shown to have decreased muscle strength after reconstructive surgery when compared with younger patients.* An awareness of this fact and emphasis on quadriceps along with hamstring strengthening may help improve outcomes in older patients. We routinely offer the option of ACL allografts to patients older than 40 years to further reduce potential extensor mechanism complications.

EFFECT OF GRAFT SELECTION ON POSTOPERATIVE REHABILITATION PROTOCOL

We currently use a single rehabilitation protocol after all ACL reconstructions regardless of graft material, with only slight weight-bearing and bracing modification, depending on the graft source (see p. 429). The current trend in rehabilitation after ACL reconstruction has been toward increasingly aggressive restoration of motion and strength, with an accelerated return to sporting activities at 4 months after surgery. A number of prospective studies have demonstrated the efficacy and safety of these accelerated programs for patients with *patellar tendon autografts.*

The benefits of *autologous hamstring grafts* have been cited as decreased donor site morbidity, improved cosmesis, and less residual anterior knee pain. However, questions have arisen regarding fixation strength, residual graft laxity, and the safety of accelerated rehabilitation protocols. Improved fixation methods for soft tissue grafts continue to be developed and currently approach the strength of patellar tendon–bone fixation. Studies comparing patellar tendon autografts with hamstring autografts show a trend toward greater laxity with the use of hamstring grafts, but this has not consistently correlated with a functional deficit. Howell and Taylor (1996) demonstrated the safety of an accelerated rehabilitation protocol with hamstring autografts. They allowed full return to sports at 4 months after brace-free rehabilitation, with clinical results similar to those with patellar tendon autografts. Results did not deteriorate between evaluations at 4 months and 2 years after surgery.

Allografts have typically been reserved for use in multiple ligament injuries or in revision surgery. Initially, fears of disease transmission and questions about weakened structural properties or delayed healing discouraged the use of allografts in primary reconstructions. Advances in screening techniques have virtually eliminated the risk of disease transmission, and abandonment of ethylene oxide and irradiation for sterilization has resulted in stronger graft properties. The advantages of allografts are no donor site morbidity, larger graft constructs, and shorter surgical time. Although questions about the increased time for graft incorporation in the host remain, comparison studies of nonirradiated, fresh frozen patellar tendon allografts and patellar tendon autografts have demonstrated few differences in outcomes after similar accelerated rehabilitation protocols.

ANTERIOR CRUCIATE LIGAMENT RECONSTRUCTION WITH MENISCAL REPAIR

A lack of firm basic science and prospective outcome studies has resulted in a wide array of opinions regarding issues such as immobilization, ROM restrictions, and weight-bearing status after meniscal repair combined with ACL reconstruction. An accelerated return to activities, with immediate weight-bearing and no ROM limitations in the early postoperative period, has produced results similar to those with more conservative rehabilitation programs. We have found little justification for modifying the standard rehabilitation protocol after meniscal repair done with ACL reconstruction. Rehabilitation after isolated meniscal repair is discussed separately later in this chapter (see pp. 484–487).

FUNCTIONAL TRAINING

Rehabilitation after ACL reconstruction is focused on the whole athlete to maintain cardiovascular conditioning, proprioception, and muscular coordination with appropriate exercises and activities that are gradually phased into the rehabilitation program. Functional training is also a useful way to maintain the patient's interest during therapy sessions because it takes some of the focus away from the knee and is often perceived as more fun than the standard rehabilitation exercises. The use of aids such as balance boards, mini-tramps, steps, balls, and the pool adds variety, breaks up the "routine" of therapy, and maintains patient motivation. Sport-specific drills can also speed the return of skills that patients will need to relearn when they return to their sports after rehabilitation. The activities used in functional training must be appropriate and safe for each recovery phase.

In the early phase of recovery, protection of the healing graft prevents significant lower extremity activities, but upper extremity ergometry and well-leg bicycling can promote aerobic conditioning, and some early proprioception training can begin. As progression to unprotected walking begins, additional proprioception drills can be added, and stair-walking exercises can be started to aid in retraining the musculature for eccentric loading patterns. When running is safely allowed, more advanced proprioception drills and plyometric exercises can be added. Figure-of-eight pattern running may be started at this time but should advance slowly, beginning first with large circles at a walking or jogging pace and progressing to smaller circles at a faster pace as the return of muscular strength and graft healing allow. Cutting and agility drills are added during the late phases of recovery. Sport-specific drills, such as dribbling and shooting drills for basketball and throwing and fielding drills for baseball, are added slowly when safely allowed and become the main focus of the late rehabilitation phases.

> **REHABILITATION PROTOCOL** — *General Guidelines for Functional Training after Anterior Cruciate Ligament Reconstruction*

PHASE 1

Aerobic Conditioning

- Upper extremity ergometry
- Well-leg bicycling

Proprioception

- Active/passive joint positioning
- Balancing activities
- Stable platform, eyes open
- Stable platform, eyes closed
- Seated ball throwing and catching

PHASE 2

Aerobic Conditioning

- Advance to two-leg bicycling
- Continue upper extremity ergometry

Plyometrics/Eccentric Exercises

Muscle Training

- Stair walking
  - Up/down, forward/backward

Aquatherapy

- Pool walking
- Pool jogging (deep-water running)

Proprioception

- Balancing activities
- Unstable platform (Kinesthetic Ability Trainer [KAT] or Biomechanical Ankle Platform System [BAPS] board) with eyes open/closed
- Mini-tramp standing
- Standing ball throwing and catching

PHASE 3

Aerobic Conditioning

- Continue bicycling/upper extremity ergometry
- Pool running/swimming
- Stair stepper/elliptical stepper
- Cross-country skiing machine

Plyometrics

- Stair jogging
- Box jumps
  - 6- to 12-inch heights

REHABILITATION PROTOCOL: *General Guidelines for Functional Training after*
Anterior Cruciate Ligament Reconstruction *Continued*

PHASE 3—cont'd

Running

- Straight-ahead jogging, progressing to running
- Figure-of-eight pattern
- Large circles, walking or slow jogging

Proprioception

- Mini-tramp bouncing
- Pogoball balancing
- Lateral slide board
- Ball throwing and catching on an unstable surface

PHASE 4

Aerobic Conditioning

- Continue as above

Agility

- Start at slow speed, advance slowly
- Shuttle run
- Lateral slides
- Carioca cross-overs

Proprioception

- Continue as above
- Add sport-specific activities ($\frac{1}{4}$ to $\frac{1}{2}$ speed)

Running

- Figure-of-eight pattern
- Small circles, running

Plyometrics

- Stair running
- Box jumps
  - 1- to 2-ft height

PHASE 5

Aerobic Conditioning

- Continue as above

Agility

- Continue as above
- Cutting drills

Continued

REHABILITATION PROTOCOL: *General Guidelines for Functional Training after Anterior Cruciate Ligament Reconstruction* *Continued*

PHASE 5—cont'd

Proprioception

• Reaction drills
• Advanced sport-specific drills (full speed)

Running

• Continue as above

Plyometrics

• Advance heights

FUNCTIONAL TESTING AFTER ANTERIOR CRUCIATE LIGAMENT RECONSTRUCTION

After ACL reconstruction and rehabilitation, clinical testing, including strength testing and laxity measurements, does not correlate well with functional ability in all patients. Functional testing was developed to help evaluate surgical and therapeutic outcomes and a patient's readiness to return to unrestricted activity. The most commonly used tests are the single hop for distance, the triple hop for distance, and the 6-m timed hop. Other proposed tests include the vertical jump, the cross-over hop for distance, and the figure-of-eight hop. The literature supporting the reliability and reproducibility of many of the functional tests is limited. No single test has been shown to be adequate for evaluating the dynamic function of the knee, and many surgeons recommend the use of a series of functional tests for testing dynamic function.

Noyes and coworkers (1991a) developed a battery of functional tests consisting of the single hop for distance, the triple hop for distance, the cross-over hop for distance, and the 6-m timed hop (Table 4-2). Independent testing has shown good reliability and reproducibility for this combination of testing. **More recently, it has been suggested that force absorption may be a more important factor in knee function than force production**. Alternative functional tests are being developed and tested, but at this time, support for these tests is limited. We currently use a battery consisting of the single-leg hop, the timed single-leg hop for 20 feet, and the vertical jump (see p. 419).

CRITERIA FOR RETURN TO SPORTS AFTER ANTERIOR CRUCIATE LIGAMENT RECONSTRUCTION

Correlation between functional testing, clinical testing, and subjective testing methods is poor when evaluating a patient after ACL reconstruction, perhaps because each method evaluates a different aspect of the recovery process. For this reason, we advocate the use of multiple criteria, drawn from each area of evaluation, in determining when a patient can return to full activity.

TABLE 4-2 Functional Testing after Anterior Cruciate Ligament Rupture

Rationale: Ruptures of the ACL result in varying amounts of functional limitations of the lower extremity. To assess these limitations quantitatively, objective testing under simulated conditions is required. Four one-legged hop function tests were devised. Their effectiveness and sensitivity in detecting limitations were assessed in two studies. These tests should be used with other clinical measuring tools (isokinetic testing, questionnaires) to verify functional limitations.

One-Legged Single Hop for Distance	One-Legged Timed Hop	One-Legged Triple Hop for Distance	One-Legged Cross-Over Hop for Distance
Method			
The patient stands on one limb, hops as far as possible, and lands on the same limb. The total distance is measured. Each limb is tested twice; the means of each are calculated and used to determine limb symmetry	The patient hops on one limb a distance of 6 m as fast as possible. The total time to cover the distance is recorded. Each limb is tested twice; the times are calculated to the nearest 0.01 sec with a stopwatch. The means of each limb are calculated and used to determine limb symmetry	The patient stands on one limb, performs three consecutive hops as far as possible, and lands on the same limb. The total distance hopped is measured; each limb is tested twice. The means of each limb are calculated and used to determine limb symmetry	A distance of 6 m with a 15-cm-long strip marked in the center of the floor is designated. The patient hops three consecutive times on one limb, crossing over the center strip on each hop. The total distance hopped is measured; each limb is tested twice. The means of each limb are calculated and used to determine limb symmetry
Calculation			
Limb symmetry = mean score of the involved limb divided by mean score of the noninvolved limb; the result is multiplied by 100: involved/noninvolved × 100	Limb symmetry = mean time of the involved limb divided by mean time of the noninvolved limb; the result is multiplied by 100: involved/noninvolved × 100	Limb symmetry = involved/noninvolved × 100	Limb symmetry = involved/noninvolved × 100

Continued

TABLE 4–2	Functional Testing after Anterior Cruciate Ligament Rupture—cont'd		
One-Legged Single Hop for Distance	One-Legged Timed Hop	One-Legged Triple Hop for Distance	One-Legged Cross-Over Hop for Distance
Study Results			
Normal limb symmetry was determined to be 85%. Approximately half of the ACL-deficient knees demonstrated abnormal test scores. Results of normal and ACL-deficient knees showed low false-positive and high specificity rates. The indicated test is of value in confirming lower limb limitations. The low sensitivity rates found exclude the use of this test as a screening tool	Normal limb symmetry was determined to be 85%. Approximately 42% to 49% of ACL-deficient knees had abnormal scores. Low false-positive and high specificity rates allow the test to be used to confirm lower limb limitations. Low sensitivity rates exclude its effectiveness in screening for limitations	Data available for 26 ACL-deficient knees only. Half the patients had abnormal symmetry scores. The low sensitivity rate excludes the test as a screening tool	Data available for 26 ACL-deficient knees only. Fifty-eight percent of the patients had abnormal symmetry scores. This test showed the highest percentage of abnormal symmetry scores of the four tests; however, the low sensitivity rate does not allow it to be used as a screening test

Conclusion/summary: The tests designed and the statistical analyses performed in these two studies attempted to correct deficiencies found in previous reports. The data collected on 93 normal knees showed no effect of gender, sports activity level, or dominance on limb symmetry. This allowed an overall normal symmetry limb score to be determined from the population as a whole, which was 85%, and simplified analysis of test scores of ACL-deficient knees. The percentage of ACL-deficient knees that had abnormal symmetry scores increased when the results of the two tests were analyzed versus just one test. Any two tests can be used; an analysis of the six possible two-test combinations failed to reveal that any one combination had a higher sensitivity rate. These tests should be used with other clinical measuring tools (isokinetic testing, questionnaires) to confirm abnormal lower limb symmetry. "Patients with normal symmetry scores should still be considered at risk for giving way during sports activities."

From Andrews JR, Zarin B, Wilk KE: Injuries in Baseball. Philadelphia, Lippincott-Raven, 1997, p 44.

> ### Criteria for Return to Sports after Anterior Cruciate Ligament Reconstruction
>
> Full painless ROM
> KT1000 side-to-side difference <3 mm
> Quadriceps strength 85% or more of the contralateral side
> Hamstring strength 100% of the contralateral side
> Hamstring-to-quadriceps strength ratio 70% or greater
> Functional testing battery 85% of the contralateral side or greater
> - Single-leg hop
> - Timed leg hop for 20 feet
> - Vertical jump
>
> No effusion
> No pain or other symptoms

COMPLICATIONS AND TROUBLESHOOTING AFTER ANTERIOR CRUCIATE LIGAMENT RECONSTRUCTION

Loss of Motion

Loss of motion is often cited as the most common complication after ACL reconstruction and can result from a number of causes. The definition of loss of motion varies in the literature. Harner and colleagues (1992) use loss of knee extension of 10 degrees or knee flexion of less than 125 degrees to define loss of motion, and Shelbourne and coworkers (1996b) define loss of motion as any symptomatic deficit of extension or flexion in comparison with that in the opposite knee. The term "arthrofibrosis" has been used when the limitation of motion is symptomatic and resistant to rehabilitative measures. Often, it is used synonymously with loss of motion in the literature.

Shelbourne and coworkers also developed a *classification system for **arthrofibrosis** or loss of motion*:

Type 1	≥10 degrees flexible extension loss and normal flexion; no capsular contracture; anterior knee pain common
Type 2	>10 degrees fixed extension loss and normal flexion; possibly mechanical block to motion and posterior capsular tightness
Type 3	>10 degrees extension loss and >25 degrees flexion loss with decreased medial and lateral movement of the patella (patellar tightness)
Type 4	10 degrees extension loss and ≥30 degrees of flexion loss and patella infra with marked patellar tightness

Patella infra, or "infrapatellar contracture syndrome" as Paulos and associates (1987) first called it, results from a hypertrophic healing response in the anterior soft tissues of the knee. The exuberant fibrosclerotic tissue entraps and tethers the patella, thereby limiting knee motion. The term "patella infra" refers to the lower position of the affected patella on a lateral radiograph when compared with the uninvolved side (Fig. 4-24). Painful restricted ROM, inflammation and induration of the peripatellar soft tissues, extensor lag, and a "shelf sign," or a step-off between

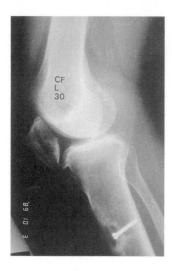

Figure 4–24 Patella infra. Note the lower position of the affected patella on the lateral radiograph.

the swollen patellar tendon and the tibial tubercle, should all raise suspicion of a developing patella infra. The most effective prevention or treatment is early quadriceps activity and knee flexion. The quadriceps maintains tension in the patellar tendon, which limits shortening or contracture of the tendon. Knee flexion stretches the tendon and surrounding soft tissues, which also prevents any shortening or contracture from developing.

Prevention of arthrofibrosis is the most effective treatment.
- Full knee extension should be obtained and maintained immediately after surgery.
- Prone heel height side-to-side difference should be less than 5 cm by 7 to 10 days after surgery.
- Knee flexion to 90 degrees should be achieved by 7 to 10 days after surgery.
- Patellar mobility should show steady progression after surgery with proper mobilization techniques.

If any of the criteria are not met, aggressive countermeasures should be implemented to prevent fixed motion loss. To improve extension, prone hangs, an extension board, manual pressure extension against a Thera-Band, and backward walking can be used (Fig. 4-25). To improve flexion, wall and heel slides, supine, prone, or sitting leg hangs, and manual pressure are used (Fig. 4-26). CPM and extension bracing, modalities to control pain and inflammation and to increase quadriceps and hamstring activity, and the judicious use of cryotherapy, NSAIDs, electrical stimulation, iontophoresis, and phonophoresis are all helpful. If inflammation is prolonged after surgery, we occasionally use methylprednisolone (Medrol Dose-Pak).

Surgical intervention is required when the motion loss becomes fixed and progress through nonoperative therapy has reached a plateau. When surgical intervention is necessary, aggressive rehabilitation to gain motion should be slowed to allow reduction of the inflammation in the knee, although strengthening should continue as tolerated. Surgery for arthrofibrosis is contraindicated in an acutely inflamed knee according to some surgeons, who believe that a better outcome is gained by waiting for the inflammation to resolve.

The first step in *surgical management of arthrofibrosis* is examination of the knee with the patient under anesthesia to delineate the extent of motion loss with the

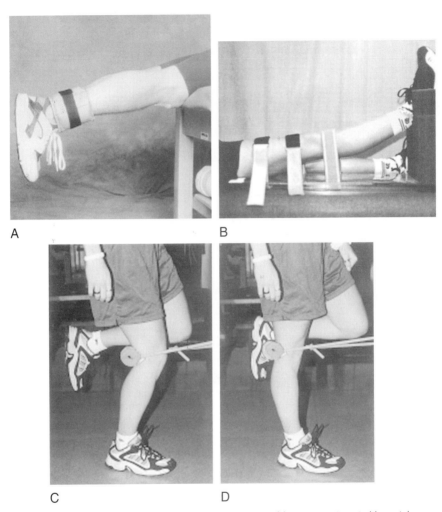

A

B

C

D

Figure 4–25 **A**, Prone extension hangs for gravity-assisted knee extension. Ankle weights may be added to increase the extension movement. **B**, A hyperextension device is used when a patient has difficulty regaining or maintaining extension. The patient lies supine to allow the hamstrings to relax. The patient's heel rests on the elevated cushion, and resistive straps are applied to the front of the knee. As the patient's leg becomes more extended and relaxed, the straps can be adjusted to apply more pressure. The device, which can be used in phases 1, 2, and 3 of rehabilitation, is used for 5 to 10 minutes several times a day. **C**, Knee extension against a padded Thera-Band (starting position). **D**, Knee extension against a Thera-Band (ending position). (**B**, From Shelbourne D: ACL rehabilitation. Physician Sports Med 28:[1]:31-44, 2000.)

patient fully relaxed. Arthroscopy in conjunction with manipulation under anesthesia allows direct examination of the knee joint to confirm the presence of a cyclops lesion, areas of exuberant scar formation, or other lesions that may be blocking motion. Any abnormal scar tissue or a hypertrophic fat pad is débrided. For more severe motion loss, medial and lateral patellar releases may be performed, and an open posterior capsular release may be necessary. Depending on the severity of the

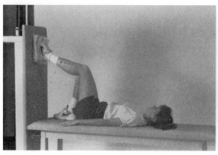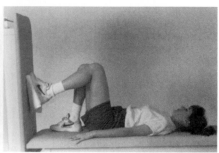

A

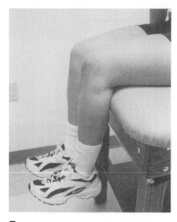

B

Figure 4–26 **A**, Wall slides. Place a socked or bare foot on a towel against the wall and slowly lower with gravity to a flexed knee position. **B**, Supine leg hang.

arthrofibrosis, multiple manipulations may be required during the arthroscopic procedure to evaluate the progress of the débridement. (Recommended reading for indications and surgical techniques for treatment of arthrofibrosis includes Shelbourne and associates [1996b].)

Rehabilitation must start immediately after surgical resection for arthrofibrosis, with emphasis on maintaining and improving ROM. Particular attention should be given to maintaining extension before directing efforts toward flexion. An extension brace may be beneficial, particularly in patients with severe arthrofibrosis.

Anterior Knee Pain

Anterior knee pain is another common problem after ACL reconstruction. Symptoms can occur anywhere along the extensor mechanism. It has been suggested that anterior knee pain after ACL reconstruction may be related to the choice of graft material. Although the literature remains mixed on this subject, most studies show a significant tendency for a decrease in anterior knee pain with the use of hamstring autografts when compared with patellar tendon autografts. Interestingly, no difference has been noted between patellar tendon autografts and allografts, thus suggesting that the relationship between donor site morbidity and anterior knee pain may not be as clear as previously thought.

Early rehabilitation to regain ROM and promote quadriceps control is important in the prevention of patellofemoral symptoms. Patellar mobilization techniques should be included to prevent contracture of the retinacular structures surrounding the patella, which may irritate the patellofemoral joint. For a patient who begins to show signs of anterior knee pain, the rehabilitation program should be modified to eliminate exercises that may place undue stress on the patellofemoral joint. Activities that increase PFJRF should be avoided, including deep squats, StairMaster use, jogging, and excessive weight during leg presses. Terminal knee extension exercises also often elicit anterior knee pain.

REHABILITATION PROTOCOL *After Anterior Cruciate Ligament Reconstruction*
D'Amato and Bach

PHASE 1: WEEKS 0-2

Goals

- Protect graft fixation
- Minimize effects of immobilization
- Control inflammation
- No CPM
- Achieve full extension, 90 degrees of knee flexion
- Educate patient about rehabilitation progress

Brace

- Locked in extension for ambulation and sleeping (drop-lock brace)

Weight-Bearing

- Weight-bearing as tolerated with two crutches
- Discontinue crutches as tolerated after 7 days (with demonstrated good quadriceps control)

Therapeutic Exercises

- Heel slides/wall slides
- Quadriceps sets, hamstring sets (electrical stimulation as needed)
- Patellar mobilization
- Non–weight-bearing gastrosoleus, hamstring stretches
- Sitting assisted flexion hangs
- Prone leg hangs for extension
- SLR in all planes with brace in full extension until quadriceps strength is sufficient to prevent extension lag
- Phase 1 functional training (see p. 416)

PHASE 2: WEEKS 2-4

Criteria for Progression to Phase 2

- Good quad set, SLR without extension lag (Fig. 4-27)
- Approximately 90 degrees knee flexion
- Full extension
- No signs of inflammation

Continued

REHABILITATION PROTOCOL: *After Anterior Cruciate Ligament*
Reconstruction   *Continued*

PHASE 2: WEEKS 2-4—cont'd

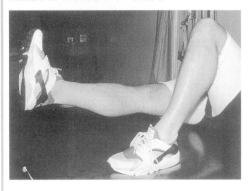

Figure 4–27   Straight leg raises. Ankle weights may be added to the ankle or thigh (1 to 5 pounds) for progressive resistance exercises.

Goals

- Restore normal gait
- Restore full ROM
- Protect graft fixation
- Improve strength, endurance, and proprioception to prepare for functional activities

Weight-Bearing

- Patellar tendon graft—continue ambulation with the brace locked in extension, may unlock the brace for sitting and sleeping, may remove the brace for ROM exercises
- Hamstring graft and allograft—may discontinue brace use when a normal gait pattern and quadriceps control are achieved

Therapeutic Exercises

- Mini-squats, 0-30 degrees
- Stationary bike (begin with a high seat, low tension)
- Closed-chain extension (leg press, 0-30 degrees)
- Toe raises
- Continue hamstring stretches, progress to weight-bearing gastrosoleus stretches
- Continue prone leg hangs with progressively heavier ankle weights until full extension is achieved
- Phase 2 functional training (see p. 416)

PHASE 3: WEEK 6-MONTH 4

Criteria for Progression to Phase 3

- Normal gait
- Full ROM
- Sufficient strength and proprioception to initiate functional activities
- Stable graft on Lachman and KT1000 testing

REHABILITATION PROTOCOL: *After Anterior Cruciate Ligament*
Reconstruction   *Continued*

PHASE 3: WEEK 6-MONTH 4—cont'd

Goals

- Improve confidence in the knee
- Avoid overstressing the graft fixation
- Protect the patellofemoral joint
- Progress strength, power, and proprioception to prepare for functional activities

Therapeutic Exercises

- Continue flexibility exercises as appropriate for the patient
- Advance closed–kinetic chain strengthening (one-leg squats; leg press, 0-60 degrees)
- Elliptical stepper, stair stepper
- Cross-country skiing machine
- Phase 3 functional training (6-12 weeks) (see p. 416)
- Phase 4 functional training (12+ weeks)

PHASE 4: MONTH 4

Criteria for Progression to Phase 4

- Full, painless ROM
- No evidence of patellofemoral joint irritation
- Sufficient strength and proprioception to progress functional activities (see p. 417)
- Physician clearance to initiate advanced closed–kinetic chain exercises and functional progression
- Stable graft on Lachman and KT1000 testing

Goal

- Return to unrestricted activities

Therapeutic Exercises

- Continue and progress flexibility and strengthening programs
- Phase 5 functional training (see p. 417)

PHASE 5: RETURN TO SPORTS

Criteria for Progression to Phase 5

- No patellofemoral joint or soft tissue complaints
- All criteria met for return to sports
- Physician clearance to resume full activity

Goals

- Safe return to athletics
- Maintenance of strength, endurance, and proprioception
- Patient education concerning any possible limitations

Continued

REHABILITATION PROTOCOL: *After Anterior Cruciate Ligament*
Reconstruction *Continued*

PHASE 5: RETURN TO SPORTS—cont'd

Brace

- Functional brace may be recommended by physician for use during sports for the first 1-2 years after surgery for psychological confidence

Therapeutic Exercises

- Gradual return to sports participation
- Maintenance program for strength and endurance
- Agility and sport-specific drills progressed

REHABILITATION PROTOCOL

After Anterior Cruciate Ligament Reconstruction
Wilk

GENERAL REHABILITATION APPROACH

- Full passive extension immediately after surgery
- Immediate motion
- Closed-chain exercises
- Emphasis on return of proprioception and neuromuscular control drills
- Drop-lock brace locked in extension during ambulation
  - 2 weeks for athletes
  - 3 weeks for general orthopaedic patients
- More gradual progression of flexion
  - Week 1—90 degrees
  - Week 2—105-115 degrees
  - Week 3—115-125 degrees
  - Week 4—beyond 125 degrees
  If restoration of flexion is too aggressive, swelling often occurs and the regimen is slowed.
- Not all closed-chain exercises produce a co-contraction; closed-chain exercises that have been shown to produce an actual co-contraction are used early
  - Vertical squats (0-45 degrees)
  - Lateral lunges
  - Balance drills
  - Slide board
  - Fitter
- Neuromuscular training and proprioception must be incorporated into every phase of the rehabilitation program

REHABILITATION PROTOCOL: *After Anterior Cruciate Ligament*
Reconstruction   Continued

GENERAL REHABILITATION APPROACH—cont'd

- Progression of proprioception and neuromuscular drills
  - Level 1 drills (immediate after surgery)
    - Joint reproduction, closed–kinetic chain drills, knee sleeve, proprioception drills, weight shifts, weight distribution
  - Level 2 drills (2-5 weeks after surgery)
    - Weight-bearing drills, squats, postural balance drills, single-leg stance, lateral lunges, pool
  - Level 3 drills (5-10 weeks after surgery)
    - Plyometrics, agility drills, neuromuscular control drills, perturbations
  - Level 4 drills (10 weeks or more after surgery)
    - Sport-specific training drills and gradual return to play
- Emphasis is placed on obtaining muscular endurance
  - Fatigued muscles result in increased translation (possible strain or tear of the graft)
  - Fatigued muscles also result in diminished proprioception
- Progression is criteria based, not time based

| REHABILITATION PROTOCOL | *Accelerated Rehabilitation after Anterior Cruciate Ligament Reconstruction with Central-Third Patellar Tendon* Wilk |

PREOPERATIVE PHASE

Goals

- Diminish inflammation, swelling, and pain
- Restore normal ROM (especially knee extension)
- Restore voluntary muscle activation
- Provide patient education to prepare the patient for surgery

Brace

- Elastic wrap or knee sleeve to reduce swelling

Weight-Bearing

- As tolerated with or without crutches

Exercises

- Ankle pumps
- Passive knee extension to 0 degrees (Fig. 4-28)
- Passive knee flexion to tolerance
- SLR—three-way: flexion, abduction, adduction
- Closed–kinetic chain exercises: 30-degree mini-squats, lunges, step-ups

Continued

REHABILITATION PROTOCOL: *Accelerated Rehabilitation after Anterior Cruciate Ligament Reconstruction with Central-Third Patellar Tendon*   *Continued*

PREOPERATIVE PHASE—cont'd

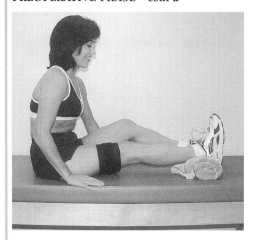

Figure 4–28   Passive knee extension to 0 degrees.

Muscle Stimulation

- Electrical muscle stimulation of the quadriceps during voluntary quadriceps exercises (4-6 hr/day)

Cryotherapy/Elevation

- Apply ice 20 minutes of every hour, elevate the leg with the knee in full extension (knee must be above the heart)

Patient Education

- Review the postoperative rehabilitation program
- Review instructional video (optional)
- Select appropriate surgical date

PHASE 1: IMMEDIATE POSTOPERATIVE PERIOD—DAYS 1-7

Goals

- Restore full passive knee extension
- Diminish joint swelling and pain
- Restore patellar mobility
- Gradually improve knee flexion
- Re-establish quadriceps control
- Restore independent ambulation

Day 1

Brace

- Transitional hinged brace locked in full extension during ambulation (Protonics Rehab System as directed by physician)

REHABILITATION PROTOCOL: *Accelerated Rehabilitation after Anterior Cruciate Ligament Reconstruction with Central-Third Patellar Tendon* Continued

---

PHASE 1: IMMEDIATE POSTOPERATIVE PERIOD—DAYS 1-7—cont'd

Weight-Bearing

- Weight-bearing as tolerated with two crutches

Exercises

- Ankle pumps
- Overpressure into full passive knee extension
- Active and passive knee flexion (90 degrees by day 5)
- SLR (flexion, abduction, adduction)
- Quadriceps isometric setting
- Hamstring stretches
- Closed–kinetic chain exercises, 30-degree mini-squats, weight shifts

Muscle Stimulation

- Used during active muscle exercises (4-6 hr/day)

Continuous Passive Motion

- As needed, 0-45/50 degrees (as tolerated by patient and directed by physician)

Ice and Elevation

- Ice 20 minutes of every hour and elevate with knee in full extension (elevated above the heart with pillows below the ankle, not the knee)

Days 2-3

Brace

- EZ Wrap brace/immobilizer, locked at 0-degree extension for ambulation and unlocked for sitting (or Protonics Rehab System as directed by physician)

Weight-Bearing

- As tolerated with two crutches

Range of Motion

- Brace removed during ROM exercises 4-6 times a day

Exercises

- Multiangle isometrics, 90 and 60 degrees (knee extension)
- Knee extension, 90-40 degrees
- Overpressure into extension
- Ankle pumps
- SLR (three-way)
- Mini-squats and weight shifts
- Standing hamstring curls
- Quadriceps isometric setting
- Proprioception and balance activities

Continued

REHABILITATION PROTOCOL: *Accelerated Rehabilitation after Anterior Cruciate Ligament Reconstruction with Central-Third Patellar Tendon* *Continued*

PHASE 1: IMMEDIATE POSTOPERATIVE PERIOD—DAYS 1-7—cont'd

Muscle Stimulation

- Continue electrical muscle stimulation 6 hr/day

Continuous Passive Motion

- 0-90 degrees as needed

Ice and Elevation

- Ice 20 minutes of every hour and elevate leg with full knee extension

PHASE 2: EARLY REHABILITATION—WEEKS 2-4

Criteria for Progression to Phase 2

- Quadriceps control (ability to perform good quad set and SLR)
- Full passive knee extension
- Passive ROM, 0-90 degrees
- Good patellar mobility
- Minimal joint effusion
- Independent ambulation

Goals

- Maintain full passive knee extension
- Gradually increase knee flexion
- Decrease swelling and pain
- Muscle training
- Restore proprioception
- Patellar mobility

Week 2

Brace

- Discontinue at 2-3 weeks

Weight-Bearing

- As tolerated (goal is to discontinue crutches 10 days after surgery)

Range of Motion

- Self-administered ROM stretching exercises 4-5 times daily, with emphasis on maintaining full passive ROM

KT2000 Testing

- 15-pound anterior-posterior test only

REHABILITATION PROTOCOL: *Accelerated Rehabilitation after Anterior Cruciate Ligament Reconstruction with Central-Third Patellar Tendon*   *Continued*

PHASE 2: EARLY REHABILITATION—WEEKS 2-4—cont'd

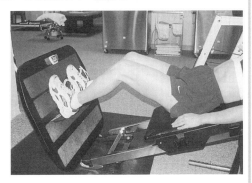

Figure 4–29   Leg press (closed-chain exercise).

Exercises

- Muscle stimulation to quadriceps exercises
- Isometric quadriceps sets
- SLR (four planes)
- Leg press (Fig. 4-29)
- Knee extension, 90-40 degrees
- Half squats, 0-40 degrees
- Weight shifts
- Front and side lunges
- Hamstring curls (Fig. 4-30)
- Bicycling
- Proprioception training
- Overpressure into extension
- Passive ROM, 0-50 degrees
- Patellar mobilization
- Well-leg exercises
- Progressive resistance program: start with 1 pound and progress 1 pound per week

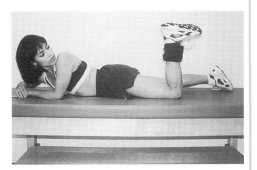

Figure 4–30   Prone hamstring curls with a 1- to 5-pound weight.

Continued

REHABILITATION PROTOCOL: *Accelerated Rehabilitation after Anterior Cruciate Ligament Reconstruction with Central-Third Patellar Tendon* Continued

PHASE 2: EARLY REHABILITATION—WEEKS 2-4—cont'd

Swelling Control

- Ice, compression, elevation

Week 3

Brace

- Discontinue

Range of Motion

- Continue ROM stretching and overpressure into extension

Exercises

- Continue all exercises as in week 2
- Passive ROM, 0-115 degrees
- Bicycling for ROM stimulus and endurance
- Pool walking program (if incision is closed)
- Eccentric quadriceps program, 40-100 degrees (isotonic only)
- Lateral lunges
- Lateral step-ups
- Front step-ups
- Lateral step-overs (cones)
- Stair stepper machine or elliptical trainer
- Progress proprioception drills, neuromuscular control drills

PHASE 3: CONTROLLED AMBULATION—WEEKS 4-10

Criteria for Progression to Phase 3

- Active ROM, 0-115 degrees
- Quadriceps strength 60% of contralateral side (isometric test at 60 degrees knee flexion)
- Unchanged KT test bilateral values (+1 or less)
- Minimal or no full joint effusion
- No joint line or patellofemoral pain

Goals

- Restore full knee ROM (0-125 degrees)
- Improve lower extremity strength
- Enhance proprioception, balance, and neuromuscular control
- Restore limb confidence and function

Brace

- No immobilizer or brace, may use knee sleeve

Range of Motion

- Self-administered ROM (4-5 times daily using the other leg to provide ROM), emphasis on maintaining 0 degrees passive extension

REHABILITATION PROTOCOL: *Accelerated Rehabilitation after Anterior Cruciate Ligament Reconstruction with Central-Third Patellar Tendon* *Continued*

PHASE 3: CONTROLLED AMBULATION—WEEKS 4-10—cont'd

KT2000 Testing

- Week 4, 20-pound anterior and posterior tests

Week 4

Exercises

- Progress isometric strengthening program
- Leg press
- Knee extension, 90-40 degrees
- Hamstring curls
- Hip abduction and adduction
- Hip flexion and extension
- Lateral step-overs
- Lateral lunges
- Lateral step-ups
- Front step-downs
- Wall squats (Fig. 4-31)
- Vertical squats
- Toe-calf raises
- Biodex Stability System (e.g., balance, squats)
- Proprioception drills
- Bicycling
- Stair stepper machine
- Pool program (backward running, hip and leg exercises)

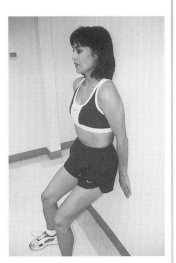

Figure 4–31 Thirty-degree wall squats performed with the back against the wall.

Continued

REHABILITATION PROTOCOL: *Accelerated Rehabilitation after Anterior Cruciate Ligament Reconstruction with Central-Third Patellar Tendon* Continued

PHASE 3: CONTROLLED AMBULATION—WEEKS 4-10—cont'd

Week 6

KT2000 Testing

- 20- and 30-pound anterior and posterior tests

Exercises

- Continue all exercises
- Pool running (forward), agility drills
- Balance on tilt boards
- Progress to balance and board throws

Week 8

KT2000 Testing

- 20- and 30-pound anterior and posterior tests

Exercises

- Continue all exercises
- Plyometric leg press
- Perturbation training
- Isokinetic exercises (90-40 degrees, 120-240 degrees/sec)
- Walking program
- Bicycling for endurance
- Stair stepper machine for endurance

Week 10

KT2000 Testing

- 20- and 30-pound and manual maximum tests

Isokinetic Test

- Concentric knee extension-flexion at 180 and 300 degrees/sec

Exercises

- Continue all exercises
- Plyometric training drills
- Continue stretching drills

PHASE 4: ADVANCED ACTIVITY—WEEKS 10-16

Criteria for Progression to Phase 4

- Active ROM, 0-125 degrees or greater
- Quadriceps strength 79% of contralateral side
- Knee extension flexor-extensor ratio, 70%-75%
- No change in KT values (comparable with contralateral side, within 2 mm)
- No pain or effusion

REHABILITATION PROTOCOL: *Accelerated Rehabilitation after Anterior Cruciate Ligament Reconstruction with Central-Third Patellar Tendon*   *Continued*

PHASE 4: ADVANCED ACTIVITY—WEEKS 10-16—cont'd

- Satisfactory clinical examination
- Satisfactory isokinetic test (values at 180 degrees)
  - Quadriceps bilateral comparison, 75%
  - Hamstrings equal bilateral
  - Quadriceps peak torque–to–body weight ratio
  - Hamstrings-quadriceps ratio, 66%-75%
- Hop test 80% of contralateral leg
- Subjective knee scoring (modified Noyes system), 80 points or better

Goals

- Normalize lower extremity strength
- Enhance muscular power and endurance
- Improve neuromuscular control
- Perform selected sport-specific drills

Exercises

- Continue all exercises

PHASE 5: RETURN TO ACTIVITY—MONTHS 16-22

Criteria for Progression to Phase 5

- Full ROM
- Unchanged KT2000 test (within 2.5 mm of opposite side)
- Isokinetic test that fulfills criteria
- Quadriceps bilateral comparison, ≥80%
- Hamstring bilateral comparison, ≥110%
- Quadriceps torque–body weight ratio, ≥70%
- Proprioceptive test 100% of contralateral leg
- Functional test ≥85% of contralateral side
- Satisfactory clinical examination
- Subjective knee scoring (modified Noyes system), ≥90 points

Goals

- Gradual return to full unrestricted sports
- Achieve maximal strength and endurance
- Normalize neuromuscular control
- Progress skill training

Tests

- KT2000 test
- Isokinetic
- Functional

Continued

REHABILITATION PROTOCOL: *Accelerated Rehabilitation after Anterior Cruciate Ligament Reconstruction with Central-Third Patellar Tendon*   *Continued*

PHASE 5: RETURN TO ACTIVITY—MONTHS 16-22

Exercises

- Continue strengthening exercises
- Continue neuromuscular control drills
- Continue plyometrics drills
- Progress running and agility program
- Progress sport-specific training

6- and 12-Month Follow-up

- Isokinetic test
- KT2000 test
- Functional test

Note: We use the **orthovid.com** patient ACL instructional videotape and handout series for these patients. This videotape was produced by the senior author of this book.

REHABILITATION PROTOCOL   *Additional Guidelines for Rehabilitation after Anterior Cruciate Ligament Reconstruction*
Wilk

AFTER RECONSTRUCTION WITH CONCOMITANT MENISCAL REPAIR

- Immediate motion
- Immediate weight-bearing
- Restrictions/limitations
  - No isolated hamstring contraction for 8-10 weeks
  - No squatting past 60 degrees knee flexion for 8 weeks
  - No squatting with rotation or twisting for 10-12 weeks
  - No lunges past 75 degrees knee flexion for 8 weeks
- Return to sports at 5-7 months

AFTER RECONSTRUCTION WITH A CONTRALATERAL PATELLAR GRAFT

Donor Leg

- Cryotherapy, ROM, and gradual strengthening exercises
- Emphasis on quadriceps strengthening
- Full ROM usually within 3 weeks

Anterior Cruciate Ligament–Reconstructed Knee

- Less painful, faster ROM
- Quadriceps weakness still present despite graft harvest from the contralateral leg
- Rehabilitation same as after the use of an ipsilateral graft
- Able to return to sports faster
- Risk for contralateral knee complications (e.g., RSD)

REHABILITATION PROTOCOL: *Additional Guidelines for Rehabilitation after Anterior Cruciate Ligament Reconstruction* *Continued*

AFTER RECONSTRUCTION AND CONCOMITANT ARTICULAR CHONDRAL INJURY

- Weight-bearing modifications
  - Microfracture technique—toe-touch weight-bearing
  - Mosaicplasty—non–weight-bearing for 6-8 weeks
- Pool program once wounds are healed (see the aqua-aerobics section)
- Immediate motion—stimulus for articular cartilage healing
- No excess loading for 3-4 months
- Return to sports in 6-9 months

REHABILITATION PROTOCOL	*After Anterior Cruciate Ligament Reconstruction Using Ipsilateral Autogenous Patellar Tendon Graft* Shelbourne

TIME FRAME	GOALS	EXERCISES	COMMENTS
Preoperative	Obtain full ROM	Prone hangs Hyperextension device (see Fig. 4-25B) Heel slides	This preoperative rehabilitation approach has decreased the incidence of postoperative ROM problems to <1%
	Reduce swelling Achieve good leg control Maintain good mental attitude Understand postoperative rehabilitation program	Cold/compression device Quad sets, step-ups, bike Explanation of program	
Surgery	Intravenous ketorolac pain prevention program Both knees moved through full ROM from full hyperextension to flexion with heel touching buttocks Cold/compression device applied over light sterile dressing		

Continued

REHABILITATION PROTOCOL: *After Anterior Cruciate Ligament Reconstruction Using Ipsilateral Autogenous Patellar Tendon Graft*   *Continued*

TIME FRAME	GOALS	EXERCISES	COMMENTS
Day 1-Week 1	Get the knee into a "quiet state" (decrease inflammation)	Bed rest except for bathroom privileges	
	Minimize hemarthrosis	Cold/compression; elevation in CPM machine	
	Full passive hyperextension	Heel prop exercise	
	Increase flexion to 110 degrees	Heel slide exercise with the use of a measuring stick: place the stick so that zero is at the heel when the leg is extended; do the heel slide exercise, and observe the number of centimeters at the level of the heel	This measurement gives the patient a point of reference to evaluate improvement
	Obtain good leg control	Quadriceps contraction exercises SLR	
Weeks 1-2	Maintain hyperextension	Heel props Prone hang Hyperextension device if needed	
	Increase flexion to 125 degrees	Heel slide (using a measuring stick for reference)	Although the physical the rapist measures ROM with a goniometer, the patient is given a flexion goal that relates to the number of centimeters of bend in the opposite, normal knee
	Achieve normal gait	Gait training in front of a mirror	

REHABILITATION PROTOCOL: *After Anterior Cruciate Ligament Reconstruction Using Ipsilateral Autogenous Patellar Tendon Graft*   *Continued*

TIME FRAME	GOALS	EXERCISES	COMMENTS
	Increase leg strength	Step-ups Step-down exercise at a low level Proper gait with stairs	
	Keep effusion to a minimum	Cold/compression continually as able	
	Resume normal daily activities (school, sedentary work)	If activities cause increased swelling or soreness, reduce activities, elevate the leg, and use the cold/compression cuff more	
Weeks 2-4	Maintain hyperextension	Heel props Prone hangs as needed	
	Increase flexion to 135 degrees	Heel slides	
	Increase leg strength	Step-down exercise at higher levels (Fig. 4-32) Stationary bike Stair-climbing machine Leg extension exercise Single-leg press Squats	Program is designed according to the type of equipment available to the patient

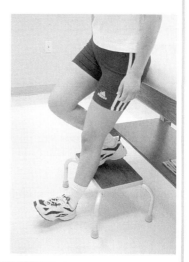

Figure 4–32   Step-down exercise using a small step.

Continued

REHABILITATION PROTOCOL: *After Anterior Cruciate Ligament Reconstruction Using Ipsilateral Autogenous Patellar Tendon Graft*   *Continued*

TIME FRAME	GOALS	EXERCISES	COMMENTS
	Maintain minimal effusion	Adjust activities as needed Cold/compression several times a day Elevation as needed	
Months 1-2	Maintain full ROM	Check for ROM each morning and perform ROM exercises as needed; should be able to sit on heels	We have observed that during this time when patients begin to increase activities, terminal flexion may decrease. Patients should monitor this daily
	Increase leg strength	Stair-climbing exercise Stationary bike Single-leg strengthening as needed Leg press Squats	
	Increase proprioception	Progression of • Functional agility program • Sport-specific drills (solo) • Sport-specific drills (controlled) • Part-time competition	Progression of these activities varies according to the patient's individual goals and the sports involved; monitor for swelling and loss of motion
Months 2 and Beyond	Maintain full ROM	Monitor daily and perform exercises as needed	
	Increase leg strength	Continue strengthening exercises	Patients sometimes need to be reminded to continue leg strengthening exercises because of theirlevel of excitement for returning to sports.

REHABILITATION PROTOCOL: *After Anterior Cruciate Ligament Reconstruction Using Ipsilateral Autogenous Patellar Tendon Graft*   Continued

TIME FRAME	GOALS	EXERCISES	COMMENTS
			Time should be devoted to single-leg strengthening to ensure that the patient does not favor the leg with sports activities
	Increase proprioception	Sport-specific drills and practice as needed, with gradual return to full participation and contact	Monitor for swelling or loss of motion

Posterior Cruciate Ligament Injuries

Michael D'Amato, MD • Bernard R. Bach, Jr., MD

Information concerning PCL injuries has expanded greatly in the past few years. Despite these advances, significant controversy still exists concerning many aspects of the evaluation and treatment of PCL injuries, especially the natural history of a PCL-injured knee. Our improved understanding of the anatomy and biomechanics of the PCL has led to a more rational and sounder basis for the design of rehabilitation programs, both in the nonoperative setting and after surgery.

REHABILITATION RATIONALE

Normal Posterior Cruciate Ligament

The normal PCL is a complex ligamentous structure with insertions on the posterior aspect of the proximal end of the tibia and the lateral aspect of the medial femoral condyle. The ligament is composed of two functional bundles, a larger anterolateral bundle, which develops tension as the knee flexes, and a smaller posteromedial bundle, which develops tension in knee extension. **The PCL functions as the primary restraint to posterior translation of the tibia and a secondary restrain to external rotation.**

Mechanism of Injury

Rupture of the PCL is usually caused by a direct blow to the proximal end of the tibia, a fall on the knee with the foot in a plantar-flexed position, or hyperflexion of the knee (Fig. 4-33). Less common causes include hyperextension or combined

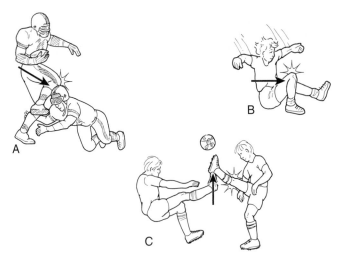

Figure 4–33 Mechanisms of posterior cruciate ligament injury. **A**, Direct posterior blow to the anterior aspect of the proximal end of the tibia. **B**, Hyperflexion of the knee with an anteriorly directed force on the femur. **C**, Hyperextension of the knee. (Adapted from Miller MD, Harner CD, Koshiwaguchi S: Acute posterior cruciate ligament injuries. In Fu FH, Harner CD, Vince KG [eds]: Knee Surgery. Baltimore, Williams & Wilkins, 1994, pp 749-767.)

rotational forces. Typically, the ligament fails in its midsubstance, but avulsions of the tibial or femoral attachments have been described. The injury may be isolated to the PCL or associated with multiple ligament injuries or knee dislocation. Isolated injuries tend to occur during athletics, and combined injuries are generally the result of high-energy trauma.

EVALUATION

A number of tests are available to clinically assess the integrity of the PCL. The *posterior drawer test* at 90 degrees of knee flexion has been shown to be the most sensitive (see Fig. 4-8). Other tests include the *posterior sag test* (see Fig. 4-9), the *quadriceps active test*, and the *reverse pivot shift test* (Fig. 4-34). In addition, rotational stability of the knee must be evaluated to rule out any associated injury to the posterolateral ligament complex. **One must also be wary when performing a Lachman test in the setting of a PCL injury. It is easy to assume that the anterior translation represents an injury to the ACL, when in fact it may be the tibia returning to a normal position from a previously abnormal posteriorly subluxated position**. The collateral ligaments and menisci should also be appropriately evaluated.

Biomechanical studies have produced several key points that should be considered in the evaluation of PCL injury:

- The PCL is the primary restraint to posterior translation at all positions of knee flexion.
- PCL tear is best detected at 70 to 90 degrees of knee flexion with posterior drawer testing.

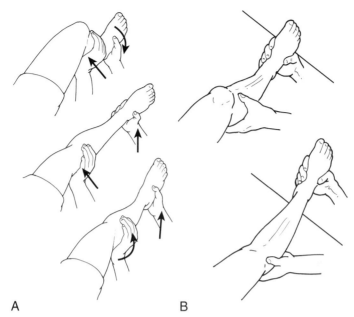

Figure 4–34 Reverse pivot shift test. **A,** With the patient in the supine position, the knee is flexed 90 degrees. External rotation, varus, and axial loads are applied as the leg is extended. With a posterior cruciate ligament (PCL) injury, the lateral tibial plateau will translate from a posterior subluxated to a reduced position as the leg is extended. **B,** In the reverse pivot shift test, which is used to identify injury to the posterolateral structures, the examiner lifts the patient's leg and sta-bilizes it with one hand on the heel against the pelvis. The other hand supports the lateral aspect of the calf with the palm on the proximal end of the fibula. *Left,* In the first step of the test, the patient's knee is flexed to 70 to 80 degrees and the foot is externally rotated, which causes the tibia on the injured side to sublux posteriorly. *Right,* In the second step, the examiner extends the patient's leg while applying valgus stress to the knee. The test is positive if the subluxation reduces. A positive test indicates that the PCL, arcuate complex, and fibular collateral ligament are torn. (**A,** Adapted from Miller MD, Harner CD, Koshiwaguchi S: Acute posterior cruciate ligament injuries. In Fu FH, Harner CD, Vince KG [eds]: Knee Surgery. Baltimore, Williams & Wilkins, 1994, pp 749-767.)

- An *isolated* PCL tear does not cause varus-valgus laxity or increased rotation.
- An *isolated* PCL tear and isolated posterolateral corner injury will produce about the same degree of posterior translation at 30 degrees of knee flexion.
- If there is varus or valgus laxity in full extension, by definition there is com-bined injury to the PCL and collateral complex.
- If the knee hyperextends asymmetrically, a combined cruciate and posterolat-eral corner injury is present.
- A posterolateral corner injury may produce mild degrees of varus laxity, but more severe degrees of varus laxity indicate PCL injury.
- The combination of a PCL tear and posterolateral corner tear produces much more severe posterior translation and external rotation than either injury does in isolation.
- It is difficult to have *severe* posterolateral corner instability without injury to the PCL, fibular collateral ligament, *and* popliteus.

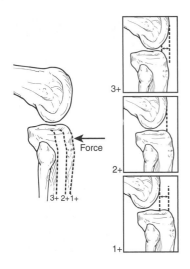

Figure 4–35   Posterior cruciate ligament injury grading. Grading is based on the relationship of the anterior aspect of the medial tibial plateau to the anterior aspect of the medial femoral condyle. In grade 1, the tibia remains anterior to the femur. In grade 2, the tibia is even with the femur. In grade 3, the tibia moves posterior to the femur.

Classification

Classification of PCL injuries is based on the relationship of the medial tibial plateau to the medial femoral condyle during a posterior drawer test (Fig. 4-35). *Grade 1* injuries have 0 to 5 mm of posterior translation and maintain the position of the medial tibial plateau anterior to the medial femoral condyle. *Grade 2* injuries have 5 to 10 mm of posterior translation, and the medial tibial plateau rests flush with the medial femoral condyle. *Grade 3* injuries have more than 10 mm of posterior translation, and the medial tibial plateau falls posterior to the medial femoral condyle.

Radiographic Evaluation

Radiographs are usually negative; however, they may identify the presence of a bony avulsion that can be reattached (Fig. 4-36). Stress radiographs have been shown to compare favorably with clinical examination techniques in the diagnosis of PCL injury. MRI is helpful in confirming the diagnosis of a PCL rupture, as well as evaluating the remaining structures of the knee (Fig. 4-37). Bone scans can be used to demonstrate increased subchondral stress resulting from changes in knee kinematics after PCL injury. The increased stress may predispose the knee to early degeneration, and some surgeons use an abnormal bone scan as an indication of the need for operative PCL stabilization (Fig. 4-38).

BIOMECHANICS OF THE POSTERIOR CRUCIATE LIGAMENT–DEFICIENT KNEE

Injury to the PCL results in changes in the kinematics of the knee. **Changes in contact pressure have been demonstrated in both the patellofemoral and the medial tibiofemoral compartments after sectioning of the PCL, with significant increases in joint forces**. This alteration in the normal kinematics may explain the tendency for the development of degenerative changes in these two compartments after PCL injury.

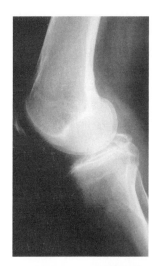

Figure 4–36 Posterior cruciate ligament (PCL) avulsion injury noted on a radiograph. The tibial insertion of the PCL is avulsed with its bony attachment from the posterior aspect of the tibia.

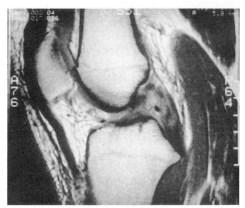

Figure 4–37 Magnetic resonance image of a posterior cruciate ligament (PCL) injury. Note the interruption of the black posterior vertical structure (PCL).

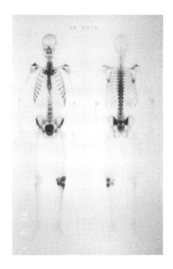

Figure 4–38 Bone scan of the knee demonstrating degenerative changes. In a chronic posterior cruciate ligament injury, degenerative changes tend to occur in the medial and patellofemoral compartments.

BIOMECHANICS OF EXERCISE

Markolf and colleagues (1997) demonstrated that passive ROM of the knee results in the generation of minimal force in the intact PCL throughout the entire motion arc. After reconstruction, no significant change in force production was noted except for a small increase at flexion angles greater than 60 degrees.

The *shear forces* generated in the knee during open– and closed–kinetic chain exercises have been closely examined. A posterior shear force occurs during closed–kinetic chain exercise throughout the entire ROM of the knee, with greater force generated as knee flexion increases. With open–kinetic chain activities, there appears to be tremendous force exerted on the PCL during flexion exercises. However, with open–kinetic chain extension, minimal or no force appears to be generated in the PCL from 0 to 60 degrees, but from 60 to 90 degrees, significant stress is produced in the PCL. It has been demonstrated that altering the position of the resistance pad can modify the force generated with open–kinetic chain exercises.

The magnitude of force generated in the PCL during exercise is much greater than that in the ACL, which may be a factor in the tendency for PCL grafts to stretch out after surgical reconstruction. The trend has been to avoid reconstruction of the PCL when possible, but it may be that proper rehabilitation can avoid the development of progressive laxity and improve the results of reconstruction.

O'Connor (1993) calculated that it is possible to unload the cruciate ligaments dynamically by co-contraction of the quadriceps, hamstrings, and gastrocnemius muscles. The role of the gastrocnemius in dynamically stabilizing the PCL is supported indirectly by the findings of Inoue and coworkers (1998), who demonstrated earlier activation of the gastrocnemius before the generation of flexion torque in PCL-deficient knees as compared with uninjured knees.

The goal should be to minimize the potentially deleterious generation of force during rehabilitation. It appears that passive motion can be safely performed through the entire range of flexion and extension. **Active closed–kinetic chain activities of any kind, in any ROM, should be used cautiously when rehabilitating the PCL, either as nonoperative therapy or after reconstruction. If these exercises are used, they should be carried out in a ROM that limits flexion of the knee to about 45 degrees or less to avoid generating higher force in the PCL.** Open–kinetic chain flexion exercises generate extremely high force in the PCL and should be avoided altogether, whereas open–kinetic chain extension appears to be safe when performed at lower flexion angles (from 60 to 0 degrees). However, in this range, patellofemoral stress is at its greatest, and the risk for development of patellofemoral symptoms is significant. Therefore, **we do not routinely recommend the use of open-chain exercises during rehabilitation after PCL injury or reconstruction**.

NATURAL HISTORY

The natural history of isolated PCL injuries remains controversial. In a number of studies, isolated PCL injuries have been shown to do well with nonoperative treatment, whereas others have shown poor outcomes after conservative measures.

Attempts have been made to determine what variables may predict the outcome of conservatively treated PCL injuries. Increased quadriceps strength has been correlated with improved outcome in some studies, but others have not found a significant relationship. Shelbourne, Davis, and Patel (1999) demonstrated that subjective and objective functional outcomes were independent of knee laxity. However, all of their patients demonstrated grade 2 laxity or less. It is unclear what effect more severe laxity has on the results of conservative treatment.

The development of degenerative changes, particularly in the medial tibiofemoral and patellofemoral compartments, is also an area of controversy. Some studies have demonstrated increased degeneration with time after conservative treatment of PCL injuries, whereas others have not.

Unlike a torn ACL and more like a torn MCL, the PCL may regain continuity with time. Shelbourne and colleagues (1999) found that at follow-up, 63 of 68 patients with PCL injuries had the same or less clinical laxity than at their initial evaluations. Athletes with isolated PCL injuries may be told that the amount of posterior laxity is likely to improve with time, but this does not mean a better knee subjectively.

Clearly, isolated PCL injuries may not be as benign as was once believed. **The problem is not one of instability, but rather one of progressive disability**. Most studies demonstrate reasonably good functional outcomes after conservative treatment of isolated PCL injuries, yet pain and early degenerative changes in the knee develop in a significant number of patients despite a good functional recovery. Unfortunately, **surgical management has not been shown to consistently alter the natural history of these injuries**.

REHABILITATION CONSIDERATIONS

In general, rehabilitation after PCL injury tends to be more conservative than after ACL injury. The severity of the PCL injury should also guide the aggressiveness of nonoperative therapy. Rehabilitation progression can be more rapid with grade 1 and 2 injuries, whereas rehabilitation after grade 3 injuries is advanced more slowly. After reconstruction a different protocol is used, and again, a more conservative approach is used than after ACL reconstruction.

Motion

Because passive motion places negligible stress on the intact PCL and only small stress on PCL grafts with knee flexion past 60 degrees, the use of CPM may be beneficial for grade 3 injuries treated nonoperatively and after reconstruction. Early active motion may expose the ligament to excessive force and lead to elongation and subsequent laxity. For grade 1 and 2 injuries treated nonoperatively, nonresisted active motion as tolerated is probably safe, but resisted motion, including weight-bearing, should be limited to a 0- to 60-degree flexion arc during the early treatment phase.

Weight-Bearing

Weight-bearing is encouraged. For mild injuries treated nonoperatively, weight-bearing should be in a brace limited to 0 to 60 degrees of motion. For more severe injuries treated nonoperatively and after PCL reconstruction, weight-bearing should be in a brace locked in extension during the early treatment phases and progressed gradually.

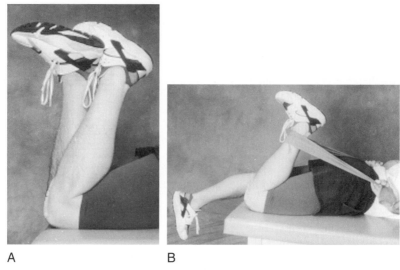

A   B

Figure 4–39 **A**, Prone flexion exercises for knee flexion. **B**, Prone knee flexion with a rubber band or towel.

External Support

After reconstruction or during nonoperative treatment of grade 3 isolated PCL injuries, **it is crucial to prevent posterior displacement of the tibia from the effects of gravity and the weight of the leg, as well as from the pull of the hamstrings**. Proper bracing is helpful to resist these forces, but the therapist must be aware of the potential for posterior sag to occur. If CPM devices are used, resistance straps must be included to support the proximal end of the tibia posteriorly. Exercises must be carried out with manual support of the tibia as well. **Alternatively, flexion exercises can be done in the prone position (Fig. 4-39) so that the posterior translational force of gravity on the tibia is eliminated**.

Limited information is available regarding the efficacy of *functional bracing* after PCL injury. At this time, use of a functional brace is commonly recommended, even though little scientific data supporting this recommendation can be found.

Muscle Training

Quadriceps strengthening is the foundation of rehabilitation after PCL injury. As noted earlier, the quadriceps functions to dynamically stabilize the tibia and counteract the posterior pull of the hamstrings. Open–kinetic chain extension activities place the lowest strain on the PCL but result in elevated patellofemoral joint force. **We recommend the use of closed–kinetic chain activities from 0 to 45 degrees as a compromise to protect both the PCL and the patellofemoral joint. Open–kinetic chain flexion activities, which produce high posterior shear force, should be avoided**.

Patellofemoral Joint

The patellofemoral joint is at particular risk for the development of symptoms during rehabilitation after PCL injury. The altered kinematics of the knee places increased force across the joint that results in early degeneration of the articular surfaces. In addition, open–kinetic chain extension exercises at low levels of knee flexion (0 to 60 degrees) create an extremely high joint reaction force across the patellofemoral joint.

TREATMENT

There is still a great deal of debate regarding the treatment of PCL injuries. Currently, most agree that combined ligamentous injuries of the knee require surgical repair or reconstruction; however, there is no clear consensus on when reconstruction is indicated for isolated PCL injuries. **For acute isolated grade 1 or 2 PCL injuries, the common recommendation is nonoperative rehabilitation. For acute isolated grade 3 injuries, the clear indication for surgery is an avulsion or "pull-off" injury of the ligament at the bony insertion site**. Less clear are the indications for surgical treatment of midsubstance rupture of the ligament. Some advocate nonoperative treatment of all acute isolated grade 3 PCL injuries, whereas others recommend reconstruction in younger, high-demand patients. For *chronic* injuries, grade 1 and most grade 2 and 3 injuries are treated by rehabilitation and modification of activity. Surgery is indicated for symptomatic chronic grade 2 and 3 injuries. The symptoms are typically pain or instability. A positive bone scan, indicating kinematic changes leading to early joint degeneration, may prompt surgical reconstruction in an attempt to forestall the progression of joint arthrosis.

Nonoperative Treatment

For grade 1 and 2 injuries, progression can proceed rapidly, with minimal immobilization, early strengthening, and return to full activity as soon as 3 to 4 weeks in some patients. Outcomes after grade 3 injuries are less predictable, and the likelihood of an undetected posterolateral corner injury is significant. Therefore, with grade 3 injuries, a more conservative approach is recommended. These injuries are generally treated with a short course of immobilization, with passive rather than active motion in the early healing phase, and a less aggressive strengthening program.

REHABILITATION PROTOCOL | *Nonoperative Treatment of Posterior Cruciate Ligament Injuries*
D'Amato and Bach

PHASE 1

Days 1-7

- ROM (0-60 degrees)
- Weight-bearing with two crutches
- Electrical muscle stimulation of the quadriceps

Continued

REHABILITATION PROTOCOL: *Nonoperative Treatment of Posterior Cruciate Ligament Injuries* *Continued*

PHASE 1—cont'd

Exercises

- Quadriceps sets
- SLR
- Hip adduction and abduction
- Mini-squats/leg press (0-45 degrees)

Weeks 2-3

- ROM (0-60 degrees)
- Weight-bearing without crutches
- Progress exercises using weights
- Bike (week 3) for ROM
- Pool program (see section on aquatic therapy in Chapter 7)
- Leg press (0-60 degrees)

PHASE 2

Week 3

- ROM to tolerance
- Discontinue brace
- Bike, StairMaster, rowing
- Progress exercises with weights
- Mini-squats (0-60 degrees)
- Leg press (0-60 degrees)
- Step-ups
- Hip abduction and adduction
- Toe-calf raises

Weeks 5-6

- Continue all exercises
- Fit functional brace
- Pool running

PHASE 3

Weeks 8-12

- Begin running program
- Continue all strengthening exercises
- Gradual return to sports activities
- Criteria to return to sports
  - No change in laxity
  - No pain, tenderness, or swelling
  - Satisfactory clinical examination
  - Functional testing 85% of contralateral knee
  - Quadriceps strength 85% of contralateral knee

Operative Treatment

The rehabilitation protocol after reconstruction of the PCL is quite conservative when compared with that after ACL reconstruction, primarily because of the greater posterior shear force generated during activity and motion of the knee. **Prevention of posterior sag and hamstring activity is paramount in avoiding residual laxity.** Despite this conservative approach, motion problems are rare after PCL reconstruction. As the biology of graft healing becomes better understood and surgical techniques improve, accelerated rehabilitation protocols may be shown to be safe, but at present, the information regarding aggressive rehabilitation is limited and protection of the graft from potentially deleterious forces must be enforced.

REHABILITATION PROTOCOL	*After Surgical Reconstruction of the Posterior Cruciate Ligament* D'Amato and Bach

GENERAL GUIDELINES

- No open-chain exercises
- Caution against posterior tibial translation (gravity, muscle action)
- No CPM
- Resistance for hip progressive resistive exercises (PREs) is placed above the knee for hip abduction and adduction; resistance may be distal for hip flexion

PHASE 1: WEEKS 0-4

Goals

- Protect healing bony and soft tissue structures
- Minimize the effects of immobilization
  - Early protected ROM (protection against posterior tibial sagging)
  - PREs for the quadriceps, hip, and calf, with emphasis on limiting patellofemoral joint compression and posterior tibial translation
- Patient education to impart a clear understanding of the limitations and expectations of the rehabilitation process and the need for supporting the proximal end of the tibia and avoiding sag

Bracing

- Brace locked at 0 degrees for 1 week
- At 1 week after surgery, the brace is unlocked for passive ROM done by a physical therapist or athletic trainer
- The patient is instructed in self-administered passive ROM with the brace on, with an emphasis on supporting the proximal end of the tibia

Weight-Bearing

- As tolerated with crutches, brace locked in extension

Special Considerations

- Pillow under the proximal posterior aspect of the tibia at rest to prevent posterior sag

Continued

REHABILITATION PROTOCOL: *After Surgical Reconstruction of the Posterior Cruciate Ligament*   *Continued*

PHASE 1: WEEKS 0-4—cont'd

Therapeutic Exercises

- Patellar mobilization
- Prone passive flexion and extension
- Quadriceps sets
- SLR
- Hip abduction and adduction
- Ankle pumps
- Hamstring and calf stretching
- Calf exercise with Thera-Band, progressing to standing calf raise with full knee extension
- Standing hip extension from neutral
- Functional electrical stimulation (may be used for trace to poor quadriceps contraction)

PHASE 2: WEEKS 4-12

Criteria for Progression to Phase 2

- Good quadriceps control (good quadriceps set, no sag with SLR)
- Approximately 60 degrees knee flexion
- Full knee extension
- No signs of active inflammation

Goals

- Increase ROM (flexion)
- Restore normal gait
- Continue quadriceps strengthening and hamstring flexibility

Bracing

- 4-6 weeks: brace is unlocked for controlled gait training only (patient may walk with brace unlocked while attending physical therapy or when at home)
- 6-8 weeks: brace is unlocked for all activities
- 8 weeks: brace is discontinued (as allowed by physician)

Weight-Bearing

- 4-8 weeks: weight-bearing as tolerated with crutches
- 8 weeks: may discontinue crutches if patient exhibits
  - No quadriceps lag with SLR
  - Full knee extension
  - Knee flexion of 90-100 degrees
  - Normal gait pattern (patient can use one crutch or cane until normal gait is achieved)

Therapeutic Exercises

Weeks 4-8

- Wall slides (0-45 degrees)
- Mini-squats (0-45 degrees)
- Leg press (0-60 degrees)

REHABILITATION PROTOCOL: *After Surgical Reconstruction of the Posterior Cruciate Ligament   Continued*

PHASE 2: WEEKS 4-12—cont'd

- Four-way hip exercises for flexion, abduction, adduction, and extension from neutral with knee fully extended
- Ambulation in pool (work on restoration of normal heel-toe gait pattern in chest-deep water)

Weeks 8-12

- Stationary bike (foot placed forward on the pedal without the use of toe clips to minimize hamstring activity, seat set slightly higher than normal)
- StairMaster, elliptical stepper, Nordic-Trac
- Balance and proprioception activities
- Seated calf raises
- Leg press (0-90 degrees)

PHASE 3: MONTHS 3-6

Criteria for Progression to Phase 3

- Full, pain-free ROM (*Note:* it is not unusual for flexion to be lacking 10-15 degrees for up to 5 months after surgery)
- Normal gait
- Good to normal quadriceps strength
- No patellofemoral complaints
- Clearance by the physician to begin more concentrated closed–kinetic chain progression

Goals

- Restore any residual loss of motion that may prevent functional progression
- Progress functionally and prevent patellofemoral irritation
- Improve functional strength and proprioception with closed–kinetic chain exercises
- Continue to maintain quadriceps strength and hamstring flexibility

Therapeutic Exercises

- Continue closed–kinetic chain exercise progression
- Treadmill walking
- Jogging in pool with a wet vest or belt
- Swimming (no frog kick)

PHASE 4: MONTH 6—FULL ACTIVITY

Criteria for Progression to Phase 4

- No significant patellofemoral or soft tissue irritation
- Presence of necessary joint ROM, muscle strength, endurance, and proprioception to safely return to athletic participation

Goals

- Safe and gradual return to athletic participation
- Maintenance of strength, endurance, and function

Continued

REHABILITATION PROTOCOL: *After Surgical Reconstruction of the Posterior Cruciate Ligament*   *Continued*

PHASE 4: MONTH 6—FULL ACTIVITY—cont'd

Therapeutic Exercises

- Continue closed–kinetic chain exercise progression
- Sport-specific functional progression, which may include but is not limited to
  - Slide board
  - Jog/run progression
  - Figure-of-eight, carioca, backward running, cutting
  - Jumping (plyometrics)

Criteria for Return to Sports

- Full, pain-free ROM
- Satisfactory clinical examination
- Quadriceps strength 85% of contralateral leg
- Functional testing 85% of contralateral leg
- No change in laxity testing

REHABILITATION PROTOCOL | *After Posterior Cruciate Ligament Reconstruction with a Two-Tunnel Graft Technique*
Wilk

IMPORTANT REHABILITATION POINTS

- Emphasize quadriceps strengthening
- Closely monitor patellofemoral and medial joint line degeneration
- Monitor capsular laxity, especially posterolateral corner
- Gradual return to sports

PHASE 1: IMMEDIATE POSTOPERATIVE PERIOD—WEEKS 1-2

Goals

- Control swelling and inflammation
- Obtain full passive knee extension
- Gradually increase flexion to 90 degrees
- Voluntary quadriceps control
- Patellar mobility

Days 1-3

Brace

- EZ Wrap locked at 0 degrees extension; patient sleeps in a brace

Weight-Bearing

- As tolerated with two crutches (50%)

Range of Motion

- Self-administered ROM (0-90 degrees) out of the brace, 4-5 times daily

REHABILITATION PROTOCOL: *After Posterior Cruciate Ligament Reconstruction with a Two-Tunnel Graft Technique* Continued

PHASE 1: IMMEDIATE POSTOPERATIVE PERIOD—WEEKS 1-2—cont'd

Exercises

- Patellar mobilization
- Stretching of hamstrings and calf
- Ankle pumps
- Quadriceps sets
- SLR (three-way) for hip flexion, abduction, and adduction
- Knee extensions (0-60 degrees)

Muscle Stimulation

- Electrical stimulation of the quadriceps (4 hr/day) during quadriceps sets

Continuous Passive Motion

- 0-60 degrees as tolerated

Ice and Elevation

- Ice 20 minutes of every hour and elevate with the knee in extension; do not allow the proximal end of the tibia to sag posteriorly

Days 4-7

Brace

- EZ Wrap locked at 0 degrees extension for ambulation and sleep only

Weight-Bearing

- Two crutches (50%)

Range of Motion

- Self-administered ROM (0-90 degrees) out of the brace, 4-5 times daily for 10 minutes
- Patellar mobilization
- Stretching of hamstrings and calf

Exercises

- Ankle pumps
- Quadriceps sets
- SLR (three-way) for hip flexion, abduction, and adduction
- Knee extensions (0-60 degrees)

Muscle Stimulation

- Electrical stimulation of the quadriceps (4 hr/day) during quadriceps sets

Continuous Passive Motion

- 0-60 degrees as tolerated

Ice and Elevation

- Ice 20 minutes of every hour and elevate with the knee in extension; do not allow the proximal end of the tibia to sag posteriorly

Continued

REHABILITATION PROTOCOL: *After Posterior Cruciate Ligament Reconstruction with a Two-Tunnel Graft Technique*   *Continued*

PHASE 2: MAXIMUM PROTECTION—WEEKS 2-6

Goals

- Control external forces to protect graft
- Restore motion
- Nourish articular cartilage
- Decrease swelling
- Decrease fibrosis
- Prevent quadriceps atrophy

Week 2

Brace

- EZ Wrap locked at 0 degrees extension

Weight-Bearing

- As tolerated (50% or more, approximately 75% of body weight), with one crutch

Range of Motion

- Self-administered ROM (0-90 degrees) out of the brace, 4-5 times daily
- Patellar mobilization
- Stretching of hamstrings and calf

Exercises

- Multiangle isometrics, 60, 40, and 20 degrees
- Quadriceps sets
- Knee extensions (0-60 degrees)
- Intermittent ROM (0-60 degrees), 4-5 times daily
- Well-leg bicycling
- Proprioception training squats (0-45 degrees) (Biodex Stability System)
- Leg press (0-60 degrees)
- Continue electrical stimulation of quadriceps
- Continue ice and elevation

Weeks 3-4

Brace

- EZ Wrap locked at 0 degrees extension

Weight-Bearing

- Full weight-bearing, no crutches

Range of Motion

- 0-100 degrees by week 3, 0-110 degrees by week 4
- Patellar mobilization
- Hamstring and calf stretching

REHABILITATION PROTOCOL: *After Posterior Cruciate Ligament Reconstruction with a Two-Tunnel Graft Technique*   *Continued*

PHASE 2: MAXIMUM PROTECTION—WEEKS 2-6

Exercises

- Weight shifts
- Mini-squats (0-45 degrees)
- Wall squats (0-50 degrees)
- Intermittent ROM (0-100/110 degrees)
- Knee extension (60-0 degrees)
- Proprioception drills (cup walking)
- Biodex Stability System
- Pool walking
- Bike for ROM and endurance

PHASE 3: CONTROLLED AMBULATION—WEEKS 5-10

Goals

- Restore full motion
- Improve quadriceps muscle strength
- Restore proprioception and dynamic stabilization
- Discontinue use of knee immobilizer

Criteria for Full Weight-Bearing with Knee Motion

- Passive ROM (0-120 degrees)
- Quadriceps strength 70% of contralateral side (isometric test)
- Decreased joint effusion

Week 5

Range of Motion

- Passive ROM (0-120 degrees)

Exercises

- Knee extension (0-60 degrees)
- Multihip machine
- Leg press (0-60/75 degrees)
- Vertical squats (0-45 degrees)
- Wall squats (0-60 degrees)
- Lateral step-ups
- Front lunges
- Side or lateral lunges
- Proprioception drills
- Single-leg balance
- Cup walking
- Heel-toe raises
- Continue stretching hamstrings and calf
- Progress pool exercises

Continued

REHABILITATION PROTOCOL: *After Posterior Cruciate Ligament Reconstruction with a Two-Tunnel Graft Technique* Continued

PHASE 3: CONTROLLED AMBULATION—WEEKS 5-10—cont'd

Week 6

Range of Motion

• Passive ROM (0-125/130 degrees)

KT2000 Test

• 15- and 20-pound anterior-posterior force at 20-35 degrees and 15- and 20-pound anterior-posterior force at the quad neutral angle (QNA) to approximately 70 degrees of flexion as tolerated

Exercises

• Continue all exercises
• Initiate swimming
• Increase closed–kinetic chain rehabilitation
• Functional exercise program

Weeks 8-10

Exercises

• Begin isokinetic ROM (60-0 degrees)
• Continue all exercises
• Initial pool running (forward only)
• Initiate hamstring curls (0-60 degrees), low weight
• Bicycle for endurance (30 minutes)
• Begin walking program
• Stair-climbing machine, ski machine

PHASE 4: LIGHT ACTIVITY—MONTHS 3-4

Goals

• Develop strength, power, and endurance
• Begin to prepare for return to functional activities

Month 3

Exercises

• Begin light running program
• Continue isokinetic exercises (light speed, full ROM)
• Continue eccentrics
• Continue mini-squats, lateral step-ups, wall squats, front step-down, knee extension
• Continue closed–kinetic chain rehabilitation
• Continue endurance exercises
• Begin light agility drills (side shuffle, cariocas)

Month 4

Tests

• Isokinetic test (week 15)
• KT2000 test (week 16)
• Functional test (before running program)

REHABILITATION PROTOCOL: *After Posterior Cruciate Ligament Reconstruction with a Two-Tunnel Graft Technique* Continued

PHASE 4: LIGHT ACTIVITY—MONTHS 3-4

Criteria for Beginning Running Program

- KT2000 test unchanged
- Functional test 70% of contralateral leg
- Isokinetic test interpretation satisfactory

Exercises

- Progress all strengthening exercises, with emphasis on quadriceps strength
- Initiate plyometrics (box jumps [Fig. 4-40], double-leg jumps)

PHASE 5: RETURN TO ACTIVITY—MONTHS 5-6

Goals

- Advance rehabilitation to competitive sports, usually at 6-7 months
- Achieve maximal strength and further enhance neuromuscular coordination and endurance

Exercises

- Closed–kinetic chain rehabilitation
- High-speed isokinetics
- Running program

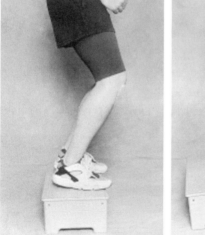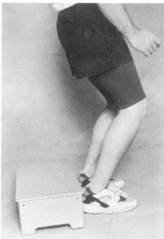

A   B

Figure 4–40 Plyometric box jumps. **A,** The patient starts on top of the box. **B,** The patient hops off the box and lands on the floor in controlled fashion. Box height is gradually increased as strength progresses. The exercise may be performed in a single-leg mode as well.

Continued

REHABILITATION PROTOCOL: *After Posterior Cruciate Ligament Reconstruction with a Two-Tunnel Graft Technique*   *Continued*

PHASE 5: RETURN TO ACTIVITY—MONTHS 5-6—cont'd

- Agility drills
- Balance and proprioception training
- Plyometrics training

Criteria for Return to Sports

- Full, nonpainful ROM
- Satisfactory isokinetic test (85% or better)
- Satisfactory KT2000 test
- Functional hop test 85% of contralateral leg
- Satisfactory clinical examination by physician

6-Month and 12-Month Follow-up

- KT2000 test
- Isokinetic test
- Functional test

REHABILITATION PROTOCOL   *After Combined Reconstruction of the Posterior Cruciate Ligament and Posterolateral Structures (Biceps Tenodesis)*
Wilk

PREOPERATIVE INSTRUCTIONS

- Gait training, weight-bearing as tolerated with crutches
- Instruction in immediate postoperative activities and hospital course
- Brace stays on for all exercises; can open brace to put on muscle stimulator and to do patellar mobilizations

PHASE 1: IMMEDIATE POSTOPERATIVE PERIOD—DAYS 1-4

Brace

- EZ Wrap locked at 0 degrees or full extension

Weight-Bearing

- Two crutches, progress to full weight-bearing as tolerated

Ice and Elevation

- Ice 20 minutes of every hour, elevate with knee in extension

Exercises

- Ankle pumps
- Patella mobilization and passive extension to 0 degrees
- Quadriceps sets, adductor sets with quadriceps setting (QS), glut sets

REHABILITATION PROTOCOL: *After Combined Reconstruction of the Posterior Cruciate Ligament and Posterolateral Structures (Biceps Tenodesis)* Continued

PHASE 2: MAXIMAL PROTECTION—DAY 5-WEEK 8

Day 5-Week 2

Brace

- Locked in full extension

Weight-Bearing

- Progress to full weight-bearing without crutches

Exercises

- Continue all exercises
- Begin PREs with leg raises

Week 6

Brace

- Discontinue brace

Exercises

- Work toward regaining full active flexion seated, not against gravity
- Start exercise bike and swimming, with emphasis on ROM
- Start PREs for the quadriceps only

Week 10

Exercises

- Begin hamstring work against gravity and then start PREs
- Continue all strengthening exercises

Week 12

- KT2000 test

Exercises

- Continue mini-squats
- Initiate lateral step-ups
- Initiate pool running (forward only)
- Hamstrings curls (0-60 degrees), low weight
- Bicycle for endurance (30 minutes)
- Begin walking program

PHASE 4: LIGHT ACTIVITY—MONTHS 3-4

Goals

- Develop strength, power, and endurance
- Begin to prepare for return to functional activities

Exercises

- Begin light running program
- Initiate isokinetics (light speed, full ROM)

Continued

REHABILITATION PROTOCOL: *After Combined Reconstruction of the Posterior Cruciate Ligament and Posterolateral Structures (Biceps Tenodesis)* *Continued*

PHASE 4: LIGHT ACTIVITY—MONTHS 3-4—cont'd

- Continue eccentrics
- Continue mini-squats and lateral step-ups
- Continue closed–kinetic chain rehabilitation
- Continue endurance exercises

Tests

- Isokinetic test (week 15)
- KT2000 test (before running program)
- Functional test (before running program)

Criteria for Running

- Isokinetic test interpretation satisfactory
- KT2000 test unchanged
- Functional test 70% of contralateral leg

PHASE 5: RETURN TO ACTIVITY—MONTHS 5-6

Goals

- Advance rehabilitation to competitive sports
- Achieve maximal strength and further enhance neuromuscular coordination and endurance

Exercises

- Closed–kinetic chain rehabilitation
- High-speed isokinetics
- Running program
- Agility drills
- Balance drills
- Plyometrics initiated
- Gradual return to sport activities

Criteria for Return to Sport Activities

- Isokinetic quadriceps torque–to–body weight ratio
- Isokinetic test 85% of contralateral side
- No change in laxity
- No pain, tenderness, or swelling
- Satisfactory clinical examination

6-Month and 12-Month Follow-up

- KT2000 test
- Isokinetic test
- Functional test

REHABILITATION PROTOCOL
After Combined Reconstruction of the Posterior and Anterior Cruciate Ligaments
Wilk

PHASE 1: IMMEDIATE POSTOPERATIVE PERIOD—DAYS 1-14

Brace

- EZ Wrap brace locked at 0 degrees extension

Weight-Bearing

- As tolerated with two crutches (50%)

Muscle Stimulation

- Electrical stimulation of quadriceps (4 hr/day) during quadriceps set

Ice and Elevation

- Ice 20 minutes out every hour and elevate with knee in extension

Continuous Passive Motion

- 0-60 degrees as tolerated

Exercises

- Ankle pumps
- Quadriceps sets
- SLR (three-way) for hip flexion, abduction, and adduction
- Knee extension (0-60 degrees)

PHASE 2: MAXIMAL PROTECTION—WEEKS 2-6

Goals

- Absolute control of external forces to protect graft
- Nourish articular cartilage
- Decrease swelling
- Decrease fibrosis
- Prevent quadriceps atrophy

Week 2

Brace

- Brace locked at 0 degrees, continue intermittent ROM exercises

Weight-Bearing

- As tolerated, 50% or more

KT Testing

- 15-pound maximal force at 70 degrees of flexion

Exercises

- Multiangle isometrics, 60, 40, and 20 degrees
- Quadriceps sets
- Knee extension (60-0 degrees)
- Intermittent ROM (0-60 degrees), 4-5 times a day

Continued

REHABILITATION PROTOCOL: *After Combined Reconstruction of the Posterior and Anterior Cruciate Ligaments*   *Continued*

PHASE 2: MAXIMAL PROTECTION—WEEKS 2-6—cont'd

- Patellar mobilization
- Well-leg bicycling
- Proprioception training squats (0-45 degrees)
- Continue electrical stimulation of quadriceps
- Leg press (0-60 degrees)
- Continue ice and elevation

Week 4

Brace

- Brace locked at 0 degrees, continue intermittent ROM exercises

Weight-Bearing

- Full weight-bearing, no crutches; one crutch if necessary

KT Testing

- 15-pound maximal force at 70 degrees of flexion

Exercises

- Weight shifts
- Mini-squats (0-45 degrees)
- Intermittent ROM (0-90 degrees)
- Knee extension (80-40 degrees) (therapist discretion)
- Pool walking
- Bike for ROM and endurance

Week 5

Brace

- Fit for functional PCL brace

Exercises

- Initiate pool exercises

PHASE 3: CONTROLLED AMBULATION—WEEKS 6-9

Criteria for Progression to Phase 3

- Active ROM (0-115 degrees)
- Quadriceps strength 60% of contralateral side (isometric test, 60-degree knee flexion angle)
- Unchanged KT test (+1 or less)

Goal

- Control forces during ambulation

Brace

- Discontinue locked brace, brace open 0-125 degrees

REHABILITATION PROTOCOL: *After Combined Reconstruction of the Posterior and*
Anterior Cruciate Ligaments   *Continued*

PHASE 3: CONTROLLED AMBULATION—WEEKS 6-9

KT Testing

- Testing at weeks 6 and 8, 20- and 30-pound test

Exercises

- Continue all exercises
- Passive ROM (0-130 degrees)
- Initiate swimming
- Initiate step-ups (start with 2 ft and gradually increase)
- Increase closed–kinetic chain rehabilitation
- Increase proprioception training

PHASE 4: MODERATE PROTECTION—WEEKS 9-14

Criteria for Progression to Phase 4

- Active ROM (0-125 degrees)
- Quadriceps strength 60% of contralateral leg (isokinetic test)
- No change in KT scores (+2 or less)
- Minimal effusion
- No patellofemoral complaints
- Satisfactory clinical examination

Goals

- Protect patellofemoral joint articular cartilage
- Maximal strengthening of quadriceps, lower extremity

Testing

- KT2000 test, week 12
- Isokinetic test, weeks 10-12

Exercises

- Emphasis on eccentric quadriceps work
- Continue closed-chain exercises, step-ups, mini-squats, leg press
- Continue knee extension (90-40 degrees)
- Hip abduction and adduction
- Hamstring curls and stretches
- Calf raises
- Bicycle for endurance
- Pool running (forward and backward)
- Walking program
- StairMaster
- Initiate isokinetic work (100-40 degrees)

PHASE 5: LIGHT ACTIVITY—MONTHS 3-4

Criteria for Progression to Phase 5

- Active ROM (0-125 degrees or more)
- Quadriceps strength 70% of contralateral side, knee flexor-extensor rated 70%-79%

Continued

REHABILITATION PROTOCOL: *After Combined Reconstruction of the Posterior and Anterior Cruciate Ligaments* *Continued*

PHASE 5: LIGHT ACTIVITY—MONTHS 3-4—cont'd

- No change in KT scores (+2 or less)
- Minimal or no effusion
- Satisfactory clinical examination

Goals

- Develop strength, power, and endurance
- Begin to prepare for return to functional activities

Tests

- Isokinetic test weeks 10-12 and 16-18

Exercises

- Continue strengthening exercises
- Initiate plyometric program
- Initiate running program
- Initiate agility drills
- Sport-specific training and drills

Criteria for Beginning Running Program

- Satisfactory isokinetic test
- Unchanged KT2000 results
- Functional test 70% of contralateral leg
- Satisfactory clinical examination

PHASE 6: RETURN TO ACTIVITY—MONTHS 5-6

Criteria for Returning to Activities

- Isokinetic test that fulfills criteria
- KT2000 test unchanged
- Functional test 80% of contralateral leg
- Satisfactory clinical examination

Goals

- Achieve maximal strength and further enhance neuromuscular coordination and endurance

Tests

- Isokinetic test before return to activity
- KT2000 test
- Functional test

Exercises

- Continue strengthening programs
- Continue closed-chain strengthening program
- Continue plyometric program

> **REHABILITATION PROTOCOL:** *After Combined Reconstruction of the Posterior and Anterior Cruciate Ligaments   Continued*
>
> **PHASE 6: RETURN TO ACTIVITY—MONTHS 5-6**
>
> - Continue running and agility program
> - Accelerate sport-specific training and drills
>
> **6-Month and 12-Month Follow-up**
>
> - KT2000 test
> - Isokinetic test
> - Functional test

Medial Collateral Ligament Injuries

Bruce Reider, MD • Kenneth J. Mroczek, MD

CLINICAL BACKGROUND

The anatomy of the medial aspect of the knee has been divided into three layers consisting of the deep investing fascia of the thigh, the superficial MCL, and the deep MCL, or the knee joint capsule. The superficial MCL is the primary restraint to valgus loading, and the deep MCL and posteromedial capsule are secondary valgus restraints to full extension.

Most isolated MCL injuries result from direct trauma to the lateral aspect of the knee in which a valgus force is created (Fig. 4-41). An indirect or noncontact mechanism, especially one involving rotation, typically produces associated injuries that usually involve the cruciate ligaments.

The patient may report a popping or tearing sensation on the medial aspect of the knee. Most injuries occur at the femoral origin or in the midsubstance over the joint line, although tibial avulsions do occur. MCL sprains may be isolated or combined with other knee injuries. Associated injuries may be diagnosed by an alert clinician who looks for clues that appear in the history and examination or while monitoring the clinical progress of the patient.

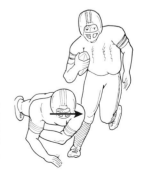

Figure 4–41   Medial collateral ligament (MCL) injury mechanism. A direct blow to the lateral aspect of the knee creates a valgus stress that disrupts the MCL. (From Baker CL Jr, Liu SH: Collateral ligament injuries of the knee: Operative and nonoperative approaches. In Fu FHJ, Harner CD, Vince KG [eds]: Knee Surgery, Baltimore, Williams & Wilkins, 1994, pp 787-808.)

PHYSICAL EXAMINATION

The physical examination begins with the patient seated. Inspection of the knee may reveal localized edema over the MCL. A visible enlargement of the normal prominence of the medial epicondyle characterizes injuries to the femoral origin. The presence of a large effusion should alert the clinician to a possible intra-articular injury, such as a fracture, meniscal tear, or cruciate ligament injury. **Because the MCL is extra-articular, isolated MCL injuries seldom produce large intra-articular swelling.** Careful palpation along the course of the MCL from the origin on the femoral epicondyle to the insertion on the proximal medial aspect of the tibia will reveal maximal tenderness over the injured portion of the ligament.

Valgus laxity should be evaluated with the patient supine and relaxed (see Fig. 4-6). The examiner supports the leg with one hand under the heel and, with the other hand, applies a gentle valgus force to the fully extended knee. In a normal knee, the examiner will feel firm resistance with virtually no separation of the femur and tibia. In an abnormal knee, the femur and tibia will be felt to separate in response to the valgus force and to "clunk" back together when the force is relaxed.

Increased laxity on valgus stress testing of the MCL in full extension (0 degrees) indicates severe injury to the MCL, the posteromedial capsule, and usually one or both cruciate ligaments.

If the valgus stress test is normal with the knee in full extension, the examiner flexes the knee about 30 degrees and repeats the test. This flexion relaxes the posterior capsule and permits more isolated testing of the MCL. With the knee flexed, the examiner again evaluates the firmness of the resistance (the "endpoint") and the amount of joint separation. The opposite knee should be examined to determine normal laxity; generalized ligamentous laxity may be incorrectly identified as abnormal opening to valgus stress.

The physical examination findings progress with higher grades of injury. In a *grade 1* sprain, the ligament is tender, but the knee is stable to valgus stress testing in 30 degrees of knee flexion. A *grade 2* sprain demonstrates abnormal valgus laxity when compared with the contralateral knee, but with a firm endpoint. The firm endpoint may be difficult to appreciate as a result of involuntary guarding. Because a *grade 3* sprain represents a complete rupture, valgus laxity is abnormal with a soft or indefinite endpoint.

	Classification of Medial Collateral Ligament Injury		
GRADE	**DAMAGE TO LIGAMENT**	**CLINICAL EXAMINATION**	**LAXITY ON EXAMINATION (mm)**
1	Microtrauma with no elongation	Tender ligament Normal valgus laxity	0-5
2	Elongated but intact	Increased valgus laxity with a firm endpoint on valgus stress at 20 degrees of knee flexion	5-10
3	Complete disruption	Increased valgus laxity with a soft endpoint on valgus stress at 30 degrees of knee flexion	>10

Differential Diagnosis

The differential diagnosis of an isolated MCL injury includes medial knee contusion, medial meniscal tear, patellar subluxation or dislocation, and physeal fracture (in a skeletally immature patient).

A careful physical examination will help differentiate an MCL sprain from other diagnostic possibilities. A *bone contusion* also produces tenderness, but it does not result in abnormal valgus laxity. Tenderness near the adductor tubercle or medial retinaculum adjacent to the patella can be caused by *patellar dislocation* or subluxation with VMO avulsion or a medial retinaculum tear. A positive patellar apprehension sign aids in distinguishing an episode of patellar instability from MCL injury. Physeal fractures in skeletally immature patients are tender over the growth plate, and the growth plate opens up on gentle stress-testing radiographs.

Joint line tenderness may be present in either a *medial meniscal tear* or an MCL sprain. Opening of the joint line on valgus laxity examination should differentiate between a meniscal tear and a grade 2 or 3 MCL sprain. Differentiation between a grade 1 MCL sprain and a medial meniscal tear is more difficult. MRI can be obtained, or the patient can be observed for a few weeks. The tenderness usually resolves with a MCL sprain but persists with a meniscal injury.

RADIOGRAPHIC EXAMINATION

Routine plain radiographs of the knee, including AP, lateral sunrise, and tunnel views, should be obtained to exclude a fracture or osteochondral injury.

Bony avulsions of the cruciates or a tibial flake avulsion of the lateral capsule (Segond sign—associated with an ACL injury) may indicate associated injuries.

The Pellegrini-Stieda sign does not indicate an avulsion fracture, but rather an ectopic calcification that may develop near the medial epicondyle after a proximal MCL sprain. Its presence on radiographs suggests a previous MCL injury. MRI is not indicated for evaluation of an isolated MCL injury but may be helpful if the examination is equivocal (Fig. 4-42). Isolated MCL sprains are rarely associated with meniscal tears.

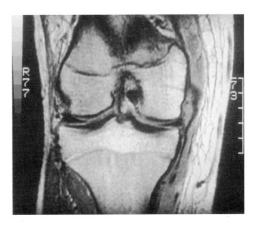

Figure 4-42 Magnetic resonance image of a medial collateral ligament injury.

TREATMENT OF ISOLATED AND COMBINED MEDIAL COLLATERAL LIGAMENT INJURIES

Treatment of all grades of isolated MCL sprain is an aggressive, nonoperative rehabilitation program. Numerous studies have shown that a functional rehabilitation treatment program allows more rapid recovery with results equal or superior to those obtained with surgery or prolonged immobilization. When abnormal MCL laxity is present, a functional hinged brace is used to support and protect the MCL while allowing full knee ROM during rehabilitation.

When an **associated cruciate ligament injury** is present, treatment of the cruciate injury assumes paramount importance, and surgery is usually recommended. For MCL sprains associated with ACL tears, surgical reconstruction of the ACL **without** direct surgical repair of the MCL is recommended by most authors. It has been shown that injuries to both ligaments (ACL and MCL) adversely affect healing of the MCL. Reconstruction of the ACL improved the healing response of the MCL. Some surgeons advocate primary repair of the MCL in association with ACL reconstruction in a knee that opens widely to valgus stress in full extension. Documentation to support this practice is scarce because these cases are relatively infrequent and difficult to compare in a controlled fashion.

For *combined PCL and MCL injuries*, primary repair of the injured medial structures and PCL reconstruction are usually recommended.

For *isolated MCL sprains*, we stress the functional rehabilitation treatment outlined later. The healing MCL is protected with a lightweight hinged brace at all times, and the patient is encouraged to return to full weight-bearing and begin an endurance activity such as cycling or stair climbing as soon as possible. This minimizes secondary muscle atrophy so that the factor limiting the patient's return to sports is the rate of healing of the MCL and not weakness or stiffness as a result of imposed restrictions. The paramount feature of this program is that progression of rehabilitation activities and return to sports are based on attainment of functional goals rather than arbitrary time periods.

When MCL injury occurs with ACL rupture, the athlete is treated with the same brace and rehabilitation program until full weight-bearing and nearly full motion are attained and swelling is minimized. ACL reconstruction is usually then carried out **without** direct repair of the MCL. Rarely, in a knee with gross increased valgus laxity at full extension, primary repair of injured medial structures is done at the time of ACL reconstruction. In this case, surgery should be performed within 7 to 10 days of injury to facilitate primary repair of the medial structures. When the superficial MCL is too compromised to permit a strong repair, it is reinforced with the semitendinosus tendon, which is left attached to the tibia and fixed at the most isometric point on the medial epicondyle. This same technique is also useful for reconstruction of the MCL in the rare case in which it does not heal primarily. Finally, for combined injuries of the PCL and MCL or the ACL, PCL, and MCL, the medial structures are generally repaired primarily during the cruciate ligament surgery.

REHABILITATION AFTER MEDIAL COLLATERAL LIGAMENT INJURY

The rehabilitation program is divided into three phases. Successful completion of each phase and progression into the next phase are based on attaining specific goals. The time in each phase varies. The average time to return to sport varies with both grade and sport.

On average, grade 1 injuries require about 10 days and grades 2 and 3 need about 3 to 6 weeks.

Sports that place more stress on the MCL, such as soccer, may require a longer period of healing before return to play.

| REHABILITATION PROTOCOL | *After Isolated Medial Collateral Ligament Injury* Reider and Mroczek |

PHASE 1

Goals

- Normal gait
- Minimal swelling
- Full ROM
- Baseline quadriceps control

Cryotherapy

- Therapeutic cold via ice packs or other means is applied to the medial aspect of the knee for 20 minutes every 3-4 hours for the first 48 hours.
- Early cryotherapy provides anesthesia and local vasoconstriction to minimize initial hemorrhage and reduce secondary edema. Leg elevation also helps limit swelling.

Weight-Bearing

- Weight-bearing is allowed as tolerated.
- Crutches are used until the patient ambulates without a limp, which takes approximately 1 week.
- For grade 2 and 3 sprains, a light-weight hinged brace is worn. The brace should protect against the valgus stress of daily living but not restrict motion or inhibit muscle function. The brace is worn at all times except when bathing during the initial 3-4 weeks.
- **Knee immobilizers and full-leg braces are discouraged because they tend to inhibit motion and prolong the period of disability.**

Exercises

- ROM exercises are begun immediately. A cold whirlpool may make these exercises easier
- Activities such as towel extension exercises and prone hangs are used to obtain extension or hyperextension equal to that on the contralateral side. A heavy shoe or light ankle weight can be used with prone hangs to aid extension.
- To promote flexion, the patient sits at the end of a table and allows gravity to aid in flexion. The uninjured limb assists by gently pushing the injured leg into further flexion.
- A similar technique of assistance by the uninjured limb can be used during supine wall slides
- To achieve greater than 90 degrees of flexion, heel slides are done with the patient sitting and grabbing the ankle to flex the knee farther.
- A stationary bicycle also aids in the restoration of motion. The bicycle seat is initially set as high as possible and gradually lowered to increase flexion.

Continued

REHABILITATION PROTOCOL: *After Isolated Medial Collateral Ligament Injury*   Continued

PHASE 1—cont'd

- Isometric quadriceps sets and SLRs are begun immediately to minimize muscle atrophy
- Electrical stimulation may be helpful by limiting reflex muscle inhibition.

PHASE 2

Goal

- Restoration of strength of the injured leg to approximately 80%-90% of the uninjured leg.

Bracing

- Continued use of the lightweight hinged brace.

Exercises

- Strengthening exercise begins with 4-inch step-ups and 30-degree squats without weights
- Light resistance exercises of knee extensions, leg presses, and curls on a standard isotonic weight bench or dedicated resistance machine. Sets with lighter weights but a higher number of repetitions are generally used.
- Recurrent pain and swelling are signs of too rapid progression. If they occur, the strengthening program should be slowed.
- Upper body, aerobic, and further lower extremity conditioning are achieved with swimming, stationary cycling, and/or a stair climber.

PHASE 3

Goals

- Completion of a running program
- Completion of a series of sport-specific activities

Bracing

- Continued use of the brace is recommended during this phase and for the rest of the athletic season. It may protect against further injury and provides at least psychological support.

Exercises

- A progressive running program commences with fast-speed walking and advances to light jogging, straight-line running, and then sprinting. Next, agility is achieved with cutting and pivoting activities such as figure-of-eight drills and cariocas.
- If pain or swelling occurs, the program is amended appropriately.
- Continued input from a trainer or physical therapist will be helpful in providing progress reports and guidance in appropriate performance of the activities.

Return to Sport

- Permitted when the athlete can complete a functional testing program, including a long run, progressively more rapid sprints, cutting and pivoting drills, and appropriate sport-specific tests.

| REHABILITATION PROTOCOL | *Progression of Rehabilitation after Medial Collateral Ligament Injury* Reider and Mroczek |

	PHASE 1	PHASE 2	PHASE 3
Bracing			
• Lightweight brace	X	X	X
Weight-Bearing			
• Full	X	X	X
• Crutches until normal gait	X		
Range of Motion			
• Cold whirlpool	X		
• Extension exercises			
• Towel extensions	X		
• Prone hangs	X		
• Flexion exercises			
• Sitting off a table	X		
• Wall slides	X		
• Heel slides	X		
Strengthening			
• Isometric quadriceps sets	X	X	
• SLRs	X	X	
• Step-ups		X	X
• Squats		X	X
• Knee extensions		X	X
• Leg presses		X	X
• Leg curls		X	X
Conditioning			
• Stationary bike	X	X	X
• Swimming		X	X
• Stair climber		X	X
Agility/Sport-Specific Training`			
• Running program			
• Fast-speed walking			X
• Light jogging			X
• Straight-line running			X
• Sprinting			X
• Figure-of-eight drills			X
• Cariocas			X
• Sport-specific drills			X

Continued

REHABILITATION PROTOCOL: *Progression of Rehabilitation after Medial Collateral Ligament Injury*   *Continued*

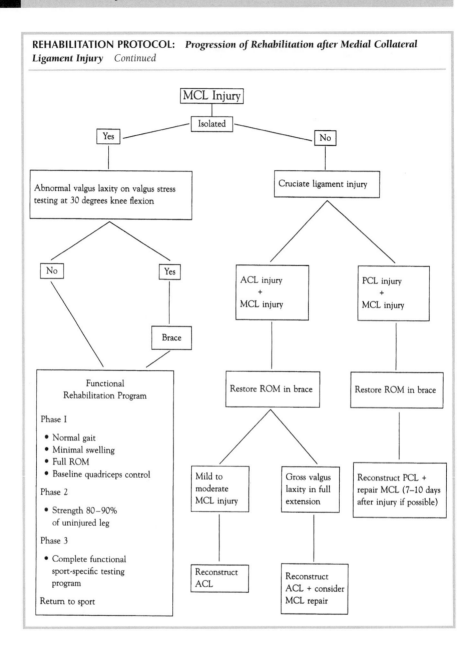

REHABILITATION PROTOCOL	*After Isolated Medial Collateral Ligament Sprains* Wilk

PHASE 1: MAXIMAL PROTECTION

Goals

- Early protected ROM
- Prevent quadriceps atrophy
- Decrease effusion and pain

Day 1

- Ice, compression, and elevation
- Knee hinge brace, nonpainful ROM, if needed
- Crutches, weight-bearing as tolerated
- Passive ROM, active-assisted ROM
- Electrical muscle stimulation of quadriceps (8 hr/day)
- Quadriceps isometrics: quad sets, SLR (flexion)
- Emphasize hamstring stretches, active-assisted ROM knee flexion stretching to tolerance

Day 2

- Continue above exercises
- Quadriceps sets
- SLR (flexion, abduction)
- Hamstring isometric sets
- Well-leg exercises
- Whirlpool for ROM (cold for first 3-4 days, then warm)
- High-voltage galvanic stimulation to control swelling

Days 3-7

- Continue above exercises
- Crutches, weight-bearing as tolerated
- ROM as tolerated
- Eccentric quadriceps work
- Bicycle for ROM stimulus
- Resisted knee extension with electrical muscle stimulation
- Initiate hip adduction and extension
- Initiate mini-squats
- Initiate leg press isotonics
- Brace worn at night, brace during day as needed
- Continue ROM and stretching exercises

PHASE 2: MODERATE PROTECTION

Criteria for Progression to Phase 2

- No increase in instability
- No increase in swelling
- Minimal tenderness
- Passive ROM (10-100 degrees)

Goals

- Full painless ROM
- Restore strength
- Ambulation without crutches

Continued

REHABILITATION PROTOCOL: *After Isolated Medial Collateral Ligament Sprains* Continued

PHASE 2: MODERATE PROTECTION—cont'd

Week 2

- Continue strengthening program with PREs
- Continue electrical muscle stimulation of quadriceps during isotonic strengthening
- Continue ROM exercises and stretching
- Emphasize closed–kinetic chain exercises (lunges, squats, lateral lunges, wall squats, lateral step-ups)
- Bicycle for endurance and ROM stimulus
- Water exercises, running in water forward and backward
- Full ROM exercises
- Flexibility exercises: hamstrings, quadriceps, iliotibial band, etc.
- Proprioception training (balance drills)
- StairMaster endurance work

Days 11-14

- Continue all exercises in week 2
- PREs with emphasis on quadriceps, hamstrings, and hip abduction
- Initiate isokinetics, progress from submaximal to maximal fast contractile velocities
- Begin running program if full painless extension and flexion are present

PHASE 3: MINIMAL PROTECTION

Criteria for Progression to Phase 3

- No instability
- No swelling or tenderness
- Full painless ROM

Goal

- Increase power and strength

Week 3

- Continue strengthening program
  - Wall squats
  - Lateral lunges
  - Knee extension
  - Vertical squats
  - Step-ups
  - Hip abduction-adduction
  - Lunges
  - Leg press
  - Hamstring curls
- Emphasize
  - Functional exercise drills
  - Fast-speed isokinetics
  - Eccentric quadriceps
  - Isotonic hip adduction, medial hamstrings
- Isokinetic testing
- Proprioception testing
- Endurance exercises

REHABILITATION PROTOCOL: *After Isolated Medial Collateral Ligament Sprains* *Continued*

PHASE 3: MINIMAL PROTECTION—cont'd

- Stationary bike (30-40 minutes)
- Nordic-Trac, swimming, etc.
- Initiate agility program, sport-specific activities

PHASE 4: MAINTENANCE

Criteria for Return to Competition

- Full ROM
- No instability
- Muscle strength 85% of contralateral side
- Satisfactory proprioception ability
- No tenderness over MCL
- No effusion
- Quadriceps strength, torque-to–body weight ratio that fulfills criteria
- Lateral knee brace (if necessary)

Maintenance Program

- Continue isokinetic strengthening exercises
- Continue flexibility exercises
- Continue proprioceptive exercises

Meniscal Injuries

Michael D'Amato, MD • Bernard R. Bach, Jr., MD

CLINICAL BACKGROUND

The importance of the menisci in preserving the health and function of the knee has been well established. Most of the functions performed by the menisci relate to protecting the underlying articular cartilage:

- By increasing the effective contact area between the femur and the tibia, the menisci lower the load per unit area borne by the articular surfaces. Total meniscectomy results in a 50% reduction in contact area.
- The menisci transmit central compressive loads out toward the periphery, thus further decreasing the contact pressure on the articular cartilage.
- Half of the compressive load in the knee passes through the menisci with the knee in full extension and 85% of the load passes through the knee with the knee in 90 degrees of flexion.

Meniscectomy has been shown to reduce the shock absorption capacity of the knee by 20%.

Meniscal Movement

The lateral meniscus has been shown to be more mobile than the medial meniscus. In each meniscus, the anterior horn has greater mobility than the posterior horn.

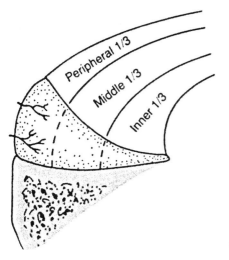

Figure 4–43 Meniscal tear zones. Peripheral meniscal tears at the red/white zone often have an intact perimeniscal capillary plexus and thus the potential for healing (blood supply present).

The reduced mobility of the posterior medial meniscus may result in greater stress in this area and thus increased vulnerability to injury, which would explain the higher rate of meniscal tears in the posterior medial meniscus.

Weight-bearing has been shown to effect few changes in the movement of the menisci, although it has been suggested that meniscal loading may lead to distraction of radial tears. ROM of the knee, especially increasing rotation and flexion of the knee past 60 degrees, results in significant changes in the AP position of the menisci. **Clinically, second-look arthroscopy has shown that extension of the knee maintains a posterior horn meniscal tear in a reduced position and knee flexion results in displacement of the tear**.

Meniscal Healing

King, in 1936, first noted that communication with the peripheral blood supply was critical for meniscal healing. Arnoczky and Warren, in 1982, described the microvasculature of the menisci. In children, the peripheral blood vessels permeate the full thickness of the meniscus. With age, penetration of the blood vessels decreases. In adults, the blood supply is limited to only the outer 6 mm, or about a third the width of the meniscus. It is in this vascular region that the healing potential of a meniscal tear is greatest (Fig. 4-43). This potential drops off dramatically as the tear progresses away from the periphery.

Meniscal healing is also influenced by the pattern of the tear (Fig. 4-44). Longitudinal tears have a more favorable healing potential than radial tears do. Simple tear patterns are more likely to heal than complex tears. Traumatic tears have higher healing rates than degenerative tears do, acute tears more so than chronic tears.

REHABILITATION CONSIDERATIONS

Weight-Bearing and Motion

Although weight-bearing has little effect on displacement patterns of the meniscus and may be beneficial in approximating longitudinal tears, weight-bearing may

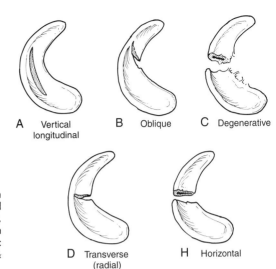

A   Vertical longitudinal   B   Oblique   C   Degenerative

D   Transverse (radial)   H   Horizontal

Figure 4–44 A-E, Variation in meniscal tear patterns. (Adapted from Ciccotti MG, Shields CL Jr, El Attrache NS: Meniscectomy. In Fu FH, Harner CD, Vince KG [eds]: Knee Surgery. Baltimore, Williams & Wilkins, 1994, pp 749-767.)

place a displacing force across radial tears. Several studies have confirmed the benefits of early motion by demonstrating meniscal atrophy and decreased collagen content in menisci after immobilization. ROM of the knee before 60 degrees of flexion has little effect on meniscal displacement, but flexion angles greater than 60 degrees translate the menisci posteriorly. This increased translation may place detrimental stress across a healing meniscus. As knee flexion increases, compressive loads across the meniscus also increase. The combination of weight-bearing and increasing knee flexion must be carefully balanced in the development of a rehabilitation protocol.

Axial Limb Alignment

Varus malalignment tends to overload the medial compartment of the knee, with increased stress placed on the meniscus, and **valgus malalignment** has the same effect on the lateral compartment and lateral meniscus. These increased stresses may interfere or disrupt meniscal healing after repair. Patients with limb malalignment tend to have more degenerative meniscal tears, which have been suggested to have an inherently poorer healing capacity. The use of an "unloader" brace has been recommended to help protect the healing meniscus, although no scientific data exist to support this approach.

Rehabilitation after Meniscectomy

Because there is no anatomic structure that must be protected during the healing phase, rehabilitation may progress aggressively. The goals are early control of pain and swelling, immediate weight-bearing, obtaining and maintaining full ROM, and regaining quadriceps strength.

Rehabilitation after Meniscal Repair

Current studies support the use of unmodified accelerated ACL rehabilitation protocols after combined ACL reconstruction and meniscal repair. In tears with decreased healing potential (such as white-white tears, radial tears, or tears with complex patterns), **limiting weight-bearing and limiting flexion to 60 degrees for the first 4 weeks have been suggested to better protect the repair and increase the healing potential of these difficult tears. However, we are unaware of any published studies that support these measures**.

Rehabilitation after isolated meniscal repair remains controversial. The healing environment is clearly inferior to that with concomitant ACL reconstruction, but good results have been obtained with accelerated rehabilitation protocols after isolated meniscal repairs.

REHABILITATION PROTOCOL

After Arthroscopic Partial Medial or Lateral Meniscectomy
Wilk

PHASE 1: ACUTE PHASE

Goals

- Diminish inflammation and swelling
- Restore ROM
- Re-establish quadriceps muscle activity

Days 1-3

- Cryotherapy
- Electrical stimulation of quadriceps
- Quadriceps sets
- SLR
- Hip adduction and abduction
- Knee extension
- $^{1}/_{2}$ squats
- Active-assisted ROM stretching, with emphasis on full knee extension (flexion to tolerance)
- Weight-bearing as tolerated (two crutches)
- Light compression wrap

Days 4-7

- Cryotherapy
- Electrical stimulation of quadriceps
- Quadriceps sets
- Knee extension (90-40 degrees)
- SLR
- Hip adduction and abduction
- $^{1}/_{2}$ squats
- Balance/proprioceptive drills
- Active-assisted and passive ROM exercises
- ROM (0-115 degrees, minimal)
- Stretching (hamstrings, gastrosoleus, quadriceps)
- Weight-bearing as tolerated (one crutch)
- Continued use of compression wrap or brace
- High-voltage galvanic stimulation/cryotherapy

REHABILITATION PROTOCOL: *After Arthroscopic Partial Medial or Lateral Meniscectomy* *Continued*

PHASE 1: ACUTE PHASE—cont'd

Days 7-10

- Continue all exercises
- Leg press (low weight)
- Toe raises
- Hamstring curls
- Bicycle (when ROM is 0-102 degrees with no swelling)

PHASE 2: INTERNAL PHASE

Goals

- Restore and improve muscular strength and endurance
- Re-establish full nonpainful ROM
- Gradual return to functional activities

Days 10-17

- Bicycle for motion and endurance
- Lateral lunges
- Front lunges
- $1/2$ squats
- Leg press
- Lateral step-ups
- Knee extension (90-40 degrees)
- Hamstring curls
- Hip abduction and adduction
- Hip flexion and extension
- Toe raises
- Proprioceptive and balance training
- Stretching exercises
- Active-assisted and passive ROM knee flexion (if necessary)
- StairMaster or elliptical trainer

Day 17-Week 4

- Continue all exercises
- Pool program (deep-water running and leg exercises)
- Compression brace may be used during activities

PHASE 3: ADVANCED ACTIVITY PHASE—WEEKS 4-7*

Criteria for Progression to Phase III

- Full, nonpainful ROM
- No pain or tenderness
- Satisfactory isokinetic test
- Satisfactory clinical examination (minimal effusion)

Goals

- Enhance muscular strength and endurance
- Maintain full ROM
- Return to sport/functional activities

Continued

REHABILITATION PROTOCOL: *After Arthroscopic Partial Medial or Lateral Meniscectomy* Continued

PHASE 3: ADVANCED ACTIVITY PHASE—WEEKS 4-7*—cont'd

Exercises

- Continue to emphasize closed–kinetic chain exercises
- May begin plyometrics
- Begin running program and agility drills
   Note: We use the **Orthovid.com** meniscectomy instructional videotape with its concomitant handouts for all postoperative patients. This videotape was produced by the senior author of this book.

*Patients can begin phase 3 when criteria are met, which may be earlier than week 4.

REHABILITATION PROTOCOL | *Accelerated Rehabilitation after Meniscal Repair* D'Amato and Bach

PHASE 1: WEEKS 0-2

Goals

- Full motion
- No effusion
- Full weight-bearing

Weight-Bearing

- As tolerated

Treatment

- ROM as tolerated (0-90 degrees)
- Cryotherapy
- Electrical stimulation as needed
- Isometric quadriceps sets
- SLR

PHASE 2: WEEKS 2-4

Criteria for Progression to Phase 2

- Full motion
- No effusion
- Full weight-bearing

Goals

- Improved quadriceps strength
- Normal gait

Therapeutic Exercises

- Closed–kinetic chain resistance exercises (0-90 degrees)
- Bike and swim as tolerated
- Early-phase functional training

REHABILITATION PROTOCOL: *Accelerated Rehabilitation after Meniscal Repair* *Continued*

PHASE 3: WEEKS 4-8

Criteria for Progression to Phase 3

- Normal gait
- Sufficient strength and proprioception for advanced functional training

Goals

- Strength and functional testing at least 85% of contralateral side
- Discharge from physical therapy to full activity

Therapeutic Exercises

- Strength work as needed
- Sport-specific functional progression
- Advanced-phase functional training

REHABILITATION PROTOCOL   *After Meniscal Repair*
Wilk

Key factors in determining progression of rehabilitation after meniscal repair:
- Anatomic site of tear
- Suture fixation (too vigorous rehabilitation can lead to failure)
- Location of tear (anterior or posterior)
- Other pathology (PCL, MCL, or ACL injury)

PHASE 1: MAXIMUM PROTECTION—WEEKS 1-6

Stage 1: Immediate Postoperative Period—Day 1-Week 3

- Ice, compression, elevation
- Electrical muscle stimulation
- Brace locked at 0 degrees
- ROM (0-90 degrees)
  - Motion is limited for the first 7-21 days, depending on the development of scar tissue around the repair site. Gradual increase in flexion ROM is based on assessment of pain (0-30, 0-50, 0-70, 0-90 degrees)
- Patellar mobilization
- Scar tissue mobilization
- Passive ROM
- Exercises
  - Quadriceps isometrics
  - Hamstring isometrics (if posterior horn repair, no hamstring exercises for 6 weeks)
  - Hip abduction and adduction
- Weight-bearing as tolerated with crutches and brace locked at 0 degrees
- Proprioception training

Stage 2: Weeks 4-6

- PREs—1-5 pounds
- Limited-range knee extension (in range less likely to impinge or pull on repair)

Continued

REHABILITATION PROTOCOL: *After Meniscal Repair* Continued

PHASE 1: MAXIMUM PROTECTION—WEEKS 1-6—cont'd

- Toe raises
- Mini-squats
- Cycling (no resistance)
- Surgical tubing exercises (diagonal patterns)
- Flexibility exercises

PHASE 2: MODERATE PROTECTION—WEEKS 6-10

Criteria for Progression to Phase 2

- ROM (0-90 degrees)
- No change in pain or effusion
- Quadriceps control ("good manual muscle testing")

Goals

- Increase strength, power, endurance
- Normalize ROM of knee
- Prepare patients for advanced exercises

Exercises

- Strength—PRE progression
- Flexibility exercises
- Lateral step-ups (30 seconds × 5 sets; 60 seconds × 5 sets)
- Mini-squats
- Isokinetic exercises

Endurance Program

- Swimming (no frog kick)
- Cycling
- Nordic-Trac
- Stair machine
- Pool running (see aquatic therapy section in Chapter 7)

Coordination Program

- Balance board
- High-speed bands
- Pool sprinting
- Backward walking

Plyometric Program

PHASE 3: ADVANCED PHASE—WEEKS 11-15

Criteria for Progression to Phase 3

- Full, nonpainful ROM
- No pain or tenderness
- Satisfactory isokinetic test
- Satisfactory clinical examination

REHABILITATION PROTOCOL: *After Meniscal Repair* *Continued*

PHASE 3: ADVANCED PHASE—WEEKS 11-15—cont'd

Goals

- Increase power and endurance
- Emphasize return-to-skill activities
- Prepare for return to full unrestricted activities

Exercises

- Continue all exercises
- Increase tubing program, plyometrics, pool program
- Initiate running program

Return to Activity: Criteria

- Full, nonpainful ROM
- Satisfactory clinical examination
- Satisfactory isokinetic test

Patellofemoral Disorders

S. Brent Brotzman, MD

CLINICAL BACKGROUND

Patellofemoral disorders (anterior knee pain) are among the most commonly treated conditions in orthopaedic and primary care practice. The patellofemoral joint is a complex articulation that depends on both dynamic and static restraints for stability. Anterior knee pain encompasses numerous underlying disorders and **cannot be treated by a single treatment algorithm**.

The key to successful treatment of patellofemoral pain is obtaining an accurate diagnosis by a thorough history and physical examination. For example, treatment of RSD is very different from that for excessive lateral pressure syndrome (ELPS), and the correct diagnosis must be made to allow appropriate treatment.

Possible Causes of Patellofemoral Pain

Acute patellar dislocation
Patellar subluxation (chronic)
Recurrent patellar dislocation
Jumper's knee (patellar tendinitis)
Osgood-Schlatter disease
Sinding-Larsen–Johansson syndrome (inferior pole of the patella)
ELPS
Global patellar pressure syndrome (GPPS)

Continued

> **Possible Causes of Patellofemoral Pain**   *Continued*
>
> Iliotibial band friction syndrome (lateral aspect of the knee at Gerdy's tubercle)
> Hoffa's disease (inflamed fat pad)
> Bursitis
> Medial patellofemoral ligament pain or tear
> Trauma
> Patellofemoral arthritis
> Sickle cell disease
> Anterior blow to the patella
> OCD
> RSD
> Hypertrophic plica (runner)
> Turf knee, wrestler's knee
> Patellar fracture
> Quadriceps rupture
> Contusion
> Tibial tubercle fracture
> Prepatellar bursitis (housemaid's knee)
> Patella baja
> Patella alta
> Medial retinaculitis
> Referred hip pain
> Gout
> Pseudogout (chondrocalcinosis)

"Chondromalacia" has been incorrectly used as an all-inclusive diagnosis for anterior knee pain. Chondromalacia is actually a pathologic diagnosis that describes articular cartilage changes seen on direct observation. This term should not be used as a synonym for patellofemoral or anterior knee pain. Frequently, the articular cartilage of the patella and femoral trochlea is normal, and the pain originates from the densely innervated peripatellar retinaculum or synovium. All peripatellar structures should be palpated and inspected. Other nociceptive input is possible from the subchondral bone, paratenon, tendon, and subcutaneous nerves in the patellofemoral joint.

Dye (1996) introduced the concept of loss of normal tissue homeostasis after overload of the extensor mechanism. The presence of excessive biomechanical load overwhelms the body's capacity to absorb energy and leads to microtrauma, tissue injury, and pain. Dye described the knee as a biologic transmission system that functions to accept, transfer, and dissipate loads. During normal ambulation, the muscles about the knee actually absorb more energy than they produce for propulsive force.

Dye also described an "envelope of function" that considers both the applied loads at the knee and the frequency of loading. This model is useful in conceptualizing both direct trauma and overuse repetitive trauma as a cause of patellofemoral pathology. Either an excessive single loading event or multiple submaximal loading variables over time could exceed the limits of physiologic function and disrupt tissue homeostasis. For healing and homeostasis to occur, the patient must keep activities and rehabilitation efforts within the available envelope of function. **Therefore, submaximal, pain-free exercise and avoidance of "flaring" activities (increased PFJRFs) are very important parts of rehabilitation of patellofemoral injuries**.

CLINICAL PEARLS FOR PATELLOFEMORAL PAIN

- Approximately 70% of patellofemoral disorders will improve with conservative (nonoperative) treatment and time.
- When thinking about and evaluating patellofemoral knee pain, first try to decide whether the problem stems from **instability or pain**. Once the diagnosis is correctly placed into one of these two categories, appropriate work-up and treatment decisions can be reached.
- **Arthroscopic release may be effective in patients with a positive lateral tilt (i.e., tight lateral structures) after failure of conservative measures. However, a lateral release should not be used to treat patellar instability.** Lateral release should never be performed in patients with a hypermobile patella (e.g., generalized ligamentous laxity). A common complication of this procedure incorrectly used for instability is iatrogenic medial patellar subluxation or instability.
- Osteochondral fractures of the lateral femoral condyle or the medial facet of the patella have been documented by arthroscopy in 40% and 50% of patellar dislocations, respectively.
- Success rates of patellar operative procedures are related to the procedure selected and the number of previous surgeries.
- PFJRFs (Fig. 4-45) increase with flexion of the knee from 0.5 times body weight during level walking to 3 to 4 times body weight during stair climbing to 7 to 8 times body weight with squatting.
- Females generally have a greater Q-angle than males do. However, critical review of available studies found no evidence that Q-angle measures correlated with the presence or severity of anterior knee pain.
- Quadriceps flexibility deficits are common in these patients, especially in chronic cases. Quadriceps stretching exercises produce dramatic improvement in symptoms in these patients.
- Restoration of flexibility (iliotibial band, quadriceps, hamstrings) is often overlooked but is extremely helpful in patients with flexibility deficits. ELPS with a tight lateral retinaculum and tight iliotibial band often responds dramatically to iliotibial band stretching and low-load, long-duration stretching of the lateral retinaculum.

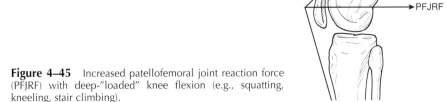

Figure 4–45   Increased patellofemoral joint reaction force (PFJRF) with deep-"loaded" knee flexion (e.g., squatting, kneeling, stair climbing).

CLASSIFICATION

Confusion over classification of patellofemoral disorders exists in the literature. Wilk and associates (1998) noted that a comprehensive patellofemoral classification scheme should (1) clearly define diagnostic categories, (2) aid in the selection of appropriate treatment, and (3) allow the comparison of treatment approaches for a specific diagnosis.

- Patellar instability
  - Acute patellar dislocation
  - Chronic patellar subluxation
  - Recurrent patellar dislocation
- Overuse syndromes
  - Patellar tendinitis (jumper's knee)
  - Quadriceps tendinitis
  - Osgood-Schlatter disease (tibial tubercle)
  - Sinding-Larsen–Johansson syndrome (inferior aspect of the patella)
- Patellar compression syndrome
  - ELPS
  - GPPS
- Soft tissue lesions
  - Iliotibial band friction syndrome (lateral aspect of the knee)
  - Symptomatic plica syndrome
  - Inflamed hypertrophic fat pad (Hoffa's disease)
  - Bursitis
  - Medial patellofemoral ligament pain
- Biomechanical linkage problems
  - Foot hyperpronation
  - Limb-length discrepancy
  - Loss of flexibility
- Direct trauma
  - Articular cartilage lesion (isolated)
  - Fracture
  - Fracture-dislocation
- OCD
- RSD syndrome

EVALUATION OF THE PATELLOFEMORAL JOINT

Signs and Symptoms

- *Instability.* Frequently, patients complain of the knee "giving way" during straight-ahead activities or stair climbing (versus instability as a result of ACL or PCL injury, which is generally associated with giving way during pivoting or changing directions). Patellar subluxation typically lacks the history of trauma found in patients with ACL-related instability. With frank episodes of patellar dislocation, the patella may spontaneously reduce or reduction may require pushing the patella medially and/or extending the knee. Dislocations are typically followed by a large bloody effusion (versus recurrent subluxation).

- *Overuse or training errors.* Training errors or overuse should be suspected in athletes, obese patients who climb stairs or squat all day, etc.
- *Localization of pain.* Pain may be diffuse or discretely localized to the patellar tendon (patellar tendinitis), medial or lateral retinaculum, quadriceps tendon, or inferior aspect of the patella (Sinding-Larsen–Johansson syndrome).
- *Crepitance.* Crepitance is often due to underlying articular cartilage damage in the patellofemoral joint, but it may be due to soft tissue impingement. Many patients describe asymptomatic crepitance with stair climbing.
- *Aggravating activities.* Painful popping with hill running may indicate only plica or iliotibial band syndrome. Aggravation of symptoms by stair climbing, squatting, kneeling, or rising from sitting to standing (movie theater sign) suggests a patellofemoral articular cartilage or retinacular source (often GPPS or ELPS).
- *Swelling.* Perceived knee swelling with patellofemoral pain is infrequently due to an actual effusion but is more commonly due to synovitis and fat pad inflammation. Large effusions are seen after patellar dislocations, but otherwise an effusion should imply other intra-articular pathology.
- *Weakness.* Though uncommon, weakness may represent quadriceps inhibition secondary to pain or may be indicative of extensive extensor mechanism damage (patellar tendon rupture, fractured patella, or patellar dislocation).
- *Night pain.* Pain at night or without relation to activity may imply tumor, advanced arthritis, infection, and the like. Unrelenting pain out of proportion to the injury, hyperesthesia, and so on implies RSD, neurogenic origin, postoperative neuroma, symptom magnification, etc.

Physical Examination

Both lower extremities should be examined with the patient in shorts only and without shoes. The patient should be examined and observed standing, walking, sitting, and lying supine. The ipsilateral knee, hip, foot, and ankle should be examined and compared with the opposite limb for symmetry, thigh muscular girth, Q-angle, and other factors.

Physical examination also should include evaluation of
- Generalized ligamentous laxity (thumb to wrist, elbow or finger hyperextension, sulcus sign of shoulder) raises a red flag for possible patellar subluxation (Fig. 4-46)
- Gait pattern
- Extensor mechanism alignment
  - Q-angle (standing and sitting) (see Fig. 4-2)
  - Genu valgum, varum, recurvatum (see Fig. 4-3)
  - Tibial torsion
  - Femoral anteversion
  - Patellar malposition (baja, alta, squinting, tilt)
  - Pes planus or foot pronation
  - Hypoplastic lateral femoral condyle
  - Patellar glide test: lateral glide, medial glide, apprehension (Fairbank sign)
  - Patellofemoral tracking
  - J sign (if present)
- Patellofemoral crepitance
- VMO atrophy, hypertrophy

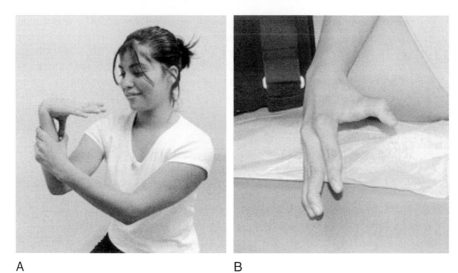

A   B

Figure 4–46   Generalized ligamentous laxity. **A,** The patient is able to place her thumb to her wrist. **B,** The patient is able to hyperextend her finger joints (i.e., "double jointed").

- Effusion (large, small, intra-articular, extra-articular)
- Peripatellar soft tissue point tenderness
  - Medial retinaculum
  - Lateral retinaculum
  - Bursae (prepatellar, pes anserine, iliotibial)
  - Quadriceps tendon
  - Patellar tendon
  - Palpable plica
  - Iliotibial band/bursa
  - Enlarged fat pad
- Atrophy of thigh, VMO, calf
- Flexibility
  - Hamstrings
  - Quadriceps
  - Iliotibial band (Ober test)
- Leg length discrepancy
- Lateral pull test
- Areas of possible referred pain (back, hip)
- RSD signs (temperature or color change, hypersensitivity)
- Hip ROM, flexion contracture

Clinical Tests for Patellofemoral Disorders

Q-Angle

The Q-angle is the angle formed by the intersection of lines drawn from the anterior superior iliac spine to the center of the patella and from the center of the patella to the tibial tubercle (see Fig. 4-2). In essence, these lines represent the lines of action

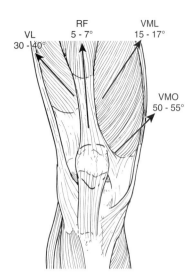

Figure 4–47 Fiber orientation of the quadriceps muscle groups. RF, rectus femoris; VL, vastus lateralis; VML, vastus medialis lateral; VMO, vastus medialis obliquus.

of the quadriceps musculature and patellar tendons, respectively, on the patella. It should be measured with the knee slightly flexed to center the patella in the trochlear groove. **Foot pronation (pes planus or flatfoot) and limb internal rotation both increase the Q-angle.** The range of normal for the Q-angle varies in the literature, and there is controversy whether the wider pelvic anatomy in women contributes to a greater Q-angle. **The reported values of normal quoted are 10 degrees for men and 15 degrees for women.** It is well accepted that patellar alignment is somewhat affected by the degree of valgus at the knee; however, the degree of valgus present is not a dependable pathologic marker for the severity of symptoms.

Soft Tissue Stabilizers of the Patella

In addition to the bony stabilizers, there are medial and lateral soft tissue restraints to the patella. The medial restraints consist of the medial retinaculum, the medial patellofemoral ligament, and the VMO. **The VMO is the most important dynamic stabilizer of the patella for resisting lateral displacement.** Its fibers are oriented at about a 50- to 55-degree angle to the long axis of the femur (Fig. 4-47). It normally inserts into the superomedial aspect of the patella along about a third to half its length. However, in some cases of instability, the muscle may be absent or hypoplastic or may insert proximal to the patella.

The lateral restraints consist of the lateral retinaculum, the vastus lateralis, and the iliotibial band. Contracture in any of these structures may exert a tethering effect (positive patellar tilt) on the patella (e.g., ELPS), and they must be appropriately assessed during evaluation of the patellofemoral region.

Standing Alignment of the Extensor Mechanism

Inspection of the entire lower extremity should be performed not only to assess the alignment of the extensor mechanism but also to look for pes planus, tibial torsion, genu varum or valgum, genu recurvatum, femoral anteversion, or limb-length discrepancy, all of which can contribute to patellofemoral dysfunction. **It is important** to evaluate the patient in a standing position. The weight-bearing position may unmask otherwise hidden deformities such as excessive forefoot pronation (which increases the relative standing Q-angle) or limb-length discrepancies. Observation of the gait pattern may reveal abnormalities in mechanics, such as foot hyperpronation, or avoidance patterns during stair descent. Muscular atrophy can be visualized qualitatively or measured quantitatively (circumferentially from a fixed point) with a tape measure. The presence of erythema or ecchymosis in a particular area may offer an additional clue to the underlying pathology.

Local Palpation

Palpation also reveals any tenderness that may be present in the soft tissues around the knee. Tenderness along the medial retinacular structures may be the result of injury occurring with patellar dislocation. As the patella dislocates laterally, the medial retinaculum has to tear to allow lateral displacement of the knee cap.

Lateral pain may be secondary to inflammation in the lateral restraints, including the iliotibial band. Joint line tenderness typically indicates an underlying meniscal tear. Tenderness secondary to tendinitis or apophysitis in the quadriceps or patellar tendon will typically be manifested as distinctly localized point tenderness at the area of involvement. Snapping or painful plicae may be felt, typically along the medial patellar border.

Range of Motion (Hip, Knee, Ankle)

ROM testing should include not only the knee but also the hip, ankle, and subtalar joints. Pathology in the hip may be manifested as referred knee pain, and abnormal mechanics in the foot and ankle can lead to increased stress in the soft tissue structures of the knee that may give rise to pain. While ranging the knee, the presence of crepitation and patellar tracking should be assessed. Palpable crepitus may or may not be painful and may or may not indicate significant underlying pathology, although it should raise suspicion of articular cartilage injury or soft tissue impingement. The *patellar grind or compression test* (Fig. 4-48) will help elucidate the cause. To perform this test, one applies a compressive force to the patella as the knee is brought through a ROM. Reproduction of pain with or without accompanying crepitus is indicative of articular cartilage damage. More experienced examiners may be able to further localize the pain to specific regions of the patella or trochlea with subtle changes in the site of compression.

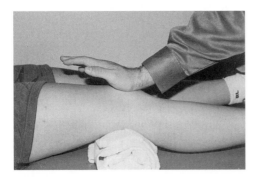

Figure 4–48   Patellar grind or compression test. The examiner evaluates articular pain and crepitus by compressing the patella into the trochlea at various angles of knee flexion. Avoid compressing the peripatellar soft tissues by pressing the patella with the thenar eminence of the hand. The flexion angles that elicit pain during compression will indicate the probable location of the lesions.

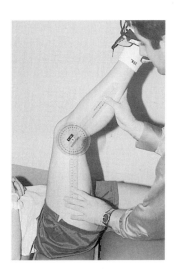

Figure 4–49 Testing hamstring flexibility. In this test, the hip is flexed with the leg extended until the pelvis begins to move or the knee begins to flex. The angle formed between the leg and the table represents the flexibility of the hamstrings (popliteal angle).

Flexibility of the Lower Extremity

Flexibility of the lower extremity must be evaluated. Quadriceps, hamstring, or iliotibial band tightness may all contribute to patellofemoral symptoms. Quadriceps flexibility may be tested with the patient in a prone or lateral position. The hip is extended and the knee progressively flexed. Limitation of knee flexion or compensatory hip flexion is indicative of quadriceps tightness. Hamstring flexibility can be tested (Fig. 4-49).

The **Ober test** (Fig. 4-50) is used to assess **iliotibial band flexibility**. The test is done with the patient in a side-lying position with the leg being measured up above the other. The lower part of the hip is flexed to flatten lumbar lordosis and stabilize the pelvis. The examiner, positioned behind the patient, gently grasps the leg proximally just below the knee, flexes the knee to apply a mild stretch on the quadriceps, and flexes the hip to 90 degrees to flatten the lumbar lordosis. The hip is then extended to neutral, and any flexion contracture is noted. With the opposite hand at the iliac crest to stabilize the pelvis and prevent the patient from rolling backward, the examiner maximally abducts and extends the hip. The abducted and extended

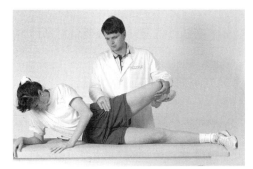

Figure 4–50 Ober test. With the patient in the lateral position and the involved leg up, the pelvis is stabilized and the hip is abducted and extended. The leg is then allowed to adduct toward the table. In a normal test, the upper part of the knee will reach the table. In an abnormal test, the knee will remain tethered by a tight iliotibial band and will fail to reach the table.

hip is then allowed to adduct by gravity while the knee is kept flexed, the pelvis stabilized, and the femur in neutral rotation. Generally, the thigh should adduct to a position at least parallel to the examining table. Palpation proximal to the lateral femoral condyle with the iliotibial band on stretch is frequently painful to patients with iliotibial band and lateral retinacular tightness. When this is found, iliotibial band stretches become a valuable part of the treatment plan. Again, bilateral comparison is important. Ober's position is useful in the treatment (stretching) as well as the diagnosis of iliotibial band tightness.

J Sign

Evaluation of patellar tracking begins with the knee in full extension. In this position, the patella typically rests just lateral to the midline. As the knee moves into flexion, at around 10 to 30 degrees, the patella centers into the trochlear groove and proceeds to track in a relatively straight path with progressive knee flexion. This normal path should progress smoothly. A sharp jump of the patella into the trochlear groove, sometimes referred to as the *J sign*, or late centering of the patella, should raise the suspicion of patellar instability.

Examination for knee instability should include a full evaluation of the cruciate and collateral ligaments to assess for any rotatory component, as well as to examine the patellar restraints. In patients with posterolateral corner knee instability, secondary patellar instability may develop as a result of a dynamic increase in the Q-angle. Similarly, secondary patellar instability may also develop in patients with chronic MCL laxity. Apprehension on medial or lateral displacement testing of the patella should raise the suspicion of *underlying instability* in the patellar restraints. Superior and inferior patellar mobility should also be assessed; they may be decreased in situations of global contracture.

Patellar Glide Test

The patellar glide test is useful to assess the medial and lateral patellar restraints. In extension, the patella lies above the trochlear groove and should be freely mobile both medially and laterally. As the knee is flexed to 20 degrees, the patella should center in the trochlear groove to provide both bony and soft tissue stability.

Lateral Glide Test

The lateral glide test evaluates the integrity of the medial restraints. Lateral translation is measured as a percentage of patellar width (Fig. 4-51). Translations of 25% of patellar width are considered normal; translations greater than 50% indicate laxity within the medial restraints. The *medial patellofemoral ligament* has been noted to provide 53% of the stabilizing force to resist lateral subluxation and normally has a solid endpoint when the lateral glide test is performed. Reproduction of the patient's symptoms with passive lateral translation of the patella by pulling on the medial structures is referred to as a *positive lateral apprehension sign*. This signals lateral patellar instability.

Medial Glide Test

The medial glide test is performed with the knee in full extension. The patella is centered on the trochlear groove, and medial translation from this "zero" point is measured in millimeters. Greater than 10 mm of translation is abnormal. The lateral retinacular laxity may be due to a hypermobile patella or, less commonly,

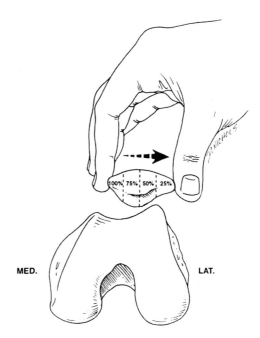

MED.   LAT.

Figure 4–51   Lateral patellar glide test.

medial instability. *Medial patellar instability is rare and is usually an iatrogenic complication after patellar realignment surgery, typically from overaggressive lateral release.* Six millimeters to 10 mm of translation is considered normal. Translation less than 6 mm medially indicates a tight lateral restraint and may be associated with ELPS.

Patellar Tilt

A *tight lateral restraint* may contribute to patellar tilt. Patellar tilt is evaluated as the knee is brought to full extension and an attempt is made to elevate the lateral border of the patella (Fig. 4-52). Normally, the lateral border should be able to be elevated 0 to 20 degrees above the medial border. Less than 0 degrees indicates tethering by a tight lateral retinaculum, vastus lateralis, or iliotibial band. The presence of clinical and radiographic lateral patellar tilt is indicative of tight lateral structures. It may be responsible for ELPS. **If extensive rehabilitation fails, the presence of a lateral patellar tilt correlates with a successful outcome after lateral release.**

Bassett Sign

Tenderness over the medial epicondyle of the femur may represent an injury to the medial patellofemoral ligament in a patient with acute or recurrent patellar dislocation.

Lateral Pull Test

This test is performed by contraction of the quadriceps with the knee in full extension and is positive (abnormal) if lateral displacement of the patella is observed. The lateral pull test demonstrates excessive dynamic lateral forces.

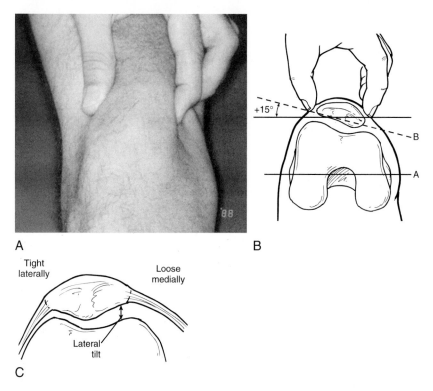

Figure 4–52 **A**, Patellar tilt test. The patella is gripped manually with the patient in the supine position and the knee extended. Gently grasp the patella, push down on its medial edge, and attempt to rotate the patella in the coronal plane to see whether lateral patellar tilt exists and, if so, whether the tilt can be corrected to "neutral." Neutral is defined as the patella's anterior surface being parallel to the examination table. Compare with the contralateral knee. **B**, Passive patellar tilt test. An excessively tight lateral restraint (lateral retinaculum) is demonstrated by a neutral or negative angle to the horizontal. This test is performed with the knee extended and the quadriceps relaxed. **C**, In excessive lateral pressure syndrome, the lateral retinaculum is excessively tight and pulls the patella laterally, which usually results in a lateral tilt and gradual stretching out of the medial retinaculum. (**B**, Adapted from Kolowich P: Lateral release of the patella: Indications and contraindications. Am J Sports Med 14:359-365, 1990.)

Radiographic Evaluation

Three views of the patella, an AP, a lateral in 30 degrees of knee flexion, and an axial image, should be obtained. The AP view can assess for the presence of any fractures, which should be distinguished from a bipartate patella, a normal variant. The overall size, shape, and gross alignment of the patella can also be ascertained. The lateral view is used to evaluate the patellofemoral joint space and to look for patella alta (see Fig. 4-2) or baja. In addition, the presence of fragmentation of the tibial tubercle or inferior patellar pole can be seen. Both the AP and the lateral views can also be used to confirm the presence and location of any loose bodies or osteochondral defects that may exist. **An axial image, typically a Merchant (knee flexed 45 degrees and the x-ray beam angled 30 degrees to the axis of the femur) or skyline view, may**

Figure 4–53 Sulcus angle and congruence angle. The sulcus angle is formed by lines BA and AC. The congruence angle is formed by a line bisecting the sulcus angle and a line drawn through the lowest point on the patella articular surface (represented by D in this diagram). A sulcus angle greater than 150 degrees indicates a shallow trochlear groove, which predisposes to patellar instability. Patellofemoral subluxation is evaluated by the congruence angle (see text).

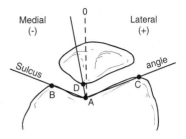

be the most important. It is used to assess patellar tilt and patellar subluxation. The anatomy of the trochlear groove is also well visualized, and the depth and presence of any condylar dysplasia can be determined. One important point deserves mention. The radiographs visualize only the subchondral bone of the patella and trochlea and do not show the articular cartilage. The articular surfaces are not necessarily of uniform thickness in these regions. Therefore, any measurements made from plain radiographs are only an indirect indication of the actual anatomic structure.

Assessment begins with the measurement of the **sulcus angle** (Fig. 4-53). A line is drawn along the medial and lateral walls of the trochlea. The angle formed between them is the sulcus angle. Greater than 150 degrees is abnormal and indicates a shallow or dysplastic groove that may have a predisposition for patellar instability.

Patellofemoral subluxation is evaluated by measurement of the **congruence angle** (see Fig. 4-53). The angle is formed by a line drawn from the apex of the trochlear groove that bisects the sulcus angle and a line drawn from the apex of the groove to the apex of the patella. A lateral position of the patellar apex relative to the apex of the trochlea is considered positive. A normal congruence angle has been described as −6 degrees ± 6 degrees.

Patellar tilt is evaluated by the patellofemoral angle (Fig. 4-54). This angle is formed by lines drawn along the articular surfaces of the lateral patellar facet and the lateral wall of the trochlear groove. The lines should be roughly parallel. Divergence is measured as a positive angle and is considered normal, whereas convergence of the lines is measured as a negative angle and indicates the presence of abnormal patellar tilt.

IMPORTANT POINTS IN REHABILITATION OF PATELLOFEMORAL DISORDERS

Patellar Instability

- Patellar instability refers to symptoms secondary to episodic lateral (rarely medial) subluxation or dislocation of the patella. Lateral patellar subluxation is very common.

Figure 4–54 Patellar tilt is evaluated by the patellofemoral angle. Lines drawn along the lateral patellar facet (*upper line*) and the trochlear groove (*lower line*) should be parallel. Convergence of these two lines indicates lateral patellar tilt.

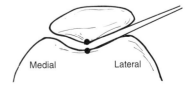

- Medial subluxation is typically rare, iatrogenic, and a result of excessive or ill-advised lateral release.
- **Predisposing risk factors** contributing to **patellar instability** include
  - Femoral anteversion
  - Genu valgum
  - Patellar or femoral dysplasia
  - Patella alta
  - High Q-angle
  - Pes planus
  - Generalized laxity
  - Over-release of the lateral retinaculum (medial instability)
  - Previous patellar dislocation
  - Atrophy of the VMO
- Patellar subluxation generally describes the transient lateral movement of the patella during early knee flexion. Frequently, this subluxation is reported as "something jumps or comes out of place" or is "hung up."
- Palpation often elicits medial retinacular tenderness.
- Patient apprehension (positive Fairbank sign) is common on displacing the patella laterally.
- Patellar mobility should be evaluated by displacing the patella medially and laterally with the knee flexed 20 to 30 degrees. If more than 50% of the total patellar width can be displaced laterally over the edge of the lateral femoral condyle, patellar instability should be suspected.
- Inspection of patellar tracking should be done with particular attention to the entrance and exit of the patella into the trochlea between 10 and 25 degrees of knee flexion. An abrupt lateral movement of the patella on terminal knee extension (extension subluxation) indicates patellar instability or subluxation.
- Conlan and coworkers (1993), in a biomechanical study of medial soft tissue restraints that prevent lateral patellar subluxation, found that the medial patellofemoral ligament provides 53% of the total restraining force (Fig. 4-55).

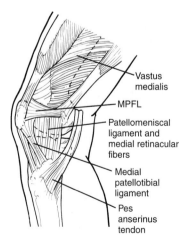

Vastus medialis

MPFL

Patellomeniscal ligament and medial retinacular fibers

Medial patellotibial ligament

Pes anserinus tendon

Figure 4–55 Anatomy of the medial aspect of the knee. The medial patellofemoral ligament (MPFL) provides 53% of the restraining force in preventing lateral displacement of the patella; the patellomeniscal ligament and medial retinacular fibers provide 22% on average. (Adapted from Boden BP, Pearsall AW, Garrett WE, Feagin JA: Patellofemoral instability: Evaluation and management. J Am Acad Orthop Surg 5:47-57, 1997.)

REHABILITATION PROTOCOL	*General Guidelines for Nonoperative Treatment of Recurrent (Not Acute) Patellar Instability (Lateral)*

GOALS

- Decrease symptoms and instability
- Increase quadriceps strength and endurance (VMO > lateral structures)
- Use of passive restraints (Palumbo-type bracing, McConnell taping) to augment stability during transition
- Enhance patellar stability by dynamic stabilization or passive mechanisms

EXERCISES/AIDS

- Modify or avoid activities that aggravate or induce symptoms (running, squatting, stair climbing, jumping, high-impact activities)
- Rest, ice, limb elevation
- Use of a cane or crutches if needed
- NSAIDs (if not contraindicated) for their anti-inflammatory effect; no steroid injection
- Modalities to modify pain, reduce effusion and edema
- Electrical stimulation
- VMO biofeedback for VMO strengthening
- External Palumbo-type lateral buttress bracing (Fig. 4-56) or McConnell taping (Fig. 4-57) based on patient preference and tolerance of the skin to taping
- Orthotics posted in subtalar neutral to control foot pronation, decrease the Q-angle, or correct leg-length discrepancy
- General conditioning and cross-training
  - Aqua exercises, deep pool running
  - Swimming
  - Avoid bicycling in the early phases
- Pain-free quadriceps strengthening exercises with VMO efficiency enhancement

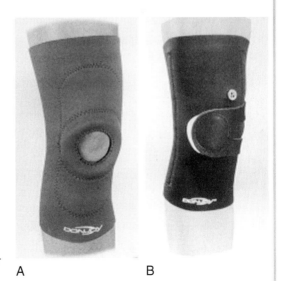

Figure 4–56 **A** and **B**, Patellar stabilizing braces. **A**   **B**

Continued

REHABILITATION PROTOCOL: *General Guidelines for Nonoperative Treatment of Recurrent (Not Acute) Patellar Instability (Lateral)* Continued

EXERCISES/AIDS—cont'd

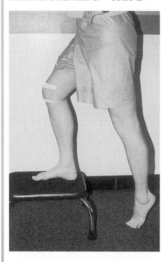

Figure 4–57 McConnell taping (patellofemoral).

- No exercises completely isolate the VMO, but several produce high EMG activity of the VMO
  - Leg press
  - Lateral step-ups
  - Isometric quadriceps setting
  - Hip adduction exercises
- Gradual restoration of flexibility (stretching) for noted deficits
  - Iliotibial band
  - Quadriceps
  - Hamstrings
  - Gastrocnemius-soleus
  - Avoid mobilization of the medial retinaculum
- Re-establish knee proprioception skills

REHABILITATION PROTOCOL	*McConnell Patellar Taping Techniques* D'Amato and Bach

- Figure 4-57 illustrates McConnell taping.
- The knee is cleaned, shaved, and prepared with an adhesive spray. If possible, try to avoid shaving immediately before taping to decrease the likelihood of skin irritation.
- Patellar taping is done with the knee in extension.
- Leukotape P is the taping material used.
- Correction is based on the individual malalignment, with each component corrected as described in the following text.

REHABILITATION PROTOCOL: *McConnell Patellar Taping Techniques*   *Continued*

CORRECTING LATERAL PATELLAR GLIDE

- The tape is started at the midlateral border.
- It is brought across the face of the patella and secured to the medial border of the medial hamstring tendons while the patella is pulled in a medial direction.
- The medial soft tissues are brought over the medial femoral condyle toward the patella to obtain more secure fixation.

CORRECTING LATERAL PATELLAR TILT

- The tape is started in the middle of the patella.
- It is brought across the face of the patella and secured to the medial border of the medial hamstring tendons to lift the lateral border of the patella.
- The medial soft tissues are brought over the medial femoral condyle toward the patella to obtain more secure fixation.

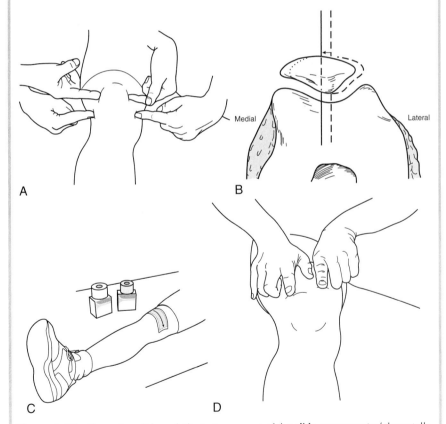

Figure 4–58   Correcting glide and tilt. **A**, Assessment of the **glide component** of the patella. **B**, Lateral glide is corrected with tape placed across the patella and pulled medially. **C**, Correction of the lateral glide component by applying a medial glide to the patella with Leukosport tape. **D**, Assessment of the tilt component of the patella.

Continued

REHABILITATION PROTOCOL: *McConnell Patellar Taping Techniques* *Continued*

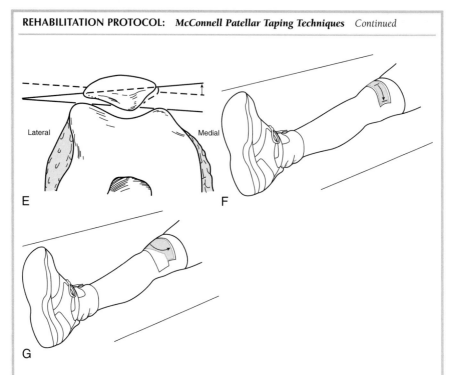

Figure 4–58, cont'd., **E**, Frequently, the lateral patellar border is pulled posteriorly (tight) by tightened lateral retinacular structures (positive presence of patellar tilt) rather than the patellar borders being horizontal. **F**, Lateral tilt correction. **G**, External rotation correction.

CORRECTING EXTERNAL ROTATION

- The tape is applied to the middle of the inferior border of the patella.
- The inferior pole of the patella is manually rotated internally.
- The tape is secured to the medial soft tissues in a superior and medial direction while the manual correction is maintained.

  Alternatively, if there is also a component of **inferior tilt**, the tape can be started on the middle of the superior pole. After manual correction of the rotational deformity, the tape is secured in a superior and lateral direction. This not only corrects patellar rotation but also lifts the inferior pole away from the fat pad. Care must be taken to not create a lateral patellar glide when using this alternative method.

CORRECTING INFERIOR PATELLAR TILT

- Correction of inferior tilt is always combined with correction of a lateral tilt or glide component.
- To correct the inferior tilt component, the starting position of the tape is shifted from the midportion of the patella to the superior portion of the patella. Correction is then carried out as above for each individual component of glide or tilt. The superior starting position of the tape lifts the inferior pole of the patella away from the fat pad.

REHABILITATION PROTOCOL: *McConnell Patellar Taping Techniques* *Continued*

TECHNICAL TAPING CONSIDERATIONS

- The tape is never left on for more than 24 hours at a time and should not be worn during nighttime sleep.
- The average duration of continuous taping treatment is 2 weeks, followed by a weaning period during which the tape is worn only during strenuous activities. Taping may be continued as long as 6 weeks if tolerated.
- The tape must be removed slowly and carefully to prevent skin irritation, which will limit further taping. Commercial solvents are available to aid in tape removal.
- The application of rubbing alcohol to the skin after tape removal helps toughen the skin and prevent skin breakdown.
- Application of a skin moisturizer overnight will nourish the skin; the moisturizer is removed before tape is applied the next day.
- Allergic reaction to the tape may occur in a few first-time patients. An itchy rash will develop on the knee, usually 7-10 days after the start of taping. Topical cortisone creams may limit the rash. Only hypoallergenic tape should be used in patients in whom an allergic reaction develops.

REHABILITATION PROTOCOL   *Principles of McConnell Taping—Protocol 2*

- Taping is used as an adjunct to exercise and muscular balancing.
- The VMO-to–vastus lateralis ratio has been shown to improve during taping.
- The ability to truly change patellar position is debated.
- To tape correctly, the position of the patella relative to the femoral condyle must be evaluated.
- Four positional relationships are evaluated statically (sitting with the legs extended and the quadriceps relaxed) and then dynamically by doing a quadriceps set.

Glide component is the relationship of the medial and lateral poles of the patella to the femoral condyles. Statically, the patella should be centered in the condyles; dynamically, this relationship should be maintained. With a quadriceps set, the patella should move superiorly without noticeable lateral movement. Most athletes require correction of the glide component for static or dynamic malalignment.

Tilt component is evaluated by comparing the anterior and posterior relationships of the medial and lateral borders of the patella. With the patient supine and the knee extended, the borders should be horizontal, both statically and dynamically. Frequently, the lateral border will be pulled posteriorly (downward) by the lateral retinaculum into the lateral condyle. This may also occur after the glide is corrected by taping.

Rotational component is the relationship between the long axis of the patella and the long axis of the femur. The ideal position is for the axes to be parallel. Frequently, the inferior pole of the patella is lateral to the axis of the femur, which would be described as lateral rotation.

Anteroposterior tilt is the anterior and posterior relationship of the superior and inferior poles of the patella. When the inferior pole of the patella is posterior, fat pad irritation is common.

Continued

REHABILITATION PROTOCOL: *Principles of McConnell Taping—Protocol 2* *Continued*

After the patella's position is evaluated, an activity is identified that consistently provokes the patient's symptoms. Observation of the patient stepping off from an 8-inch step is often effective. After taping, the test should be performed again to ensure the effectiveness of taping in eliminating pain.

TAPING PROCEDURE

- Corrections are typically done in the order of evaluation, but the most significant alteration in position should be corrected first.
- Leukosport tape (Beiersdorf, Inc.) is commonly used.
- Tape that is strong and tacky enough to be effective requires a protective cover next to the skin, such as "Cover Roll Stretch."
- To correct the **glide component**, the tape is anchored on the lateral pole of the patella, and the patella is manually glided medially and taped in this position.
- The **tilt component** is corrected by starting the tape in the middle of the patella, pulling the medial pole of the patella posteriorly, and anchoring over the tape used for the glide correction.
- A **rotational fault** is corrected by anchoring on the lateral aspect of the inferior pole of the patella and pulling toward the medial joint line.
- If an **anteroposterior tilt** is present, it is corrected by taping the glide or tilt on the superior aspect of the patella to pull the inferior aspect of the patella out of the fat pad.
- Not all components have to be corrected if the pain is eliminated with one or two corrections.
- A provocation test should be done after each stage of taping to check its effectiveness.
- Tape is worn during activities that produce pain: just with athletics or with all activities of daily living.
- Once muscular control of the patella is improved, the patient is weaned from the tape; it is not intended for long-term use.

PATELLAR EXCESS PRESSURE SYNDROMES (GLOBAL PATELLAR PRESSURE SYNDROME, EXCESSIVE LATERAL PRESSURE SYNDROME)

The most important clinical finding differentiating GPPS from ELPS is patellar mobility. In GPPS, mobility is restricted in both the medial and lateral directions. Frequently, superior mobility is also restricted. With ELPS, tightness is present **only** in the lateral retinacular structures.

The rehabilitation program for **ELPS** focuses on stretching the tight lateral retinacular structures and includes medial mobilization with medial glides and tilts, McConnell taping to "medialize" or normalize the patella (correct the tilt), and low-load long-duration stretching of the tight lateral structures. Musculotendinous stretching should include the hamstrings, quadriceps, and iliotibial band. Improving quadriceps strength, especially the VMO, is emphasized. Open-chain knee extension and bicycling are not used in early rehabilitation. NSAIDs can be taken for synovitis and inflammation, in addition to modalities such as high-voltage galvanic stimulation and cryotherapy. Daily home exercises are done, and the patient is educated about which activities to avoid (stairs, squatting, kneeling, jumping, running) and counseled about changing sports.

GPPS is treated in a similar manner, with a few important changes. **Patellar mobility in all planes must be re-established or improved before initiation of any aggressive rehabilitation to decrease inflammation and cartilage degeneration.** Modalities such as a warm whirlpool and ultrasound can be used before mobilization of the patella. The glide is held for at least 1 to 2 minutes, 10 to 12 minutes if possible, during mobilization. Mobilization of the quadriceps insertion is used. The patient performs unrestricted knee motion several times a day to maintain soft tissue mobility. Restoration of full passive knee extension is vital to preserve the integrity of patellofemoral articular cartilage. Initially, multiangle quadriceps isometric contraction, SLRs, and 40-degree mini-squats are performed until patellar mobilization improves. Leg press, lunge, and wall squat can be added. Bicycling, deep knee bends, deep squats, and resisted knee extension **should be avoided** until patellar mobility is restored. Bracing or taping is not used in patients with GPPS because it restricts and compresses the patella.

REHABILITATION PROTOCOL	***Patellofemoral Compression Syndromes: Excessive Lateral Pressure Syndrome (ELPS) and Global Patellar Pressure Syndrome (GPPS)*** D'Amato and Bach

PHASE 1

Goals

- Reduce pain and inflammation
- Increase patellar mobility, mobilize contracted peripatellar structures
- Regain quadriceps control
- Improve patellofemoral movements

Taping/Bracing

- ELPS: McConnell taping to correct tilt
- GPPS: no bracing or taping

Therapeutic Exercises

- Ice, electrical stimulation, and NSAIDs to decrease inflammation and pain
- Quadriceps sets and SLRs, multiangle quadriceps isometrics
- Hip adduction and abduction, flexion and extension exercises
- Begin patellar mobilization techniques
  - ELPS: mobilize tight lateral patellar tissue
  - GPPS: mobilize medial, lateral, and superior peripatellar tissue

PHASE 2

Criteria for Progression to Phase 2

- Minimal pain
- Minimal inflammation

Goals

- Good quadriceps set with no extension lag
- Improve ROM
- Increase patellar mobility (*Note:* Avoid aggressive strengthening with GPPS until patellar mobility is significantly improved)

Continued

REHABILITATION PROTOCOL: *Patellofemoral Compression Syndromes: Excessive Lateral Pressure Syndrome (ELPS) and Global Patellar Pressure Syndrome (GPPS)*   *Continued*

PHASE 2—cont'd

Therapeutic Exercises

- Continue patellar mobilization
- Fit a patella stabilizing brace or use McConnell taping (ELPS) to correct patellar tilt
- Continue ice and electrical stimulation (especially after exercise) and NSAIDs
- SLRs, quadriceps sets
- Flexibility exercises for the quadriceps, hamstrings, iliotibial band, gastrocnemius, soleus
- Closed-chain exercises: mini-lunges, wall slides, lateral step-ups, mini-squats
- Avoid bicycling, deep knee bends, deep squats, resisted knee extension
- Pool exercises, swimming
- Advance exercises for the hip flexors and extensors, abductors and adductors, and muscles of the lower part of the leg and foot by increasing weight as tolerated; do 3-10 sets and increase weight by 2 pounds

PHASE 3

Criteria for Progression to Phase 3

- No increase in pain or inflammation
- Good quadriceps strength

Goals

- Full knee motion
- Improved strength and flexibility

Bracing

- Continue using brace or taping if helpful

Therapeutic Exercises

- Advance hamstring-strengthening exercises
- Bicycling, swimming, stair stepping, or walking for cardiovascular and muscle endurance; increase duration, then speed
- Continue flexibility exercises
- Progress closed-chain activities

PHASE 4

Criteria for Progression to Phase 4

- Full knee motion
- Quadriceps strength 80% of normal

Goal

- Return to full activity

Brace

- Brace or tape is worn for sports participation if desired. Tape up to 6 weeks, then discontinue. Continue brace as needed

REHABILITATION PROTOCOL: *Patellofemoral Compression Syndromes: Excessive Lateral Pressure Syndrome (ELPS) and Global Patellar Pressure Syndrome (GPPS)* *Continued*

PHASE 4—cont'd

Therapeutic Exercises

- Add slow return to running if desired; increase distance, then speed
- Warm up well
- Use ice after workout
- Continue aerobic cross-training
- Start jumping, cutting, and other sport-specific exercises

Return to Full Activity

- Full pain-free motion
- Strength and functional tests 85% of normal

REHABILITATION PROTOCOL

After First-Time Acute Lateral Patellar Dislocation
D'Amato and Bach

PHASE 1

Goals

- Decrease pain and avoid recurrent dislocation
- Return of muscle function
- Decrease swelling
- Limit ROM to protect healing tissues
- Limit weight-bearing to protect healing tissues
- Avoid leading the patient into a pain dysfunction syndrome with overaggressive therapy

Bracing

- Limited-range brace set at 0 degrees with ambulation initially; lateral buttress doughnut pad in brace
- Patella stabilizing brace or McConnell taping
- Light compressive dressing

Weight-Bearing

- Partial weight-bearing with crutches

Therapeutic Exercises

- Cryotherapy
- Electrical stimulation to promote quadriceps activity, with emphasis on the VMO (high-voltage galvanic stimulation)
- Supine SLR when pain level allows
- Passive ROM in pain-free range
- Ankle pumps if swelling is present
- Isometric hamstrings
- Aspiration of blood if effusion is inhibiting quadriceps

Continued

REHABILITATION PROTOCOL: *After First-time Acute Lateral Patellar Dislocation*   *Continued*

PHASE 2

Criteria for Progression to Phase 2

- No significant joint effusion
- No quadriceps extension lag
- Avoid performing apprehension to patellar mobility test
- Little or no pain with activities of daily living

Goals

- Improve quadriceps muscle function
- Obtain full pain-free ROM
- Begin low-level functional activities
- Initiate conditioning program
- Avoid patellofemoral symptoms or instability

Bracing

- Continue patellar bracing or taping

Weight-Bearing

- As tolerated
- Discard crutches when quadriceps control with no extension lag is achieved

Therapeutic Exercises

- Continue electrical stimulation as needed
- Continue supine SLR and add PREs, adduction and abduction SLR
- Toe raises with equal weight-bearing bilaterally
- Modalities as needed
- Closed–kinetic chain exercises (wall sitting, toe raises)
- Low-level endurance training (well-leg cycling)
- Low-level pool activities

PHASE 3

Criteria for Progression to Phase 3

- Full active ROM
- Good to normal quadriceps function
- Full weight-bearing without gait deviation

Goals

- Improve functional capabilities
- Gradual return to sports activity or other high-level activity

Bracing

- Wean from patellar brace or taping as quadriceps strength improves

Therapeutic Exercises

- Four-way hip exercises (i.e., SLR with adduction, abduction, flexion, extension)
- Aqua therapy, walking progressing to running in water

REHABILITATION PROTOCOL: *After First-time Acute Lateral Patellar*
Dislocation   Continued

PHASE 3—cont'd

- Sport- and skill-specific training
- Proprioceptive training
- Patient education

Criteria for Return to Full Activity (8-12 Weeks)

- ROM equal to that of opposite limb
- No pain or effusion
- Strength 85% of opposite limb
- Satisfactory 1-minute hop test, two-legged hop test
- Patellar stability on clinical examination

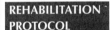
After Lateral Retinacular Release
D'Amato and Bach

INDICATIONS FOR LATERAL RELEASE

- Recalcitrant patellofemoral pain with a positive lateral tilt of the patella (see p. 498)
- Tight lateral retinaculum—positive ELPS
- Lateral retinacular pain with positive lateral tilt

PHASE 1: IMMEDIATELY AFTER SURGERY—2 WEEKS

Goals

- Protect healing soft tissue structures
- Improve knee flexion and extension
- Increase lower extremity strength, including quadriceps muscle re-education
- Education of patient regarding limitations and rehabilitation process

Weight-Bearing

- As tolerated with two crutches

Therapeutic Exercises

- Quadriceps sets and isometric adduction with biofeedback for the VMO
- Heel slides
- Ankle pumps
- Non–weight-bearing gastrosoleus and hamstring exercises
- SLR in flexion with turnout, adduction, and extension; begin hip abduction at approximately 3 weeks
- Functional electrical stimulation can be used for trace to poor quadriceps contraction
- Begin aquatic therapy at 2 weeks (when wound is healed), with emphasis on normalization of gait
- Stationary bike for ROM when sufficient knee flexion is present

Continued

REHABILITATION PROTOCOL: *After Lateral Retinacular Release*   *Continued*

PHASE 2: WEEKS 2-4

Criteria for Progression to Phase 2

- Good quadriceps set
- Approximately 90 degrees active knee flexion
- Full active knee extension
- No signs of active inflammation

Goals

- Increase flexion
- Increase lower extremity strength and flexibility
- Restore normal gait
- Improve balance and proprioception

WEIGHT-BEARING

- Ambulation as tolerated without crutches if the following criteria are met
  - No extension lag with SLR
  - Full active knee extension
  - Knee flexion of 90-100 degrees
  - Nonantalgic gait pattern
- May use one crutch or cane to normalize gait before walking without assistive device

Therapeutic Exercises

- Wall slides from 0-45 degrees knee flexion, progressing to mini-squats
- Four-way hip exercises for flexion, extension, and adduction
- Calf raises
- Balance and proprioception activities (including single-leg stance, KAT, and BAPS board)
- Treadmill walking with emphasis on normalization of gait pattern
- Iliotibial band and hip flexor stretching

PHASE 3: WEEKS 4-8

Criteria for Progression to Phase 3

- Normal gait
- Good to normal quadriceps strength
- Good dynamic control with no evidence of patellar lateral tracking or instability
- Clearance by physician to begin more concentrated closed–kinetic chain progression

Goals

- Restore any residual loss of ROM
- Continue improvement of quadriceps strength
- Improve functional strength and proprioception

Therapeutic Exercises

- Quadriceps stretching when full knee flexion has been achieved
- Hamstring curl
- Leg press from 0-45 degrees knee flexion
- Closed–kinetic chain progression
- Abduction on four-way hip exercises

REHABILITATION PROTOCOL: *After Lateral Retinacular Release* Continued

PHASE 3: WEEKS 4-8—cont'd

- StairMaster or elliptical trainer
- Nordic-Trac
- Jogging in pool with a wet vest or belt

PHASE 4: RETURN TO FULL ACTIVITY—WEEK 8

Criteria for Progression to Phase 4

- Release by physician to resume full or partial activity
- No patellofemoral or soft tissue complaints
- No evidence of patellar instability
- Necessary joint ROM, muscle strength and endurance, and proprioception to safely return to athletic participation

Goals

- Continue improvements in quadriceps strength
- Improve functional strength and proprioception
- Return to appropriate activity level

Therapeutic Exercises

- Functional progression, which may include but is not limited to
  - Slide board
  - Walk/jog progression
  - Forward and backward running, cutting, figure-of-eight, and carioca
  - Plyometrics
  - Sport-specific drills

REHABILITATION PROTOCOL
After Distal and/or Proximal Patellar Realignment Procedures
D'Amato and Bach

GENERAL GUIDELINES

- No closed–kinetic chain exercises for 6 weeks
- Same rehabilitation protocol is followed for proximal and distal realignments, except for weight-bearing limitations as noted
- After combined proximal and distal realignment, the protocol for distal realignment is used

PHASE 1: IMMEDIATE POSTOPERATIVE PERIOD—WEEKS 1-6

Goals

- Protect fixation and surrounding soft tissues
- Control inflammatory process
- Regain active quadriceps and VMO control
- Minimize adverse effects of immobilization through CPM and heel slides in the allowed ROM
- Full knee extension
- Patient education regarding the rehabilitation process

Continued

REHABILITATION PROTOCOL: *After Distal and/or Proximal Patellar Realignment Procedures*   *Continued*

PHASE 1: IMMEDIATE POSTOPERATIVE PERIOD—WEEKS 1-6—cont'd

Range of Motion

- 0-2 weeks: 0-30 degrees of flexion
- 2-4 weeks: 0-60 degrees of flexion
- 4-6 weeks: 0-90 degrees of flexion

Brace

- 0-4 weeks: locked in full extension for all activities except therapeutic exercises and CPM use; locked in full extension for sleeping
- 4-6 weeks: unlocked for sleeping, locked in full extension for ambulation

Weight-Bearing

- As tolerated with two crutches for a proximal realignment procedure, 50% with two crutches for a distal realignment procedure

Therapeutic Exercises

- Quadriceps sets and isometric adduction with biofeedback and electrical stimulation for the VMO (no electrical stimulation for 6 weeks with proximal realignment)
- Heel slides from 0-60 degrees of flexion for proximal realignment, 0-90 degrees for distal realignment
- CPM for 2 hours, twice daily, from 0-60 degrees of flexion for proximal realignment, 0-90 degrees of flexion for distal realignment
- Non–weight-bearing gastrocnemius-soleus, hamstring stretches
- SLR in four planes with the brace locked in full extension (can be done standing)
- Resisted ankle ROM with Thera-Band
- Patellar mobilization (begin when tolerated)
- Begin aquatic therapy at 3-4 weeks with emphasis on gait

PHASE 2: WEEKS 6-8

Criteria for Progression to Phase 2

- Good quadriceps set
- Approximately 90 degrees of flexion
- No signs of active inflammation

Goals

- Increase range of flexion
- Avoid overstressing the fixation
- Increase quadriceps and VMO control for restoration of proper patellar tracking

Brace

- Discontinue use for sleeping, unlock for ambulation as allowed by physician

Weight-Bearing

- As tolerated with two crutches

Therapeutic Exercises

- Continue exercises, with progression toward full flexion with heel slides
- Progress to weight-bearing gastrocnemius-soleus stretching

REHABILITATION PROTOCOL: *After Distal and/or Proximal Patellar*
Realignment Procedures *Continued*

PHASE 2: WEEKS 6-8

- Discontinue CPM if knee flexion is at least 90 degrees
- Continue aquatic therapy
- Balance exercises (single-leg standing, KAT, BAPS board)
- Stationary bike: low resistance, high seat
- Wall slides progressing to mini-squats, 0-45 degrees flexion

PHASE 3: 8 WEEKS-4 MONTHS

Criteria for Progression to Phase 3

- Good quadriceps tone and no extension lag with SLR
- Nonantalgic gait pattern
- Good dynamic patellar control with no evidence of lateral tracking or instability

Weight-Bearing

- May discontinue use of crutches when following criteria are met
  - No extension lag with SLR
  - Full extension
  - Nonantalgic gait pattern (may use one crutch or cane until gait is normalized)

Therapeutic Exercises

- Step-ups, begin at 2 inches and progress toward 8 inches
- Stationary bike, add moderate resistance
- Four-way hip exercises for flexion, adduction, abduction, extension
- Leg press for 0-45 degrees of flexion
- Swimming, StairMaster for endurance
- Toe raises
- Hamstring curls
- Treadmill walking with emphasis on normalization of gait
- Continue proprioception exercises
- Continue flexibility exercises for gastrocnemius-soleus and hamstrings; add iliotibial band and quadriceps as indicated

PHASE 4: 4-6 MONTHS

Criteria for Progression to Phase 4

- Good to normal quadriceps strength
- No evidence of patellar instability
- No soft tissue complaints
- Clearance from physician to begin more concentrated closed–kinetic chain exercises and resume full or partial activity

Goals

- Continue improvements in quadriceps strength
- Improve functional strength and proprioception
- Return to appropriate activity level

Therapeutic Exercises

- Progression of closed–kinetic chain activities
- Jogging/running in pool with a wet vest or belt
- Functional progression, sport-specific activities

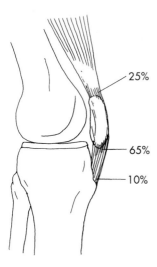

25%

65%

10%

Figure 4–59 Typical locations of pain in a jumper's knee.

OVERUSE SYNDROMES OF THE KNEE

Overuse syndromes involving the extensor mechanism are commonly grouped together under the term "**jumper's knee.**" **Patellar tendinitis** is the most common and is typically manifested as pain near the insertion of the tendon at the inferior pole of the patella (Fig. 4-59). Less commonly, symptoms may be localized to the distal tendon insertion at the tibial tubercle or the quadriceps tendon insertion at the proximal pole of the patella. In adolescents, it is typically manifested as a form of apophysitis and occurs at the tibial tubercle (**Osgood-Schlatter disease**) or distal patellar pole (**Sinding-Larsen–Johansson disease**) (Fig. 4-60).

History of Patellar Tendinitis (Jumper's Knee)

The typical history is that of an insidious onset of anterior knee pain, localized to the site of involvement, that develops during or soon after repetitive running or jumping activities. The pain usually resolves after a short period of rest but recurs with renewed activity. It occurs most often in basketball, volleyball, and track-and-field

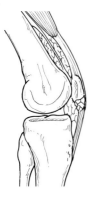

Figure 4–60 Sinding-Larsen–Johansson disease is osteochondritis of the inferior pole of the patella in the skeletally immature. Conservative treatment leads to healing in 3 to 12 months. (Adapted from Colosimo A, Bassett FH 3rd: Jumper's Knee: Diagnosis and treatment. Orthop Rev 19:139, 1990.)

athletes. One theory is that it results from the accumulation of damage after recurrent episodes of microtrauma to the tendon. It has been shown that when compared with asymptomatic athletes, athletes with jumper's knee have an ability to generate greater force during jumping activities, which is indicative of an overload phenomenon as a possible cause. The type of playing surface may also play a role, with activities on hard surfaces leading to an increased incidence of tendinitis symptoms.

Classification

The classification of tendinitis by Blazina and associates (1973) is the most commonly cited and is useful in organizing a treatment plan.

Classification of Patellar Tendinitis

Phase 1   Pain only after participation
Phase 2   Pain during participation that does not limit performance
Phase 3   Pain during participation that limits performance
Phase 4   Complete tendon disruption

Patients in phases 1 and 2 typically respond to nonoperative therapy. Patients with phase 3 symptoms have a more variable response to conservative treatment. Surgery is indicated for patients in phase 1, 2, or 3 in whom at least 3 to 6 months of conservative therapy fails and for all patients with phase 4 involvement.

REHABILITATION PROTOCOL — *Patellar Tendinitis*
D'Amato and Bach

PHASE 1

Goals

- Patient education
- Promote healing time
- Resolve or control pain

Therapeutic Treatments

- Rest
- NSAIDs
- Cryotherapy, electrical stimulation, iontophoresis, phonophoresis
- Flexibility exercises, with specific focus on hamstrings
- Lower extremity strengthening in pain-free range (closed-chain only)
- General conditioning, hip strengthening of flexors, abductors, and adductors
- SLR with progressive resistance

PHASE 2

Criteria for Progression to Phase 2

- No pain at rest
- Decreased tenderness to palpation

Continued

REHABILITATION PROTOCOL: *Patellar Tendinitis*   *Continued*

PHASE 2—cont'd

- No pain with activities of daily living
- Decreased swelling

Goals

- Increase strength
- Increase flexibility
- Control inflammation
- Promote healing

Therapeutic Treatments

- Use of a Cho-Pat "counterforce" strap
- Continue flexibility exercises
- Closed–kinetic chain exercises
- Four-position hip strengthening
- Start endurance training (pool, bike, cross-country ski machine)
- Balance training

PHASE 3

Criteria for Progression to Phase 3

- No pain with activities of daily living
- No pain with running
- Quadriceps strength 70%-80% of contralateral extremity

Goals

- Pain-free return to activity
- Patient education to prevent recurrent episodes and modify activities
- Maintain strength and flexibility

Therapeutic Treatments

- Continue flexibility exercises
- Continue strengthening
- Running program and skill-specific activities
- Aerobic conditioning
- Patient education

ILIOTIBIAL BAND FRICTION SYNDROME

Repetitive activity can also lead to irritation of soft tissues, such as in the iliotibial band friction syndrome, which is common in runners. The iliotibial band is a thick fibrous tissue band that runs along the **lateral** aspect of the thigh and inserts at Gerdy's tubercle on the anterolateral aspect of the proximal end of the tibia. It has small attachments to the lateral patellar retinaculum and to the biceps femoris. As the knee moves from full extension to flexion, the iliotibial band shifts from a position anterior to the lateral femoral epicondyle to a position posterior to the epicondyle (Fig. 4-61). The transition occurs at about 30 degrees of knee flexion. The repetitive flexion and extension of the knee in running can lead to irritation of the

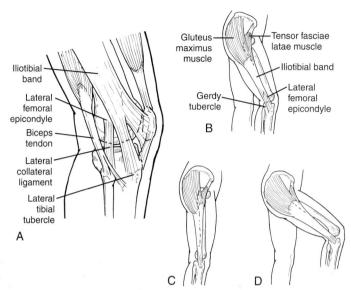

Figure 4–61   **A**, Anatomy of the lateral aspect of the knee showing the location of the iliotibial band. **B**, With the knee in approximately 30 degrees of flexion, the iliotibial band lies over the lateral femoral epicondyle. **C**, With the knee between 30 degrees of flexion and full extension, the iliotibial band is anterior to the lateral femoral epicondyle and assists in extension. **D**, With knee flexion greater than 30 degrees, the iliotibial band is posterior to the lateral femoral epicondyle and assists in flexion. (Adapted from Lineger JM, Christensen CP: Is the iliotibial band syndrome often overlooked? Physician Sports Med 20:98-108, 1992; and Aronen JG, Chronister R, Regan K, Hensien MA: Practical conservative management of iliotibial band syndrome. Physician Sports Med 21:[9]:59-69, 1993.)

iliotibial band as it passes back and forth over the lateral femoral epicondyle. Subsequently, the surrounding tissues and bursa become inflamed and painful.

History and Examination

Patients typically complain of a gradual onset of pain, tightness, or burning at the lateral aspect of the knee that develops during the course of a run. Symptoms usually resolve with rest. Examination reveals tenderness and possibly localized swelling at the lateral femoral epicondyle or at Gerdy's tubercle, and when the knee is put through ROM, pain, snapping, popping, or crepitation may be felt as the iliotibial band crosses the epicondyle. Iliotibial band contracture is associated with the presence of symptoms and can be evaluated by the Ober test.

Predisposing Factors

Factors that predispose runners to iliotibial band friction syndrome include inexperience, a recent increase in distance, and running on a track. Other potential causes include leg-length discrepancies, hyperpronation of the foot, and running repetitively in one direction on a pitched surface.

Treatment of Iliotibial Band Friction Syndrome

The basic progression of treatment is early reduction of the acute inflammation, followed by stretching of the iliotibial band, strengthening of the hip abductors to alleviate soft tissue contracture, and finally, education in proper running techniques and institution of an appropriate running program to prevent recurrence (see the following rehabilitation protocol).

REHABILITATION PROTOCOL	*Iliotibial Band Friction Syndrome in Runners* Brotzman

- Rest from running until asymptomatic
- Ice area before and after exercise
- Oral NSAIDs
- Relative rest from running and high–flexion-extension activities of the knee (cycling, running, stair descent, skiing)
- Avoid downhill running
- Avoid running on pitched surfaces with a pitched drainage grade of the road
- Use of soft, new running shoes rather than hard shoes

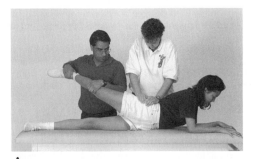

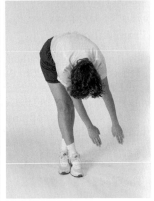

Figure 4–62 **A**, Two-person Ober stretch. **B**, Self-administered Ober stretch. **C**, Cross-over lateral fascial stretch (the involved leg crosses behind the uninvolved leg).

REHABILITATION PROTOCOL: *Iliotibial Band Friction Syndrome in Runners*   Continued

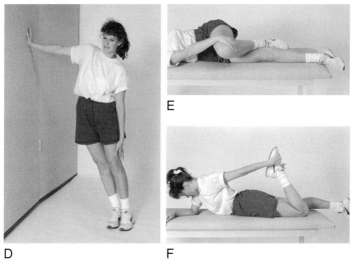

Figure 4–62, cont'd., **D**, Leaning lateral fascial stretch (the involved leg is closer to the wall). **E**, Posterior fascial stretch, including the gluteus maximus and piriformis. **F**, Quadriceps self-stretch.

- Use of iontophoresis if helpful
- Steroid injection into the bursa if required
- Stretching exercises (Fig. 4-62)
  - Two-man Ober stretch
  - Self-administered Ober stretch
  - Lateral fascial stretch
  - Posterior fascial stretch plus gluteus maximus and piriformis self-stretch
  - Standing wall lean for lateral fascial stretch
  - Rectus femoris self-stretch
  - Iliopsoas with rectus femoris self-stretch
- Possible use of lateral heel wedge in shoe, especially for iliotibial band tightness
- Built-in correction in the shoe for leg-length discrepancy

Articular Cartilage Procedures of the Knee

G. Kelley Fitzgerald, PhD, PT • James J. Irrgang, PhD, PT, ATC

CLINICAL BACKGROUND

Designing successful rehabilitation programs after surgical procedures on articular cartilage requires careful consideration of the healing process and a thorough understanding of the potential stress applied to the articular surfaces during therapeutic exercise. Although it is important to begin early rehabilitation to promote tissue healing and to restore joint motion, muscular strength, and functional capacity, rehabilitation procedures must be applied in a manner that does not interfere with or disrupt the healing articular lesion.

TYPES OF MOTION

Evidence from animal studies suggests that early active and passive motion exercises after articular cartilage lesions can enhance the quality of tissue healing, limit the adverse effects of joint immobilization on the remaining healthy articular cartilage, and reduce the risk for adhesions. **Complete immobilization is not recommended after surgical procedures that involve the articular cartilage.**

However, the application of shear stress while the healing articular lesion is under compression may have adverse effects on the healing process. ROM exercises should be done in a controlled manner to avoid excessive shear loads while the joint is under compression. This can be accomplished by emphasizing passive, active-assisted, and unloaded active ROM exercises in the early postoperative period (0 to 6 weeks).

MUSCLE STRENGTHENING

Muscle performance training is an essential component of postoperative rehabilitation after surgical procedures on articular cartilage. Muscles need to be strong enough to assist in absorbing shock and dissipating loads across the joint. The resistance exercise program should be tailored to minimize shear loading across the lesion during the healing period. In general, exercises that have the potential for producing high shear stress coupled with compression, such as closed-chain exercises, should be avoided in the early phases of rehabilitation.

We believe that isometric exercises are the safest option for restoring muscle strength during early rehabilitation.

Isometric quadriceps exercises in full knee extension may be effective in preventing or resolving knee extensor lag, and most articular lesions will not be engaged with the knee in full extension. Isometric exercise at 90 degrees of flexion may also be a safe option because it is unlikely to result in excessive compression or shear loads across most articular cartilage lesions. In addition, it has been shown that isometric quadriceps training at 90 degrees of flexion can result in increased production of muscle force at other joint angles. Isometric exercises at angles between 20 and 75 degrees should be used with caution because most articular lesions would be engaged in this arc of motion. If open-chain leg extension exercises are to be performed, it is essential that the arc of motion be limited to ranges that do not engage the lesion. This requires effective communication between the surgeon and the therapist regarding ROM limitations for resistive exercises.

WEIGHT-BEARING PROGRESSION

Progression of weight-bearing and functional activities is a gradual process that begins in the intermediate phase of postoperative rehabilitation. Weight-bearing status after surgery is dependent on the size, nature, and location of the lesion, as well as the surgical procedure that has been used to treat it. Progression of weight-bearing is also dependent on resolution of impairments in joint motion and muscular strength in the early rehabilitation period.

After **arthroscopic débridement**, patients are usually permitted to bear weight as tolerated with crutches. Weight-bearing can be progressed as long as increased loading does not result in increased pain or effusion. Crutches can be discontinued when the patient has full passive knee extension and at least 100 degrees of knee flexion, can perform an SLR without an extensor lag, and can walk without pain or a limp.

When patients have undergone **abrasion arthroplasty, a microfracture procedure, fixation of an articular cartilage defect, or osteochondral grafting**, weight-bearing is usually delayed for 6 weeks to allow adequate initial healing of the lesion. Non–weight-bearing or touch-down weight-bearing with crutches is allowed in the immediate postoperative period. In some cases, depending on the location of the lesion or the stability of the fixation, partial weight-bearing or weight-bearing as tolerated with crutches may be permitted in conjunction with use of a rehabilitation brace locked in full knee extension. Progressive weight-bearing is usually initiated 6 weeks after surgery. At this time, fibrocartilage should have begun to fill in the articular defect, and an osteochondral graft or articular cartilage fragment should have united with adjacent subchondral bone. Crutches can be discontinued when the patient has full passive knee extension and at least 100 degrees of knee flexion, can perform an SLR without an extensor lag, and can walk without pain or a limp. Therapists should monitor patients for increases in pain or effusion during progressive weight-bearing and reduce the progression if these iatrogenic effects arise.

Progression from protected weight-bearing to full weight-bearing can be facilitated by using techniques that gradually increase the load on the knee. Deweighting devices can be used for treadmill ambulation and running. Unloading of body weight by the deweighting device is increased to the point that the activity can be performed without pain or gait abnormalities. The unloading is then gradually reduced over time until the patient can perform the activity in full weight-bearing without pain. A pool can also be used to unload body weight for ambulation and running activities. These activities can be initiated in shoulder-deep water and then gradually progressed by decreasing the depth of the water.

Once the patient has progressed to pain-free full weight-bearing, a variety of low-impact aerobic activities, such as walking, cycling, and the use of step or cross-country ski machines, can be performed to improve local muscular and cardiovascular endurance. Returning to sports activities may not be possible for some patients, depending on the severity of joint damage. These patients should be counseled with respect to appropriate activity modifications. For patients who wish to return to recreational or sports activities, a functional retraining program involving agility training and sport-specific skill training should be incorporated into the program. These activities should be delayed until the patient can perform low-impact aerobic activities without recurrent pain or effusion. Agility and sport-specific skill training should be progressed gradually from 50% to full effort. The therapist should continue to monitor the patient for changes in pain and effusion as these activities are progressed.

IMPORTANT REHABILITATION CONSIDERATIONS

- The surgeon should include on the physical therapy referral form the type of surgical procedure, the location of the lesion, and restrictions in ROM during exercise. A diagram of the lesion site is also helpful. Therapists must adhere to the surgeon's ROM limitations so that the lesion is not engaged during exercise.

- Unloaded passive or active-assisted ROM exercises should begin as soon as possible after surgery. Closed-chain exercises should be avoided in the first 6 weeks after surgery.
- Isometric exercises with the knee in full extension or 90 degrees of flexion should be emphasized for early strength training. Open-chain exercises can be performed in arcs of motion that do not engage the lesion.
- Protected weight-bearing with the use of crutches and, in some cases, a rehabilitation brace should be incorporated in the first 6 weeks after surgery. Assistive devices can be discontinued when the patient has full knee extension and 100 degrees of knee flexion, can perform an SLR without an extensor lag, and can walk without pain or a limp.
- Progression of weight-bearing activities can be made easier by gradually increasing the load on the knee. This can be accomplished with the use of deweighting devices or pool activities. A gradual progression of agility and sport-specific skill training should be completed before the patient is allowed to return to full sports activity.

REHABILITATION PROTOCOL

Our rehabilitation protocol is divided into three phases: early postoperative phase (0 to 6 weeks), intermediate phase (6 to 12 weeks), and return to activity phase (12 weeks and beyond). The time frames for these phases are only estimated guidelines. Progression to each phase depends on meeting criteria based on the type of surgical procedure, estimated periods of healing, restoration of joint mobility and strength, and potential recurrence of pain and joint effusion. Individual patients are able to progress at different intervals, and the surgeon and therapist are required to use their clinical judgments in determining when progression should be delayed or can be accelerated.

REHABILITATION PROTOCOL | *After Articular Cartilage Procedures*
Fitzgerald and Irrgang

EARLY POSTOPERATIVE PHASE (0-6 WEEKS)

	JOINT MOBILITY	MUSCLE PERFORMANCE	WEIGHT-BEARING
Arthroscopic Débridement	Passive and active-assisted ROM with no restrictions on ROM. Full knee extension should be obtained in 1 week and full flexion in 3 weeks	Initiate training with isometric exercises. May progress to open-chain resisted exercises* when tolerated. Closed-chain resisted exercises† are initiated when the patient meets criteria for full weight-bearing	Weight-bearing as tolerated with crutches until the patient has full extension, 100 degrees of flexion, and no knee extensor lag and ambulates without pain or effusion. Initiate low-impact aerobic

REHABILITATION PROTOCOL: *After Articular Cartilage Procedures*   Continued

EARLY POSTOPERATIVE PHASE (0-6 WEEKS)—cont'd

	JOINT MOBILITY	MUSCLE PERFORMANCE	WEIGHT-BEARING
			activities (walking program, stationary cycling, swimming) at 3-6 weeks, when the patient meets full weight-bearing status
Abrasion Arthroplasty, Subchondral Drilling, Microfracture Procedures	Passive and active-assisted ROM in pain-free range for 6 weeks. Full extension should be achieved in 1 week, full flexion in 3 weeks	Isometric exercises in ROM that does not engage the lesion site. Open-chain exercises with light resistance may be initiated at 4-6 weeks in ROM that does not engage the lesion site. Avoid closed-chain exercises	Non–weight-bearing or toe-touch weight-bearing with crutches
Osteochondral Grafts	Passive and active-assisted ROM in range restrictions that do not engage the lesion site. Full knee extension should be obtained in 1 week, full flexion in 6 weeks	Isometric exercises in ROM that does not engage the lesion site. Open-chain exercises with light resistance may be initiated at 4-6 weeks in ROM that does not engage the lesion site. Avoid closed-chain exercises	Non–weight-bearing or toe-touch weight-bearing with crutches
Osteotomy	Passive and active ROM exercises in pain-free ROM. Full knee extension should be achieved in 1 week, full flexion in 8 weeks	Isometric exercises for 4-6 weeks. No open- or closed-chain resisted exercises for 4-6 weeks to avoid loading across the full extension osteotomy site	Touch-down weight-bearing for the first 2 weeks, partial weight-bearing in 2-4 weeks, weight-bearing as tolerated with crutches in 4-8 weeks. Rehabilitation brace locked in full extension

Continued

REHABILITATION PROTOCOL: *After Articular Cartilage Procedures* *Continued*

INTERMEDIATE PHASE (6-12 WEEKS)

	JOINT MOBILITY AND MUSCLE PERFORMANCE	WEIGHT-BEARING AND FUNCTIONAL RETRAINING
Arthroscopic Débridement	Full motion should be achieved at this time. Continue with maintenance active ROM. Progress open- and closed-chain resistance exercises‡§ as tolerated	Agility‖ and sport-specific skill training initiated at 50% effort and progressed to full effort as tolerated. Initiate return to full activity when these activities to do not induce recurrent pain or effusion
Abrasion Arthroplasty, Subchondral Drilling, Microfracture Procedures	Progress to full-range active ROM. Progress loading of resistive exercises. May initiate closed-chain exercise when full weight-bearing is achieved. Restrict to ranges that do not engage the lesion site	Discontinue use of crutches at 6-8 weeks when the patient has achieved full knee extension, 100 degrees of flexion, and no extensor lag and can ambulate without pain or effusion. May use deweighting device or pool activities in making the transition to full weight-bearing
Osteochondral Grafts	Progress to full-range active ROM. Progress loading of resistive exercises. May initiate closed-chain exercise when full weight-bearing is achieved. Restrict to ranges that do not engage the lesion site	Discontinue use of crutches at 6-8 weeks when the patient has achieved full knee extension, 100 degrees of flexion, and no extensor lag and can ambulate without pain or effusion. May use deweighting device or pool activities in making the transition to full weight-bearing. Low-impact aerobic activities may be initiated when the patient achieves full weight-bearing status
Osteotomy	Progress to full-range active ROM. Progress loading of resistive exercises. May initiate closed-chain exercise when full weight-bearing is achieved. Restrict to ranges that do not engage the lesion site	Discontinue rehabilitation brace. Progress to full weight-bearing without crutches when the patient has achieved full knee extension, 100 degrees of flexion, and no extensor lag and can ambulate without pain or effusion. May use deweighting device or pool activities in making the transition to full weight-bearing. Low-impact aerobic activities may be initiated when the patient achieves full weight-bearing status

REHABILITATION PROTOCOL: *After Articular Cartilage Procedures* Continued

RETURN-TO-ACTIVITY PHASE (12 WEEKS AND BEYOND)

	JOINT MOBILITY AND MUSCLE PERFORMANCE	FUNCTIONAL RETRAINING AND RETURN TO ACTIVITY
Arthroscopic Débridement		Patients should have returned to full activity by this time
Abrasion Arthroplasty, Subchondral Drilling, Microfracture Procedures	Continue with maintenance full active ROM exercise. Continue with progression of resistance for open- and closed-chain exercises as tolerated in ranges that do not engage the lesion site	Initiate agility and sport-specific skill training when tolerating low-impact aerobic activities without recurrent pain or effusion. Agility and sport-specific skill training should be initiated at 50% effort and progressed to full effort as tolerated. Running should be delayed until 6 months after surgery. May initiate return to activity when tolerating running and agility and sport-specific skill training without recurrent pain or effusion
Osteochondral Grafts	Continue with maintenance full active ROM exercise. Continue with progression of resistance for open- and closed-chain exercises as tolerated in ranges that do not engage the lesion site or effusion	Initiate agility and sport-specific skill training when tolerating low-impact aerobic activities without recurrent pain or effusion. Agility and sport-specific skill training should be initiated at 50% effort and progressed to full effort as tolerated. Running should be delayed until 6 months after surgery. May initiate return to activity when tolerating running and agility and sport-specific skill training without recurrent pain
Osteotomy	Continue with maintenance full active ROM exercise. Continue with progression of resistance for open- and closed-chain exercises as tolerated in ranges that do not engage the lesion site	Initiate agility and sport-specific skill training when tolerating low-impact aerobic activities without recurrent pain or effusion. Agility and sport-specific skill training should be initiated at 50% effort and progressed to full effort as tolerated. Running should be delayed until 6 months after surgery.

Continued

REHABILITATION PROTOCOL: *After Articular Cartilage Procedures* Continued

---

RETURN-TO-ACTIVITY PHASE (12 WEEKS AND BEYOND)—cont'd

Joint Mobility and Muscle Performance	Functional Retraining and Return to Activity
	May initiate return to activity when tolerating running and agility and sport-specific skill training without recurrent pain or effusion

*Resisted open-chain exercises refer to non–weight-bearing leg extensions for quadriceps strengthening and leg curls for hamstring strengthening.
†Resisted closed-chain exercises include leg press, partial-range squats, wall slides, and step-ups.
‡Resisted open-chain exercises refer to non–weight-bearing leg extensions for quadriceps strengthening and leg curls for hamstring strengthening.
§Resisted closed-chain exercises include leg press, partial-range squats, wall slides, and step-ups.
‖Agility training includes activities such as side slides, cariocas, shuttle runs, cutting and pivoting drills, and figure-of-eight running.
¶A deweighting device is a pelvic harness that is suspended above the treadmill from a frame. Cables attached to the harness are connected to an electric motor that can be programmed to apply an upward-lifting load on the pelvis through the harness, which in turn will reduce the loading effect of the patient's body weight on the lower extremities while the patient is ambulating on the treadmill. The upward-lifting load is set high enough to allow performance of walking on the treadmill without reproducing the patient's pain. Treatment is progressed over a period of several sessions by gradually reducing the upward-lifting load as tolerated by the patient until the patient is able to ambulate in full weight-bearing on the treadmill without pain.

TROUBLESHOOTING TECHNIQUES AFTER ARTICULAR CARTILAGE PROCEDURES

Pain and Effusion with Exercise or Activity Progression

Monitoring of pain and effusion in response to exercise or activity progression is important to maintain a safe and effective rehabilitation process. Pain and effusion in response to exercise may indicate that the articular lesion is being harmed or the intensity of exercise is too rigorous. Therapists should reconsider the ROM restrictions that are being used and perhaps modify them to re-establish pain-free ranges. The frequency and duration of joint mobility exercises or the magnitude of loading during resistance exercises may also have to be reduced.

Recurrence of pain and effusion during progression of weight-bearing or functional retraining activities indicates that the joint is not ready to progress to higher levels of activity. Progression of activity may need to be delayed in these circumstances.

Footwear and activity surface types should also be considered. Patients may need to obtain footwear that provides better cushioning or biomechanical foot orthotics to compensate for faulty foot mechanics. Activities may need to be begun on softer surfaces to acclimate to more rigorous ground reaction forces as higher activity levels are introduced.

Persistent effusion in the early postoperative period may result in quadriceps inhibition (reduced ability to voluntarily activate the quadriceps muscles). This can significantly retard progress with the rehabilitation program. Use of cold treatments, compression bandaging, limb elevation, and intermittent isometric contractions of the thigh and leg muscles may help resolve problems with effusion. If significant effusion persists more than 1 or 2 weeks after surgery, the therapist should notify the surgeon.

Quadriceps Inhibition or Persistent Knee Extensor Lag

Some patients may have difficulty with voluntary activation of the quadriceps muscles after surgery. This problem may be indicated by an inability to perform a full, sustained, isometric quadriceps contraction or the presence of a knee extensor lag on SLR. If patients exhibit this problem, they may not respond well to voluntary exercises alone. In addition, prolonged inability to actively achieve full knee extension may result in a knee flexion contracture that could, in turn, result in gait abnormalities and excessive loading of the knee during weight-bearing activities. Other treatment adjuncts to enhance quadriceps muscle activation, such as *neuromuscular electrical stimulation or EMG biofeedback*, may need to be incorporated into the program. If these treatment adjuncts are administered, the intensity of the treatment stimulus should be great enough to produce a full, sustained contraction of the quadriceps as evidenced by superior glide of the patella during the quadriceps contraction. Superior glide of the patella is important to prevent patellar entrapment in the intercondylar groove, which may sometimes be a causative factor in knee extensor lag.

Baker's (Popliteal) Cyst

S. Brent Brotzman, MD

CLINICAL BACKGROUND

Popliteal cysts are often referred to by the eponym "Baker's cyst." In 1877, Baker described an enlarged popliteal cyst formed by trapping of fluid in a bursa related to the semimembranosus tendon. He noted *communication between the cyst and the joint* synovium with fluid that leaks into the bursa but cannot flow back in the reverse direction (see Fig. 4-4).

Wilson, in 1938, noted that the bursa under the medial head of the gastrocnemius and the bursa under the semimembranosus often had connections and concluded that a popliteal cyst arose from distention of the gastrocnemius-semimembranosus bursa. In a dissection study, Taylor and Rana (1973) found that a large number of popliteal cysts had a valvular communication between the medial gastrocnemius bursa and the knee joint. Lindgren (1977) demonstrated that with increased age, the frequency of communication of the bursa with the joint increased, which he believed to be secondary to thinning of the posterior joint capsule.

The term "Baker's cyst" describes cysts that occur on the posteromedial aspect of the knee between the medial head of the gastrocnemius and the semimembranosus tendon.

Popliteal cysts are frequently associated with intra-articular pathology. Meniscal tears, rheumatoid arthritis, osteoarthritis, conditions causing synovitis, Charcot joints, and tuberculosis have all been reported to be associated with the formation of popliteal cysts. Fielding and coworkers (1991) found that 82% of popliteal cysts were associated with a meniscal tear, commonly a tear of the posterior portion of the medial meniscus. Only 38% of tears involved the lateral meniscus. ACL tears were present in 13% of subjects. They also found that the overall prevalence of popliteal cysts was 5% and increased with older age.

CLINICAL FINDINGS

Popliteal cysts are typically manifested as a mass in the posteromedial aspect of the knee. In the rare pediatric patient with a popliteal cyst, the mass is generally asymptomatic and is noticed by the patient, who is concerned about the prominence of the posterior popliteal fossa. In adults, the complaint is typically an achy sensation and fullness in the back of the knee that is exacerbated with exercise or activities that involve significant flexion and extension. These symptoms are often accompanied by symptoms from the underlying pathologic condition, such as a meniscal tear, torn ACL, or degenerative arthritis.

Rupture of a popliteal cyst may occur suddenly and cause severe pain and swelling in the calf region. This combination has been called the "**pseudothrombophlebitis syndrome**" because the signs and symptoms of a ruptured popliteal cyst are identical to those of thrombophlebitis, with a positive Homans sign and tenderness in the posterior aspect of the calf.

Venous Doppler sonography or venography should be used to rule out thrombophlebitis. On clinical examination, a hard cord corresponding to the thrombosed vein may be palpable in patients with thrombophlebitis but is not present in those with a ruptured popliteal cyst; however, it is not easily palpated in some patients.

The differential diagnosis of popliteal cysts includes fibrosarcoma, synovial sarcoma, malignant fibrohistiocytoma, and degenerative meniscal cysts.

Because of the associated high incidence of intra-articular pathology with Baker's cysts, MRI is recommended in the evaluation of popliteal cysts.

On MRI, *degenerative meniscal cysts* typically have a communicating peripheral tear and are more medial or lateral than a true popliteal cyst. MRI can also distinguish popliteal cysts from solid lesions or tumors in the popliteal area. Because of the cyst's high content of free water, MRI typically shows features of a low signal intensity on T1-weighted images and high signal intensity on T2-weighted images. Septa are often present within popliteal cysts, as well as hemorrhage, loose bodies, and debris.

TREATMENT

In *children*, popliteal cysts are generally benign, asymptomatic, self-limited, and rarely associated with intra-articular pathology. MRI is typically recommended to confirm the diagnosis and rule out a soft tissue tumor. Because most popliteal cysts in children resolve spontaneously, surgery is not indicated.

In *adults*, injection of steroids into the cyst has been recommended. This is usually just a temporizing measure, and the cyst recurs unless the associated intra-articular disorder is corrected.

If MRI is negative for intra-articular pathology, the cyst is treated symptomatically and monitored conservatively. *Arthroscopic evaluation* is indicated if MRI reveals an intra-articular lesion causing mechanical symptoms that do not respond to nonsurgical management (anti-inflammatory agents, compression sleeves, and physical therapy). If pain or persistent swelling interferes with activities of daily living despite conservative measures, surgical treatment is indicated. If arthroscopic intervention does not relieve the symptoms, open excision may be necessary. The stalk leading from the joint to the cyst is located and sutured or cauterized, and the cyst is removed. The reported recurrence rate after open popliteal cyst excision varies widely, with some studies reporting frequent recurrences.

Treatment of the intra-articular disorder often leads to resolution of the popliteal cyst. Jayson (1972) reported good results with anterior synovectomy in patients with rheumatoid arthritis and popliteal cysts.

Open Surgical Technique

Hughston and colleagues (1991) described a surgical procedure in a series of 30 patients with only two recurrences. The procedure is performed via a posteromedial approach through a medial hockey-stick incision with the knee flexed at 90 degrees (Fig. 4-63). The capsular incision begins between the medial epicondyle and the adductor tubercle and is extended distally along the posterior edge of the tibial

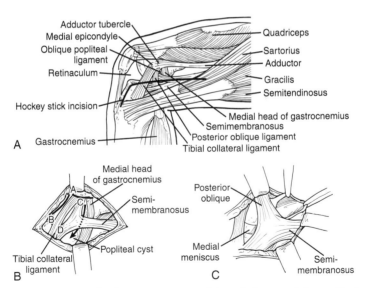

Figure 4–63 Hughston and colleagues' posteromedial surgical approach for popliteal cyst incision. **A,** Medial hockey-stick incision and the underlying anatomic structures in the right knee. **B,** Area exposed by the incision. The skin and subcutaneous tissues have been removed to demonstrate the relationship of the popliteal cyst to the anterior medial retinacular incision (A-B) and the posterior capsular incision (C-D). The posterior oblique ligament can be retracted posteriorly for inspection of the medial meniscus and the intra-articular aspect of the posterior capsule. **C,** Opening plus retraction of the cyst demonstrates adherence to the surrounding tissues. The cyst can then be isolated and excised in its entirety. (Adapted from Curl WW: Popliteal cysts: historical background and current knowledge. J Am Acad Orthop Surg 4[3]129-133, 1996.)

collateral ligament (anterior to the popliteal oblique ligament). The popliteal oblique ligament is retracted posteriorly. The cyst is found between the semimembranosus tendon and the medial head of the gastrocnemius. The cyst is dissected free of its surrounding adhesions and excised with the capsular origin of the cyst identified. The rent in the capsule is repaired with nonabsorbable suture and can be reinforced with a pedicle flap from the medial head of the gastrocnemius as described by Rauschning (1980).

POSTOPERATIVE REHABILITATION

After the wound is closed, the knee is immobilized in a large hinged cast, which is worn for 2 to 3 days with crutch-assisted weight-bearing as tolerated. For the first few days after surgery, SLR and gentle ankle pumps are done and icing is used for edema and pain control. Gentle active ROM of the knee is begun between postoperative days 3 and 7, with care taken to *avoid excess tension* on the medial hockey-stick incision.

Patellar Fractures

S. Brent Brotzman, MD

ANATOMY AND BACKGROUND

- The patella is the largest human sesamoid bone and a very important *functional* component of the extensor mechanism.
- The patella serves to increase the magnitude of the quadriceps moment arm. The contribution to the increase in extension "strength" made by the patella is enhanced with progressive extension of the knee, being almost 30% at full extension.

For this reason, total patellectomy should be avoided in the treatment of patellar fractures if possible.

- The patella is subject to complex loading. In knee *extension*, the patella is loaded primarily in tension. However, in knee *flexion*, the articular surface contacts the distal end of the femur and is subject to compressive force, termed *patellofemoral joint reactive force* (PFJRF) (see Fig. 4-45).

EVALUATION

- A history of a direct blow, a severe muscle contraction, or an unexpected, rapid knee flexion while the quadriceps was contracted is often elicited.
- The examiner should look for a possible palpable defect of the patella, localized contusion or tenderness over the patella, weak extension of the knee, or inability to actively extend the knee (i.e., perform an SLR).

Inability to perform active extension of the knee with radiographic evidence of a displaced patellar fracture is an absolute indication for surgical open reduction and internal fixation or surgical repair of a patellar fracture in an operative candidate. Operative intervention may include open reduction with internal fixation and partial patellectomy.

Bipartite Patella

- Secondary ossification centers that never fused to the body of the patella may sometimes be confused with the rare marginal or peripheral fracture. **Obtaining radiographs of the opposite patella** is often helpful in this differentiation **because bipartite patellas almost never occur unilaterally**. Bipartite patellas are typically *not tender on palpation* of the suspicious area, in contrast to a marginal or peripheral fracture.

CLASSIFICATION

Patellar fractures are classified according to their *mechanism of injury* (direct and indirect) and *fracture morphology*.

Direct blows (e.g., dashboard) usually cause significant comminution but often little displacement. The important articular cartilage of the contact area is typically significantly injured by this type of mechanism.

Indirect blows (e.g., jumping) are usually less comminuted than those from direct blows, but they are often displaced and transverse. The articular cartilage is less damaged than with direct blows.

To help in treatment planning, patellar fractures are classified morphologically (Fig. 4-64).

- *Transverse* fractures occur in the medial-lateral direction. They are usually found in the central or distal third of the patella. Displaced transverse patella fractures typically require open reduction and internal fixation; nondisplaced transverse fractures are generally treated nonoperatively.
- *Vertical* fractures are rare and occur in the superior-inferior direction. Usually, the extensor mechanism remains intact (nonoperative treatment).
- *Marginal* fractures occur at the edge of the patella and do not disrupt the function of the extensor mechanism (nonoperative).

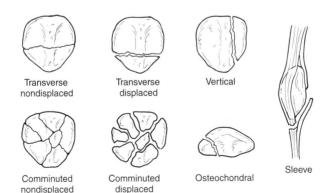

Figure 4–64 Patellar fractures are classified according to their radiographic pattern. Displaced fractures are treated surgically. Nondisplaced fractures in patients with the ability to perform a straight-leg raise are generally treated nonoperatively. (Adapted from Carpenter JE, Matthews LS: When the kneecap and kneecap extensors are injured. J Musculoskel Med 14[2]:83-90, 1997. Artist: Charles H. Boyter.)

- *Sleeve* fractures typically occur in children. The inferior (or occasionally superior) pole of the patella is pulled off (avulsion) with a large amount of important articular cartilage that is very hard to identify radiographically. The diagnosis of a sleeve fracture is generally made by clinical findings of local pain and tenderness, inability to fully actively extend the knee, and radiographs showing a high-riding patella (alta) in comparison to the uninjured side. We follow Houghton and Ackroyd's (1979) recommendation of operative treatment of these fractures.
- *Osteochondral* fractures include sleeve fractures (see above) and osteochondral fragments as a result of a patellar dislocation or direct blow. The latter types may result in a displaced fragment that becomes a troublesome loose body (surgical excision or transosseous fixation of large fragments) or result in a fracture fragment that never becomes displaced (nonoperative treatment).

RADIOGRAPHS

AP, lateral, and "sunrise" views of the knee should be taken. On the lateral view, Insall's method (see Fig. 4-2B) of assessing patellar height should be used to rule out associated patellar tendon rupture with its resultant "patella alta" as the unopposed quadriceps pulls the patella superiorly.

The length of the patellar tendon (from the distal pole of the patella to the tibial tubercle) is measured and compared with the height of the patella. If the ratio of patella to patellar tendon height is less than 0.8, the patella is too high (i.e., patella alta) and a patellar tendon rupture with proximal retraction is suspected.

The sunrise view most commonly used is Merchant's (45 degrees of knee flexion).

TREATMENT

Restoration of articular congruity of the articular portion of the patella is very important to avoid post-traumatic arthritis.

- The most important factors in the treatment of patella fractures are restoration of articular congruity and retaining the ability to actively extend the knee.

Patellar fractures with articular incongruity (step-off) of more than 2 mm or separation (displacement) of the two fragments (inferior and superior pole) of more than 3 mm require surgical treatment. Lack of ability to actively extend the knee (disruption of the extensor mechanism) is also a surgical indication.

Nonoperative Treatment

- Nonoperative treatment is indicated for most vertical fractures, nondisplaced fractures, and fractures with less than 2 mm of articular incongruity of the articular surface (step-off) and an intact extensor mechanism on SLR testing. For example, a patient with a nondisplaced, transverse fracture who can perform an SLR is treated nonoperatively.
- Frequently, a few degrees of extreme flexion are lost with nonoperative treatment, but patient satisfaction is high (>95%). Bostrom (1972) reported slight or no pain in 89% of these patients and normal or slightly impaired function in 91%. Ninety percent of nonoperative patients had 0 to 120 degrees of ROM.

- Four to 6 weeks of immobilization in extension in a cast or large hinged brace followed by gentle, progressive ROM exercises and, later, quadriceps strengthening exercises.

REHABILITATION PROTOCOL   *Nonoperative Patellar Fracture*

WEEKS 0-6

- Continue icing until the effusion resolves.
- Wear a straight-leg cylinder cast for 2-3 weeks or controlled motion brace locked at 0 degrees in a very compliant patient.
- Allow weight-bearing to tolerance with crutches.
- Employ a $1/4$-inch heel lift (shoe insert) on the *contralateral* extremity to help with ground clearance of the involved "stiff" leg.
- Begin quadriceps sets, gluteal sets, hamstring sets, and SLR in all planes (supine and standing) before discharge from the hospital (quadriceps sets help decrease adhesion formation during the healing process).
- May begin open- and closed-chain exercises with the cast on, especially for hip strengthening.
- Replace the cast with a controlled motion brace at 2-3 weeks.
- Begin electrical muscle stimulation for quadriceps re-education.
- Progress weight-bearing to tolerance with crutches to weight-bearing with the use of a cane.
- In general, begin strengthening and ROM exercises at week 3 or 4 (open- and closed-chain exercises).
- Begin gentle patellar mobilization; the patient should be independent with this exercise.
- At approximately 6 weeks, begin stationary bicycling with the seat elevated and no resistance for ROM and strengthening.
- Begin isokinetic exercises at speeds of 60-120 degrees/sec to strengthen the quadriceps musculature and decrease the forces on the patellofemoral joint that occur at lower speeds.
- Use stool scoots for hamstring strengthening.

WEEKS 6-12

- Begin and progress closed-chain exercises, such as 40-degree mini-squats and step-ups.
- May use a Thera-Band for resistance in hip exercises and mini-squats.
- Start BAPS board exercises.
- Begin lunges (usually in 8-10 weeks).
- Can use stationary bicycling with the affected leg only, with resistance added to aid strengthening.
- Because some degree of chondromalacia eventually develops in most patients with patellar fractures, emphasize that restoration of quadriceps strength is essential to assist in the absorption of body weight load that is transmitted up the kinetic chain.
- The exercise program should emphasize restoration of lower extremity strength and flexibility. After this is achieved, implement a maintenance program with emphasis on closed-chain exercises. All exercises should be performed in pain-free ROM.
- Evaluate the entire lower extremity, especially for excessive pronation of the feet, which adds stress to the knee and exacerbates patellofemoral-type symptoms. Use orthotics if excessive pronation is noted.

Operative Treatment

Most patellar fractures will be treated operatively.

Treatment is aimed at preservation of patellar function whenever possible, preferably through open reduction and internal fixation if bone quality allows. Restoring articular congruity is key to avoiding post-traumatic arthritis.

- It is important to obtain secure, stable fixation for anticipated knee motion during rehabilitation. If significant or poor bone quality exists, a major (usually superior) fragment with a large amount of articular cartilage is retained and a partial patellectomy is performed (Fig. 4-65).

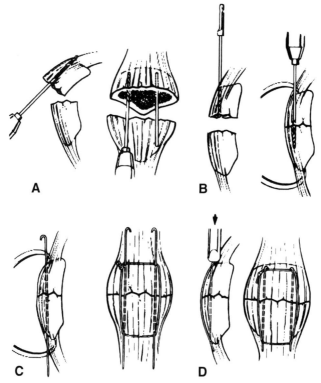

Figure 4–65 Modified AO tension band technique for patellar fracture fixation (see text). **A,** Retrograde drilling of the proximal fragment. K-wires mark the proximal ends of the holes during reduction. **B,** Reduction, clamping, and antegrade partial drilling of the distal fragment. K-wires with prebent proximal ends are then hammered through the remaining bone of the distal pole. **C,** With a large-bore needle, the 1.2-mm tension band wire is placed deep to the proximal and distal ends of the K-wires immediately adjacent to the patella, through the stout soft tissue attachments of the quadriceps tendon and patellar ligament. Medially and laterally, the tension band wire lies anterior to the patella and usually is not crossed. It is tightened and twisted securely, and the "pigtail" end is bent flush with the bone surface. A twist or a square knot is reliable. The AO bent wire fastening technique is not secure enough for definitive fixation. **D,** The prebent proximal ends of the K-wires are driven into the proximal pole, and the distal ends are trimmed if necessary. (From Sanders R, Gregory PR: Patellar fractures and extensor mechanism injuries. In Browner BD, Jupiter JB, Levine AM, Trafton PG [eds]: Skeletal Trauma, 2nd ed. Philadelphia, WB Saunders, 1998.)

Patellar Operative Technique (General Principles)

- Minimize further soft tissue trauma caused by excess knee flexion, direct contact with ice, or splints with excessive compression.
- If a tense hematoma is stretching the anterior skin, consider hematoma aspiration.
- Use of a *longitudinal* incision (not transverse). Although transverse incisions are better from a cosmetic standpoint, this incision can seldom be used in future procedures (slough possible later).
- Avoid excess retractor tension or prolonged retraction during surgery.
- Often, comminution (especially inferior pole) is underestimated on radiographs, and thus intraoperative reassessment is vital.
- **Partial patellectomy with patellar tendon repair is preferable to tenuous open reduction and internal fixation of comminuted soft bone.**
- Fractures with some comminution may frequently be converted to a simple transverse fracture by lag screw fixation of the comminuted fragments.

The most important goal is restoration of articular congruity under direct visualization and palpation.

- Extension of the exposure with a small medial parapatellar capsular incision to allow *direct* visualization and palpation of the articular congruity is recommended.
- A modified tension band technique is currently the most widely accepted operative technique.
- The anterior tension band (18-gauge wire looped over Kirschner wires and over the anterior aspect of the patella) acts to neutralize the large distraction force across the patella with quadriceps contraction and knee flexion.
- Avoid making the most common error in the tension band technique: failure to bring the tension board *directly* into contact with the distal and proximal poles of the patella so that intervening soft tissue is left.
- Irrigate and remove all comminuted fragments and debris that may later act as loose bodies intra-articularly.
- Place the knee through gentle ROM intraoperatively after operative fixation to observe the stability of the surgical construct. Document the degree of flexion at which the repair is stable (e.g., 90 degrees) and inform the therapist.

Partial Patellectomy

- No. 2 braided polyester suture is used to reattach the patellar tendon to the patella through multiple drill holes.
- Preserve as much of the length of the patellar tendon as possible.
- The holes drilled through the patella should enter as close to the articular surface as possible so that there is minimal step-off between the tendon and the remaining patellar articular cartilage.
- Postoperative complications can be minimized by careful attention to wound care, accurate fracture reduction, secure fixation, and early ROM.

Postoperative Management (General Principles)

- Monitor the wound closely postoperatively.
- It is essentially impossible to completely unload the patella postoperatively. The fracture is loaded with each quadriceps contraction.
- **Weight-bearing itself does not increase quadriceps force; therefore, weight-bearing with the use of a brace locked in extension is permitted.**

REHABILITATION PROTOCOL	*After Open Reduction and Internal Fixation of Patellar Fracture*

S. Brent Brotzman, MD

Note: Rehabilitation protocols vary depending on the type of fracture, the surgical technique, and the rehabilitation philosophy of the surgeon. Gentle ROM intraoperatively after tension band wiring (or partial patellectomy) is often performed to observe the stability of the fracture and construct. This information (e.g., stable to 90 degrees of flexion) is helpful for timing of postoperative ROM progression. Document the degrees of flexion reached intraoperatively with good stability of the construct and give to the therapist.

POSTOPERATIVE DAYS 1-7

- Weight-bearing as tolerated with crutches or a walker with a long-leg straight-leg cylinder cast or commercial full-length knee brace locked in extension (0 degrees). The brace may be unlocked during ambulation at approximately 3 weeks if good quadriceps control is present.
- Maximal elevation plus ice for 3-5 days.
- Gentle quad sets, SLR if the surgeon believes that the construct is *very* stable.
- Use heel elevation for the *contralateral* shoe to help ground clearance of the involved straight-leg cast during ambulation.

WEEKS 2-6

- Begin gentle patellar mobilization exercises; the patient should become independent in this exercise.
- Electrical muscle stimulation for quadriceps re-education.
- Stationary bicycling with the seat elevated and no resistance. Begin at 5-6 weeks.

WEEK 6

- Ensure radiographic evidence of fracture healing before progression.
- Progress isometric exercises with 1- to 2-pound weights on the thigh for SLR.
- Perform stool scoots.
- Increase bicycling distance, speed, and endurance.
- Begin gentle closed-chain exercises.
  - 30-degree mini-squats
  - Wall sits
  - Stool scoots
  - Lateral step-ups (4-inch platform)
- Perform hamstring curls with 2-5 pounds at the ankle.
- We use a hinged brace until the patient reaches 90 degrees of flexion and has excellent quadriceps control.

Bibliography

KNEE LIGAMENTS/MENISCAL/ANTERIOR KNEE PAIN

Aglietti P, Insall JN, Cerulli G: Patellar pain and incongruence. I: Measurements of incongruence. Clin Orthop 176:217-224, 1983.

Ahmed AM: The load-bearing role of the knee menisci. In Mow VC, Arnoczky SP, Jackson DW (eds): Knee Meniscus: Basic and Clinical Foundations. New York, Raven Press, 1992, pp 59-73.

Ahmed AM: Burke DL, Hyder A: Force analysis of the patellar mechanism. J Orthop Res 5:69-85, 1987.

Anderson AF, Lipscomb AB: Analysis of rehabilitation techniques after anterior cruciate reconstruction. Am J Sports Med 17:154-160, 1989.

Anderson DR, Weiss JA, Takai S, et al: Healing of the MCL following a triad injury: A biomechanical and histological study of the knee in rabbits. J Orthop Res 10:485-495, 1992.

Arms S, Boyle J, Johnson R, Pope M: Strain measurement in the medial collateral ligament of the human knee: An autopsy study. J Biomech 16:491-496, 1983.

Arnoczky SP: Meniscus. In Fu FH, Harner CD, Vince KG (eds). Knee Surgery. Baltimore, Williams & Wilkins, 1994, pp 131-140.

Arnoczky SP, Tarvin GB, Marshall JL: Anterior cruciate ligament replacement using patellar tendon: An evaluation of graft revascularization in the dog. J Bone Joint Surg Am 64:217-224, 1982.

Arnoczky SP, Warren RF: Microvasculature of the human meniscus. Am J Sports Med 10:90-95, 1982.

Bach BR Jr, Levy ME, Bojchuk J, et al: Single-incision endoscopic anterior cruciate ligament reconstruction using patellar tendon autograft—minimum two year follow-up evaluation. Am J Sports Med 26: 30-40, 1998.

Bach BR Jr, Tradonsky S, Bojchuk J, et al: Arthroscopically assisted anterior cruciate ligament reconstruction using patellar tendon autograft. Am J Sports Med 26:20-29, 1998.

Ballock RT, Woo SL-Y, Lyon RM, et al: Use of patellar tendon autograft for anterior cruciate ligament reconstruction in the rabbit: A long term histological and biomechanical study. J Orthop Res 7: 474-485, 1989.

Barber FA: Accelerated rehabilitation for meniscus repairs. Arthroscopy 10:206-210, 1994.

Barber FA, Click SD: Meniscus repair rehabilitation with concurrent anterior cruciate reconstruction. Arthroscopy 13:433-437, 1997.

Barber FA, Elrod BF, McGuire DA, Paulos LE: Is an anterior cruciate ligament reconstruction outcome age dependent? Arthroscopy 12:720-725, 1996.

Barber-Westin SD, Noyes FR, Heckmann TP, Shaffer BL: The effect of exercise and rehabilitation on anterior-posterior knee displacements after anterior cruciate ligament autograft reconstruction. Am J Sports Med 27:84-93, 1999.

Barrack RL, Skinner HB, Buckley SL: Proprioception in the anterior cruciate deficient knee. Am J Sports Med 17:1-6, 1989.

Barratta R, Solomonow M, Zhou BH, et al: Muscular coactivation: The role of the antagonist musculature in maintaining knee stability. Am J Sports Med 16:113-122, 1988.

Barrett DS: Proprioception and function after anterior cruciate ligament reconstruction. J Bone Joint Surg Br 73:833-837, 1991.

Beard DJ, Kyberd PJ, Ferguson CM, Dodd CAF: Proprioception enhancement for ACL deficiency: A prospective randomized trial of two physiotherapy regimens. J Bone Joint Surg Br 76:654-659, 1994.

Bell DG, Jacobs I: Electro-mechanical response times and rate of force development in males and females. Med Sci Sports Exerc 18:31-36, 1986.

Bellemans J, Cauwenberghs F, Brys P, et al: Fracture of the proximal tibia after Fulkerson anteromedial tibial tubercle transfer. Am J Sports Med 26:300-302, 1998.

Beynnon BD, Fleming BC: Anterior cruciate ligament strain in-vivo: A review of previous work. J Biomech 31:519-525, 1998.

Beynnon BD, Johnson RJ: Anterior cruciate ligament injury rehabilitation in athletes: Biomechanical considerations. Sports Med 22:54-64, 1996.

Beynnon BD, Johnson RJ, Fleming BC, et al: The effect of functional knee bracing on the anterior cruciate ligament in the weightbearing and nonweightbearing knee. Am J Sports Med 25:353-359, 1997.

Blazina ME, Kerlan RK, Jobe FW, et al: Jumper's knee. Orthop Clin North Am 4:665-673, 1973.

Bockrath K, Wooden C, Worrell T, et al: Effects of patella taping on patella position and perceived pain. Med Sci Sports Exerc 25:989-992, 1993.

Bolgla LA, Keskula DR: Reliability of lower extremity functional performance tests. J Orthop Sports Phys Ther 26:138-142, 1997.

Bose K, Kanagasuntheram R, Osman MBH: Vastus medialis obliquus: An anatomic and physiologic study. Orthopedics 3:880-883, 1980.

Boynton MD, Tietjens BR: Long-term followup of the untreated isolated posterior cruciate ligament–deficient knee. Am J Sports Med 24:306-310, 1996.

Brody LT, Thein JM: Nonoperative treatment for patellofemoral pain. J Orthop Sports Phys Ther 28: 336-344, 1998.

Bush-Joseph CA, Bach BR Jr: Arthroscopic assisted posterior cruciate ligament reconstruction using patellar tendon autograft. Sports Med Arthrosc Rev 2:106-119, 1994.

Butler DL, Grood ES, Noyes FR, Sodd AN: On the interpretation of our ACL data. Clin Orthop 196: 26-34, 1985.

Butler DL, Guan Y, Kay MD, et al: Location-dependent variations in the material properties of the anterior cruciate ligament. J Biomech 25:511-518, 1992.

Butler DL, Noyes FR, Grood ES: Ligamentous restraints to anterior-posterior drawer in the human knee. J Bone Joint Surg Am 62:259-270, 1980.

Bylski-Austrow DI, Ciarelli MJ, Kayner DC, et al: Displacements of the menisci under joint load: An in vitro study in human knees. J Biomech 27:421-431, 1994.

Caborn DNM, Coen M, Neef R, et al: Quadrupled semitendinosus-gracilis autograft fixation in the femoral tunnel: A comparison between a metal and a bioabsorbable interference screw. Arthroscopy 14:241-245, 1998.

Caborn DNM, Urban WP Jr, Johnson DL, et al: Biomechanical comparison between BioScrew and titanium alloy interference screws for bone–patellar tendon–bone graft fixation in anterior cruciate ligament reconstruction. Arthroscopy 13:229-232, 1997.

Caylor D, Fites R, Worrell TW: The relationship between the quadriceps angle and anterior knee pain syndrome. J Orthop Sports Phys Ther 17:11-16, 1993.

Cerny K: Vastus medialis oblique/vastus lateralis muscle activity ratios for selected exercises in persons with and without patellofemoral pain syndrome. Phys Ther 75:672-683, 1995.

Chang PCC, Lee LKH, Tay BK: Anterior knee pain in the military population. Ann Acad Med Singapore 26:60-63, 1997.

Clancy WG Jr, Shelbourne KD, Zoellner GB, et al: Treatment of knee joint instability secondary to rupture of the posterior cruciate ligament: Report of a new procedure. J Bone Joint Surg Am 65:310-322, 1983.

Cohn BT, Draeger RI, Jackson DW: The effects of cold therapy in the postoperative management of pain in patients undergoing anterior cruciate ligament reconstruction. Am J Sports Med 17:344-349, 1989.

Colby SM, Hintermeister RA, Torry MR, Steadman JR: Lower limb stability with ACL impairment. J Orthop Sports Phys Ther 29:444-451, 1999.

Conlan T, Garth WP Jr, Lemons JE: Evaluation of the medial soft-tissue restraints of the extensor mechanism of the knee. J Bone Joint Surg Am 75:682-693, 1993.

Cooper DE, Xianghua HD, Burstein AL, Warren RF: The strength of the central third patellar tendon graft. Am J Sports Med 21:818-824, 1993.

Corry IS, Webb JM, Clingeleffer AJ, Pinczewski LA: Arthroscopic reconstruction of the anterior cruciate ligament: A comparison of patellar tendon autograft and four-strand hamstring tendon autograft. Am J Sports Med 27:444-454, 1999.

Cosgarea AJ, Sebastianelli WJ, DeHaven KE: Prevention of arthrofibrosis after anterior cruciate ligament reconstruction using the central third patellar tendon autograft. Am J Sports Med 23:87-92, 1995.

Cross MJ, Powell JF: Long-term followup of posterior cruciate ligament rupture. Am J Sports Med 12: 292-297, 1984.

Denham RA, Bishop RED: Mechanics of the knee and problems in reconstructive surgery. J Bone Joint Surg Br 60:345-351, 1978.

Doucette SA, Child DP: The effect of open and closed chain exercise and knee joint position on patellar tracking in lateral patellar compression syndrome. J Orthop Sports Phys Ther 23:104-110, 1996.

Doucette SA, Goble EM: The effect of exercise on patellar tracking in lateral patellar compression syndrome. Am J Sports Med 20:434-440, 1992.

Dowdy PA, Miniaci A, Arnoczky SP, et al: The effect of cast immobilization on meniscal healing: An experimental study in the dog. Am J Sports Med 23:721-728, 1995.

Dye SF: The knee as a biologic transmission with an envelope of function: A theory. Clin Orthop 325: 10-8, 1996.

Eng JJ, Pierrynowski MR: Evaluation of soft foot orthotics in the treatment of patellofemoral pain syndrome. Phys Ther 73:62-70, 1993.

Engle CP, Noguchi M, Ohland KJ, et al: Healing of the rabbit medial collateral ligament following an O'Donoghue triad injury: The effects of anterior cruciate ligament reconstruction. J Orthop Res 12:357-364, 1994.

Escamilla RF, Fleisig GS, Zheng N, et al: Biomechanics of the knee during closed kinetic chain and open kinetic chain exercises. Med Sci Sports Exerc 30:556-569, 1998.

Falconiero RP, DiStefano VJ, Cook TM: Revascularization and ligamentization of autogenous anterior cruciate ligament grafts in humans. Arthroscopy 14:197-205, 1998.

Feretti A: Epidemiology of jumper's knee. Sports Med 3:289-295, 1986.

Fetto JF, Marshall JL: Medial collateral ligament injuries of the knee: A rationale for treatment. Clin Orthop 132:206-218, 1978.

Frank CB, Jackson DW: The science of reconstruction of the anterior cruciate ligament. J Bone Joint Surg Am 79:1556-1576, 1997.

Fukibayashi T, Torzilli PA, Sherman MF, Warren RF: An in-vitro biomechanical evaluation of anterior-posterior motion of the knee. J Bone Joint Surg Am 64:258-264, 1982.

Fulkerson JP, Kalenak A, Rosenberg TD, Cox JS: Patellofemoral pain. Instr Course Lect 41:57-70, 1992.

Gerrard B: The patellofemoral pain syndrome in young, active patients: A prospective study. Clin Orthop 179:129-133, 1989.

Gilleard W, McConnell J, Parsons D: The effect of patellar taping on the onset of vastus medialis obliquus and vastus lateralis muscle activity in persons with patellofemoral pain. Phys Ther 78:25-31, 1998.

Giove TP, Miller SJ III, Kent BE, et al: Non-operative treatment of the torn anterior cruciate ligament. J Bone Joint Surg Am 65:184-192, 1983.

Giurea M, Zorilla P, Amis AA, Aichroth P: Comparative pull-out and cyclic-loading strength tests of anchorage of hamstring tendon grafts in anterior cruciate ligament reconstruction. Am J Sports Med 27:621-625, 1999.

Goldfuss AJ, Morehouse CA, LeVeau BF: Effect of muscular tension on knee stability. Med Sci Sports Exerc 5:267-271, 1973.

Gollehon DL, Torzilli PA, Warren RF: The role of the posterolateral and cruciate ligaments in the stability of the human knee: A biomechanical study. J Bone Joint Surg Am 69:233-242, 1987.

Gomez MA, Woo SL-Y, Amiel D, et al: The effects of increased tension on healing medial collateral ligaments. Am J Sports Med 19:347-354, 1991.

Goodfellow J, Hungerford DS, Zindel M: Patello-femoral mechanics and pathology. I: Functional anatomy of the patello-femoral joint. J Bone Joint Surg Br 58:287-290, 1976.

Grabiner MD, Koh TJ, Draganich LF: Neuromechanics of the patellofemoral joint. Med Sci Sports Exerc 26:10-21, 1994.

Greenwald AE, Bagley AM, France EP, et al: A biomechanical and clinical evaluation of a patellofemoral knee brace. Clin Orthop 324:187-195, 1996.

Grelsamer RP, Klein JR: The biomechanics of the patellofemoral joint. J Orthop Sports Phys Ther 28:286-298, 1998.

Grood ES, Noyes FR, Butler DL, et al: Ligamentous and capsular restraints preventing straight medial and lateral laxity in intact human cadaver knees. J Bone Joint Surg Am 63:1257-1269, 1981.

Grood ES, Stowers SF, Noyes FR: Limits of movement in the human knee: Effect of sectioning the posterior cruciate ligament and posterolateral structures. J Bone Joint Surg Am 70:88-97, 1988.

Grood ES, Suntay WJ, Noyes FR, Butler DL: Biomechanics of the knee-extension exercise. J Bone Joint Surg Am 66:725-734, 1984.

Habata T, Ishimura M, Ohgushi H, et al: Axial alignment of the lower limb in patients with isolated meniscal tear. J Orthop Sci 3:85-89, 1998.

Hakkinen K: Force production characteristics of leg extensor, trunk flexor, and extensor muscles in male and female basketball players. J Sports Med Phys Fitness 31:325-331, 1991.

Hardin GT, Bach BR Jr: Distal rupture of the infrapatellar tendon after use of its central third for anterior cruciate ligament reconstruction. Am J Knee Surg 5:140-143, 1992.

Hardin GT, Bach BR Jr, Bush-Joseph CA: Extension loss following arthroscopic ACL reconstruction. Orthop Int 1:405-410, 1993.

Harner CD, Hoher J: Evaluation and treatment of posterior cruciate ligament injuries. Am J Sports Med 26:471-482, 1998.

Harner CD, Irrgang JJ, Paul J, et al: Loss of motion after anterior cruciate ligament reconstruction. Am J Sports Med 20:499-506, 1992.

Harner CD, Olson E, Irrgang JJ, et al: Allograft versus autograft anterior cruciate ligament reconstruction. Clin Orthop 325:134-144, 1996.

Hewett TE, Lindenfeld TN, Riccobene JV, Noyes FR: The effect of neuromuscular training on the incidence of knee injury in female athletes. Am J Sports Med 27:699-706, 1999.

Hewett TE, Noyes FR, Lee MD: Diagnosis of complete and partial posterior cruciate ligament ruptures: Stress radiography compared with KT-1000 Arthrometer and posterior drawer testing. Am J Sports Med 5:648-655, 1997.

Hewett TE, Stroupe AL, Nance TA, Noyes FR: Plyometric training in female athletes: Decreased impact forces and increased hamstring torques. Am J Sports Med 24:765-773, 1996.

Holmes SW, Clancy WG: Clinical classification of patellofemoral pain and dysfunction. J Orthop Sports Phys Ther 28:299-306, 1998.

Howell SM, Taylor MA: Brace-free rehabilitation, with early return to activity, for knees reconstructed with a double-looped semitendinosus and gracilis graft. J Bone Joint Surg Am 78:814-825, 1996.

Huberti HH, Hayes WC: Contact pressures in chondromalacia patellae and the effects of capsular reconstructive procedures. J Orthop Res 6:499-508, 1988.

Huberti HH, Hayes WC, Stone JL, Shybut GT: Force ratios in the quadriceps tendon and ligamentum patellae. J Orthop Res 2:49-54, 1984.

Hull ML, Berns GS, Varma H, Patterson HA: Strain in the medial collateral ligament of the human knee under single and combined loads. J Biomech 29:199-206, 1996.

Huston LJ, Wojtys EM: Neuromuscular performance characteristics in elite female athletes. Am J Sports Med 24:427-436, 1996.

Indelicato PA: Non-operative treatment of complete tears of the medial collateral ligament of the knee. J Bone Joint Surg Am 65:323-329, 1983.

Ingersoll C, Knight K: Patellar location changes following EMG biofeedback or progressive resistive exercises. Med Sci Sports Exerc 23:1122-1127, 1991.

Inoue M, Yasuda K, Ohkoshi Y, et al: Factors that affect prognosis of conservatively treated patients with isolated posterior cruciate ligament injury. Paper presented at the 64th Annual Meeting of the American Academy of Orthopaedic Surgeons, 1997, San Francisco, p 78.

Inoue M, Yasuda K, Yamanaka M, et al: Compensatory muscle activity in the posterior cruciate ligament–deficient knee during isokinetic knee motion. Am J Sports Med 26:710-714, 1998.

Insall J, Falvo KA, Wise DW: Chondromalacia patellae. A prospective study. J Bone Joint Surg Am 58:1-8, 1976.

Itoh H, Kurosaka M, Yoshiya S, et al: Evaluation of functional deficits determined by four different hop tests in patients with anterior cruciate ligament deficiency. Knee Surg Sports Traumatol Arthrosc 6:241-245, 1998.

Jenkins WL, Munns SW, Jayaraman G, et al: A measurement of anterior tibial displacement in the closed and open kinetic chain. J Orthop Sports Phys Ther 25:49-56, 1997.

Juris PM, Phillips EM, Dalpe C, et al: A dynamic test of lower extremity function following anterior cruciate ligament reconstruction and rehabilitation. J Orthop Sports Phys Ther 26:184-191, 1997.

Jurist KA, Otis JC: Anteroposterior tibiofemoral displacements during isometric extension efforts. Am J Sports Med 13:254-258, 1985.

Karst GM, Willett GM: Onset timing of electromyographic activity in the vastus medialis oblique and vastus lateralis muscles in subjects with and without patellofemoral pain syndrome. Phys Ther 75:813-837, 1995.

Kartus J, Magnusson L, Stener S, et al: Complications following arthroscopic anterior cruciate ligament reconstruction. Knee Surg Sports Traumatol Arthrosc 7:2-8, 1999.

Keller PM, Shelbourne KD, McCarroll JR, Rettig AC: Nonoperatively treated isolated posterior cruciate ligament injuries. Am J Sports Med 21:132-136, 1993.

King D: The healing of semilunar cartilages. J Bone Joint Surg 18:333-342, 1936.

Klein L, Heiple KG, Torzilli PA, et al: Prevention of ligament and meniscus atrophy by active joint motion in a non–weight-bearing model. J Orthop Res 7:80-85, 1989.

Kleipool AEB, Zijl JAC, Willems WJ: Arthroscopic anterior cruciate ligament reconstruction with bone–patellar tendon–bone allograft or autograft. Knee Surg Sports Traumatol Arthrosc 6:224-230, 1998.

Klingman RE, Liaos SM, Hardin KM: The effect of subtalar joint posting on patellar glide position in subjects with excessive rearfoot pronation. J Orthop Sports Phys Ther 25:185-191, 1997.

Kolowich PA, Paulos LE, Rosenberg TD, Farnsworth S: Lateral release of the patella: Indications and contraindications. Am J Sports Med 18:359-365, 1990.

Komi PV, Karlsson J: Physical performance, skeletal muscle enzyme activities, and fibre types in monozygous and dizygous twins of both sexes. Acta Physiol Scand Suppl 462:1-28, 1979.

Kowall MG, Kolk G, Nuber GW, et al: Patellofemoral taping in the treatment of patellofemoral pain. Am J Sports Med 24:61-66, 1996.

Kvist J, Gillquist J: Anterior tibial translation during eccentric, isokinetic quadriceps work in healthy subjects. Scand J Med Sci Sports 9:189-194, 1999.

Kwak SD, Colman WW, Ateshian GA, et al: Anatomy of the human patellofemoral joint articular cartilage: A surface curvature analysis. J Orthop Res 15:468-472, 1997.

Laprade J, Culham E, Brouwer B: Comparison of five isometric exercises in the recruitment of the vastus medialis oblique in persons with and without patellofemoral pain. J Orthop Sports Phys Ther 27:197-204, 1998.

Larsen B, Andreasen E, Urfer A, et al: Patellar taping: A radiographic examination of the medial glide technique. Am J Sports Med 23:465-471, 1995.

Larsen NP, Forwood MR, Parker AW: Immobilization and re-training of cruciate ligaments in the rat. Acta Orthop Scand 58:260-264, 1987.

Laurin CA, Levesque HP, Dussault R, et al: The abnormal lateral patellofemoral angle. A diagnostic roentgenographic sign of recurrent patellar subluxation. J Bone Joint Surg Am 60:55-60, 1978.

Lephart SM, Kocher MS, Fu FH, et al: Proprioception following anterior cruciate ligament reconstruction. J Sports Rehabil 1:188-196, 1992.

Lephart SM, Pincivero DM, Rozzi SL: Proprioception of the ankle and knee. Sports Med 3:149-155, 1998.

Lian O, Engebretsen L, Ovrebo RV, Bahr R: Characteristics of the leg extensors in male volleyball players with jumper's knee. Am J Sports Med 24:380-385, 1996.

Lieb FJ, Perry J: Quadriceps function: An anatomical and mechanical study using amputated limbs. J Bone Joint Surg Am 53:749-758, 1971.

Lieber RL, Silva PD, Daniel DM: Equal effectiveness of electrical and volitional strength training for quadriceps femoris muscles after anterior cruciate ligament surgery. J Orthop Res 14:131-138, 1996.

Lipscomb AB Jr, Anderson AF, Norwig ED, et al: Isolated posterior cruciate ligament reconstruction: Long-term results. Am J Sports Med 21:490-496, 1993.

Lundberg M, Messner K: Long-term prognosis of isolated partial medial collateral ligament ruptures. Am J Sports Med 24:160-163, 1996.

Lutz GE, Palmitier RA, An KN, Chao EYS: Comparison of tibiofemoral joint forces during open-kinetic-chain and closed-kinetic-chain exercises. J Bone Joint Surg Am 75:732-739, 1993.

MacDonald P, Miniaci A, Fowler P, et al: A biomechanical analysis of joint contact forces in the posterior cruciate deficient knee. Knee Surg Sports Traumatol Arthrosc 3:252-255, 1996.

Magen HE, Howell SM, Hull ML: Structural properties of six tibial fixation methods for anterior cruciate ligament soft tissue grafts. Am J Sports Med 27:35-43, 1999.

Mangine RE, Eifert-Mangine M, Burch D, et al: Postoperative management of the patellofemoral patient. J Orthop Sports Phys Ther 28:323-335, 1998.

Marder RA, Raskind JR, Carroll M: Prospective evaluation of arthroscopically assisted anterior cruciate ligament reconstruction: Patellar tendon versus semitendinosus and gracilis tendons. Am J Sports Med 19:478-484, 1991.

Mariani PP, Santori N, Adriani E, Mastantuono M: Accelerated rehabilitation after arthroscopic meniscal repair: A clinical and magnetic resonance imaging evaluation. Arthroscopy 12:680-686, 1996.

Markolf KL, Burchfield DM, Shapiro MM, et al. Biomechanical consequences of replacement of the anterior cruciate ligament with a patellar ligament allograft. Part II: Forces in the graft compared with forces in the intact ligament. J Bone Joint Surg Am 78:1728-1734, 1996.

Markolf KL, Mensch JS, Amstutz HC: Stiffness and laxity of the knee: The contributions of the supporting structures. J Bone Joint Surg Am 58:583-593, 1976.

Markolf KL, Slauterbeck JR, Armstrong KL, et al: A biomechanical study of replacement of the posterior cruciate ligament with a graft. Part II: Forces in the graft compared with forces in the intact ligament. J Bone Joint Surg Am 79:381-386, 1997.

McConnell J: The management of chondromalacia patellae: A long term solution. Aust J Physiother 32:215-223, 1986.

McDaniel WJ, Dameron TB: Untreated ruptures of the anterior cruciate ligament. J Bone Joint Surg Am 62:696-705, 1980.

McDaniel WJ, Dameron TB: The untreated anterior cruciate ligament rupture. Clin Orthop 172:158-163, 1983.

McKernan DJ, Paulos LE: Graft selection. In Fu FH, Harner CD, Vince KG (eds): Knee Surgery. Baltimore, Williams & Wilkins, 1994.

McLaughlin J, DeMaio M, Noyes FR, Mangine RE: Rehabilitation after meniscus repair. Orthopedics 17:463-471, 1994.

Merchant AC: Classification of patellofemoral disorders. Arthroscopy 4:235-240, 1988.

Merchant AC, Mercer RL, Jacobsen RH, Cool CR: Roentgenographic analysis of patellofemoral congruence. J Bone Joint Surg Am 56:1391-1396, 1974.

Mirzabeigi E, Jordan C, Gronley JK, et al: Isolation of the vastus medialis oblique muscle during exercise. Am J Sports Med 27:50-53, 1999.

Mok DWH, Good C: Non-operative management of acute grade III medial collateral ligament injury of the knee. Injury 20:277-280, 1989.

Moller BN, Krebs B: Dynamic knee brace in the treatment of patellofemoral disorders. Arch Orthop Trauma Surg 104:377-379, 1986.

Morgan CD, Wojtys EM, Casscells CD, Cassells SW: Arthroscopic meniscal repair evaluated by second-look arthroscopy. Am J Sports Med 19:632-637, 1991.

Muhle C, Brinkmann G, Skaf A, et al: Effect of a patellar realignment brace on patients with patellar subluxation and dislocation. Am J Sports Med 27:350-353, 1999.

Muneta T, Sekiya I, Ogiuchi T, et al: Effects of aggressive early rehabilitation on the outcome of anterior cruciate ligament reconstruction with multi-strand semitendinosus tendon. Int Orthop 22:352-356, 1998.

Neeb TB, Aufdemkampe G, Wagener JH, Mastenbroek L: Assessing anterior cruciate ligament injuries: The association and differential value of questionnaires, clinical tests, and functional tests. J Orthop Sports Phys Ther 26:324-331, 1997.

Nissen CW, Cullen MC, Hewett TE, Noyes FR: Physical and arthroscopic examination techniques of the patellofemoral joint. J Orthop Sports Phys Ther 28:277-285, 1998.

Nogalski MP, Bach BR Jr: Acute anterior cruciate ligament injuries. In Fu FH, Harner CD, Vince KG (eds): Knee Surgery. Baltimore, Williams & Wilkins, 1994.

Novak PJ, Bach BR Jr, Hager CA: Clinical and functional outcome of anterior cruciate ligament reconstruction in the recreational athlete over the age of 35. Am J Knee Surg 9:111-116, 1996.

Noyes FR: Functional properties of knee ligaments and alterations induced by immobilization: A correlative biomechanical and histological study in primates. Clin Orthop 123:210-242, 1977.

Noyes FR, Barber SD, Mangine RE: Abnormal lower limb symmetry determined by function hop tests after anterior cruciate ligament rupture. Am J Sports Med 19:513-518, 1991a.

Noyes FR, Butler DL, Grood ES, et al: Biomechanical analysis of human ligament grafts used in knee-ligament repairs and replacements. J Bone Joint Surg Am 66:344-352, 1984.

Noyes FR, DeMaio M, Mangine RE: Evaluation-based protocol: A new approach to rehabilitation. J Orthop Res 14:1383-1385, 1991b.

Noyes FR, Wojtys EM, Marshall MT: The early diagnosis and treatment of developmental patella infra syndrome. Clin Orthop 265:241-252, 1991c.

Nyland J: Rehabilitation complications following knee surgery. Clin Sports Med 18:905-925, 1999.

O'Connor JJ: Can muscle co-contraction protect knee ligaments after injury or repair. J Bone Joint Surg Br 75:41-48, 1993.

Odensten M, Hamberg P, Nordin M, et al: Surgical or conservative treatment of the acutely torn anterior cruciate ligament. Clin Orthop 198:87-93, 1985.

O'Donoghue DH: Surgical treatment of fresh injuries to the major ligaments of the knee. J Bone Joint Surg Am 32:721-738, 1950.

Ohno K, Pomaybo AS, Schmidt CC, et al: Healing of the MCL after a combined MCL and ACL injury and reconstruction of the ACL: Comparison of repair and nonrepair of MCL tears in rabbits. J Orthop Res 13:442-449, 1995.

Ostenberg A, Roos E, Ekdahl C, Roos H: Isokinetic knee extensor strength and functional performance in healthy female soccer players. Scand J Med Sci Sports 8:257-264, 1998.

Osteras H, Augestad LB, Tondel S: Isokinetic muscle strength after anterior cruciate ligament reconstruction. Scand J Med Sci Sports 8:279-282, 1998.

Otero AL, Hutcheson L: A comparison of the doubled semitendinosus/gracilis and central third of the patellar tendon autografts in arthroscopic anterior cruciate ligament reconstruction. Arthroscopy 9:143-148, 1993.

Palumbo PM: Dynamic patellar brace: A new orthosis in the management of patellofemoral pain. Am J Sports Med 9:45-49, 1981.

Papagelopoulos PJ, Sim FH: Patellofemoral pain syndrome: Diagnosis and management. Orthopedics 20:148-157, 1997.

Parolie JM, Bergfeld JA: Long-term results of nonoperative treatment of isolated posterior cruciate ligament injuries in the athlete. Am J Sports Med 14:35-38, 1986.

Paulos LE, Rosenberg TD, Drawbert J, et al: Infrapatellar contracture syndrome: An unrecognized cause of knee stiffness with patella entrapment and patella infra. Am J Sports Med 15:331-341, 1987.

Pincivero DM, Lephart SM, Henry TJ: The effects of kinesthetic training on balance and proprioception in anterior cruciate ligament injured knee. J Athletic Train 31(Suppl 2):S52, 1996.

Pope MH, Johnson RJ, Brown DW, Tighe C: The role of the musculature in injuries to the medial collateral ligament. J Bone Joint Surg Am 61:398-402, 1979.

Popp JE, Yu JS, Kaeding CC: Recalcitrant patellar tendinitis: Magnetic resonance imaging, histologic evaluation, and surgical treatment. Am J Sports Med 25:218-222, 1997.

Powers CM: Rehabilitation of patellofemoral joint disorders: A critical review. J Orthop Sports Phys Ther 28:345-354, 1998.

Powers CM, Landel R, Perry J: Timing and intensity of vastus muscle activity during functional activities in subjects with and without patellofemoral pain. Phys Ther 76:946-966, 1996.

Race A, Amis AA: The mechanical properties of the two bundles of the human posterior cruciate ligament. J Biomech 27:13-24, 1994.

Radin EL, Rose RM: Role of subchondral bone in the initiation and progression of cartilage damage. Clin Orthop 213:34-40, 1986.

Reider B: Medial collateral ligament injuries in athletes. Sports Med 21:147-156, 1996.

Reider B, Sathy MR, Talkington J, et al: Treatment of isolated medial collateral ligament injuries in athletes with early functional rehabilitation. Am J Sports Med 22:470-477, 1993.

Reinold MM, Fleisig GS, Wilk KE: Research supports both OKC and CKC activities. Biomechanics 2(2 Suppl):27-32, 1999.

Risberg MA, Holm I, Steen H, et al: The effect of knee bracing after anterior cruciate ligament reconstruction. Am J Sports Med 27:76-83, 1999.

Roberts D, Friden T, Zatterstrom R, et al: Proprioception in people with anterior cruciate ligament–deficient knees: Comparison of symptomatic and asymptomatic patients. J Orthop Sports Phys Ther 29:587-594, 1999.

Rodeo SA: Arthroscopic meniscal repair with use of the outside-in technique. J Bone Joint Surg Am 82:127-141, 2000.

Sachs RA, Daniel DM, Stone ML, Garfein RF: Patellofemoral problems after anterior cruciate ligament reconstruction. Am J Sports Med 17:760-765, 1989.

Schutzer SF, Ramsby GR, Fulkerson JP: Computed tomographic classification of patellofemoral pain patients. Orthop Clin North Am 144:16-26, 1986.

Schutzer SF, Ramsby GR, Fulkerson JP: The evaluation of patellofemoral pain using computerized tomography: A preliminary study. Clin Orthop 204:286-293, 1986.

Seitz H, Schlenz I, Muller E, Vecsei V: Anterior instability of the knee despite an intensive rehabilitation program. Clin Orthop 328:159-164, 1996.

Sernert N, Kartus J, Kohler K, et al. Analysis of subjective, objective, and functional examination tests after anterior cruciate ligament reconstruction. Knee Surg Sports Traumatol Arthrosc 7:160-165, 1999.

Shelbourne KD, Davis TJ: Evaluation of knee stability before and after participation in a functional sports agility program during rehabilitation after anterior cruciate ligament reconstruction. Am J Sports Med 27:156-161, 1999.

Shelbourne KD, Davis TJ, Patel DV: The natural history of acute, isolated, nonoperatively treated posterior cruciate ligament injuries. Am J Sports Med 27:276-283, 1999.

Shelbourne KD, Foulk AD: Timing of surgery in anterior cruciate ligament tears on the return of quadriceps muscle strength after reconstruction using an autogenous patellar tendon graft. Am J Sports Med 23:686-689, 1995.

Shelbourne KD, Nitz P: Accelerated rehabilitation after anterior cruciate ligament reconstruction. Am J Sports Med 18:292-299, 1990.

Shelbourne KD, Patel DV: Treatment of limited motion after anterior cruciate ligament reconstruction. Knee Surg Sports Traumatol Arthrosc 7:85-92, 1999.

Shelbourne KD, Patel DV, Adsit WS, Porter DA: Rehabilitation after meniscal repair. Clin Sports Med 15:595-612, 1996a.

Shelbourne KD, Patel DV, Martini DJ: Classification and management of arthrofibrosis of the knee after anterior cruciate ligament reconstruction. Am J Sports Med 24:857-862, 1996b.

Shelbourne KD, Wilckens JH, Mollabaashy A, DeCarlo MS: Arthrofibrosis in acute anterior cruciate ligament reconstruction: The effect of timing of reconstruction and rehabilitation. Am J Sports Med 9:332-336, 1991.

Shellock FG, Mink JH, Deutsch AL, Foo TK: Kinematic MR imaging of the patellofemoral joint: Comparison of passive positioning and active movement techniques. Radiology 184:574-577, 1992.

Shelton WR, Papendick L, Dukes AD: Autograft versus allograft anterior cruciate ligament reconstruction. Arthroscopy 13:446-449, 1997.

Skyhar MJ, Warren RF, Oritz GJ, et al: The effects of sectioning of the posterior cruciate ligament and the posterolateral complex on the articular contact pressures within the knee. J Bone Joint Surg Am 75:694-699, 1993.

Snyder-Mackler L, Ladin Z, Schepsis AA, Young JC: Electrical stimulation of thigh muscles after reconstruction of anterior cruciate ligament. J Bone Joint Surg Am 73:1025-1036, 1991.

Steinkamp LA, Dillingham MF, Markel MD, et al: Biomechanical considerations in patellofemoral joint rehabilitation. Am J Sports Med 21:438-444, 1993.

Stetson WB, Friedman MJ, Fulkerson JP, et al: Fracture of the proximal tibia with immediate weightbearing after a Fulkerson osteotomy. Am J Sports Med 25:570-574, 1997.

Thompson WO, Thaete FL, Fu FH, Dye SF: Tibial meniscal dynamics using three-dimensional reconstruction of magnetic resonance images. Am J Sports Med 19:210-216, 1991.

Torg JS, Barton TM, Pavlov H, Stine R: Natural history of the posterior cruciate ligament–deficient knee. Clin Orthop 246:208-216, 1989.

Tyler TF, McHugh MP, Gleim GW, Nicholas SJ: The effect of immediate weightbearing after anterior cruciate ligament reconstruction. Clin Orthop 357:141-148, 1998.

Vedi V, Williams A, Tennant SJ, et al: Meniscal movement: An in-vivo study using dynamic MRI. J Bone Joint Surg Br 81:37-41, 1999.

Voloshin AS, Wosk J: Shock absorption of the meniscectomized and painful knees: A comparative in vivo study. J Biomed Eng 5:157-161, 1983.

Vos EJ, Harlaar J, van Ingen-Schenau GJ: Electromechanical delay during knee extensor contractions. Med Sci Sports Exerc 23:1187-1193, 1991.

Weiss JA, Woo SL-Y, Ohland KJ, Horibe S: Evaluation of a new injury model to study medial collateral ligament healing: Primary repair versus non-operative treatment. J Orthop Res 9:516-528, 1991.

Wilk KE: Rehabilitation of isolated and combined posterior cruciate ligament injuries. Clin Sports Med 13:649-677, 1994.

Wilk KE, Andrews JR: The effects of pad placement and angular velocity on tibial displacement during isokinetic exercise. J Orthop Sports Phys Ther 17:24-30, 1993.

Wilk KE, Arrigo C, Andrews JR, Clancy WG: Rehabilitation after anterior cruciate ligament reconstruction in the female athlete. J Athletic Train 34:177-193, 1999.

Wilk KE, Davies GJ, Mangine RE, Malone TR: Patellofemoral disorders: A classification system and clinical guideline for nonoperative rehabilitation. J Orthop Sports Phys Ther 28:307-322, 1998.

Williams JS Jr, Bach BR Jr: Rehabilitation of the ACL deficient and reconstructed knee. Sports Med Arthrosc Rev 3:69-82, 1996.

Woo SL-Y, Chan SS, Yamaji T: Biomechanics of knee ligament healing, repair, and reconstruction. J Biomech 30:431-439, 1997.

Woo SL-Y, Gomez MA, Sites TJ, et al: The biomechanical and morphological changes of the MCL following immobilization and remobilization. J Bone Joint Surg Am 69:1200-1211, 1987.

Woo SL-Y, Hollis JM, Adams DJ, et al: Tensile properties of the human femur–anterior cruciate ligament complex. Am J Sports Med 19:217-225, 1991.

Woo SL-Y, Inoue M, McGurck-Burleson E, Gomez M: Treatment of the medial collateral ligament injury II. Structure and function of canine knees in response to differing treatment regimens. Am J Sports Med 15:22-29, 1987.

Woodland LH, Francis RS: Parameters and comparisons of the quadriceps angle of college-aged men and women in the supine and standing positions. Am J Sports Med 20:208-211, 1992.

Yack HJ, Collins CE, Whieldon TJ: Comparison of closed and open kinetic chain exercises in the anterior cruciate ligament–deficient knee. Am J Sports Med 21:49-54, 1993.

Yamaji T, Levine RE, Woo SL-Y, et al: MCL healing one year after a concurrent MCL and ACL injury: An interdisciplinary study in rabbits. J Orthop Res 14:223-227, 1996.

Yasuda K, Erickson AR, Beynnon BD, et al: Dynamic elongation behavior in the medial collateral and anterior cruciate ligaments during lateral impact loading. J Orthop Res 11:190-198, 1993.

Zavetsky AB, Beard DJ, O'Connor JJ: Cruciate ligament loading during isometric muscle contractions. Am J Sports Med 22:418-423, 1994.

Zheng N, Fleisig GS, Escamilla RF, Barrentine SW: An analytical model of the knee for estimation of the internal forces during exercise. J Biomech 31:963-967, 1998.

ARTICULAR CARTILAGE REPAIR

Bandy WD, Hanten WP: Changes in torque and electromyographic activity of the quadriceps femoris muscles following isometric training. Phys Ther 73:455-465, 1993.

Buckwalter J: Effects of early motion on healing musculoskeletal tissues. Hand Clin 12:13-24, 1996.

Rosenberg TD, Paulos LE, Parker RD, et al: The forty five degree posteroanterior flexion weight bearing radiograph of the knee. J Bone Joint Surg Am 70:1479-1483, 1988.

Salter RB, Minster R, Bell R, et al: Continuous passive motion and the repair of full-thickness articular cartilage defects: A 1-year follow-up [abstract]. Trans Orthop Res Soc 7:167, 1982.

Salter RB, Simmonds DF, Malcolm BW, et al: The biological effect of continuous passive motion on healing of full-thickness defects in articular cartilage: An experimental study in the rabbit. J Bone Joint Surg Am 62:1232-1251, 1980.

Suh J, Aroen A, Muzzonigro T, et al: Injury and repair of articular cartilage: Related scientific issues. Oper Tech Orthop 7:270-278, 1997.

BAKER'S (POPLITEAL) CYST

Burleson RJ, Bickel WH, Dahlin DC: Popliteal cyst: A clinicopathological survey. J Bone Joint Surg Am 38:1265-1274, 1956.

Bogumill GP, Bruno PD, Barrick EF: Malignant lesions masquerading as popliteal cysts: A report of three cases. J Bone Joint Surg Am 63:474-477, 1981.

Curl WW: Popliteal cysts: Historical background and current knowledge. J Am Acad Orthop Surg 4:129-133, 1996.

Dinham JM: Popliteal cysts in children: The case against surgery. J Bone Joint Surg Br 57:69-71, 1975.

Fielding JR, Franklin PD, Kustan J: Popliteal cysts: A reassessment using magnetic resonance imaging. Skeletal Radiol 20:433-435, 1991.

Hermann G, Yeh HC, Lehr-Janus C, et al: Diagnosis of popliteal cyst: Double-contrast arthrography and sonography. AJR Am J Roentgenol 137:369-372, 1981.

Hughston JC, Baker CL, Mello W: Popliteal cyst: A surgical approach. Orthopedics 14:147-150, 1991.

Janzen DL, Peterfy CG, Forbes JR, et al: Cystic lesions around the knee joint: MR imaging findings. AJR Am J Roentgenol 163:155-161, 1994.

Jayson MI, Dixon AS, Kates A, et al: Popliteal and calf cysts in rheumatoid arthritis. Treatment by anterior synovectomy. Ann Rheum Dis 31:9-15, 1972.

Katz RS, Zizic TM, Arnold WP, et al: The pseudothrombophlebitis syndrome. Medicine (Baltimore) 56:151-164, 1977.

Lantz B, Singer KM: Meniscal cysts. Clin Sports Med 9:707-725, 1990.

Lindgren PG, Willen R: Gastrocnemius-membranosus bursa and its relation to the knee joint. I. Anatomy and histology. Acta Radiol Diagn (Stockh) 18:497-512, 1977.

Rauschning W: Popliteal cysts (Baker's cysts) in adults II. Acta Orthop Scand 51:547-555, 1980.

Taylor AR, Rana NA: A valve. An explanation of the formation of popliteal cysts. Ann Rheum Dis 32:419-421, 1973.

PATELLA FRACTURES

Bostrom A: Fracture of the patella. A study of 422 patella fractures. Acta Orthop Scand Suppl 143:1-80, 1972.

Houghton GR, Ackroyd CE: Sleeve fractures of the patella in children: a report of three cases. J Bone Joint Surg Br 61:165-168, 1979.

5 | Foot and Ankle Injuries

KEN STEPHENSON, MD • CHARLES L. SALTZMAN, MD •
S. BRENT BROTZMAN, MD

Ankle Sprains

Ken Stephenson, MD

Ankle sprains account for about 15% of all athletic injuries, with a reported 23,000 ankle ligament injuries occurring each day in the United States. They are particularly common in basketball, volleyball, soccer, modern dance, and ballet. Most patients recover fully, but chronic symptoms of pain and instability develop in an estimated 20% to 40%.

RELEVANT ANATOMY

The stability of any joint depends on the inherent constraints provided by the bony configuration and the active and passive soft tissue restraints. The ankle joint is quite stable in the neutral position because the wider anterior portion of the talus fits snugly into the ankle mortise. Plantar flexion of the ankle rotates the narrower posterior talus into the mortise, which results in a much looser fit with a particular tendency toward inversion. Active soft tissue restraint depends on the muscle-tendon units involved in movement and support of the joint. The talus, however, has no tendinous insertions and must rely in an indirect way on muscular actions on other bones adjacent to the ankle joint. Passive support of the ankle is provided by the medial, lateral, and posterior ligaments and the syndesmosis. The lateral ankle ligament complex is the structure most commonly involved in ankle sprains.

The three main components of the lateral ligament complex are the anterior talofibular ligament (ATFL), the calcaneofibular ligament (CFL), and the posterior talofibular ligament (Fig. 5-1). The ATFL is relaxed in neutral and taut in plantar flexion. It is the primary restraint against inversion while the foot is plantar-flexed. The CFL is also relaxed in neutral, but it is taut in dorsiflexion.

The **most common ankle injury** involves an isolated tear of the ATFL, followed by a combined tear of the ATFL and CFL. The mechanism of injury is usually inversion of a plantar-flexed foot (Fig. 5-2).

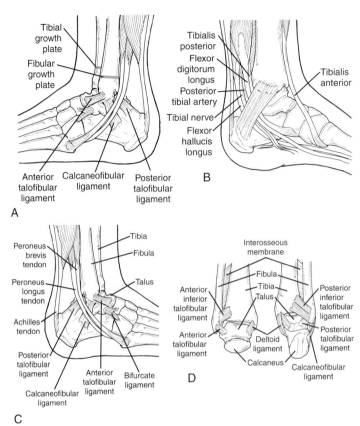

Figure 5–1 **A,** Ankle stability is provided by the peroneus longus and brevis tendons on the posterolateral side and by the tibialis posterior, flexor digitorum longus, and flexor hallucis longus on the medial side. When the foot is plantar-flexed, the anterior talofibular ligament tightens and is more likely to become injured than the calcaneofibular and posterior talofibular ligaments. The growth plate in children is particularly vulnerable to fracture because it is weaker than the surrounding ligaments, bone, and periosteum. **B,** Structures crossing the medial aspect of the ankle anteriorly include the tibialis anterior tendon and the saphenous vein and nerve. Behind the medial malleolus lie the important tibialis posterior, flexor digitorum longus, posterior tibial artery and veins, tibial nerve, and the posteriorly located flexor hallucis longus. **C,** Lateral view of the ankle showing its chief musculotendinous and ligamentous stabilizers. **D,** Anterior (*left*) and posterior (*right*) views of the syndesmotic ligaments. The interosseous ligament is deep to the anterior inferior and posterior inferior tibiofibular ligaments. Syndesmotic sprains are usually produced by high-impact external or internal rotational forces. Low-grade syndesmotic injury can occur alone or in conjunction with other ligamentous injury of the ankle or foot. Severe syndesmotic sprain can cause destabilization of the ankle mortise, which is usually accompanied by fracture.

CLASSIFICATION OF LATERAL COLLATERAL LIGAMENT SPRAINS

A *grade 1*, or mild, ankle sprain is a stretch of the ligament with no macroscopic tear, little swelling or tenderness, minimal or no functional impairment, and no joint instability. A *grade 2*, or moderate, ankle sprain involves a partial tear of the ligament with moderate swelling and tenderness, some loss of joint function, and mild joint instability. A *grade 3*, or severe, sprain involves a complete tear of the ligaments

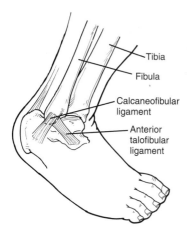

Tibia

Fibula

Calcaneofibular ligament

Anterior talofibular ligament

Figure 5–2 The most typical injury mechanism in an ankle sprain is plantar flexion, inversion, and adduction. The anterior talofibular ligament is most commonly torn in a plantar flexion–inversion mechanism. (Adapted from Lane SE: Severe ankle sprains. Physician Sports Med 19[11]:43, 1990.)

(ATFL and CFL) with severe swelling, ecchymosis and tenderness, inability to bear weight on the extremity, and mechanical joint instability (Fig. 5-3).

DIAGNOSIS

An inversion injury is commonly associated with a tearing sensation or a pop felt by the patient over the lateral aspect of the ankle. Swelling can occur immediately in grade 2 and 3 sprains, and the initial intense pain subsides after a few hours, only to return more intensely as the hemorrhage continues 6 to 12 hours after the injury.

Physical Examination

Physical examination reveals mild swelling in grade 1 sprains and moderate to severe swelling in a diffuse pattern in grade 2 and 3 sprains. Tenderness is usually elicited at the anterior edge of the fibula with ATFL injuries and at the tip of the fibula with CFL injuries. The region of the syndesmosis and the base of the fifth metatarsal should also be palpated to rule out injuries to these structures.

The anterior drawer test and the talar tilt test are commonly used to identify signs of joint instability (Fig. 5-4A and B). The anterior drawer test is performed by stabilizing the distal end of the tibia anteriorly with one hand and pulling the slightly

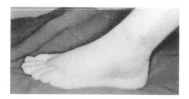

Figure 5–3 Grade 3 ankle sprain. Note the significant ecchymosis and swelling associated with a grade 3 injury. (From Lane SE: Severe ankle sprains. Physician Sports Med 18[11]:43, 1990.)

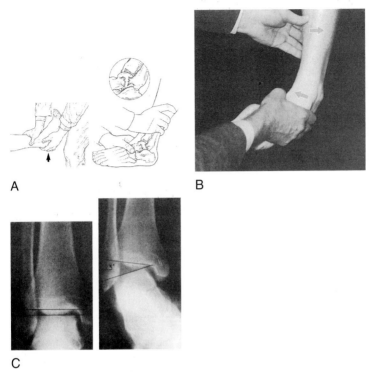

Figure 5–4 **A**, *Left*, Test for ligamentous instability with the **anterior drawer test**. Grasp the patient's foot at the heel and pull forward while maintaining the tibia in a fixed position with the other hand at the anterior distal aspect of the tibia. Translation greater than 3 mm or a difference in anterior translation from the asymptomatic ankle suggests a tear of the anterior talofibular ligament (ATFL). *Right*, Excessive anteroposterior (AP) translation of the tibia on the talus during the anterior drawer test indicates that the patient has an ATFL injury. **B**, The **talar tilt test** (**inversion stress test**) assesses the integrity of the calcaneofibular ligament. This test may be performed with a commercial jig or leaded hands during radiographic imaging. Invert the foot while stabilizing the tibia with one hand and the subtalar joint with the other. **C**, *Left*, AP view of the ankle before stress. *Right*, AP view of the ankle with inversion stress revealing marked lateral ligament injury. (**A**, *Left*, From Ganley TJ, Flynn JM, Pill SG, Hanlon PA: Ankle injury in the young athlete: Fracture or sprain? J Musculoskel Med 17:311, 2000. Artist: Teri J. McDermott; *Right*, from Baker CL, Todd JL: Intervening in acute ankle sprain and chronic instability. J Musculoskel Med 12[7]:51, 1995; **B**, from Meisterling RC: Recurrent lateral ankle sprains. Physician Sports Med 21[3]:123, 1993; **C**, from Lassiter TE, Malone TR, Garrett WE: Injuries to the lateral ligaments of the ankle. Orthop Clin North Am 20:632, 1989.)

plantar-flexed foot forward with the other hand from behind the heel. A positive finding of more than 5 mm of anterior translation indicates a tear of the ATFL. The talar tilt test is performed by stabilizing the distal end of the tibia with one hand and inverting the talus and calcaneus as a unit with the other hand. A positive finding of more than 5 mm with a soft endpoint indicates a combined injury to the ATFL and CFL (see Fig. 5-4C). It is important to always compare the affected ankle with the contralateral side because some patients are naturally very flexible (generalized ligamentous laxity), which could result in a false-positive test.

Examination of the Ankle after an Inversion Injury

Palpation of the lateral collaterals (ATFL and CFL)

Medial palpation of the deltoid ligament

Palpation of the proximal end of the fibula (close to the knee) to rule out a Maisonneuve fracture (tearing of the interosseous membrane and migration of forces proximally to cause a proximal fibula fracture)

Squeeze test to rule out tearing of the ankle syndesmosis with resultant instability of the ankle mortise (Fig. 5-5A)

External rotation (Cotton) test (see Fig. 5-5B and C) to test for injury to the syndesmosis

Palpation of the proximal (base) end of the fifth metatarsal to rule out avulsion fracture from pull of the peroneus brevis

Anterior drawer and inversion (talar tilt) stress testing

Motor testing of the posterior tibial (inversion) and peroneal (eversion) tendons, including the single-raise heel test

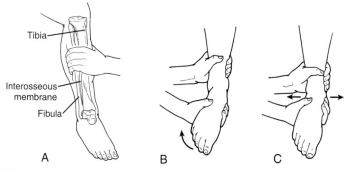

Figure 5–5   A, The **squeeze test** is used to evaluate the syndesmotic ligaments of the ankle. It is performed by grasping the anterior of the leg proximally and squeezing the fibula and tibia to compress the interosseous ligaments. If syndesmotic injury exists, the player complains of distal ankle pain at the joint. **B,** The **external rotation stress test** is performed with the patient's foot in neutral position and the knee flexed 90 degrees. While stabilizing the tibia and fibula with one hand, the physician externally rotates the ankle with the other hand. Pain in the syndesmotic area indicates injury to the syndesmosis. **C,** In the **tibiotalar shuck test (Cotton test),** the examiner holds the lower part of the patient's leg with one hand while alternately applying medial and lateral force to the talus with the other. Pain in the syndesmosis or a feeling of looseness (comparison with the normal side may help) indicates syndesmotic ligament injury. (Adapted from Crosby LA, Davick JP: Managing common football injuries on the field. J Musculoskel Med 17:651, 2000; and Bassewitz HL, Shapiro MS: Persistent pain after ankle sprain. Physician Sports Med 25[12]:58, 1997.)

SYNDESMOSIS INJURY

Disruption of the syndesmosis ligament complex (tibiofibular ligaments and interosseous membrane) may occur in as many as 10% of all ankle ligament injuries (Fig. 5-6). The examiner should always test for this injury (see the squeeze test and external rotation test, above). Rupture of the syndesmosis is often associated with deltoid (medial) ligament rupture, and concomitant fracture of the fibula is common (see the ankle fracture section). The mechanism may be pronation and eversion of

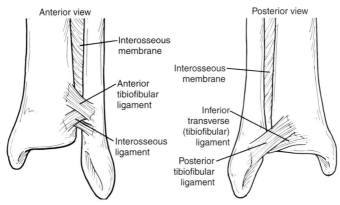

Figure 5–6 Components of the distal lower extremity syndesmosis. The syndesmosis comprises four ligaments and the interosseous membrane. The ligaments are the anterior tibiofibular, posterior tibiofibular, transverse tibiofibular, and interosseous.

the foot combined with internal rotation of the tibia on a fixed foot, such as occurs in football players who have an external rotation force applied to the foot (stepped on) while lying prone on the field.

Point tenderness and pain are located primarily on the anterior aspect of the syndesmosis (not over the lateral collaterals as with an ankle sprain), and the patient is usually unable to bear weight. These injuries are typically more severe than ankle sprains, with more pain, swelling, and difficulty bearing weight. Stress radiographs taken with the ankle in external rotation (in both dorsiflexion and plantar flexion) often display the diastasis (gap) between the tibia and fibula. Bone scanning is useful if the diagnosis is suspected but difficult to confirm.

Partial isolated syndesmosis tears are typically treated nonoperatively in a removable cast for 6 to 8 weeks (partial weight-bearing with crutches). With complete syndesmosis rupture, the fibula may shorten and externally rotate. A complete tear is treated by suture of the ligament and temporary fixation of the tibia and fibula with a syndesmosis screw or use of the "tightrope" (Arthrex, Naples, FL). The tightrope uses EndoButton-type fixation medially at the tibia with strong suture fixation over a metal button at the fibula. The syndesmosis screw must be placed with the ankle dorsiflexed to neutral (the widest portion of the talus) to avoid limited dorsiflexion postoperatively. A walking boot is used (touch-down weight-bearing) for 6 to 8 weeks after surgery. Early active and passive motion out of the boot is encouraged from day 7, and full weight-bearing is allowed at 6 weeks. An aggressive rehabilitation program stressing vigorous range of motion (ROM), strengthening, and proprioception exercises is undertaken (see the ankle sprain rehabilitation protocol, p. 557). The patient should be informed about the longer recovery than needed for ankle sprains and the potential for pain and late sequelae, such as heterotopic ossification.

Factors crucial for a good outcome after injuries to the syndesmosis are recognition of the injury and obtaining and maintaining anatomic reduction of the ankle mortise and the distal lower extremity syndesmosis. Fixation of the syndesmosis is usually indicated to avoid the more catastrophic complications of mortise widening and joint incongruity (e.g., early post-traumatic arthritis).

Radiographic Evaluation

Radiographs are taken to rule out fractures of the medial and lateral malleoli, the talus, and the fifth metatarsal base. Radiographs should include three views of the ankle on long cassettes that include the entire length of the fibula (anteroposterior [AP], lateral, and mortise views [Fig. 5-7A]) and three views of the foot (AP, lateral, and oblique) (see Fig. 5-7B-D). Stress radiographs can be used to quantify instability during the anterior drawer and talar tilt stress tests. More than 10 mm of anterior talar subluxation or more than a 5-mm difference from the contralateral ankle indicates a positive anterior drawer stress test. Talar tilt of 15 degrees or a 10-degree difference from the contralateral ankle indicates a positive talar tilt test.

Treatment of Lateral Collateral Sprains

The current literature supports functional rehabilitation as the preferred method of treatment of ankle sprains instead of cast immobilization because it allows earlier return to work and physical activity without a higher rate of late symptoms (ankle instability, pain, stiffness, or muscle weakness).

Immediately after injury in the **acute phase**, the PRICE (protection, rest, ice, compression, and elevation) principle is followed (see the rehabilitation protocol). The goal is to reduce hemorrhage, swelling, inflammation, and pain. A period of immobilization is initiated, depending on the severity of the injury. Some authors stress the importance of immobilizing the ankle in neutral rather than in plantar flexion because the ATFL is stretched out during plantar flexion. For grade 1 and 2 sprains, an ankle brace (Fig. 5-8) is used for immobilization. For grade 3 sprains, a removable

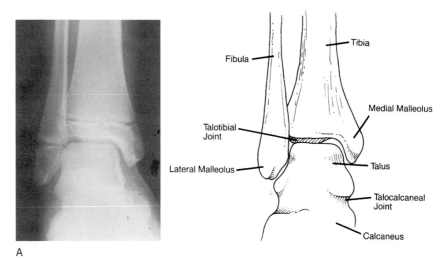

A

Figure 5–7 **A,** Anteroposterior (AP) views of the ankle. *Left,* Radiograph illustrating the relationships of the ankle joint, including the medial mortise. *Right,* Anatomic drawing for correlation. Typically, three views of the ankle are taken (AP, lateral, and mortise).

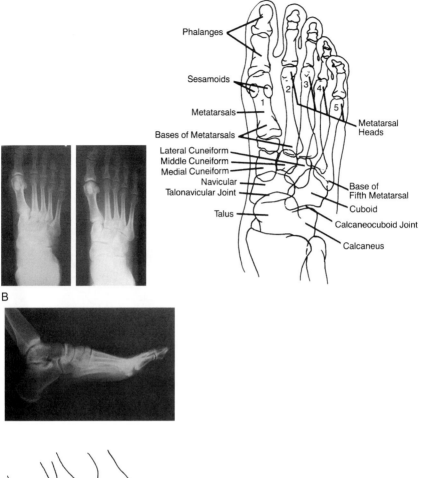

Phalanges

Sesamoids

Metatarsals

Bases of Metatarsals

Lateral Cuneiform
Middle Cuneiform
Medial Cuneiform
Navicular
Talonavicular Joint

Talus

Metatarsal
Heads

Base of
Fifth Metatarsal

Cuboid

Calcaneocuboid Joint

Calcaneus

B

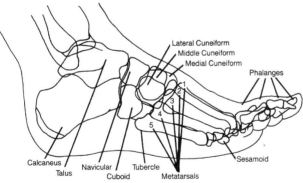

C

Lateral Cuneiform
Middle Cuneiform
Medial Cuneiform

Phalanges

Calcaneus
Talus
Navicular
Cuboid
Tubercle
Metatarsals

Sesamoid

Figure 5–7 **B**, AP projections of the foot. *Left*, A perpendicular x-ray beam demonstrates the forefoot anatomy, particularly the phalanges and metatarsophalangeal (MTP) joints. Note the distal third and fourth metatarsal fractures. *Center*, An angled x-ray beam provides improved detail of the midfoot anatomy, particularly the normal alignment of the lateral border of the first MTP joint and the medial border of the second MTP joint. *Right*, Anatomic drawing for correlation. **C**, Lateral projection of the foot. *Top*, Radiograph illustrating the anatomic relationships of the midfoot and hindfoot. *Bottom*, Anatomic drawing for correlation.

(Figure continues on next page)

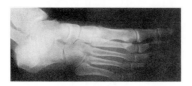

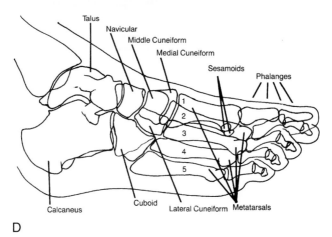

D

Figure 5–7, cont'd **D**, Medial oblique projection of the foot. *Top*, Radiograph demonstrating the normal medial border alignment of the third and fourth MTP joints. It also allows evaluation of the talonavicular and calcaneocuboid relationships. *Bottom*, Anatomic drawing for correlation. (From Mann R, Coughlin M: Surgery of the Foot and Ankle. Philadelphia, CV Mosby, 1997).

cast boot offers more stability and protection and allows earlier weight-bearing with less pain. Immobilization is continued for several days with mild sprains and for up to 3 weeks with severe grade 3 sprains. As grade 3 sprains improve, the cast boot is replaced with an ankle brace.

In the **subacute phase**, goals include continued reduction of swelling, inflammation, and pain and initiation of some motion, strengthening, and appropriate controlled weight-bearing. This is the period of collagen fiber proliferation, and too much stress on the ligaments at this point could result in weaker tissue.

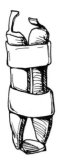

Standard
ankle brace

Figure 5–8 Aircast ankle brace (1-800-526-8785). (From DeLee JC, Drez D Jr: Orthopaedic Sports Medicine: Principles and Practice. Philadelphia, WB Saunders, 1994.)

The **rehabilitative phase** focuses on improving strength, endurance, balance, and weight-bearing proprioception. During this maturation phase of the healing ligament, about 3 weeks after the injury, controlled stretching of the muscles and movement of the joint promote a more normal orientation of the collagen fibers, parallel with the stress lines. Repeated exercise during this phase has been shown to increase the mechanical and structural strength of the ligaments.

REHABILITATION PROTOCOL *After Ankle Sprains (Lateral Collateral Ligament)*
Stephenson

PHASE 1: ACUTE PHASE

Timing

- Grade 1 sprain: 1-3 days
- Grade 2 sprain: 2-4 days
- Grade 3 sprain: 3-7 days

Goals

- Decrease swelling
- Decrease pain
- Protect from reinjury
- Maintain appropriate weight-bearing status

Protection Options

- Taping
- Functional bracing
- Removable cast boot (some grade 2 and most grade 3 sprains)
- Rest (crutches to promote ambulation without gait deviation)

Ice

- Cryocuff ice machine
- Ice bags
- Ice with other modalities (interferential [Fig. 5-9A], high-voltage galvanic stimulation, ultrasound)

Light Compression

- Elastic (Ace) wrap
- TED (thromboembolic disease) hose
- Vasopneumatic pump

Elevation

- Above the heart (combined with ankle pumps)

PHASE 2: SUBACUTE PHASE

Timing

- Grade 1 sprain: 2-4 days
- Grade 2 sprain: 3-5 days
- Grade 3 sprain: 4-8 days

Continued

REHABILITATION PROTOCOL: *After Ankle Sprains (Lateral Collateral Ligaments)*   Continued

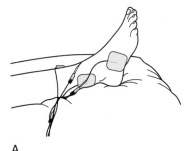

A

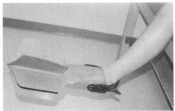

B

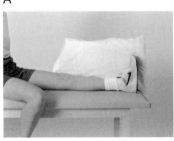

C

Figure 5–9   **A**, Interferential electrical stimulation. **B**, Aqua ankle. Ankle resistance training is performed with this device in a cold whirlpool and then eventually in warm water (1-877-272-2376 or www.kineticinnovations.com). **C**, Isometric strengthening: eversion against a fixed object (wall) with a pillow as a cushion.

Goals

- Decrease swelling
- Decrease pain
- Increase pain-free ROM
- Begin strengthening
- Begin non–weight-bearing proprioceptive training
- Provide protective support as needed

Modalities to Decrease Pain and Swelling

- Ice or contrast baths
- Electrical stimulation (high-voltage galvanic or interferential)
- Ultrasound
- Cross-friction massage (gently)
- Soft orthotics with a ⅛- to ³⁄₁₆-inch lateral wedge if needed

Weight-Bearing

- Progress weight-bearing as symptoms permit
- Partial weight-bearing to full weight-bearing if no signs of an antalgic gait are present

Therapeutic Exercises

- Active ROM exercises
  - Dorsiflexion
  - Inversion

REHABILITATION PROTOCOL: *After Ankle Sprains (Lateral Collateral Ligaments)* Continued

PHASE 2: SUBACUTE PHASE—cont'd

- Foot circles
- Plantar flexion
- Eversion
- Alphabet
- Use of the Aqua Ankle in cold water for gentle strengthening and ROM (see Fig. 5-9B)
- Strength exercises
  - Isometric in a pain-free range (see Fig. 5-9C)
  - Toe curls with a towel (place weight on the towel to increase resistance)
  - Pick up objects with the toes (tissue, marbles)
- Proprioceptive training
  - Seated Biomechanical Ankle Platform System (BAPS board) (Fig. 5-10)
  - Wobble board
  - Ankle disk
- Stretching
  - Passive ROM—only dorsiflexion and plantar flexion in a pain-free range, *not* eversion or inversion
  - Achilles stretch (gentle)
  - Joint mobilization (grades 1-2 for dorsiflexion/plantar flexion)

PHASE 3: REHABILITATIVE PHASE

Timing

- Grade 1 sprain: 1 week
- Grade 2 sprain: 2 weeks
- Grade 3 sprain: 3 weeks

Goals

- Increase pain-free ROM
- Progress strengthening
- Progress proprioceptive training

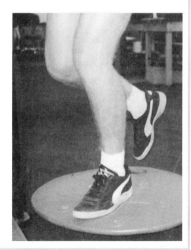

Figure 5–10 Patients can perform balancing exercises on a circular tilt board to improve proprioception while sitting or standing. (From Meisterling RC: Recurrent lateral ankle sprains. Physician Sports Med 21[5]:123, 1993.)

Continued

REHABILITATION PROTOCOL: *After Ankle Sprains (Lateral Collateral Ligaments)* *Continued*

PHASE 3: REHABILITATIVE PHASE—cont'd

- Increase pain-free activities of daily living
- Pain-free full weight-bearing and uncompensated gait

Therapeutic Exercises

- Stretching
  - Gastrocnemius and soleus with increased intensity
  - Joint mobilization (grades 1, 2, and 3 for dorsiflexion, plantar flexion, and eversion; hold inversion)
- Strengthening
  - Weight-bearing exercises
    - Heel raises (see Fig. 5-11A)
    - Toe raises (see Fig. 5-11B)
    - Stair steps
    - Quarter squats
  - Eccentric/concentric exercises and isotonics (Thera-Band and cuff weights)
    - Inversion (Fig. 5-12A)
    - Eversion (see Fig. 5-12B)
    - Plantar flexion (see Fig. 5-12C)

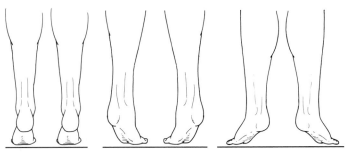

A

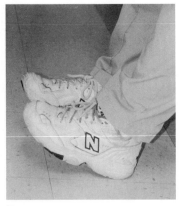

B

Figure 5–11 **A**, Standing heel raises. The raises are done with the foot in neutral position (*left*), inversion (*center*), and eversion (*right*). **B**, Toe raise. (**A**, Adapted from Kovan JR, McKeag DB: Lower extremity overuse injuries in aerobic dancers. J Musculoskel Med 9[4]:33, 1992.)

REHABILITATION PROTOCOL: *After Ankle Sprains (Lateral Collateral Ligaments)*   *Continued*

PHASE 3: REHABILITATIVE PHASE—cont'd

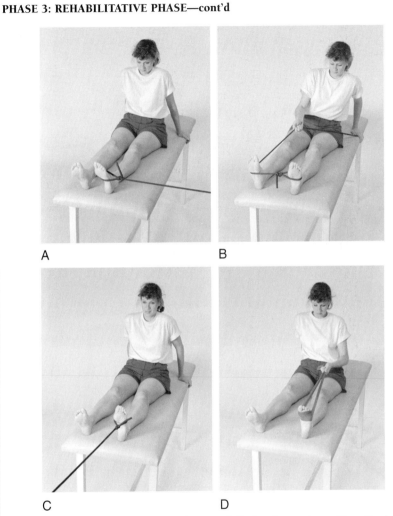

A   B

C   D

Figure 5–12   **A**, Inversion against a Thera-Band. **B**, Eversion against a Thera-Band. This is probably the most important of the Thera-Band exercises. **C**, Dorsiflexion against a Thera-Band. **D**, Plantar flexion against a Thera-Band.

- Dorsiflexion (see Fig. 5-12D)
- Peroneal strengthening
- Isokinetics
- Proprioceptive training (progress from the non–weight-bearing/controlled weight-bearing stage to full weight-bearing
  - Standing BAPS board
  - Standing wobble board

Continued

REHABILITATION PROTOCOL: *After Ankle Sprains (Lateral Collateral Ligaments)* *Continued*

PHASE 3: REHABILITATIVE PHASE—cont'd

- Kinesthetic Ability Trainer (KAT) system
- Single-leg balance activities (stable to unstable surfaces, without to with distractions) (Fig. 5-13)

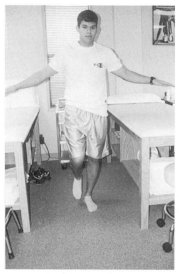

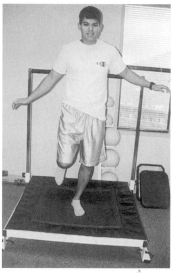

Figure 5–13 **A**, Single-leg balance. **B**, Single-leg balance on a trampoline. **C**, Single-leg balance with distraction.

REHABILITATION PROTOCOL: *After Ankle Sprains (Lateral Collateral Ligaments)*   *Continued*

PHASE 3: REHABILITATIVE PHASE—cont'd

- Continue modalities as needed, specifically after exercises to prevent recurrence of pain and swelling
- Supportive taping, bracing, and orthotics used as needed. Typically, we finish the athletic season with supportive bracing in an effort to avoid reinjury

PHASE 4: RETURN TO ACTIVITY OR FUNCTIONAL PHASE

Timing

- Grade 1 sprain: 1-2 weeks
- Grade 2 sprain: 2-3 weeks
- Grade 3 sprain: 3-6 weeks

Goals

- Regain full strength
- Normal biomechanics
- Return to participation
- Protection and strengthening of any mild residual joint instability

Therapeutic Exercises

- Continue progression of ROM and strengthening exercises
- Sport-specific strengthening and training are imperative
- Running progression
  - Unloaded jogging on ZUNI (Fig. 5-14)
  - Unloaded running on ZUNI
  - Alternate jog-walk-jog on smooth, straight surfaces

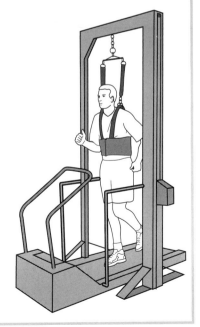

Figure 5–14   Unloaded jogging.

Continued

REHABILITATION PROTOCOL: *After Ankle Sprains (Lateral Collateral Ligaments)* *Continued*

PHASE 4: RETURN TO ACTIVITY OR FUNCTIONAL PHASE—cont'd

- Alternate sprint-jog-sprint on smooth, straight surfaces
- Figure-of-eights
- Zigzag cutting
- Agility drills
  - Back pedaling
  - Side stepping
  - Carioca
- Plyometrics specific to each sport
- Progress weight-bearing multidirectional balance exercises and movement activities (Fig. 5-15)

Return to Competition

- When the above skills are accomplished at full speed, the athlete may return to practice
- When full practice is tolerated, competition can be resumed
- Some type of ankle support is recommended for the first several months. We typically use a low-profile Aircast or the Bledsoe Ultimate Ankle Brace

PHASE 5: PROPHYLACTIC PHASE

Goal

- Prevent injury

Therapeutic Exercises

- Functional drills
- Multidirectional balance board activities
- Prophylactic strengthening (emphasis on peroneal eversion)
- Prophylactic protective support as needed

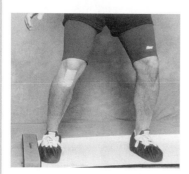

Figure 5–15   Use of a slide board.

PREVENTION OF ANKLE SPRAINS

Proper strengthening and rehabilitation are critical to help prevent inversion ankle injuries; however, some patients require additional biomechanical support. We routinely use ankle braces in athletes prone to ankle injuries in high-risk sports such as basketball and volleyball. We prefer a lace-up brace with figure-of-eight straps or a functional stirrup brace that is placed beneath the insole of the shoe.

The "Ultra" ankle brace (Bregg, San Diego, CA) effectively limits inversion injuries but still allows the ankle to dorsiflex and plantar-flex. However, some athletes, such as ballet dancers, may not be able to perform in a brace, which limits its usefulness in certain activities. Another effective means of preventing inversion injuries is to apply a slight lateral flare to the sole of the tennis shoe or a lateral wedge to an insole. This, again, is effective only for certain sports in which a tennis shoe is worn.

Ankle taping may be of some benefit, but much of the strength is lost because of loosening of the tape within the first 10 minutes. We use a closed basket weave technique (Fig. 5-16).

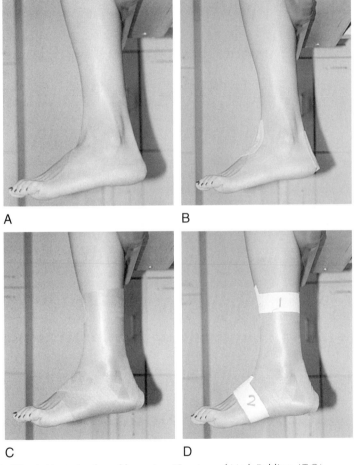

Figure 5–16   Ankle taping for ankle sprains. (Courtesy of Mark Bohling, AT-C.)
1. Have the seated athlete position the ankle at 90 degrees (**A**).
2. Spray a tape adherent (e.g., Tuf-Skin, QDA) over the area to be taped.
3. Apply a heel and lace pad with skin lubricant on the anterior and posterior aspects of the ankle (**B**).
4. Apply pre-wrap, starting at the midfoot and continuing up the leg, and overlap by half until approximately 5 to 6 inches above the medial malleolus (**C**).
5. Apply an anchor strip at the proximal (#1) and distal (#2) ends of the pre-wrap, with half of the tape covering the pre-wrap and the other half adhering to the skin (**D**).

Continued

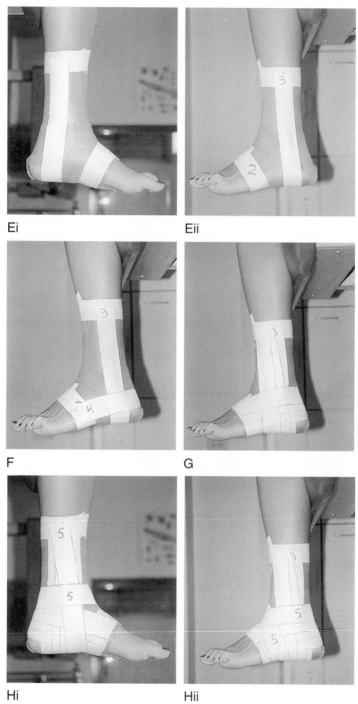

Ei

Eii

F

G

Hi

Hii

Figure 5–16, cont'd Ankle taping for ankle sprains.
For legend see opposite page.

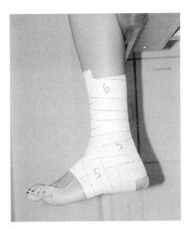

I

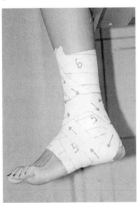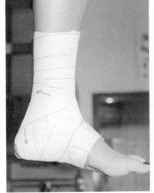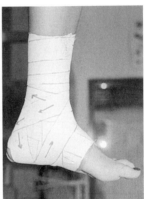

Ji   Jii   Jiii

Figure 5–16, cont'd   Ankle taping for ankle sprains.

6. Starting posteromedially on the proximal anchor, apply a stirrup covering the posterior third of the medial malleolus and then under the foot and up the lateral side to the proximal anchor (#3) (**Ei** and **Eii**).

7. Starting at the distal anchor (#4), apply a horseshoe around the heel (approximately 2 inches from the plantar surface) to the other side of the distal anchor (**F**).

8. Repeat steps 6 and 7 twice. Each time, overlap the previous strip by half the width of the tape (**G**).

9. To apply a figure-of-eight, start medially (**Hi**) at the position of the first stirrup (#5) and pull the tape at an angle toward the medial longitudinal arch (approximately where the third stirrup goes under the foot), across the anterior aspect of the ankle, and around the ankle (just above the third horseshoe strip) (**Hii**).

10. Close up the tape by applying single strips of tape around the leg and overlapping by half until the area from the ankle to the proximal anchor is covered (#6) (**I**).

11. To apply a heel lock, start at the anterior aspect of the proximal anchor laterally. Pull the tape at an angle (*arrows*) toward the posterior aspect of the lateral malleolus, around the posterior aspect of the ankle, under the heel, up the lateral side of the foot, and across the anterior aspect of the ankle (**Ji-Jiii**).

Continued

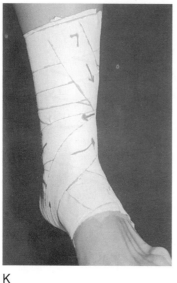

K

Figure 5–16, cont'd   Ankle taping for ankle sprains. To apply a continuous double-heel lock, make one complete loop around the ankle (#7); continue around the ankle, down around the posterior aspect of the ankle, under the heel, up the medial side of the foot (**K**), and across the anterior aspect of the ankle; and complete with another full loop around the ankle.

Chronic Lateral Ankle Instability: Rehabilitation after Lateral Ankle Ligament Reconstruction

Mark Colville MD • Ken Stephenson, MD

It is estimated that long-term sequelae such as pain, swelling, or instability develop in 20% to 40% of patients with ankle sprains. Interestingly, the severity of the ankle sprain does not seem to correlate with the development of chronic symptoms. If a patient has received appropriate treatment of an ankle sprain and has completed a rehabilitation program but continues to have significant symptoms, another etiology of the symptoms must be sought. Causes to be considered in patients with chronic ankle pain include occult bony injuries such as fractures, osteochondral defects, or bone contusions; cartilage damage; ankle, subtalar, or syndesmosis instability secondary to ligament rupture; tendon pathology such as a peroneal tendon or posterior tibial tendon (PTT) longitudinal tear; neuropraxia of the superficial peroneal or sural nerves; or soft tissue problems such as anterolateral ankle soft tissue impingement.

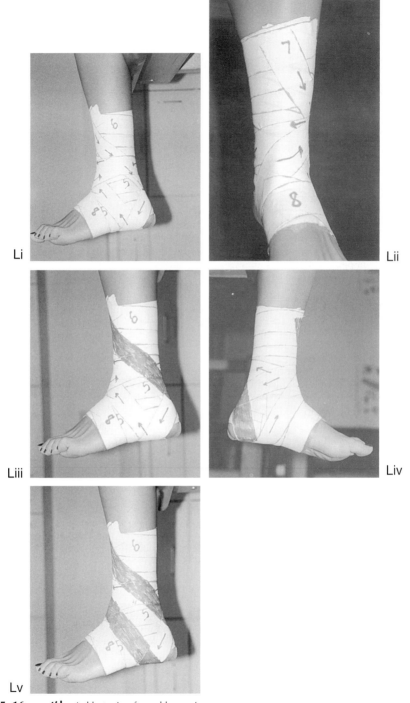

Li

Lii

Liii

Liv

Lv

Figure 5–16, cont'd Ankle taping for ankle sprains.
12. Apply one or two closure strips (*dark tape*) around the foot (#8) to hold the horseshoes down to the foot and the anchor strip (**Li-Lv**).

Possible Causes of Chronic Ankle Pain

Chronic ankle ligament instability (instability with minor provocation, such as stepping off a curb)

Reflex sympathetic dystrophy

Undetected syndesmotic sprain or diastasis (see p. 552)

Undetected tear of the deltoid ligament (medially)

Stress fracture

PTT injury

Osteochondral fracture or osteochondritis dissecans of the talus or tibial plafond

Os trigonum fracture (posterior pain, clicking, positive radiograph)

Subtalar joint sprain or instability

Tibiotalar synostosis (ossification of the syndesmosis impairing normal tibiofibular motion with restricted dorsiflexion on examination)

Midfoot sprain of the transverse tarsal (midtarsal), intertarsal, or tarsometatarsal joints

Bony impingement from osteophytes off the anterior surface of the tibia, with soft tissues trapped between the spur and the talus during dorsiflexion

Ankle arthrosis

Undetected fractures
- Lateral, medial, or posterior malleolus
- Posterior or lateral process of the talus
- Anterior process of the calcaneus
- Fifth metatarsal
- Navicular or other midtarsal bone

Nerve injuries
- Superficial peroneal nerve stretch after ankle sprain
- Common peroneal nerve entrapment
- Tarsal tunnel syndrome (entrapment of the posterior tibial nerve)

Tumor

RADIOGRAPHIC EXAMINATION

If the patient has a history or examination consistent with instability, stress radiographs (talar tilt and anterior drawer) are indicated. Although there is some controversy in the literature regarding normal values for stress radiographs, in general, a *positive talar tilt* is more than 15 degrees or more than a 10-degree difference from the contralateral side. A *positive anterior drawer* is 5- to 10-mm anterior subluxation of the talus or more than a 5-mm difference from the contralateral side. Magnetic resonance imaging (MRI) is useful for delineating bone contusions, avascular necrosis, osteochondral defects, and tendon or ligament injuries. The diagnosis of chronic lateral ankle ligament instability is based on a history of multiple inversion ankle sprains, often with fairly minor provocation (such as stepping off a curb). Instability, not pain alone, should be the primary criterion for ligament reconstruction.

ANKLE LIGAMENT RECONSTRUCTION

Numerous surgical procedures have been described for correction of lateral ankle instability, but the most commonly used is the modified Broström procedure. It involves anatomic repair of the ATFL and CFL augmented by suture of the superior edge of the inferior peroneal retinaculum to the anterior edge of the fibula. This procedure is particularly indicated in ballet dancers or patients whose livelihood depends on full ROM and in most patients undergoing reconstruction for the first time.

The Gould modification of the Broström ligament reconstruction procedure allows augmentation of the ligament repair by suturing the inferior extensor retinaculum to the fibula. Mechanical testing of fresh cadaver feet showed a mean 58% increase in torque to failure in feet treated with the Gould modification as compared with those treated without augmentation (Aydogan et al., 2004).

Currently, the editors use autograft gracilis or allograft anatomic reconstruction (anterior tibial tendon) for **revision** of failed Broström procedures. We prefer this type of anatomic reconstruction and revision in patients with little or no native tissue left instead of peroneus brevis–sacrificing procedures (Chrisman-Snook, Evans, etc.). These latter nonanatomic repairs have a good success rate (80%) but limit subtalar and ankle motion, a nondesirable result in the athletic population.

The goal of ankle ligament reconstruction in an unstable ankle is to restore stability while preserving normal ankle and subtalar motion whenever possible. Most patients with chronic instability have laxity of the ATFL and CFL and increased subtalar joint motion.

GENERAL PRINCIPLES OF REHABILITATION AFTER ANKLE LIGAMENT RECONSTRUCTION

Postoperatively, a short leg, well-padded splint is applied with the ankle in slight eversion, and the patient remains non–weight-bearing. One to 2 weeks after surgery, the patient is placed in a removable cast boot or a short leg walking cast with the foot in neutral position and is allowed to begin partial weight-bearing, with progression to full weight-bearing as tolerated. Four weeks postoperatively, the patient is placed in a functional brace or removable cast boot, and active rehabilitation is started with gentle ROM exercises and isometric strengthening exercises. Usually at 6 weeks, proprioception and balancing exercises are started. In athletes, sport-specific exercises are started at about 8 weeks postoperatively. Return to sports or dancing is allowed when peroneal strength is normal and the patient is able to perform multiple single-leg hops on the injured side without pain. A lace-up brace or functional stirrup brace should be worn for at least the first season, and most athletes prefer bracing or taping for sports indefinitely.

REHABILITATION PROTOCOL	*After Modified Broström Ankle Ligament Reconstruction* Modified Hamilton Protocol

DAYS 0-4

• Place the ankle in anterior-posterior plaster splints in neutral dorsiflexion and discharge the patient as non–weight-bearing.

DAYS 4-7

• When swelling has subsided, apply a short leg walking cast with the ankle in neutral.
• Allow weight-bearing as tolerated in the cast.

Continued

REHABILITATION PROTOCOL: *After Modified Broström Ankle Ligament*
Reconstruction   Continued

WEEK 4

- Remove the cast.
- Apply an air splint for protection, to be worn for 6-8 weeks after surgery.
- Begin gentle ROM exercises of the ankle.
- Begin isometric peroneal strengthening exercises.
- Avoid adduction and inversion until 6 weeks postoperatively.
- Begin swimming.

WEEK 6

- Begin proprioception/balancing activities.
  - Unilateral balancing for timed intervals
  - Unilateral balancing with visual cues
  - Balancing on one leg and catching a #2 plyoball
  - Slide board, increasing distance
  - Fitter activity, catching ball
  - Side-to-side bilateral hopping (progress to unilateral)
  - Front-to-back bilateral hopping (progress to unilateral)
  - Diagonal patterns, hopping
  - Mini-tramp jogging
  - Shuttle leg press and rebounding, bilateral and unilateral
  - Positive deceleration, ankle everters, Kin-Com
- Complete rehabilitation of the peroneals is essential.
- Dancers should perform peroneal exercises in full plantar flexion, the position of function in these athletes (Fig. 5-17A).
- Early in rehabilitation, pool exercises may be beneficial (see Fig. 5-17B).
- Dancers should perform plantar flexion/eversion exercises with a weighted belt (2-20 pounds).

WEEKS 8-12

- Patient can return to dancing or sports if peroneal strength is normal.

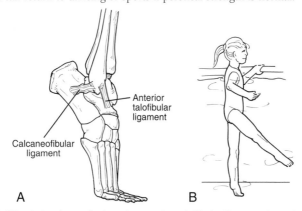

Figure 5–17   A, In plantar flexion, the anterior talofibular ligament is vertically oriented and is particularly vulnerable to inversion forces. Plantar flexion is the position of function for ballet dancers. **B**, During rehabilitation, Barre exercises may also be performed in a pool to take advantage of the buoyancy in water. (Adapted from Malone T: Rehabilitation of the foot and ankle injuries in ballet dancers. J Orthop Sports Phys Ther 11:8, 1990.)

Inferior Heel Pain (Plantar Fasciitis)

S. Brent Brotzman, MD

CLINICAL BACKGROUND

Heel pain is best classified by anatomic location (see the differential diagnosis box). This section discusses plantar fasciitis (inferior heel pain). Posterior heel pain is discussed in the section on Achilles tendinitis.

Differential Diagnosis of Heel Pain

Plantar (inferior) signs and symptoms

    Plantar fasciitis/plantar fascia rupture/partial plantar fascia rupture

    Calcaneal spur or heel spur (misnomer)

    Fat pad syndrome

    Calcaneal periostitis

    Compression of the nerve to the abductor digiti quinti (rare)

    Calcaneal apophysitis (skeletally immature patients), called Sever's disease

Medial

    PTT disorders (insufficiency, tenosynovitis, or rupture)

    Tarsal tunnel syndrome

    Jogger's foot (medial plantar neuropraxia)

    Medial calcaneal neuritis (very rare)

Lateral

    Peroneal tendon disorders (tendinitis, rupture)

    Lateral calcaneal nerve neuritis

Posterior

    Retrocalcaneal bursitis

    Haglund's deformity (pump bump)

    Calcaneal exostosis

    Achilles tendinitis/tendinosis/partial rupture/complete rupture

Diffuse

    Calcaneal stress fracture

    Calcaneal fracture

Other

    Systemic disorders (often bilateral heel pain present)

    Reiter's syndrome

Continued on following page

Ankylosing spondylitis

Lupus

Gouty arthropathy

Pseudogout (chondrocalcinosis)

Rheumatoid arthritis

Systemic lupus erythematosus

Modified from Doxey GE: Calcaneal pain: A review of various disorders. J Orthop Sports Phys Ther 9:925, 1987.

ANATOMY AND PATHOMECHANICS

The plantar fascia is a dense, fibrous connective tissue structure originating from the medial tuberosity of the calcaneus (Fig. 5-18). Of its three portions—medial, lateral, and central bands—the largest is the central portion. The central portion of the fascia originates from the medial process of the calcaneal tuberosity superficial to the origin of the flexor digitorum brevis, quadratus plantae, and abductor hallucis muscles. The fascia extends through the medial longitudinal arch into individual bundles and inserts into each proximal phalanx.

The medial calcaneal nerve supplies sensation to the medial aspect of the heel. The nerve to the abductor digiti minimi may rarely be compressed by the intrinsic muscles of the foot. Some studies, such as those by Baxter and Thigpen (1984), suggest that nerve entrapment (abductor digiti quinti) does on rare occasion play a role in inferior heel pain (Fig. 5-19).

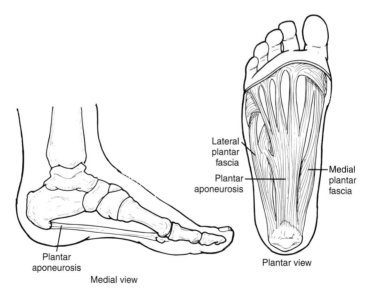

Figure 5–18 From its origin at the calcaneal tubercle, the plantar fascia extends distally and attaches to the metatarsophalangeal joints and the base of the toes. It is functionally divided into contiguous medial, central, and lateral bands. The fascia covers the intrinsic musculature and neurovascular anatomy of the plantar surface of the foot. (Adapted from McGarvey WC: Heel pain: Front line management of a bottom line problem. J Musculoskel Med 15[4]:14, 1998.)

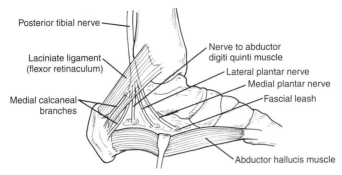

Figure 5–19   Site of entrapment of the posterior tibial nerve and its branches. Note the nerve to the abductor digiti minimi, which on rare occasion may be entrapped with resultant burning and neurogenic pain in the inferior aspect of the heel.

The plantar fascia is an important static support for the longitudinal arch of the foot. Strain on the longitudinal arch exerts its maximal pull on the plantar fascia, especially its origin on the medial process of the calcaneal tuberosity. The plantar fascia elongates with increased loads to act as a shock absorber, but its ability to elongate is limited (especially with the decreasing elasticity common with age). Passive extension of the metatarsophalangeal (MTP) joints pulls the plantar fascia distally and also increases the height of the arch of the foot (Fig. 5-20).

The plantar aponeurosis is essential to foot biomechanics. It transmits Achilles tendon forces from the hindfoot to the forefoot during the stance phase of gait (Erdemir et al., 2004).

Riddle and Schappert (2004) reported that approximately 1 million patient visits per year are made to medical doctors because of plantar fasciitis. Sixty-two percent of these visits were made to primary care physicians and 31% were made to orthopaedic surgeons. Podiatry visits were not included in the estimates.

In an examination of the factors associated with disability related to plantar fasciitis, Riddle et al. (2004) found that an increased body mass index was the only variable that was significantly associated with increased disability.

The activities most affected in this study were running-related activities and the patients' usual work and hobbies. Non–weight-bearing activities and household activities were least affected.

MYTH OF THE HEEL SPUR

The bony spur at the bottom of the heel does not cause the pain of plantar fasciitis. Rather, this pain is caused by inflammation and microtears of the plantar fascia.

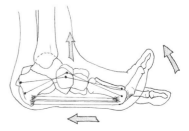

Figure 5–20   The windlass effect. Dorsiflexion of the metatarsophalangeal joints results in increased arch height. (From Mann RA, Coughlin MJ: Survey of the Foot and Ankle, 6th ed. St Louis, CV Mosby, 1993.)

The spur is actually the origin of the short flexors of the toes. Nonetheless, the misnomer persists among the lay public and in the literature.

Heel spurs have been found in approximately 50% of patients with plantar fasciitis. This exceeds the 15% prevalence of radiographically visualized spurs in normal asymptomatic patients noted by Tanz (1963). However, spur formation is related to progression of age. The symptomatic loss of elasticity of the plantar fascia with the onset of middle age suggests that this subset of patients would be expected to show an increased incidence of spurs on radiographs.

ETIOLOGY

Inferior (subcalcaneal) pain may well represent a spectrum of pathologic entities, including plantar fasciitis, nerve entrapment of the abductor digiti quinti nerve, periostitis, and subcalcaneal bursitis.

Plantar fasciitis is more common in sports that involve running and long-distance walking and is also frequent in dancers, tennis players, basketball players, and nonathletes whose occupations require prolonged weight-bearing. Direct repetitive microtrauma to the ligamentous and nerve structures with heel strike has been implicated, especially in middle-aged, overweight, nonathletic individuals who stand on hard, unyielding surfaces, as well as in long-distance runners.

Some anatomic features seem to make plantar fasciitis more likely. Campbell and Inman (1974) noted that in patients with *pes planus*, *heel pronation* increased tension on the plantar fascia and thereby predisposed the patient to heel pain. Pronation of the subtalar joint everts the calcaneus and lengthens the plantar fascia. A *tight gastrocnemius* (with increased compensatory pronation) also predisposes patients to plantar fasciitis. Cavus feet with relative rigidity have been noted to place more stress on the loaded plantar fascia. Several studies have shown an association between plantar fasciitis and obesity. However, other researchers have not demonstrated similar findings.

Bone spurs may be associated with plantar fasciitis, but they are not believed to be the cause of it. Many studies show no clear association between spurs and plantar fasciitis. Studies of patients with plantar fasciitis report that 10% to 70% have an associated ipsilateral calcaneal spur; however, most also have a spur on the contralateral asymptomatic foot. Anatomic studies have shown that the spur is located at the origin of the short toe flexor tendon rather than at the plantar fascia origin, thus further casting doubt on its role in contributing to heel pain.

NATURAL HISTORY

Although plantar fasciitis can seem quite debilitating during the acute phase, it rarely causes lifelong problems. It is estimated that 90% to 95% of patients who have true plantar fasciitis recover with nonoperative treatment. However, recovery frequently takes 6 months to 1 year, and patients often require much encouragement to continue stretching, wearing appropriate and supportive shoes, and avoiding high-impact activities or prolonged standing on hard surfaces. Operative treatment can be very helpful in selected "failed" patients, but the success rate of surgery is only 50% to 85%.

Orthotripsy (extracorporeal shock wave treatment) has shown some promise, with less risk for post-treatment longitudinal arch collapse than after plantar fascia release (see page 589).

BILATERAL HEEL INVOLVEMENT

Diagnosis of bilateral plantar fasciitis requires ruling out systemic disorders such as Reiter's syndrome, ankylosing spondylitis, gouty arthropathy, and systemic lupus erythematosus. A high index of suspicion for a systemic disorder should accompany bilateral heel pain in a young male aged 15 to 35 years.

Causes of Inflammation of the Heel

PRIMARY INFLAMMATION

Idiopathic
Local factors
  Abnormal foot alignment
  Cavus foot (high arch)
  Planovalgus foot
  Pronated foot (flatfoot)
  Leg-length discrepancy
  Externally rotated lower limb
Increased loading on the plantar fascia
  Tight Achilles tendon
  Fat pad atrophy
  Osteopenia of the calcaneus
Systemic factors
  Overweight
  Systematic disease
  Inflammatory arthritis
  Gout
  Sarcoidosis
Hyperlipoproteinemia
Training errors
  Overuse
  Incorrect training
  Incorrect footwear
  Hard surface
Middle age

SECONDARY INFLAMMATION

Local inflammatory conditions
Sprain of the foot
Nerve entrapment
  Medial branch of the posterior tibial nerve (rare)
  Nerve to the abductor digiti quinti (rare)
Bony disorders
  Accessory coalition
  Tarsal coalition
  Subtalar instability
  Calcaneal periostitis
  Fracture
  Haglund's deformity
Subcalcaneal bursitis
Retrocalcaneal bursitis

Continued

Causes of Inflammation of the Heel   *Continued*

SECONDARY INFLAMMATION—cont'd

Systemic inflammatory conditions
  Inflammatory arthritis
  Gout
  Infection
  Gonorrhea
  Tuberculosis

Modified from Noyes FE, Demaio M, Mangine RE: Heel pain. Orthopedics 16:1154, 1993.

SIGNS AND SYMPTOMS

The classic findings of plantar fasciitis include a gradual, insidious onset of inferomedial heel pain at the insertion of the plantar fascia (Fig. 5-21). Pain and stiffness are worse with rising in the morning or after prolonged ambulation and may be exacerbated by climbing stairs or doing toe raises. It is rare for patients with plantar fasciitis to not have pain or stiffness with the first few steps in the morning or after prolonged rest.

EVALUATION OF PATIENTS WITH INFERIOR HEEL PAIN

- History and examination
- Biomechanical assessment of the foot
  - Pronated or pes planus foot
  - Cavus-type foot (high arch)
  - Assessment of the fat pad (signs of atrophy)
  - Presence of a tight Achilles tendon
- Squeeze test of the calcaneal tuberosity (medial and lateral sides of the calcaneus) to evaluate for a possible calcaneal stress fracture
- Evaluation for possible training errors in runners (e.g., rapid increase in mileage, running on steep hills, poor running shoes, improper techniques)
- Radiographic assessment with a 45-degree oblique view and standard three views of foot
- Bone scan if recalcitrant pain (>6 weeks after initiation of treatment) or a stress fracture is suspected from the history
- Rheumatologic work-up (Table 5-1) for patients with a suspected underlying systemic process (patients with bilateral heel pain, recalcitrant symptoms, or associated sacroiliac joint or multiple joint pain)
- Electromyographic (EMG) studies if clinical suspicion of nerve entrapment
- Establish the correct diagnosis and rule out other possible causes (Tables 5-2 and 5-3).

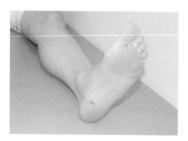

Figure 5–21   Plantar fasciitis pain is inferior, located at the origin of the plantar fascia.

TABLE 5-1	Rheumatologic Findings in Patients with a Suspected Underlying Systemic Process Associated with Heel Pain				
	Rheumatoid Arthritis	**Reiter's Syndrome**	**Ankylosing Spondylitis**	**Hyperlipoproteinemia Type II**	**Gout**
Signs	Retrocalcaneal bursitis, most common Cocking-up of toes Subluxation of metatarsal heads Fibular deviation of toes 2-5 Swelling of tibiotalar joint Loss of subtalar motion	Plantar fasciitis Acute diffuse swelling of digits Pain at medial calcaneal tuberosity or swelling over Achilles insertion Low back pain	Plantar fasciitis May follow Reiter's syndrome Limited chest expansion Low back pain Painful sacroiliac joints	Plantar nodules and fasciitis Xanthomatous nodules in plantar fascia	Plantar fasciitis Tophi Swelling of ankle Pain Metatarsal pain and swelling
Radiographic signs	Changes at metatarsal and interphalangeal joints of great toe	Enthesopathy Periostitis	Enthesopathy Periostitis Spine radiographs characteristic	Asymmetrical arthritis of small and large joints	Bony erosion Calcific tophi

From Noyes FE, DeMaio M, Mangine RE: Heel pain. Orthopedics 16:1154, 1993.

TABLE 5–2	Helpful Findings in Evaluating the Etiology of Heel Pain
Etiology	**Findings**
Plantar fasciitis	Pain and tenderness located **inferiorly** at the plantar fascia origin (not posteriorly)
	Almost all patients complain of inferior heel pain in the mornings with the first few steps and may complain of pain after prolonged walking or standing
Plantar fascia rupture	Typically antecedent plantar fasciitis symptoms, with a pop or "crunch" during push-off or pivoting, then severe pain with subsequent inability to bear weight (or only with difficulty)
	Most commonly follows iatrogenic weakening of the fascia after cortisone injection
Calcaneal stress fracture	Much more common in athletes and runners with overuse history and repetitive high-impact activity or osteoporotic elderly females with overuse in their walking or exercise regimen (e.g., 4 miles/day, 7 days/wk)
	Pain is **more diffuse** than that of plantar fasciitis, with a **positive squeeze test** (see Fig. 5-22), rather than discrete, localized inferior heel pain
	Bone scan is positive for a linear fracture rather than increased tracer uptake at the plantar fascia origin as in plantar fasciitis.
	Unless a calcaneal stress fracture is suspected, bone scanning is not part of routine work-up (see Fig. 5-23)

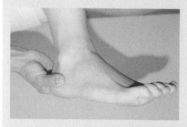

Figure 5–22 The squeeze test of the calcaneus is positive when the patient has a stress fracture. Palpation of the calcaneal tuberosity is painful on squeeze testing.

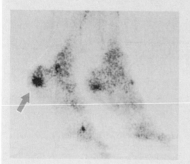

Figure 5–23 A bone scan of the feet of a 40-year-old male runner demonstrates increased tracer uptake at the right medial calcaneal tuberosity (*arrow*), typical of acute plantar fasciitis. (From Batt T: Overuse injuries in athletes. Physician Sports Med 23[6]:63, 1995.)

TABLE 5–2	Helpful Findings in Evaluating the Etiology of Heel Pain—cont'd

Etiology	Findings
Sever's disease (calcaneal apophysitis)	Symptoms almost identical to those of plantar fasciitis, except that tenderness is not inferior, with more symptoms at the physis Occurs only in skeletally immature patients with inflammation or apophysitis at the physis Treatment is the same as for plantar fasciitis, except that a well-padded UCBL orthotic is used
Achilles tendinitis or rupture, Haglund's deformity	Pain is **posterior** rather than inferior In Haglund's deformity (pump bump), tenderness is present over the prominent bony deformity, which often rubs or is irritated by the heel counter of the shoe Patients with a complete rupture of the Achilles tendon describe a feeling of being "shot" in the tendon while pushing off and have a positive Thompson squeeze test (see Fig. 5-39) and a lack of active plantar flexion except a small flicker from the long toe flexors
Posterior tibial tendon (PTT) insufficiency	Pain is **medial** rather than inferior or posterior Often, difficulty or inability to perform a unilateral heel raise (see the PTT section) Frequently, point tender and boggy along the course of the PTT medially
Tarsal tunnel syndrome	Pain and numbness or tingling in the medial aspect of the ankle radiating to the **plantar** aspect of the foot only. No dorsal foot numbness or tingling (consider peripheral neuropathy if dorsal numbness is present) Positive Tinel sign medially in the tarsal tunnel. Electromyography is 90% accurate in identifying well-established tarsal tunnel syndrome Decreased sensation in the distribution of the medial plantar or lateral plantar nerve, or both (plantar distribution only)
Reiter's syndrome, seronegative spondyloarthropathies	Bilateral plantar fasciitis in a young male is often one of the first symptoms of an inflammatory arthritis Consider an HLA-B27 test and rheumatoid profile if other joint involvement is noted
Jogger's foot	Jogger's foot (as described by Rask) consists of local nerve entrapment of the medial plantar nerve at the fibromuscular tunnel formed by the abductor hallucis muscle and its border with the navicular tuberosity Most often associated with a valgus hindfoot deformity (pronator) and long-distance running Characterized by running-induced neuritic pain (medial arch) radiating into the medial aspect of the toes along the distribution of the medial plantar nerve. This distribution is medial and on the plantar aspect of the foot

TABLE 5–3	Palpatory Signs of Heel Pain Syndrome
Diagnosis	**Anatomic Location of Pain**
Plantar fasciitis	Origin of the plantar aponeurosis at the medial calcaneal tubercle
Fat pad syndrome	Plantar fat pad (bottom and sides)
Calcaneal periostitis	Diffuse plantar and medial and lateral calcaneal borders
Posterior tibial tendon disorders	Over the medial midtarsal area at the navicular; may radiate proximally behind the medial malleolus
Peroneal tendon disorders	Lateral calcaneus and peroneal tubercle
Tarsal tunnel syndrome	Diffuse pain involving the plantar surface of the foot; may radiate distally with tingling, burning, and numbness in the bottom of the foot only (not dorsal)
Medial calcaneal neuritis	Well localized to the anterior half of the medial plantar heel pad and medial side of the heel; does not radiate into the distal part of the foot
Lateral calcaneal neuritis	Heel pain that radiates laterally, more poorly localized
Calcaneal stress fracture	Diffuse pain over the entire calcaneus; positive squeeze test of the calcaneal tuberosity
Calcaneal apophysitis	Generalized over the posterior aspect of the heel, especially the sides, in skeletally immature patients (apophysis)
Generalized arthritis	Poorly localized but generally involving the entire heel pad

Modified from Doxey GE: Calcaneal pain: A review of various disorders. J Orthop Sports Phys Ther 9:925, 1987.

REHABILITATION PROTOCOL

Treatment of Plantar Fasciitis
Brotzman

GENERAL PRINCIPLES

- Examine the lower extremity for possible contributing factors: pes cavus (high arch), pes planus (flat arch), leg-length discrepancy, fat pad atrophy, signs of systemic inflammatory arthritis, morbid obesity, etc.
- Review and question for possible training errors or overuse in runners and athletes (see Chapter 7, Special Topics).
- Identify poor shoe wear, hard walking or running surface, supinator- or pronator-like wear of running shoes.
- Treatment phases are progressively more aggressive, or more invasive measures are used if the first phase is unsuccessful in relieving symptoms.
- Repetitive daily plantar fascia stretches plus Achilles tendon stretching has been shown to provide the **most effective relief** of plantar fasciitis (83% successful results). Stretching should be done each morning before ambulation and four or five times throughout the day. One to 2 months of daily stretching may be required for significant pain relief.
- The key to successful treatment is **patient education** to convey to the patient that 95% of patients with plantar fasciitis eventually have resolution of symptoms in 6-12 months with conservative treatment despite the intense pain often encountered initially.
  We use a patient educational tape and handout from www.orthovid.com (Fig. 5-24).

REHABILITATION PROTOCOL: *Treatment of Plantar Fasciitis* *Continued*

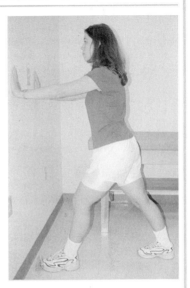

Figure 5–24 The www.orthovid.com Plantar Fasciitis patient instructional video series (25 minutes) is used to give the patient all the background, anatomy, rehabilitation exercises, and other information that are difficult to cover in the office. These tapes were created in coordination with physicians from this text (www.orthovid.com).

PHASE 1

Plantar Fascia Stretching

- Done 4-5 times a day, 5-10 repetitions.
- Done before the first steps in morning, before standing after a long period of rest.
- Seated plantar fascia stretching:
  - While sitting, grab all five toes and pull the toes back toward the knee (Fig. 5-25). Hold for 30 seconds and repeat five times. An alternative method is to crouch with the toes curled (extension at the MTP joints) under the feet. Sit back on the heels until tension is felt in plantar fascia origin (Fig. 5-26). Hold for 30 seconds *without* bouncing. Repeat 5 times.
  - While seated, place the foot as shown in Figure 5-27, and then begin applying downward pressure on the calf. Hold for 30 seconds. Repeat 5 times.
- Plantar fascia stretches against the wall:
  - Place the foot against the wall as shown in Figure 5-28. Gently lean forward slowly and hold for 30 seconds. Repeat 3-5 times.

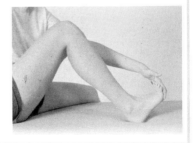

Figure 5–25 Plantar fascia stretch. The patient sits with the knees bent and the heel flat on the floor. The tops of the toes are gently bent upward with the hand. With the ankle dorsiflexed, pull the toes toward the ankle. Hold the stretch in a sustained fashion for 10 seconds; repeat 10 times a day. The stretch should be felt in the plantar fascia.

Continued

REHABILITATION PROTOCOL: *Treatment of Plantar Fasciitis* Continued

PHASE 1—cont'd

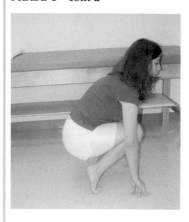

Figure 5–26 Alternative plantar fascia stretches. The patient crouches with the toes curled up under the feet (metatarsophalangeal joint extension). The buttocks are gently lowered to the heels until mild tension is felt in the bottom of the feet. Hold for 30 seconds and repeat five times per session. Do not bounce.

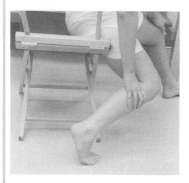

Figure 5–27 Seated plantar fascia stretches. While seated, the patient places the metatarsophalangeal (MTP) joints into hyperextension and gently presses the calf to further stretch the MTP joints. Hold for 30 seconds; repeat five times per session.

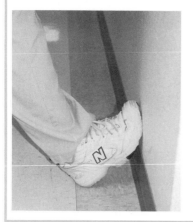

Figure 5–28 Plantar fascia stretch against the wall.

REHABILITATION PROTOCOL: *Treatment of Plantar Fasciitis*   *Continued*

PHASE 1—cont'd

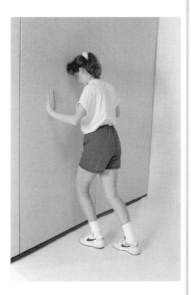

Figure 5–29   Bent-knee runner's stretch (soleus stretch).

Runner's Stretches for the Achilles Tendon

- A tight Achilles tendon is often implicated as an exacerbating or causative factor in plantar fasciitis. For this reason, much attention is given to Achilles tendon stretching exercises.
- Soleus runner's stretch:
  - Slowly stretch (no bobbing) the Achilles tendon by placing the affected leg back (Fig. 5-29) and slowly bending the knee into a flexed position. Hold for 30 seconds and repeat 5 times.
- Gastrocnemius runner's stretch:
  - Keep the knee straight and slowly stretch the affected leg for 30 seconds (Fig. 5-30).

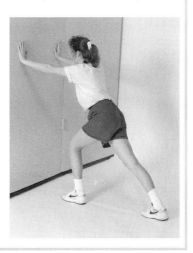

Figure 5–30   Runner's stretch (gastrocnemius).

Continued

REHABILITATION PROTOCOL: *Treatment of Plantar Fasciitis* *Continued*

PHASE 1—cont'd

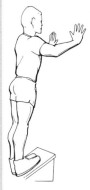

Figure 5–31 Runner's stretch on an incline board. (From DeLee JC, Drez D Jr: Orthopaedic Sports Medicine: Principles and Practice. Philadelphia, WB Saunders, 1994.)

- Achilles stretching on an incline board:
  - Place the feet as shown in Figure 5-31 and hold for 30 seconds while slowly leaning forward to stretch the Achilles tendon.

Relative Rest

- Discontinue running and activities until asymptomatic for 6 weeks. Switch to
  - Low-impact exercise
  - Stationary bicycling
  - Swimming
  - Deep-water "running" with an aqua belt (see the aquatic therapy section, Chapter 7)
- Weight loss.
- Modification of hard surfaces (cement) to soft surfaces (grass or cinder).

Cushioned Heel Inserts

- The American Orthopaedic Foot and Ankle Society (AOFAS) in a multicenter study found that inexpensive, over-the-counter cushioned heel inserts were **more effective** for plantar fasciitis than expensive, rigid, custom orthotics.
- We typically use well-cushioned running shoes and Viscoheel inserts (Fig. 5-32) or PPT/Plastazote inserts (Alimed) initially.
- Patients with abnormal biomechanics of the lower extremity, such as pes cavus or pes planus, may benefit from the eventual use of custom cushioned orthotics (see phase 2).

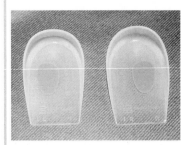

Figure 5–32 Viscoheels. Soft cushions are placed in whatever shoe the patient is wearing (1-800-423-3405).

REHABILITATION PROTOCOL: *Treatment of Plantar Fasciitis*   *Continued*

PHASE 1—cont'd

Shoe Wear Modification (Running Shoes)

- Flared, stable heel to help control heel stability.
- Firm heel counter to control the hindfoot.
- Soft cushioning to raise the heel 12-15 mm higher than the sole.
- Well-molded Achilles pad.
- Avoid rigid leather dress shoes that increase torque on the Achilles tendon.

Low-Dye Taping

- Some patients obtain relief with low-dye taping, but from a practicality standpoint, daily taping is difficult to maintain.
- The science behind low-dye taping has not been effectively studied.

Ice Massage

- Ice to the area of inflammation for an anti-inflammatory effect.
- Use ice in a paper or Styrofoam cup (peeled away) for 5-7 minutes; make sure to avoid frostbite.

ANTI-INFLAMMATORIES

- Oral anti-inflammatories have variable results. A brief trial of a cyclooxygenase-2 (COX-2) inhibitor (e.g., celecoxib [Celebrex]) is initiated. If response is not dramatic, this therapy is discontinued because of possible side effects.

PHASE 2

- If phase 1 measures fail to relieve symptoms after several months, phase 2 treatments are instituted.
- Before initiation of these measures, re-evaluate the patient for other causes of heel pain:
  - Consider a bone scan if a calcaneal stress fracture is suspected.
  - Consider an HLA-B27 and rheumatoid/seronegative spondyloarthropathy laboratory work-up if other systemic signs or symptoms are evident.

Casting

- Casting has been shown to be helpful in about 50% of patients.
- A short-leg walking cast can be used for 1 month, with the foot placed in neutral.
- A removable cast (cam boot) is used if the right foot is involved (to allow the patient to remove the cam boot to drive).
- Evaluate progress at 1 month; consider an additional month of removable cast wear if necessary.
- Complete the second month of cast wear in a removable boot to allow a gradual transition from the boot back into running shoes.

Orthotics

- Patients with very high or very low arches may benefit from orthotic inserts.
- A less rigid, accommodative insert is applicable to a more rigid cavus type of foot (high arch), which requires more cushion and less hindfoot control.
- A padded but rigid insert is indicated for a more unstable foot with compensatory pronation (pes planus or low arch), which requires more control.

Cortisone Injection (Fig. 5-33)

- Injection of cortisone into the area close to the plantar fascia often improves pain, **but it may weaken the plantar fascia and lead to rupture and eventual collapse of the arch**.

Continued

REHABILITATION PROTOCOL: *Treatment of Plantar Fasciitis*   *Continued*

ANTI-INFLAMMATORIES—cont'd

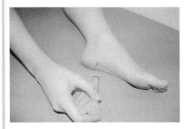

Figure 5–33   Technique for a cortisone injection (plantar fasciitis).

- The possible risks associated with injection (rupture, fat pad atrophy, infection) must be discussed with the patient and the possible long-term sequelae weighed against short-term benefits.
- One or possibly two steroid injections may be given in a 3- to 6-month period, and only after failure of phase 1 treatment measures.

Night Splints

- A 5-degree dorsiflexion night splint worn at night has been reported to be beneficial. The splint holds the plantar fascia in a continuously tensed state. The theory behind the use of a night splint is to minimize the change in tension on the fascia that occurs with each day's new activities. Other commercial night splints are manufactured at neutral (0 degrees) and are available through AliMed (1-800-225-2610) (Fig. 5-34).

Modalities

- Ultrasound (Fig. 5-35).
- Deep friction massage (Fig. 5-36).
- Modalities may be beneficial for selected patients, but the literature on their efficiency is inconclusive.

PHASE 3

- A recent form of treatment of recalcitrant plantar fasciitis involves the use of high-energy extracorporeal shock wave treatment with an OssaTron device (Healthtronics, Marnetta, GA). This treatment, known as orthotripsy, is used in patients who have failed multiple phase 1 and phase 2 nonoperative measures.

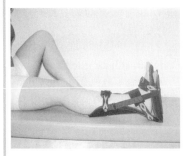

Figure 5–34   Position of the splint for use at night.

REHABILITATION PROTOCOL: *Treatment of Plantar Fasciitis*   *Continued*

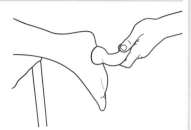

Figure 5–35   Ultrasound of the plantar fascia.

PHASE 3

- Alvarez et al. (2003), in a study involving the use of orthotripsy, reported a satisfactory result in 83% of patients at 1 year after one or two treatments. The duration of pretreatment symptoms had minimal impact on the orthotripsy results. A 76% satisfaction rate was obtained for patients with symptoms present more than 2 years before orthotripsy. Placebo treatment had a 55% success rate. The rate of satisfactory results was 82% for patients with plantar fasciitis and a heel spur. Seventy-nine percent was reported for those with plantar fasciitis and no heel spur.
- The editors like to try this form of treatment before surgical plantar fascia release because of the significant incidence of longitudinal arch collapse and recalcitrant calcaneocuboid pain associated with plantar fascia release.
- Haake et al. (2003), however, performed a randomized double-blind trial of 137 patients treated by extracorporeal shock wave therapy for chronic plantar fasciitis. At 12 weeks the success rate was only 35% for orthotripsy and 30% in the placebo group. Similar results were present in both groups at 1 year, which led the authors to conclude that extracorporeal shock wave therapy was ineffective for the treatment of plantar fasciitis.
- Thus there remains significant controversy in the literature on the efficacy of orthotripsy in the treatment of plantar fasciitis.
- Patients in whom all phase 1 and 2 measures have failed may also be candidates for surgical intervention (plantar fascia release).
- Because of the high complication rate from this surgery and the self-limited nature of plantar fasciitis in 90% to 95% of patients, we extend our operative indications to failure of all phase 1 and 2 treatments for 18 months. Much of the literature recommends 12 months of conservative therapy.
- We **never** perform endoscopic release because of the increased complication rate and poor visualization in comparison to open release and the inability to identify the nerve to the abductor digiti quinti.

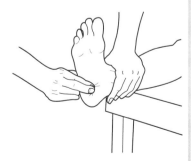

Figure 5–36   Deep friction massage of the plantar fascia.

<table>
<tr><td></td><td>

***American Orthopaedic Foot and Ankle Society
Position on Endoscopic and Open Heel Surgery***
</td></tr>
</table>

Nonsurgical treatment is recommended for a minimum of 6 months and preferably 12 months.

More than 90% of patients respond to nonsurgical treatment within 6-10 months.

When surgery is being contemplated, medical evaluation should be considered before surgery.

Patients should be advised of complications and risks if an endoscopic or open procedure is indicated.

If nerve compression is coexistent with fascial or bone pain, an endoscopic or closed procedure should not be attempted.

The AOFAS does not recommend surgical procedures before nonoperative methods have been used.

The AOFAS supports responsible, carefully planned surgical intervention when nonsurgical treatment fails and work-up is complete.

The AOFAS supports cost constraints in the treatment of heel pain when the outcome is not adversely altered.

The AOFAS recommends heel padding, medications, and stretching before prescribing custom orthoses or extended physical therapy.

This position statement is meant as a guide to the orthopaedist and is not intended to dictate a treatment plan.

RUPTURE OF THE PLANTAR FASCIA

Background

Though not commonly reported in the literature, partial or complete plantar fascia rupture may occur in jumping or running sports. Frequently, it is missed or misdiagnosed as an acute flare-up of plantar fasciitis. Complete rupture of the plantar fascia usually results in permanent loss of the medial (longitudinal) arch of the foot. Such collapse is typically quite disabling for athletes.

Examination

Patients generally complain of a pop or crunch in the inferior heel area, with immediate pain and inability to continue playing. It usually occurs during push-off, jumping, or initiation of a sprint. After an antecedent cortisone injection, the trauma may be much more minor (e.g., stepping off a curb).

Weight-bearing is very difficult, and swelling and ecchymosis in the plantar aspect of the foot occur fairly rapidly. Palpation along the plantar fascia elicits marked point tenderness. Dorsiflexion of the toes and foot often causes pain in the plantar fascia area.

Radiographic Evaluation

Diagnosis of a plantar fascia rupture is a clinical one. Pain radiographs are taken (three views of the foot) to rule out a fracture. MRI may be used but is not necessary for diagnosis (Fig. 5-37). MRI may miss the area of the actual rupture but does typically pick up the associated hemorrhage and swelling surrounding the rupture.

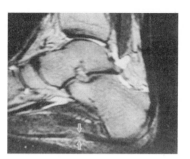

Figure 5–37 In this sagittal magnetic resonance image of the right foot of a male college basketball player, increased signal intensity and discontinuity of the plantar fascia (*arrows*) are consistent with edema, hemorrhage, and complete rupture. (Courtesy of the Radiology Department of the Medical College of Ohio at Toledo. From Kruse RJ: Diagnosing plantar fasciitis. Physician Sports Med 23[1]:117, 1995.)

REHABILITATION PROTOCOL | *After Rupture of the Plantar Fascia*
Brotzman

PHASE 1: DAYS 0-14

- Immediate non–weight-bearing with crutches
- Light compression wrap changed several times a day for 2-3 days
- Ice therapy with ice massage of the swollen/ecchymotic area several times a day
- Maximal elevation on 4-5 pillows above the level of the heart for 72 hours, then elevation for 8-12 hr/day (sleeping with pillows under the foot)
- Non–weight-bearing, light, fiberglass cast on day 3, worn for 1-2 weeks, depending on the resolution of pain
- Nonsteroidal anti-inflammatory drugs (NSAIDs) (if not contraindicated) for 2-3 weeks
- Gentle active toe extension and flexion exercises while still in the cast

PHASE 2: WEEKS 2-3

- Removal of the fiberglass cast
- Use of a ⅛-inch felt pad placed from the heel to the heads of the metatarsals (Fig. 5-38) and lightly wrapped with bandage (Coban, Unna boot, Ace bandage). We use a cotton sock or Coban to keep the felt in place
- The foot and felt wrapping are placed in a removable walking cast, which allows the foot to be taken out daily for therapy and pool exercises
- Weight-bearing is progressed from as tolerated in the boot with crutches to weight-bearing in the boot only. Pain is the guiding factor for progression of weight-bearing
- Exercises are begun as pain allows:
  - Swimming
  - Deep-water running with an Aquajogger.com flotation belt
  - Stationary bicycling with no resistance
  - Gentle Achilles stretches with a towel looped around the foot

PHASE 3: WEEKS 3-8

- Proprioception exercises with a BAPS board as pain allows
- Removable cast and felt typically worn for 4-6 weeks
- Active ankle strengthening exercises are progressed
- High-impact exercises are held until patient has been completely asymptomatic (with ambulation in a tennis shoe) for 2-3 weeks
- Use of a custom orthotic layered with an overlying soft substance (such as Plastazote) is often helpful for eventual athletic participation

Continued

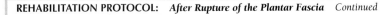

REHABILITATION PROTOCOL: *After Rupture of the Plantar Fascia*   *Continued*

PHASE 3: WEEKS 3-8—cont'd

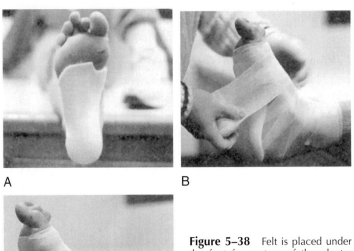

A

B

C

Figure 5–38   Felt is placed under the foot for rupture of the plantar fascia. **A,** To allow mobility on a torn plantar fascia after the initial cast is removed, a ⅛-inch felt pad is placed from the heel to the heads of the metatarsals. **B** and **C,** The pad is held in place with a Coban or Unna boot dressing. (From Kruse RJ, McCoy RL, Erickson ATC: Diagnosing plantar fascia rupture. Physician Sports Med 23[1]:65, 1995.)

- It is not uncommon to have permanent impairment in high-impact athletes who have suffered a plantar fascia rupture. For this reason, cortisone injections should rarely, if ever, be used in high-impact athletes.

Achilles Tendon Dysfunction

Robert C. Greenberg, MD • Charles L. Saltzman, MD

The Achilles tendon is the largest and strongest tendon in the body. The tendon has no true synovial sheath but is encased in a paratenon of varying thickness. The vascular supply to the tendon comes distally from intraosseous vessels from the calcaneus and proximally from intramuscular branches. There is a relative area of avascularity 2 to 6 cm from the calcaneal insertion that is more vulnerable to degeneration and injury. Achilles tendon injuries are commonly associated with repetitive impact loading as a result of running and jumping. *The primary factors resulting in damage to the Achilles tendon are training errors such as a sudden increase in activity, a sudden increase in training intensity (distance, frequency), resumption of training after a long period of inactivity, and running on uneven or loose terrain.* Achilles dysfunction can also be related to postural problems (e.g., pronation), poor footwear (generally poor hindfoot support), and a tight gastrosoleus complex.

ACHILLES TENDINITIS

Important Practitioner Pearls about the Achilles Tendon

1. The Achilles tendon is the largest tendon in the human body. It can withstand forces across it of up to 1000 pounds. Nonetheless, it is the most frequently ruptured tendon.
2. Because of its size and unique anatomy, the Achilles tendon is susceptible to both acute (or sudden) and chronic (nagging and ongoing) injuries. Sudden injuries generally include partial or complete rupture of the Achilles tendon. Chronic injuries are usually Achilles tendinitis (inflammation of the tendon) or tendinosis (degeneration of the tendon) or paratenonitis (inflammation of the sleeve surrounding the Achilles tendon tissue, called the paratenon).
3. Achilles tendonitis is a very common overuse injury and is characterized by inflammation and pain in the Achilles tendon.
4. This large tendon serves to connect the calf musculature to the heel bone. The more rigorous the activity, the greater the stress exerted across the Achilles tendon. This translates to up to 10 times body weight repetitively exerted on the Achilles tendon during running.
5. Rupture of the Achilles tendon usually occurs 2 to 6 cm proximal (or up) from where the tendon inserts into the heel bone (calcaneus).
6. The Achilles tendon is surrounded by a structure called the paratenon, a sleeve of tissue that allows it to glide smoothly. This paratenon is able to stretch 2 to 3 cm with movement of the tendon. If the paratenon becomes contracted (tight), it can also be a source of inflammation and pain.
7. Lagergren and Lindholm (1958), in a classic blood supply study, found that the most poorly supplied region of blood flow to the Achilles is located in a region 2 to 6 cm proximal to (above) the insertion of the Achilles tendon into the heel. This poor blood supply explains why this is the most common area of rupture or tearing with a sudden injury to the Achilles.
8. Achilles tendonitis is an **overuse injury** found most often in middle-aged men and is very commonly associated with running sports and high impact.

How Common Is Achilles Tendinitis?

1. The incidence of Achilles tendinitis in runners is reported to vary from 6.5% to 18% (Clain and Baxter, 1992).
2. Clement et al. (1984) found a disproportionately high number of Achilles injuries in male runners as compared with women (7.9% of men and 3.2% of women).

Common Causes of Achilles Tendinitis

The following are *very common training errors*:

1. **Overuse with high-impact sports** involving running and/or repetitive jumping. Overuse injuries of the Achilles tendon most commonly occur in individuals who are active and subject the tendon to repetitive large forces beyond its ability to heal.
2. **A rapid increase** in either **mileage** or **intensity** (speed) or running.
3. **Inadequate Achilles stretching** before and after a high-impact exercise.
4. **Resuming** previous mileage **too quickly** after a period of rest or layoff from exercise.
5. Adding **hill running** or stair climbing to a running regimen.
6. Poorly made, worn-out, or **rigid shoe wear** placing increased stress on the Achilles tendon.
7. Poor natural flexibility of the calf muscles and lower extremity musculature.

Classification (Types) of Achilles Tendinitis

Insertional Achilles Tendinitis

- Pain is located where the tendon physically inserts into the heel bone (calcaneus).
- Pain and tenderness are located at the tendon-bone junction (low at the very end of the actual tendon).
- The pain is frequently worse after exercise but may ultimately become constant.
- Insertional Achilles tendonitis can be aggravated by running uphill or activities performed on hard surfaces.
- Frequently the patient reports a history of poor stretching, running up on the heels, excessive distance in running, or a sudden increase in training intensity (speed, hills, distance, etc.).

Noninsertional Achilles Tendinitis

- Puddu and colleagues (1976) devised a classification system for noninsertional tendonitis in which three possible entities were described: peritendinitis, peritendinitis with tendinosis of the Achilles, and pure tendinosis.
- These three entities all occur 2 to 6 cm proximal to the insertion of the Achilles tendon into the heel bone.
- In peritendinitis (peri meaning around), the inflammation is limited only to the lining surrounding the Achilles tendon.
- In peritendinitis *with* tendinosis, a portion of the tendon also becomes involved in the disease process, with inflammation of the Achilles tendon (tendinosis) occurring as well as inflammation of the lining of the Achilles.
- In pure tendinosis, the tendon eventually degenerates in an area 2 to 6 cm proximal (above) to the insertion into the heel bone. This degeneration leads to localized tenderness with a large nodule that can be felt and, on occasion, crunching/grinding and a thickened tendon in this area. This degenerative tendon in an area of poor blood supply is thought by many to be a precursor/causative factor in a complete rupture (tearing) of the tendon with rapid push-off (e.g., sprinting) of the involved leg.

"Vascular Wringing" Theory

Many experts (Clement et al., 1984; James et al., 1978) have implicated functional "overpronation" as a causative factor for noninsertional Achilles tendinitis. To understand the term "pronation," think of a flat-footed person running and the foot collapsing even flatter when the heel strikes the ground (pronation). This abnormal rotatory force places extremely high force on the tendon, essentially "wringing out" blood flow that is trying to reach the tendon. Eventually, this leads to Achilles tendonitis (inflammation) and then tendinosis (degeneration). A flat-footed "pronator" is encouraged to get orthotics and appropriate running shoes (often with an antipronation segment built into the shoe, and to cross-train with low-impact activities (swimming, cycling, etc.)

General Treatment Strategies for Achilles Tendonitis (Insertional and Noninsertional)

1. **Rest** from the aggravating/flaring exercise or activity. An avid runner is encouraged to swim or "run" in the deep end of the pool in a flotation belt (www.aquajogger.com) without the feet striking the bottom. This "deweights" the forces normally generated when the heel strikes the pavement. Complete rest is a good option in a recreational runner.

2. Application of **"wet ice"** to the inflamed area several times a day and after activity. Ice has an anti-inflammatory effect by constricting the blood vessels that bring in inflammatory cells. By "wet ice" we mean by an ice bag or cold pack placed on a wet towel on the location to be iced. This allows the ice to cool the area faster while still protecting the skin from frostbite.

3. **Oral anti-inflammatories** to decrease inflammation. The authors use Celebrex, 200 mg orally per day, but numerous NSAIDs exist, and clinicians will recommend their favorite.

4. **Custom-made orthotic devices (inserts)** in the shoes often help. Heel lifts placed in the running shoe take some pressure off the Achilles. Custom orthotics are helpful if the patient has underlying "abnormal" foot biomechanics (high arch, flatfoot, etc) that place added stress on the Achilles.

5. **Stretching**. Achilles/calf stretching (30 seconds per stretch) several times a day before and after activity. Stretch all other tight lower extremity structures (e.g., quad, hip flexors, hamstrings).

6. **Activity modification** such as decreasing the speed or mileage and hill running. Stop interval training or sprinting. Alternate days (Monday, Wednesday, Friday) with a day of rest in between. Cross-train with low-impact activities that decrease the stress on the Achilles. Such activities include swimming, cycling, and walking. Failure to respond to activity modification requires complete cessation of running with rest from high-impact activity.

7. *Never* allow a physician to inject cortisone around or in the Achilles tendon. This often results in a tendon **rupture** because the cortisone temporarily weakens the tendon.

8. Avoidance of rigid (leather) dress shoes that place more stress on the Achilles or hard rigid shoe counters (back of the shoe) that rub or irritate the Achilles tendon.

9. **New** well-cushioned **running shoes** fit to the patient by a person knowledgeable about runners, foot types, pronation, supination, etc.

10. Failure to eventually respond to these nonoperative measures may lead to complete rest and use of a removable walking boot (with a rocker bottom) worn during ambulation to "cool down" the tendonitis for 6 weeks.

How Long Should a Patient Endure Nonsurgical Treatment before Considering Surgical Intervention?

Recommendations on this topic vary widely from 6 weeks (Marcus et al., 1989) to 12 weeks (Scioli 1994) of nonsurgical treatment up to 6 months or 1 year if some improvement is noted with the nonoperative treatment (Leach et al., 1992; Schepsis et al., 1994).

The authors recommend 4 to 6 months of nonoperative treatment in patients younger than 35 years unless the symptoms significantly worsen.

Differential Diagnosis of Achilles Tendinitis

Partial rupture of the Achilles tendon

Retrocalcaneal bursitis (of the retrocalcaneal bursa)

Haglund's deformity (pump bump)

Calcaneal apophysitis (skeletally immature—Sever's apophysitis)

Calcaneal exostosis

Calcaneal stress fracture (positive squeeze test)

Calcaneal fracture (acute fall or motor vehicle accident)

PTT tendinitis (medial pain)

Plantar fasciitis (inferior heel pain)

Examination

Examination is performed with the patient placed prone and the feet hanging off the edge of the table. Palpate the entire substance of the gastrocnemius-soleus myotendinous complex while the ankle is put through active and passive ROM. Evaluate for tenderness, warmth, swelling or fullness, nodularity, or substance defect. The **Thompson test** is performed to evaluate the continuity of the Achilles tendon (Fig. 5-39). A positive Thompson test (no plantar flexion of the foot with squeezing of the calf) indicates a complete rupture of the Achilles tendon. Note the resting position of the forefoot with the ankle and talonavicular joints held in the neutral position. Ankle and subtalar mobility may often be decreased. Calf atrophy is common in any Achilles tendon dysfunction.

While seated on the examination table, the patient's foot should be passively dorsiflexed, first with the knee flexed and then with the knee fully extended. This will tell the examiner how tight the Achilles tendon is. Many females who have worn high-heeled shoes for years will not be able to dorsiflex the foot to neutral with the knee in full extension.

Figure 5–39 Thompson squeeze test. This test evaluates the Achilles tendon for complete rupture. In a normal patient placed prone with the knee flexed at 90 degrees, squeezing the calf muscle will cause the foot to plantar-flex (*arrow*) because the tendon is intact. With a complete rupture of the tendon, squeezing of the calf will not cause plantar flexion of the foot (i.e., a positive Thompson test indicates a complete rupture). This test is important because most patients with a completely ruptured Achilles tendon can still weakly plantar-flex the foot on request by "cheating" with the long toe flexors. (Adapted from Kovan JR, McKeag DB: Lower extremity overuse injuries in aerobic dancers. J Musculoskel Med 9[4]:43, 1992.)

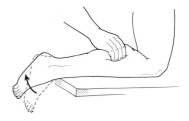

Do not be fooled by the patient's ability to weakly plantar-flex the foot during evaluation for a potential complete rupture of the Achilles. The long toe flexors can still weakly plantar-flex the foot despite a complete Achilles rupture.

Imaging

Most Achilles problems can be diagnosed with a thorough history and physical examination. Imaging helps confirm the diagnosis, assist with surgical planning, or rule out other diagnoses.
- *Routine radiographs* are generally normal. Occasionally, calcification in the tendon or its insertion is noted. Inflammatory arthropathies (erosions) and Haglund's deformity (pump bump) can be ruled out on radiographs.
- *Ultrasound* is inexpensive and fast and allows dynamic examination, but it requires substantial interpreter experience. It is the most reliable method for determining the thickness of the Achilles tendon and the size of a gap after a complete rupture.
- *MRI* is not used for dynamic assessment, but it is superior in the detection of partial tears and evaluation of various stages of chronic degenerative changes, such as peritendinous thickening and inflammation. MRI can be used to monitor tendon healing when recurrent partial rupture is suspected and is the best modality for surgical planning (location, size).

ACHILLES PARATENONITIS

Background

Inflammation is limited to the paratenon without associated Achilles tendinosis. Fluid often accumulates next to the tendon, and the paratenon is thickened and adherent to normal tendon tissue. Achilles paratenonitis most commonly occurs in mature athletes involved in running and jumping activities. It does not generally progress to degeneration. Histologic evaluation of paratenonitis shows inflammatory cells and capillary and fibroblastic proliferation in the paratenon or peritendinous areolar tissue.

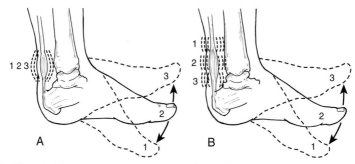

Figure 5–40   Painful arc sign. **A,** In peratenonitis, the tenderness remains in one position despite moving the foot from dorsiflexion to plantar flexion. **B,** In the case of partial tendon rupture or tendinitis, the point of tenderness moves as the foot goes from dorsiflexion to plantar flexion. (Adapted from Williams JG: Achilles tendon lesions in sport. Sports Med 3:114, 1986.)

Clinical Signs and Symptoms

Pain starts with initial morning activity. The discomfort is well-localized tenderness and sharp, burning pain with activity. The discomfort is present 2 to 6 cm proximal to the insertion of the Achilles tendon into the calcaneus. Pain is primarily aggravated by activity and relieved by rest. Pain is elicited with single-heel raises and absent on the Thompson test. Significant heel cord contracture will exacerbate symptoms.

Swelling, local tenderness, warmth, and tendon thickening are common. Calf atrophy and weakness and tendon nodularity can be present in chronic cases. Crepitation is rare.

The *painful arc sign* (Fig. 5-40) is negative in paratenonitis. It is important to localize the precise area of tenderness and fullness. In paratenonitis, the area of tenderness and fullness stays fixed with active ROM of the ankle. Here the inflammation involves only the paratenon, which is a fixed structure, unlike pathology of the Achilles tendon itself, which migrates superiorly and inferiorly with ROM of the ankle.

In the acute setting, symptoms are typically transient, present only with activity, and last less than 2 weeks. Later, symptoms start at the beginning of exercising or at rest, and tenderness increases. The area of tenderness is well localized and reproducible by side-to-side squeezing of the involved region.

Partial rupture may be superimposed on chronic paratenonitis and can result in an acute episode of pain and swelling.

REHABILITATION PROTOCOL   *Treatment of Achilles Paratenonitis*

PHASE 1: 0-6 WEEKS

- Rest and/or activity modification is required to reduce symptoms to a level that can achieve pain-free activity.
- If pain is severe, a walking boot or cast is worn for 3-8 weeks to allow pain-free activities of daily living.
- Crutch-assisted ambulation is added when there is persistent pain with a boot or cast.

REHABILITATION PROTOCOL: *Treatment of Achilles Paratenonitis*   Continued

PHASE 1: 0-6 WEEKS—cont'd

- Most patients have chronic pain that requires an initial period of complete rest until symptoms subside, followed by rehabilitation and gradual return to activities.
- NSAIDs and ice massage decrease pain and inflammation, particularly in the acute phase.
- A stretching program is essential. Gentle calf, Achilles, and hamstring stretching is done 3-4 times a day.
- Acute pain usually resolves in the first 2 weeks.
- Footwear is changed or modified if overpronation or poor hindfoot support is present.
- Athletic activity:
  - Gradual return to activity
  - Adequate warm-up and cool-down periods
  - Stretching of the gastrocnemius-soleus complex before and after exercise
  - Decrease in duration and intensity
  - Decreased training on hard surfaces
  - Avoidance of hill and incline training
  - Replacement of inadequate or worn-out footwear
- Progress to gentle strengthening with low-impact exercises.

PHASE 2: 6-12 WEEKS

- Indicated for failed phase 1 or recurrent symptoms after previous resolution.
- Repeat or continue phase 1 immobilization and stretching.
- Add modalities:
  - Contrast baths
  - Ultrasound
- Footwear:
  - Small heel lift for severe pain
  - Arch support orthotic if overpronation present
- Persistent heel cord tightness is treated by stretching exercises and the use of a 5-degree dorsiflexion night ankle-foot orthosis worn for 3 months while sleeping.
- Staged cross-training program for most athletes, especially runners.
- Aqua jogging and swimming, stationary cycling, exercise on stair-climbing and cross-country skiing machines. Avoid repetitive impact loading (e.g., running).

PHASE 3: 3 MONTHS AND BEYOND

- **Brisement** (only for paratenonitis):
  - Dilute local anesthetic and sterile saline injected into the paratenon sheath to break up adhesion between the inflamed paratenon and the Achilles tendon (preferable to steroid injection). Can be done with ultrasound to confirm correct placement
- Corticosteroid injections:
  - Generally avoided
  - Rarely indicated, only for recalcitrant cases to inhibit inflammation and prevent scar formation
  - The risk for adverse effects if injected into the tendon or if overused is generally worse than any known benefit

Operative Treatment of Paratenonitis

Operative treatment is generally indicated if 4 to 6 months of conservative treatment fails to relieve the symptoms. Preoperative MRI is usually obtained primarily to evaluate for associated tendinosis and confirm the diagnosis.

Technique

The patient is positioned prone and a thigh tourniquet is applied. A longitudinal incision is made posteromedially along the Achilles tendon. Full-thickness flaps are raised, with very gentle soft tissue handling. The thickened paratenon and adhesions are removed posteriorly, medially, and laterally as needed. **Anterior dissection is avoided because the blood supply of the tendon is primarily within the anterior mesotenon and fat pad**. The tendon is inspected for thickening and degeneration (tendinosis); if noted intraoperatively or on MRI, surgical treatment is as described for tendinosis.

Postoperative Protocol

- A padded splint is applied in neutral position.
- Non–weight-bearing motion is initiated immediately, both active ROM and gentle passive dorsiflexion with rubber tubing.
- Crutch-assisted weight-bearing as tolerated is initiated after 7 to 10 days, when pain permits and swelling has decreased. If the wound is healing uneventfully at 2 to 3 weeks, ambulation is allowed as tolerated.
- Exercises are begun on a stationary bike and stair climber when the patient can walk without pain. Swimming and aqua jogging are allowed, as tolerated by the patient and when the wound is healed.
- Running can be resumed 6 to 10 weeks postoperatively.
- Return to competition is allowed after 3 to 6 months; calf strength must be at least 80% of the normal side.

ACHILLES TENDINOSIS

Background

Achilles tendinosis is characterized by intratendinous or mucoid degeneration of the Achilles tendon without evidence of paratenonitis (inflammation). The process starts with interstitial microscopic failure, which leads to central tissue necrosis and subsequent mucoid degeneration. Achilles tendinosis most commonly occurs in mature athletes as a result of accumulated repetitive microtrauma from training errors. It is associated with an increased risk for Achilles tendon rupture.

Achilles tendinosis may be insertional (commonly associated with ossification on plain films) or may occur in the avascular zone (2 to 6 cm proximal to the insertion).

The histology is generally noninflammatory, with decreased cellularity and fibrillation of collagen fibers within the tendon. Along with the collagen fiber disorganization, there is scattered vascular ingrowth and occasional areas of necrosis and rare calcification.

Initially, the paratenon sheath may become inflamed, and with overuse, the tendon itself becomes inflamed or hypovascular because of restriction of blood flow through the scarred paratenon.

Clinical Signs and Symptoms

Achilles tendinosis is often asymptomatic and remains subclinical until the tendon ruptures. It may elicit low-grade discomfort related to activities, and a palpable pain-less mass or nodule may be present 2 to 6 cm proximal to the insertion of the tendon (i.e., in the avascular area). This can progress to gradual thickening of the entire tendon substance.

The painful arc sign is positive in patients with Achilles tendinosis. The thickened portion of tendon moves with active plantar flexion and dorsiflexion of the ankle (in contrast to paratenonitis, in which the area of tenderness remains in one position despite dorsiflexion and plantar flexion of the foot).

Paratenonitis and tendinosis can coexist when inflammation involves the paratenon and intratendinous focal degeneration is present. It gives the clinical appearance of paratenonitis because the symptoms associated with tendinosis are absent or very subtle. Most patients seek treatment of symptoms related to the paratenonitis, and usually, the tendinosis is unrecognized until both processes are noted on MRI or at surgery (most commonly after a rupture). Conservative treatment is the same as for paratenonitis. MRI is very useful in preoperative planning, which must consider both entities.

Treatment

The initial treatment of Achilles tendinosis is always conservative and progresses as described for paratenonitis. If symptoms are severe, initial treatment may include 1 to 2 weeks of immobilization and crutch ambulation, in addition to NSAIDs, ice, and heel cord stretching. Foot and leg alignment should be carefully evaluated, with orthotic correction if necessary.

Topical glyceryl trinitrate patches applied for 6 months were found to be more effective in the treatment of noninsertional Achilles tendinopathy than placebo in a double-blind study from Australia (Paoloni et al., 2004). Patients who received the medicated patch had significantly reduced pain with activity at 6 months. Seventy-eight percent of the 36 tendons in the medicated group were asymptomatic with activities of daily living, versus 49% of the 41 tendons in the control group. Conservative treatment is continued for 4 to 6 months; surgery is indicated if such treatment fails to relieve the symptoms.

Operative Treatment

MRI is used to confirm the diagnosis and plan the operative procedure.

Technique.
The patient is placed prone with a thigh tourniquet and the foot hanging off the end of the table. The incision is placed posteromedially just off the edge of the tendon (avoids the sural nerve). Full-thickness flaps are created with very careful soft tissue handling. The paratenon is inspected and any hypertrophic paratenon adherent to the tendon is excised. A longitudinal incision is made within the body of the tendon over the thickened, nodular parts to expose areas of central tendon necrosis. Degenerative areas are excised (should correspond with MRI). Débridement is followed by side-to-side closure to repair any defect. If the defect is too large to be closed prima-rily or lacks adequate substance after débridement, the Achilles tendon is recon-structed with the plantaris tendon, flexor digitorum longus, or a turn-down flap.

REHABILITATION PROTOCOL	*After Débridement of Achilles Tendinosis*

- A padded splint is applied in neutral position.
- Gentle non–weight-bearing motion is begun in first week; active ROM and passive dorsiflexion with rubber tubing are done several times a day.
- A removable walking boot with an adjustable heel is used for 2-4 weeks. Crutch-assisted ambulation for the first 10-14 days. At 2 weeks, weight-bearing without crutches is allowed in the boot as tolerated.
- Stationary bicycling is begun when the patient is ambulating comfortably.
- Swimming and aqua jogging are started when the wound is completely healed.
- Running is typically allowed 8-10 weeks after surgery.
- Return to competition is allowed at 4-6 months.
- If significant reconstruction is done along with débridement, rehabilitation must progress more slowly, similar to that following tendon repair after rupture.

REHABILITATION PROTOCOL	*General Guidelines for Achilles Tendinitis, Paratenonitis, and Tendinosis in High-Impact Athletes* Brotzman

- Establish the correct diagnosis.
- Correct underlying training and biomechanical problems.
  - Stop any rapid increase in mileage.
  - Stop hill running.
  - Correct improper intensity of training, duration, schedule, hard surface, poor shoe wear.
  - Decrease mileage significantly and/or initiate cross-training (pool, bicycle), depending on the severity of symptoms at initial evaluation.
  - Correct functional overpronation and resultant vascular wringing of the tendon (Fig. 5-41) with a custom orthotic that usually incorporates a medial rear foot post.
  - Stop interval training.

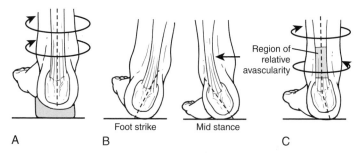

Figure 5–41 **A**, Correction of functional overpronation by a medial rear foot post minimizes the potential for postulated vascular wringing. **B**, Whipping action of the Achilles tendon produced by overpronation. **C**, External tibial rotation produced by knee extension conflicting with internal tibial rotation as a result of prolonged pronation. This results in "wringing out" of vessels in the zone of relative avascularity. (Adapted from Clement DB, Taunton JF, Smart GW: Achilles tendinitis and peritendinitis: Etiology and treatment. Am J Sports Med 12[3]:181, 1984.)

REHABILITATION PROTOCOL: *General Guidelines for Achilles Tendinitis, Paratenonitis, and Tendinosis in High-Impact Athletes   Continued*

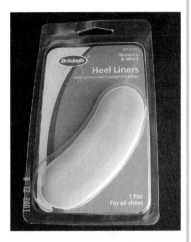

Figure 5–42   Soft heel counter inserts (Dr. Scholl's: www.DrScholls.com) to lessen rubbing of the posterior heel counter on the Achilles tendon.

- Soften a hard heel counter or use shoe counter heel cushions (Fig. 5-42) to minimize posterior "rubbing" symptoms.
- Begin a runner's stretching program before and after exercises (see p. 595).
- Oral anti-inflammatories (over-the-counter medications or COX-2 inhibitors, e.g., Celebrex).
- **Avoid cortisone injection, which will cause weakening or rupture of the tendon. Hugate et al. (2004), in a rabbit study, reported that intratendinous injections of corticosteroid significantly weakened the Achilles tendon, as did injections into the retrocalcaneal bursa.**
- Use cryotherapy (ice massage) after exercise for its anti-inflammatory effect.
- Correct leg-length discrepancy if noted. First try ¼-inch heel insert for a ½-inch leg-length discrepancy; if not improved, go to ½-inch insert. "Overcorrection" (too rapid an orthotic correction of a long-standing leg-length discrepancy) may worsen the symptoms.
- If symptoms persist after 4-6 weeks of conservative measures, immobilization in a removable cam boot or cast may be required for 3-6 weeks.
- Slow, painless progression to preinjury activities:
  - Swimming
  - Deep-water "running" with an Aquajogger.com flotation belt
  - Bicycling
  - Walking
  - Eccentric exercises for Achilles strengthening
  - Light jogging
- Eccentric strengthening of the Achilles tendon should condition the tendon and make it less susceptible to overuse injuries; however, such exercises are not performed until the patient is asymptomatic and painless for 2-3 weeks:
  - Toe raises in pool
  - Plantar flexion against progressively harder Thera-Bands
  - Multiple sets of very light (20-pound) total gym or slider board exercises (Fig. 5-43)

Continued

REHABILITATION PROTOCOL: *General Guidelines for Achilles Tendinitis, Paratenonitis, and Tendinosis in High-Impact Athletes* Continued

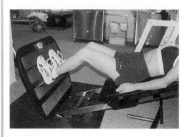

Figure 5–43 Slider board or total gym exercises for strengthening the Achilles tendon.

HAGLUND'S DEFORMITY

- Haglund's deformity, which is a bone prominence emanating from the superior portion of the posterior calcaneal tuberosity, should be differentiated from Achilles tendinosis.
- Haglund's deformity causes pain in the retrocalcaneal bursa that is often increased in association with shoe wear and activity.
- Lietze et al. (2003) reported good success with endoscopic decompression as an alternative to open decompression for the treatment of Haglund's deformity and retrocalcaneal bursitis.
- A hooded burr via a medical portal was used. The average AOFAS ankle-hindfoot score improved from 61.8 preoperatively to 87.5 points postoperatively. The endoscopic procedure had fewer complications than the open technique did.

ACHILLES TENDON RUPTURE

Background

Complete ruptures tend to occur in middle-aged patients and those without preexisting complaints. Partial ruptures occur in well-trained athletes and involve the lateral aspect of the tendon. Acute ruptures commonly result from acute eccentric overload on a dorsiflexed ankle that has chronic tendinosis. Patients should be questioned about previous steroid injection and fluoroquinolones (possible association with tendon weakening and rupture).

Clinical Signs and Symptoms

Sharp pain and a pop heard at the time of complete rupture are commonly reported. Patients often describe a sensation of being kicked in the Achilles tendon. Most have an immediate inability to bear weight or return to activity. A palpable defect may be present in the tendon initially.

Partial rupture is associated with an acutely tender, localized swelling that occasionally involves an area of nodularity.

The Thompson test (see Fig. 5-39) is positive with a complete Achilles tendon rupture. A positive test occurs when squeezing the calf fails to plantar-flex the foot because of lack of continuity of the tendon (rupture).

Thompson Test

The patient is placed prone, with both feet extended off the end of the table. Both calf muscles are squeezed by the examiner. If the tendon is intact, the foot will plantar-flex when the calf is squeezed. If the tendon is ruptured, normal plantar flexion will not occur (a positive Thompson test).

In some patients, accurate diagnosis of a complete rupture is difficult by physical examination alone. The tendon defect can be disguised by a large hematoma. A false-negative Thompson test can occur because of plantar flexion of the ankle caused by the extrinsic foot flexors when the accessory ankle flexors are squeezed together with the contents at the superficial posterior leg compartment. It is important to critically compare the test with results on the normal side.

The long toe flexors can also weakly plantar-flex the foot when examining for a complete Achilles rupture. The examiner should not be fooled by weak plantar flexion on active ROM testing. Patients with a complete rupture of the Achilles can still have weak active plantar flexion via the long toe flexors.

Partial Achilles ruptures are also difficult to accurately diagnose, and MRI should be used to confirm the diagnosis.

Treatment of Acute Rupture of the Achilles Tendon

Both conservative therapy and operative treatment are commonly used to restore length and tension to the tendon to optimize strength and function. Both methods are reasonable, and treatment should be individualized according to operative candidacy. High-level and competitive athletes usually undergo primary repair. Operative repair is associated with lower re-rupture rates, quicker return to full activity, and a theoretically higher level of function. However, the difference in outcomes between conservative and operative treatment is variable. The main surgical risk is wound breakdown. An increased risk for wound problems is noted with tobacco use, steroid use, and female gender. A trend toward an increased risk was seen in diabetic patients (Bruggeman and Turner, 2004). A wound complication occurred in 8 (42%) of 19 patients with two or more of the aforementioned risk factors versus 6.2% of 146 patients without risk factors.

Regardless of the definitive treatment, initial treatment consists of a short leg splint in a comfortable position of plantar flexion, ice, elevation, and crutch ambulation.

Nonoperative treatment of a complete Achilles tendon rupture in a 20-degree plantar-flexed cast is usually reserved for chronically ill patients, poor operative candidates, elderly patients, and low-demand patients. The re-rupture rate is much higher in patients treated nonoperatively (with a plantar-flexed cast for 8 weeks of non–weight-bearing) than in those treated operatively. A review of multiple studies found an average re-rupture rate of 17.5% in nonoperative patients versus 1.2% in operatively treated patients. However, major and minor complications were more frequent with operative treatment.

Josey et al. (2003), in a study of nonoperatively treated Achilles tendon rupture, reported a 95% satisfaction rate. These patients were managed with an equinus cast with a heel buildup and immediate weight-bearing as tolerated.

After 2 months the patients went to a shoe with a heel-rise. At follow-up there was no difference in plantar flexion strength between the injured and uninjured limbs. The rate of re-rupture was 8.3% (4 of 48 patients).

Gorschewsky et al. (2004) reviewed 66 patients managed by percutaneous repair of an acute Achilles rupture and reported no wound complications but 1 re-rupture (with trauma) 3 weeks after the procedure.

Nonoperative Treatment of Acute Achilles Tendon Rupture

Nonoperative treatment in poor operative candidates requires immobilization to allow hematoma consolidation. Ultrasound is used to confirm that apposition of the tendon ends occurs with 20 degrees or less of plantar flexion. Nonoperative treatment is best for small partial ruptures. Surgical repair is indicated if a diastasis or gap remains with the leg placed in 20 degrees of plantar flexion.

A 20-degree, non–weight-bearing, plantar-flexed short leg cast (preference) or a removable boot (not to be removed by the patient) with an elevated heel is worn for 8 weeks. The patient remains non–weight-bearing in the cast for 8 weeks.

At 6 to 8 weeks, plantar flexion of the cast is slowly decreased (most easily done in a commercial cam boot with adjustable ankle angle setting). An initial heel lift of 2 to 2.5 cm should be worn for 1 month when progressive weight-bearing is initiated. Gentle non–weight-bearing active ROM exercises and gentle passive stretching with rubber tubing are begun. At 10 to 12 weeks, the heel lift is decreased to 1 cm and, over the next month, is progressively decreased so that the patient is walking without a heel lift by 3 months.

Progressive resistance exercises for the calf muscles should be started between 8 and 10 weeks. Running may be resumed after 4 to 6 months if strength is 70% of the uninvolved leg. Maximal plantar flexion power may not return for 12 months or more.

Operative Treatment of Complete Achilles Tendon Rupture

Operative treatment is generally preferred for young, athletic, and active patients. The incision and approach are the same as for paratenonitis and tendinosis. A medial approach is used to expose the tendon ends, and a modified Bunnell technique is used to repair the rupture.

REHABILITATION PROTOCOL

After Surgical Repair of Acute Achilles Tendon Rupture in Athletes
Brotzman

- Well-padded 20-degrees equinus posterior splint with a plaster *ankle stirrup* initially postoperatively.
- Non–weight-bearing with crutches for 4 weeks.
- Progress to partial weight-bearing with crutch-assisted ambulation in a short-leg fiberglass cast.

FOR HIGH-LEVEL COMPLIANT ATHLETES

- Initially use a cam boot with 15-20 degrees of equinus (plantar flexion) dialed in, a heel lift, and an ankle angle boot setting of 20 degrees of plantar flexion.
- Active non–weight-bearing ROM exercises can be started as early as 7 days after surgery. The incision must be well healed before initiation of exercises.

REHABILITATION PROTOCOL: *After Surgical Repair of Acute Achilles Tendon Rupture in Athletes*   *Continued*

FOR HIGH-LEVEL COMPLIANT ATHLETES—cont'd

- Initial exercise consists of very gentle passive plantar flexion and active dorsiflexion limited to 20 degrees, 2 sets of 5 performed 3 times a day.
- At 1 month, start to slowly bring the ankle toward neutral by decreasing the heel lift in the boot by 1 cm. Wean out of the heel lift over a 6- to 8-week period.
- Use a walking boot for 6-8 weeks, and then make the transition to normal shoes when using the smaller heel lifts.
- Stationary bicycling (no resistance) and swimming are initiated at 6 weeks.
- Gradual return to competition as with conservative treatment. Must have full strength (versus the nonoperative side) and full endurance and have completed the running program.

FOR LOWER-DEMAND ATHLETES

- Use a short leg, non–weight-bearing, gravity equinus cast for 6-8 weeks, followed by 1-cm heel lift in a removable boot for 1 month.
- Progressive non–weight-bearing resistance exercises are started at 8-10 weeks.
- Stationary bicycling and swimming at approximately 8 weeks.
- Return to some athletic activity (light running) at 5-6 months if strength is 70% of the uninvolved leg.
- Generally, return to full activity takes 1 year, but up to 18 months may be required.

Posterior Tibial Tendon Insufficiency

S. Brent Brotzman, MD

PTT insufficiency is the most common cause of acquired flatfoot deformity in adults.

PTT injuries and insufficiency are among the most commonly missed diagnoses in primary care and orthopaedics. Failure to perform an examination with the patient standing often results in the physician missing collapse of the medial longitudinal arch, hindfoot valgus, and inability to perform a unilateral heel raise, findings that usually characterize PTT injuries. This diagnosis must be remembered in the evaluation of medial ankle and foot pain and unilateral arch collapse with flatfoot deformity.

ANATOMY AND PATHOPHYSIOLOGY

The PTT functions as a plantar flexor of the foot and as an inverter of the subtalar joint. It originates on the posterior aspect of the tibia, interosseous membrane, and fibula. It courses posteriorly along the medial aspect of the ankle, adjacent and posterior to the medial malleolus. The PTT then inserts in the midfoot at the navicular tuberosity and sends bands that attach to the plantar aspect of the cuneiforms, the second, third, and fourth metatarsals, and the sustentaculum tali (Fig. 5-44).

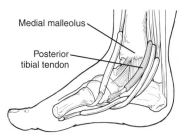

Figure 5–44   Posterior tibial tendon.

The PTT and its opposing tendon, the peroneus brevis, function during the midstance phase of gait. The PTT is very large (cross-sectional area of 16.9 mm^2) in comparison to any of the available tendons that can be transferred to replace it (e.g., the flexor digitorum longus is only 5.5 mm^2).

Loss of the PTT's force of inversion is evidenced in patients with PTT insufficiency by a limited ability or complete inability to perform a unilateral heel raise.

With progressive dysfunction of the PTT, the medial longitudinal arch of the foot collapses, the subtalar joint everts, the heel assumes a valgus position (Fig. 5-45A), and the foot eventually abducts at the talonavicular joint (see Fig. 5-45B).

ETIOLOGY

The etiology of PTT insufficiency ranges from inflammatory synovitis (leading to degeneration, lengthening, and rupture) to acute trauma. Holmes and Mann (1992) reported that 60% of those who suffered a PTT rupture had a history of obesity, diabetes, hypertension, previous surgery or trauma to the medial foot, or previous

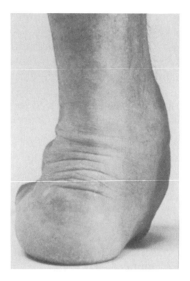

Figure 5–45   Hindfoot valgus and arch collapse of the foot as a result of insufficiency of the posterior tibial tendon. The forefoot is also "abducted" (pointing away from the midline) at the talonavicular joint. (From Mann RA, Coughlin MJ: Surgery of the Foot and Ankle. St Louis, CV Mosby, 1993.)

treatment with steroids. Acute traumatic PTT rupture is very rare. Most ruptures and insufficiency of the PTT are due to gradual failure or intrinsic abnormality rather than extrinsic trauma.

Frey and coworkers (1990) demonstrated a zone of hypovascularity in the tendon beginning 1 to 1.5 cm distal to the medial malleolus and extending 1 cm farther. This area is where most ruptures and degenerative changes are found intraoperatively.

PTT dysfunction may be associated with seronegative inflammatory disorders, including ankylosing spondylitis, psoriasis, and Reiter's syndrome. Other conditions that may be associated with PTT dysfunction include rheumatoid arthritis and pes planus. Injection of steroids (cortisone) around the PTT appears to significantly increase the potential for rupture.

Injection of the PTT with cortisone is contraindicated because of the risk for weakening and rupture of the tendon.

DIAGNOSIS

The diagnosis of PTT insufficiency is primarily a clinical one. MRI of the course of the tendon in the foot and ankle may be of some value if the diagnosis is uncertain. MRI is not routinely recommended and its clinical usefulness is questionable.

Signs and Symptoms

In the early stages of PTT insufficiency, most patients complain of fatigue, aching, and pain of the plantar-medial aspect of the foot and ankle just proximal to the tendon insertion onto the navicular tuberosity (Fig. 5-46). Discomfort is located medially along the course of the tendon. Swelling or bogginess along the tendon is common if the dysfunction is associated with tenosynovitis. Pain is exacerbated by activity, weight-bearing, and calf raises. The patient's ability to walk distances usually decreases.

Examination

Both feet should be examined with the patient standing and both lower extremities entirely visible. The feet should also be viewed from behind to appreciate hindfoot valgus on standing. The too-many-toes sign as described by Johnson (1983) should

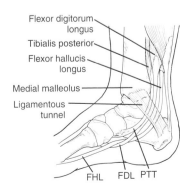

Figure 5–46 Tenderness of the posterior tibial tendon (PTT) proximal to its insertion onto the navicular tuberosity. FDL, flexor digitorum longus; FHL, flexor hallucis longus. (Adapted from Hunter-Griffin LY (ed): Athletic Training and Sports Medicine. Park Ridge, IL, American Academy of Orthopaedic Surgeons, 1991.)

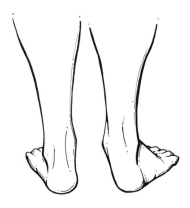

Figure 5–47 The "too-many-toes" sign. More toes are visible lateral to the heel on the patient's right leg. The sign is found with posterior tibial tendon insufficiency and resultant collapse, forefoot abduction, and hindfoot valgus. (From DeLee JC, Drez D Jr: Orthopaedic Sports Medicine: Principles and Practice. Philadelphia, WB Saunders, 1994.)

also be looked for from behind the patient: abduction of the forefoot relative to the hindfoot allows more of the lateral toes to be seen on the symptomatic foot than on the unaffected foot (Fig. 5-47).

Patients with early (stage 1) PTT insufficiency may have only swelling and tenderness medially. As the insufficiency progresses, the longitudinal arch collapses. Hindfoot valgus is initially flexible (hindfoot correctable to subtalar neutral) and eventually becomes fixed.

A single-limb or "unilateral" heel raise should be attempted while the patient is standing (Fig. 5-48). This test is an excellent determinant of the function of the PTT. With support for balance by the examiner, the patient is asked to first suspend the unaffected leg in the air and then attempt to perform a heel raise on the affected foot. With dysfunction of the PTT, inversion of the heel is weak, and the patient is unable to rise onto the forefoot or the heel remains in valgus rather than being swung into varus on heel raise.

While the patient is seated, the examiner should test PTT strength (inversion) against resistance. During the test, the hindfoot should first be positioned in plantar flexion and eversion and the forefoot in abduction (Fig. 5-49) to eliminate the synergistic action of the anterior tibial tendon, which would otherwise fire and mask strength loss in the PTT. The patient is asked to invert the foot against the examiner's hand, and strength is graded. This test is less sensitive than the unilateral heel raise.

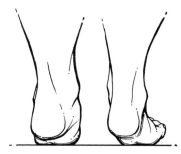

Figure 5–48 Single-heel raise test. The affected (posterior tibial tendon–deficient) right heel does not assume a stable (varus) position (as seen on the *left*) when the patient attempts to stand on the toes (for details of the test, see text). (From DeLee JC, Drez D Jr: Orthopaedic Sports Medicine: Principles and Practice. Philadelphia, WB Saunders, 1994.)

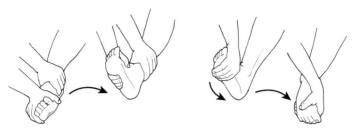

Figure 5–49   Testing of the posterior tibial tendon (PTT). The PTT is an inverter. During testing of a weak PTT, the anterior tibial tendon is often recruited. To test the "isolated" PTT, first bring the foot into plantar flexion and eversion (to eliminate the anterior tibial tendon). Then gauge the strength of inversion against the examiner's hand. (Adapted from McKeag DB, Dolan C: Overuse syndromes of the lower extremity. Physician Sports Med 17[2]:108, 1989.)

Areas of tenderness, swelling, and bogginess should be palpated. In the later stages of collapse, the patient may complain of lateral pain and tenderness in the sinus tarsi region (Fig. 5-50) as a result of impingement of the talus under the fibula. This is referred to as "sinus tarsi impingement."

The hindfoot (heel) should also be tested to see whether the subtalar joint can be reduced to neutral (flexible hindfoot) or not (fixed-deformity hindfoot). The Achilles tendon often becomes contracted or shortened in the later stages, and its passive ankle ROM in dorsiflexion should be compared with that of the other extremity.

Radiographic Evaluation

Radiographic evaluation should include four weight-bearing views: AP of both ankles, AP of both feet, lateral of both ankles, and lateral of both feet. On the weight-bearing lateral radiograph of the foot with longitudinal collapse, the talus inclines plantarward when compared with the normal foot. AP foot films often demonstrate abduction of the midfoot by revealing an "uncovered" talar head at the talonavicular joint.

CLASSIFICATION OF POSTERIOR TIBIAL TENDON INSUFFICIENCY

Johnson and Strom (1989) described a classification of PTT insufficiency that is helpful in developing treatment algorithms, but it does not consider the contracted gastrocnemius that is evident in some patients (shortened Achilles) (Table 5-4).

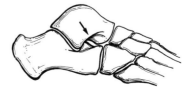

Figure 5–50   Sinus tarsi impingement. (From DeLee JC, Drez D Jr: Orthopaedic Sports Medicine: Principles and Practice. Philadelphia, WB Saunders, 1994.)

TABLE 5–4	Classification of Posterior Tibial Tendon Dysfunction/ Insufficiency
Stage 1	Absence of a fixed foot or ankle deformity (except Achilles contracture) Normal foot alignment on standing Pain, tenderness, or swelling medially along the course of the PTT
Stage 2	Dynamic (correctable) hindfoot valgus deformity Weakness of the PTT on resistance testing Too-many-toes sign Inability to perform a unilateral heel-rise Relatively normal arc of subtalar motion
Stage 3	Fixed hindfoot valgus deformity The talonavicular joint cannot be reduced with the hindfoot in a fixed valgus position Usually, fixed forefoot supination deformity compensating for hindfoot valgus to allow a plantigrade foot No obvious ankle deformities
Stage 4	Stage 3 plus ankle deformity

From Myerson MS: Adult acquired flat foot deformity: Treatment of dysfunction of the posterior tibial tendon. Instr Course Lect. 46:393, 1997.

TREATMENT

The initial treatment for patients with any stage of PTT insufficiency is nonoperative, which includes relative rest (cast, splint, or orthotic) for 6 to 8 weeks, use of NSAIDs, and assessment of the degree of improvement (Table 5-5).

For acute tenosynovitis, a removable walking cast is worn for 6 to 8 weeks, with weight-bearing as tolerated with a cane or crutch. NSAIDs are given, and ice massage is applied to the tendon for 1 to 2 weeks. If improvements are noted in symptoms and on examination, the cast is removed and replaced by an orthotic with a supportive medial longitudinal arch and a stiff-soled shoe. Some authors recommend a stiff-soled shoe with a medial heel-and-sole wedge. Low-impact activities (swimming, cycling) are substituted for former high-impact activities (jogging, long-distance walking). If there is no improvement with nonoperative treatment, surgical tenosynovectomy is indicated (see later).

For PTT insufficiency (stages 1 to 4), a custom-molded ankle-foot orthosis, double upright brace with a medial T-strap (Fig. 5-51), or an ankle brace (Fig. 5-52) can help control deformity and alleviate symptoms. Sedentary or elderly patients can be treated with bracing if symptoms are tolerable in the brace. The brace will not "correct" the deformity, but it acts as a stabilizer. If conservative measures fail or the patient is unwilling to wear the bulky brace, operative treatment is indicated. Operative treatment often includes Achilles lengthening because the Achilles is usually contracted and shortened in patients with PTT insufficiency.

TABLE 5–5	Treatment of Dysfunction of the Posterior Tibial Tendon		
Stage	**Characteristics**	**Nonoperative Treatment**	**Operative Treatment**

Tenosynovitis	Acute medial pain and swelling
	Can perform a heel-rise
	Seronegative inflammation
	Extensive tearing
		NSAIDs
		Immobilization for 6-8 wk
		If symptoms improve, ankle
		  stirrup brace
		If symptoms do not improve,
		  operative treatment
			Tenosynovectomy
			Tenosynovectomy + calcaneal osteotomy
			Tenodesis of FDL to PTT

Stage I rupture	Medial pain and swelling Hindfoot correctable Can perform a heel-rise	Medial heel-and-sole wedge Hinged AFO Orthotic arch supports	Débridement of PTT FDL transfer FDL transfer + calcaneal osteotomy

Stage II rupture	Valgus angulation of heel
	Lateral pain
	Hindfoot correctable
	Cannot perform heel-rise
		Medial heel-and-sole wedge
		Stiff orthotic support
		Hinged AFO
		Injection of steroids into
		  sinus tarsi
			FDL transfer + calcaneal medializing
			  osteotomy
			FDL transfer + bone block arthrodesis
			  at the calcaneocuboid joint
			  (lateral column lengthening)

Stage III rupture	Valgus angulation of the heel Lateral pain Hindfoot rigid Cannot perform a heel-rise	Rigid AFO	Triple arthrodesis
Stage IV rupture	Hindfoot rigid Valgus angulation of the talus Ankle involvement	Rigid AFO	Tibiotalocalcaneal arthrodesis

AFO, ankle-foot orthosis; FDL, flexor digitorum longus; NSAIDs, nonsteroidal anti-inflammatory drugs; PTT, posterior tibial tendon.
From Myerson MS: Adult acquired flat foot deformity: Treatment of dysfunction of the posterior tibial tendon. Instr Course Lect 46:393, 1997.

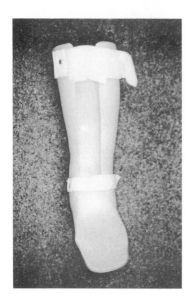

Figure 5–51 Polypropylene ankle-foot orthosis with a molded Plastazote lining. (From Mann RA, Coughlin MJ: Surgery of the Foot and Ankle. St Louis, CV Mosby, 1993.)

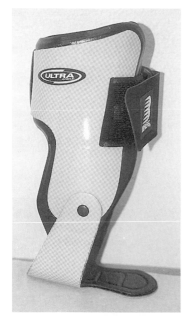

Figure 5–52 Ankle brace.

Metatarsalgia

Brett R. Fink, MD • Mark S. Mizel, MD

BACKGROUND

Metatarsalgia describes an assortment of conditions that cause plantar pain in the forefoot around the MTP joints.

Metatarsalgia is not, in itself, a diagnosis, but rather an anatomic description of where the patient is experiencing discomfort. *Successful treatment of this condition hinges on identifying the underlying cause*. A clear understanding of its causes and a systematic approach to examination are therefore necessary for a successful outcome. **Metatarsalgia is best characterized by pain under the metatarsal heads exacerbated by weight-bearing**.

The fatty cushion of the forefoot is a highly specialized tissue. Fibrous septa beneath the dermis compartmentalize the subcutaneous fat. When weight is applied, hydrostatic pressure builds within the compartments and dampens and disperses force on the plantar skin. This mechanism acts as a cushion to protect the area from potentially damaging focal concentrations in pressure.

Inflammatory arthritis, trauma, or neuromuscular disorders can cause an imbalance in flexion and extension forces around the small joints of the toes. Toe deformity is a consequence of this imbalance. Hyperextension at the MTP joint is a common component of these deformities and draws the fatty cushion of the forefoot distally and dorsally with the proximal phalanx (Fig. 5-53). When this occurs, the weight transferred through the metatarsal heads is applied to the thinner proximal skin without the intervening fatty cushion. Increases in local pressure result in a hyperkeratotic reaction of the plantar skin, which causes further increases in pressure and, eventually, a **painful intractable plantar keratosis (IPK)** (Fig. 5-54).

IPKs are often confused with plantar warts. Both cause hyperkeratotic lesions of the plantar surface of the skin, which can be painful. However, plantar warts occur as a result of infection of the epidermis with papillomavirus. Whereas treatment of IPKs is mechanical (shaving, cushioning, relief pads), treatment of symptomatic plantar warts is directed toward eradicating the infected tissue. Care should be taken to ensure that the sometimes-caustic plantar wart preparations do not cause scarring of the plantar skin, which can be more painful than the initial wart. IPKs, unlike plantar warts, are almost always found directly below a weight-bearing area of the foot (e.g., metatarsal head). Plantar warts bleed in a characteristic "punctate" fashion when shaved, with multiple punctate areas of bleeding.

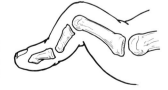

Figure 5–53 With a claw toe, the metatarsophalangeal joint is hyperextended, essentially driving the metatarsal head into the ground. (Adapted from Coady CM, Gow MD, Stanish W: Foot problems in middle-aged patients: Keeping active people up to speed. Physician Sports Med 26[5]:107, 1998.)

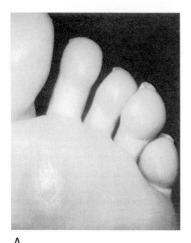

A

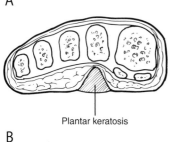

Plantar keratosis

B

Figure 5–54 **A**, Intractable plantar keratosis under the second metatarsal head. **B**, Cross section of the foot showing a discrete plantar keratosis beneath the prominent fibular condyle of a metatarsal head. (**A**, From Gould JS: Painful feet. In McCarthy DJ [ed]: Arthritis and Allied Conditions: A Textbook of Rheumatology, 11th ed. Philadelphia, Lea & Febiger, 1989, p 1406.)

Synovitis and *instability* (Fig. 5-55) of the MTP joints can also cause pain along the metatarsal heads. Although *inflammatory arthritides* can incite this, the etiology of the instability is commonly mechanical. Chronic hyperextension of the MTP joints (claw toes) and flexion at the interphalangeal joints can occur in an attempt to accommodate a *shoe toe box that is too small* (Fig. 5-56). Eventually, the plantar plate and collateral ligaments become attenuated, and instability and subluxation ensue (Fig. 5-57). Varus or valgus malalignment of the toes can develop as a result. Dorsal MTP joint dislocation is sometimes seen in severe cases.

Extra-articular causes of pain in the metatarsal region should also be considered. *Morton's neuroma* is hypertrophy and subsequent irritation of the common interdigital nerve as it passes between the metatarsal heads. Inflammation of the intermetatarsal bursa and impingement by the intermetatarsal ligament are thought to contribute to the development of this condition. It most commonly affects the

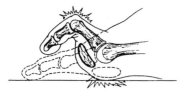

Figure 5–55 Synovitis leads to subluxation of the metatarsophalangeal (MTP) joint. The fatty cushion is displaced dorsally with subluxation of the MTP joint. Pain occurs at the plantar aspect of the metatarsal. (From Mann RA, Coughlin MJ: Surgery of the Foot and Ankle, 6th ed. St Louis, CV Mosby, 1993.)

Figure 5–56 Intractable plantar keratosis (IPK) under the metatarsal head (plantar) and a callosity at the proximal interphalangeal (PIP) joint (dorsally) from toe-box rub. A buckling effect may occur with concomitant hammertoe formation at the PIP joint and the development of IPK beneath the second metatarsal head (cross section of a shoe). The same pressure that causes this callosity increases pain under the metatarsal heads, or metatarsalgia. (From DeLee JC, Drez D Jr: Orthopaedic Sports Medicine: Principles and Practice. Philadelphia, WB Saunders, 1994.)

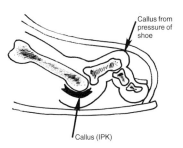

Callus from pressure of shoe

Callus (IPK)

nerve of the third web space. It is often mistaken for synovitis (see the Morton neuroma section) and can coexist with it. Morton's neuroma rarely involves more than one common digital nerve. *Tenderness* from a **stress fracture of the metatarsal** typically occurs in the metatarsal neck or shaft. Such fractures can be invisible on radiographs for several weeks *after onset*. Finally, pain from a herniated **lumbar disk**, **tarsal tunnel**, or other neurologic problem can be referred to the forefoot and is often mistaken for pain from a disorder *originating in the foot*.

HISTORY AND PHYSICAL EXAMINATION

A careful history and physical examination are the most important tools for differentiating the causes of metatarsalgia. **The examination should begin with an evaluation of the suitability of footwear in relation to the size of the foot**. Measure the patient's true shoe size and width, and then see what size shoe the patient wears into the office. A complete evaluation of the foot and ankle can disclose problems in other areas of the foot that may make the forefoot painful. For instance, medial foot disorders can cause lateral forefoot pain because of lateral weight shifting. Weakness in the anterior tibial tendon can cause toe deformity through adaptive overuse of the extrinsic toe extensors and result in forefoot pain.

The **plantar skin** should be inspected for plantar keratoses. Paring these lesions is important, not only to decrease pressure but also to differentiate them from plantar warts. Plantar warts, unlike plantar keratoses, contain vessels within the keratinized tissue that are easily seen open and bleeding after paring. The interdigital spaces should also be inspected for soft corns. **Sensation** should be tested and **pulses** palpated. Careful palpation of the metatarsal heads and intermetatarsal spaces to localize the exact area of tenderness narrows the differential diagnosis.

Manual compression of the interspace (**Mulder's click**) can elicit crepitus, tenderness, and radiating pain from a Morton neuroma (see the Morton neuroma section). A **drawer maneuver** of the MTP joint (Fig. 5-58) can detect articular stability problems.

Figure 5–57 **A,** Medial deviation of the second toe (as a result of synovitis and subsequent alteration of the collateral ligaments and plantar plate) may be associated with the development of acute pain in the second intermetatarsal space. **B,** Hyperextension of the second metatarsophalangeal joint may be associated with plantar capsular pain. (From Coughlin MJ: The crossover second toe deformity. Foot Ankle 8[1]:29, 1987.)

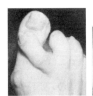

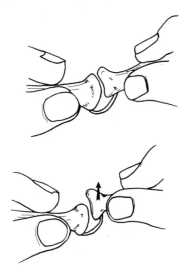

Figure 5–58   Drawer sign of the toe. **A,** The toe is grasped between the examiner's thumb and index finger. **B,** The toe is manipulated at the metatarsophalangeal joint in a plantar and dorsal direction. Instability is characterized by excess laxity (positive drawer) in the dorsal direction. (From DeLee JC, Drez D Jr: Orthopaedic Sports Medicine: Principles and Practice. Philadelphia, WB Saunders, 1994.)

It is done by applying dorsally directed pressure to the plantar base of the proximal phalanx while stabilizing the metatarsal with the opposite hand.

The contralateral toes, as well as the other toes on the ipsilateral foot, should be evaluated to establish a baseline degree of normal translation on MTP joint drawer testing for each patient. MTP joint tenderness, swelling, and bogginess usually signify synovitis of the MTP joint, whereas pain with a relative increase in translation during MTP drawer testing generally signifies joint instability.

RADIOGRAPHIC EVALUATION

Radiographs are important to define forefoot deformities and identify neoplasms, fractures, dislocations, and arthritic joints that may contribute to pain in the metatarsal area. *The relative lengths of adjacent metatarsals should be compared because discrepancies in metatarsal length can cause concentration of stress. Patients with significant shortening of the first metatarsal after a bunion operation sometimes have pain under the second metatarsal (transfer metatarsalgia).* When combined with lead markers placed on the IPK skin, radiographs help identify prominent condyles or sesamoids under the metatarsal head that can cause plantar keratoses. Isolated second metatarsal pain may be caused by **Freiberg's infraction** (Fig. 5-59).

Other imaging techniques, such as MRI and computed tomography (CT), are helpful only when specifically indicated and are not a routine part of the evaluation of metatarsalgia.

Although exercise and stretching offer little relief for most patients with metatarsalgia, **pedorthic management can figure prominently in the initial treatment.** For most patients who wear inappropriate (high heels) or tight shoes, a discussion of the fit of the shoes should focus on the shape and room in the toe box for the toes. In addition, shoes with laces, stiff soles, and low heels help disperse and reduce the pressure on the forefoot. Occasionally, patients have severe fixed forefoot deformities that require prescription extra-depth shoe wear.

Full-length PPT and Plastazote or silicone insoles are very helpful in dispersing the pressure on tender areas in the forefoot. If this is unsuccessful, more sophisticated

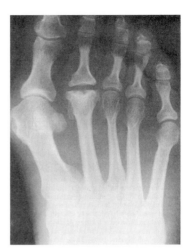

Figure 5–59 Freiberg's infraction. This patient demonstrates deformity of the second metatarsal head. It is broadened, flattened, and somewhat sclerotic with osteophytes. Osteophytes have also developed at the base of the second proximal phalanx (degenerative changes superimposed on Freiberg's infraction). Note the thickened cortex of the shaft of the second metatarsal and the hallux valgus deformity. (From Brower A: Orthopaedic radiology. Orthop Clin North Am 14:112, 1983.)

orthotic devices may be necessary. Soft metatarsal pads made of felt or silicone (Fig. 5-60A), by themselves or added to a Spenco insert, can be used to relieve pressure. Correct placement of the pad is crucial. The crest of the pad should be approximately 1 cm *proximal to the tender area* (see Fig. 5-60B). To help position the insert, lipstick or a marker can be applied to the tender area on the foot and the patient

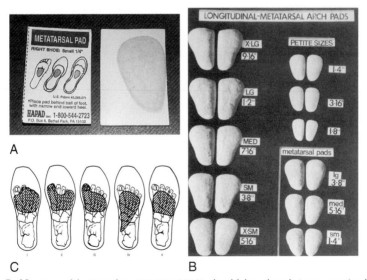

Figure 5–60 **A**, A felt Hapad (1-800-544-2733) should be placed 1 cm proximal to the metatarsal head or heads to "push" the metatarsal head or heads dorsally and decrease the pressure on them. We apply this pad onto a full-length, {1/8}-inch PPT, Plastazote, or Spenco insole. **B**, Examples of felt supports that are extremely useful in alleviating areas of pressure beneath the metatarsal heads. **C**, Commonly used shoe pads for relief of painful conditions of the foot. **i**, Pad designed to relieve pressure on the sesamoids. **ii**, Pad to support various metatarsal heads (in this case, for treatment of Morton's neuroma). **iii**, Pad to support the short first metatarsal and relieve pressure on the lesser metatarsal heads. **iv**, Pad to support the longitudinal arch and relieve pressure on the metatarsal heads. **v**, Pad to relieve pressure on the metatarsal heads. (**B** and **C**, From Mann RA, Coughlin MJ: Surgery of the Foot and Ankle. St Louis, CV Mosby, 1993.)

asked to step on the insole to identify where to place the pad (1 cm proximal). A custom-molded accomodative insert can also be fabricated with a well-excavated well beneath the tender metatarsal to unload it (relief well).

Metatarsal bars can be built onto the shoe to unload the forefoot, but such bars tend to wear out quickly and resistance is encountered from patients for cosmetic reasons. A rocker-bottom sole, along with a stiffener placed into the sole, helps reduce toe motion and disperse pressure away from the metatarsal heads.

Steroid injections combined with 1% lidocaine have a definite, but limited role in diagnosing and treating pain caused by synovitis or irritation of a Morton neuroma from intermetatarsal bursitis.

Surgery is offered to patients in whom nonoperative treatment fails to relieve the pain.

Differential Diagnosis of Metatarsalgia of the Foot

Brotzman

Metatarsalgia. Plantar pain under the lesser metatarsal heads exacerbated by weight-bearing. It may be exacerbated by hyperextension of the MTP joint (claw toe) "driving" the metatarsal head plantarward, fat pad atrophy, and the like. Transfer metatarsalgia occurs when a shortened metatarsal (e.g., iatrogenically or naturally "short" or incompetent first metatarsal [bunion]) does not allow well-distributed weight-bearing and excess pressure is transferred laterally to the second, third, and possibly the fourth and fifth metatarsals.

MTP joint synovitis. Inflammation of the MTP joints may occur (synovitis) with rheumatoid arthritis, a cross-over toe deformity (see Fig. 5-57), and the like. This synovitis is typically boggy, swollen, and tender to palpation of the MTP joint, both plantar and dorsal.

Arthritis of the MTP joints. This is confirmed on radiographs of the foot.

Morton's neuroma. Pain, numbness, burning, and tingling are localized to a discrete interspace (third or second) and not the MTP joint. Mulder's click and tenderness in the interspace are evident, *without* tenderness on palpation of the MTP joints (see the section on Morton's neuroma).

Soft tissue tumor. Ganglion, synovial cyst, lipoma, neoplasm, and rheumatoid nodule are examples.

IPK. A callosity is formed directly under a weight-bearing portion of the foot (e.g., metatarsal head). Usually a result of fat pad atrophy, claw toe, or excess pressure. The callosity (IPK) is formed by the body in response to repetitive excess pressure (see Fig. 5-54).

Continued on following page

Abscess. This is usually hot, red, swollen, and fluctuant.

Stress fracture of the metatarsal(s). This may be confirmed by a positive bone scan and/or eventual plain radiographic evidence of bone callus formation (≥2 weeks after fracture).

Inflammatory arthritis may be differentiated by involvement of multiple joints, a marker (HLA-B27), or systemic symptoms.

Neurogenic pain or burning:

Morton's neuroma

Tarsal tunnel–positive Tinel sign at the tibial nerve at the medial aspect of the ankle and follows the medial and/or lateral plantar nerve distribution(s)

Lumbar disk

Peripheral neuropathy

Reflex sympathetic dystrophy

Freiberg's infraction of the second metatarsal. Pain occurs under the second metatarsal with radiographic findings compatible with Freiberg's (see Fig. 5-59).

Hallux Rigidus

Mark M. Casillas, MD • Margaret Jacobs, PT

CLINICAL BACKGROUND

The term *hallux rigidus* describes a limited arthrosis of the first MTP joint. The first MTP joint and the great toe (hallux) provide significant weight transfer from the foot to the ground, as well as active push-off. An intact first MTP joint implies complete and pain-free ROM, in addition to full intrinsic and extrinsic motor strength.

The first MTP joint ROM is variable. The neutral position is described by 0 (or 180) degrees angulation between a line through the first metatarsal and a line through the hallux (Fig. 5-61). Dorsiflexion, or ROM above the neutral position, varies between 60 and 100 degrees (Fig. 5-62A). Plantar flexion, or ROM below the neutral position, varies between 10 and 40 degrees (see Fig. 5-62B). ROM is noncrepitant and pain-free in the uninjured joint.

Two sesamoid bones (the medial, or tibial, sesamoid and the lateral, or fibular, sesamoid) provide mechanical advantage to the intrinsic plantar flexors by increasing the distance between the empirical center of the joint and the respective tendons.

Hallux rigidus is an arthritic condition limited to the dorsal aspect of the first MTP joint. Also known as a dorsal bunion or hallux limitus, the condition is most commonly idiopathic (but may be associated with post-traumatic osteochondritis dissecans of the metatarsal head) and is characterized by an extensive dorsal

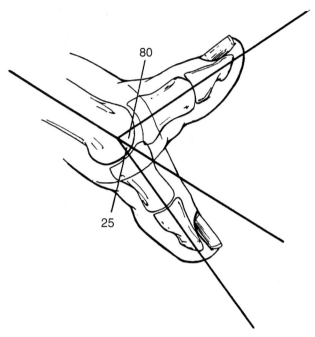

Figure 5–61 Hallux dorsiflexion and plantar flexion are determined by referencing the longitudinal axis of the first metatarsal. (From Coughlin MJ: Conditions of the forefoot. In DeLee JC, Drez D Jr: Orthopaedic Sports Medicine: Principles and Practice. Philadelphia, WB Saunders, 1994, p 1861.)

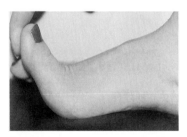

A

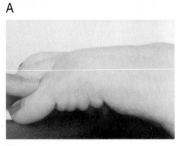

B

Figure 5–62 Passive hallux dorsiflexion (**A**) and plantar flexion (**B**).

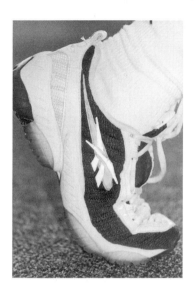

Figure 5–63 Excessive shoe flexibility at the forefoot increases the potential for hyperdorsiflexion of a hallux metatarsophalangeal joint.

osteophyte and dorsal third cartilage damage and loss. An associated synovitis may further aggravate the limited and painful ROM.

A foot with increased first ray ROM and increased pronation may be predisposed to the condition. Excessive flexibility of the shoe forefoot increases the potential for hyperdorsiflexion of the hallux MTP joint (Fig. 5-63). For this reason, this type of shoe wear should be avoided.

CLASSIFICATION OF HALLUX RIGIDUS

A useful classification system grades clinical and radiographic findings from mild to end stage (Table 5-6).

TABLE 5–6	Classification of Hallux Rigidus	
Grade	**Findings**	**Treatment**
Mild	Near-normal ROM, pain with forced hyperdorsiflexion, tender dorsal joint, minimal dorsal osteophyte	Symptomatic
Moderate	Painful, limited dorsiflexion, tender dorsal joint, osteophyte on lateral radiograph	Symptomatic; consider early surgical repair
Severe	Painful, severely limited dorsiflexion, tender dorsal joint, large osteophyte on lateral radiograph, decreased joint space on AP radiograph	Symptomatic; consider surgical repair, dorsiflexion osteotomy
End stage	Severe pain and limited motion, global arthrosis and osteophyte formation, loss of joint space on all radiograph projections	Symptomatic; consider arthrodesis

AP, anteroposterior; ROM, range of motion.

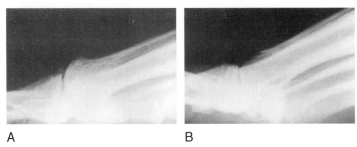

A   B

Figure 5–64   Lateral views of the foot before (**A**) and after (**B**) excision of a dorsal spur of the first metatarsal.

DIAGNOSIS

Clinical Examination

Patients with hallux rigidus complain of dorsal pain, swelling, and stiffness localized to the hallux MTP joint. The sitting examination may reveal decreased ROM in dorsiflexion and, to a lesser degree, in plantar flexion. ROM becomes more and more painful as the condition advances. *Forced dorsiflexion reveals an abrupt dorsal bony block associated with pain.* In addition, forced plantar flexion produces pain as the dorsal capsule and the extensor hallucis longus tendon are stretched across the dorsal osteophyte. The dorsal osteophyte is easily palpable and typically exquisitely tender.

Radiographic Evaluation

Standard radiographic evaluation includes AP and lateral views of the weight-bearing foot (Fig. 5-64). Bone scan, CT, and MRI are capable of demonstrating the condition but are not part of a routine work-up.

The differential diagnosis of hallux rigidus is shown in Table 5-7.

TABLE 5–7	Differential Diagnosis of First Ray Pain
Differential Diagnosis	**Significant Findings**
Hallux rigidus	Chronic condition
	Limited dorsiflexion
	Dorsal osteophyte on lateral radiograph
Hallux valgus (bunion)	Chronic condition
	Lateral deviation of great toe
	Tender medial eminence (not dorsal spur)
	Increased hallux valgus angle on radiograph
Hallux arthrosis	Chronic condition
(arthritic first	Painful and limited ROM
MTP joint)	**Loss of entire joint space on radiograph**
Gout	Acute severe pain
	Tenderness, erythema, joint irritability localized to first MTP
	Elevated uric acid
	Sodium urate crystals

MTP, metatarsophalangeal; ROM, range of motion.

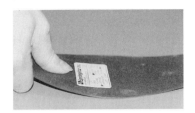

Figure 5–65 Low-profile carbon plate shoe inserts increase shoe stiffness and decrease dorsiflexion of the first metatarsophalangeal joint.

TREATMENT

Treatment of hallux rigidus is based on the symptom. ***Acute exacerbations*** are treated with the RICE (rest, ice, compression, and elevation) method, followed by a gentle ROM program and protected weight-bearing. ***Chronic*** conditions are treated with a ROM program and protected weight-bearing. The hallux MTP joint is supported by shoe modifications (e.g., rocker-bottom sole), a rigid shoe insert (Fig. 5-65), a stiff-soled shoe, or various taping methods that resist forced dorsiflexion (Fig. 5-66). A soft upper and deep toe box reduce pressure over the dorsal osteophyte. The joint is also protected by reducing activity levels, increasing rest intervals and duration, and avoiding excessively firm play surfaces. Occasionally, a patient with excessive pronation will benefit from an antipronation orthotic. NSAIDs and cold therapy are used to reduce swelling and inflammation. Occasionally, injection of corticosteroid into the MTP joint is used as adjunctive therapy.

Operative treatment is indicated for symptoms that fail to respond to a reasonable period of well-supervised conservative management (Fig. 5-67). Hallux MTP débridement and exostectomy are standard treatment of hallux rigidus. **Ideally, intraoperative**

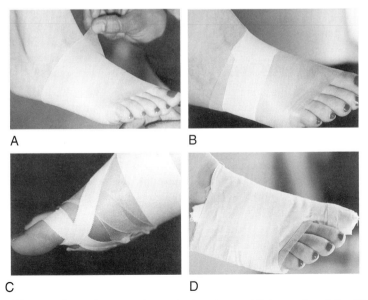

Figure 5–66 Dorsiflexion-limiting taping method: underwrap (**A**), base or foundation (**B**), 1-inch strips crossing on the plantar side of the joint (**C**), and a circumferential cover to complete and secure the tape (**D**).

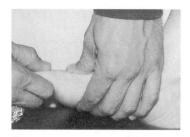

A

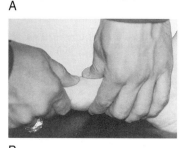

B

Figure 5–67 Hallux metatarsophalangeal joint mobilization: gentle dorsal (**A**) and plantar (**B**) translation of the proximal phalanx relative to the metatarsal head.

and postoperative passive ROM should approach 90 degrees of dorsiflexion. If the arthrosis is extensive and such ROM not obtainable, a **dorsiflexion osteotomy** may be added to the surgical repair. The osteotomy is designed to place the functional ROM of the hallux within the newly established pain-free arc of motion. Patients with severe findings must be warned that outcomes become less predictable with advanced stages. CT images are useful in discriminating between severe hallux rigidus and frank degenerative joint disease. Hallux arthrodesis (fusion) is a more predictable reconstruction method for the most advanced cases of hallux rigidus. Pain relief is provided at the expense of permanent loss of joint motion.

Authors' Recommended Treatment

An acutely swollen and painful hallux rigidus is treated with the RICE method for several days (Fig. 5-68). For chronic conditions, a stiff-soled shoe with a soft upper is prescribed along with a rigid low-profile carbon insert. We often rocker-bottom the shoe. NSAIDs and ice are used as an adjunct to reduce inflammation. Adequate rest and recovery are scheduled with increasing frequency and duration. If symptoms persist or if the patient has moderate to severe findings, hallux rigidus repair is considered. Adequate débridement and soft tissue release are performed to achieve 90 degrees of intraoperative dorsiflexion. If the joint is globally affected (hallux arthrosis), hallux arthrodesis is performed.

Nonoperative Rehabilitative Treatment of Hallux Rigidus

Occasionally, hallux rigidus is associated with a synovitis that can be improved by nonoperative treatment. Fundamental to the protocol is prevention of recurrent injury by limiting dorsiflexion of the hallux MTP with appropriate shoe wear, rigid shoe inserts, or taping. Taping (by the trainer) is useful in athletic events but is

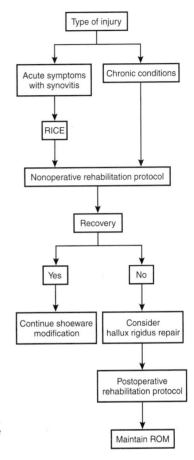

Figure 5–68 Treatment algorithm for hallux rigidus. RICE, rest, ice, compression, and elevation; ROM, range of motion.

limited by time-related failure and the poor results with self-application. Off-the-shelf devices are readily available, and custom devices can be used for difficult sizes or specialty shoe wear. The phases of rehabilitation are variable in length and depend completely on re-establishment of ROM and resolution of pain. Flexibility is emphasized throughout the protocol.

REHABILITATION PROTOCOL | *Nonoperative Treatment of Hallux Rigidus*
Casillas and Jacobs

PHASE 1: ACUTE PHASE—DAYS 0-6

- Rest, ice bath, contrast bath, whirlpool, and ultrasound for pain, inflammation, and joint stiffness
- Joint mobilization (see Fig. 5-67), followed by gentle passive and active ROM
- Isometrics around the MTP joint as pain allows
- Isolated plantar fascia stretches with a can (Fig. 5-69) or golf ball
- Cross-training activities, such as water activities and cycling, for aerobic fitness
- Protective taping and shoe modifications for continued weight-bearing activities

Continued

REHABILITATION PROTOCOL: *Nonoperative Treatment of Hallux Rigidus* *Continued*

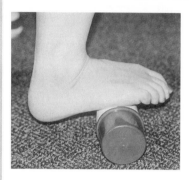

Figure 5–69 Plantar fascia stretches are accomplished with a can rolled beneath the foot with varying amounts of force.

PHASE 2: SUBACUTE PHASE—WEEKS 1-6

- Modalities to decrease inflammation and joint stiffness
- Emphasis on increasing flexibility and ROM, with both passive and active methods and joint mobilization
- Plantar fascia stretching
- Gastrocnemius stretching (Fig. 5-70)
- Progressive strengthening
  - Towel scrunches (Fig. 5-71)
  - Toe pick-up activities (Fig. 5-72)

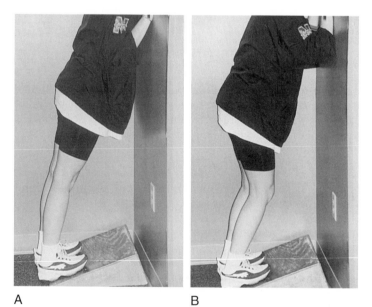

A   B

Figure 5–70 **A,** Gastrocnemius stretching on an inclined box with the knee extended. **B,** The soleus is stretched more effectively by flexing the knee and relaxing the gastrocnemius muscle.

REHABILITATION PROTOCOL: *Nonoperative Treatment of Hallux Rigidus*   *Continued*

PHASE 2: SUBACUTE PHASE—WEEKS 1-6—cont'd

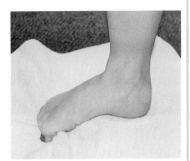

Figure 5–71   Towel scrunches. The towel is gathered by the toes.

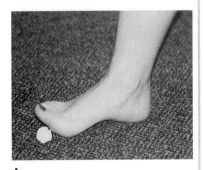

A

Figure 5–72   Toe pick-ups. A small object, in this case a ball of adhesive tape (**A**), is grasped by the toes (**B**).

B

- • Seated toe and ankle dorsiflexion with progression to standing (Fig. 5-73)
  - • Seated isolated toe dorsiflexion with progression to standing
  - • Seated supination-pronation with progression to standing
- • Balance activities, with progression of difficulty to include a BAPS board (Fig. 5-74)
- • Cross-training activities (slide board, water running, cycling) to maintain aerobic fitness

Continued

REHABILITATION PROTOCOL: *Nonoperative Treatment of Hallux Rigidus*   *Continued*

PHASE 3: RETURN-TO-SPORT PHASE—WEEK 7

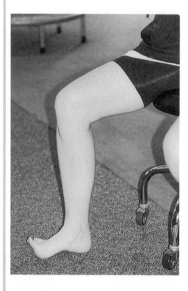

Figure 5–73   Seated toe and ankle dorsiflexion.

- Continued use of protective inserts or taping
- Continued ROM and strength exercises
- Running, to progress within limits of a pain-free schedule
- Monitored plyometric and cutting program, with progression of difficulty

Care should be taken to avoid reinjury during these activities.

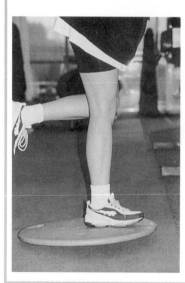

Figure 5–74   Biomechanical Ankle Platform System (BAPS) board.

After Hallux Rigidus Cheilectomy (Removal of a Dorsal Spur)
Casillas and Jacobs

GENERAL PRINCIPLES

- Fundamental to postoperative rehabilitation is re-establishment of hallux MTP ROM in **dorsiflexion**
- The surgical dressing is left undisturbed for 7-14 days
- Full weight-bearing in a rigid postoperative shoe is allowed on the first postoperative day
- Rehabilitation begins as soon as the wound appears stable, not necessarily before suture removal
- The phases of rehabilitation are arbitrary in length and depend completely on re-establishment of ROM and resolution of pain
- Flexibility is emphasized throughout the protocol

PHASE 1: ACUTE PHASE—DAYS 6-13

- Rest and ice for pain, inflammation, and joint stiffness
- Joint mobilization followed by gentle passive and active ROM
- Isometric around the MTP joint as pain allows
- Isolated plantar fascia stretches with a can roll or frozen golf ball
- Cross-training activities (such as cycling) to maintain aerobic fitness
- Postoperative rigid shoe for continued weight-bearing for first 3 postoperative weeks

PHASE 2: SUBACUTE PHASE—WEEKS 2-6

- Ice, contrast bath, whirlpool, ultrasound to decrease inflammation and joint stiffness
- Emphasis on increasing flexibility and ROM with both active and passive methods, with addition of joint and scar mobilization
- Continued plantar fascia stretching
- Gastrosoleus stretching
- Progressive strengthening
  - Towel scrunches
  - Toe pick-up activities
  - Manual resistive hallux MTP dorsiflexion and plantar flexion (Fig. 5-75)
  - Seated toe and ankle dorsiflexion, with progression to standing
  - Seated isolated toe dorsiflexion, with progression to standing
  - Seated supination-pronation, with progression to standing
- Balance activities, with progression of difficulty to include a BAPS board
- Cross-training activities (slide board, water running, cycling) to maintain aerobic fitness

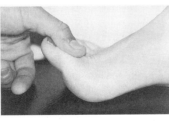 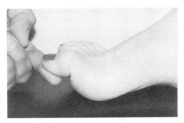

A   B

Figure 5–75   Manual resistive hallux metatarsophalangeal joint dorsiflexion (**A**) and plantar flexion (**B**).

Continued

REHABILITATION PROTOCOL: *After Hallux Rigidus Cheilectomy (Removal of a Dorsal Spur)* Continued

PHASE 3: RETURN-TO-SPORT PHASE—WEEK 7
- Continued ROM and strength activities
- Running, with progression within limits of pain-free schedule
- Monitored plyometric and cutting program, with progression of difficulty

Care must be taken to avoid exacerbation of postoperative pain and swelling.

First Metatarsophalangeal Joint Sprain (Turf Toe)

Mark M. Casillas, MD • Margaret Jacobs, PT

CLINICAL BACKGROUND

A first MTP joint sprain (turf toe) is capable of producing significant impairment and disability in running athletes. Turf toe describes a range of injuries to the capsuloligamentous complex of the first MTP joint.

The first MTP joint ROM is variable. The neutral position is described by 0 (or 180) degrees angulation between a line through the first metatarsal and a line through the hallux (see Fig. 5-61). Dorsiflexion, or ROM above the neutral position, varies between 60 and 100 degrees. Plantar flexion, or ROM below the neutral position, varies between 10 and 40 degrees. The ROM is noncrepitant and pain-free in the uninjured joint.

The power to move the MTP joint is provided by both intrinsic (flexor hallucis brevis, extensor hallucis brevis, abductor hallucis, adductor hallucis) and extrinsic (flexor hallucis longus, extensor hallucis longus) muscle groups. Two sesamoid bones (medial, or tibial, sesamoid and lateral, or fibular, sesamoid) provide mechanical advantage to the intrinsic plantar flexors by increasing the distance between the empirical center of joint rotation and the respective tendons (Fig. 5-76). The sesamoid

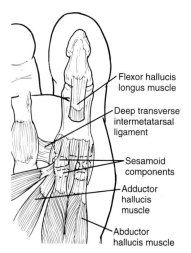

Flexor hallucis longus muscle

Deep transverse intermetatarsal ligament

Sesamoid components

Adductor hallucis muscle

Abductor hallucis muscle

Figure 5–76 Anatomy of a metatarsophalangeal (MTP) joint affected by a turf toe injury. The tendons of the flexor hallucis brevis, adductor hallucis, and abductor hallucis muscles combine with the deep transverse metatarsal ligaments to form the fibrocartilaginous plate on the plantar aspect of the MTP joint capsule. The two sesamoid bones are contained within the fibrocartilaginous plate. (Adapted from Rodeo SA, O'Brien SJ, Warren RF, et al: Turf toe: Diagnosis and treatment. Physician Sports Med 17[4]:132, 1989.)

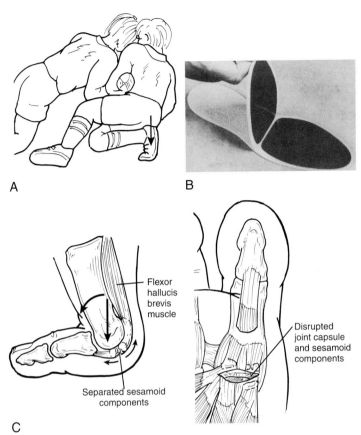

Figure 5–77   **A**, The primary mechanism of turf toe occurs when the player's forefoot is fixed on the ground and the metatarsophalangeal (MTP) joint is forced into hyperextension when another player falls across the dorsal surface of the first player's leg. **B**, A 0.51-mm spring steel shoe insert provides rigidity along the distal part of the shoe for preventing hyperextension of the MTP joint. The insert has a bilaminar construction. **C**, Disruption of the joint capsule in turf toe may result in separation of the components of a multipartite sesamoid. (Adapted from Rodeo SA, O'Brien SJ, Warren RF, et al: Turf toe: Diagnosis and treatment. Physician Sports Med 17[4]:132, 1989.)

complex articulates with facets on the plantar aspect of the first metatarsal head and is stabilized by a plantar capsule (plantar plate), as well as by a ridge (or crista) on the metatarsal head that separates the two sesamoids.

The mechanism of a first MTP joint sprain is forced dorsiflexion of the MTP joint (Fig. 5-77). The typical football-associated injury occurs when a player firmly plants his forefoot and is then struck from behind. Continued forward motion of the leg over the fixed forefoot produces hyperdorsiflexion of the first MTP joint and increased tension on the plantar plate and capsule. Taken to an extreme, these forces may continue and produce a dorsal impaction injury of the cartilage and bone of the metatarsal head.

The extreme motion required to produce an acute injury is more likely to occur in an **overly flexible shoe** as opposed to a relatively stiff-soled shoe (see Fig. 5-63). The **playing surface** has also been implicated as an associated factor. The hard playing surface of an artificial turf field may result in an increased incidence of first MTP joint sprains, hence the term "turf toe." A chronic, cumulative injury mechanism is associated with similar risk factors.

The mechanism of injury for a first MTP joint sprain is by no means specific. A multitude of afflictions of the first MTP joint and its contiguous structures must be ruled out (Table 5-8).

CLASSIFICATION

Acute first MTP joint sprains are classified according to the degree of capsular injury (Clanton's classification) (Table 5-9).

DIAGNOSIS

Signs and Symptoms

First MTP joint sprains are associated with acute localized pain, swelling, ecchymosis, and guarding. Increasing degrees of swelling, pain, and loss of joint motion are noted as the severity of the injury increases. An antalgic gait may be present, as well a tendency to avoid loading of the first ray by foot supination.

Radiographic Evaluation

The standard radiographic evaluation includes AP and lateral views of the weight-bearing foot, as well as a sesamoid projection (Fig. 5-78). The diagnosis is confirmed

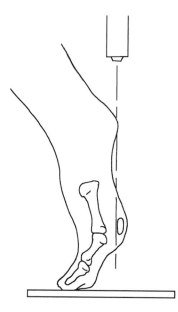

Figure 5–78   Radiographic view of the sesamoid.

TABLE 5–8	Pathology of the First Metatarsophalangeal Joint

Differential Diagnosis	Significant Findings
First MTP joint sprain (turf toe)	Acute or chronic injury Tender MTP joint Limited motion
Hallux fracture	Acute injury Tenderness isolated to the MTP joint or phalanx Fracture seen on radiograph, bone scan, CT, or MRI
Hallux dislocation	Acute injury Severe deformity on examination, verified by radiograph
Hallux rigidus	Chronic condition Limited dorsiflexion, painful ROM Dorsal osteophyte on lateral radiograph
Hallux arthrosis (arthritic first MTP joint)	Chronic condition Painful and limited ROM Loss of joint space on radiograph
Sesamoid fracture	Acute injury Tenderness isolated to the sesamoid Fracture seen on radiograph, bone scan, CT, or MRI
Sesamoid stress fracture	Chronic injury Tenderness isolated to the sesamoid Stress fracture seen on radiograph, bone scan, CT, or MRI
Sesamoid nonunion	Acute or chronic injury Tenderness isolated to the sesamoid Nonunion seen on radiograph, bone scan, CT, or MRI
Bipartite sesamoid	Congenital lack of fusion of the two ossicles of the sesamoid with a radiolucent line (cartilage) left between the two ossicles; often mistaken for a fracture Nontender to palpation, asymptomatic Comparison radiographs of the opposite foot may reveal a similar bipartite sesamoid High incidence of bilaterality, so take a comparison radiograph to differentiate bipartite from a sesamoid fracture
Sesamoid arthrosis	Acute or chronic injury Painful ROM Tenderness isolated to the sesamoid Arthrosis seen on radiograph, bone scan, CT, or MRI
Sesamoid avascular necrosis	Acute or chronic injury Tenderness isolated to the sesamoid Fragmentation seen on radiograph, CT, or MRI
Stenosing flexor	Overuse syndrome tenosynovitis Trigger phenomenon Painful flexor hallucis longus excursion Tenosynovitis seen on MRI
Gout	Acute severe pain Tenderness, erythema, and joint irritability localized to the first MTP joint Often elevated uric acid, sodium urate crystals on aspiration of joint

CT, computed tomography; MRI, magnetic resonance imaging; MTP, metatarsophalangeal; ROM, range of motion.

TABLE 5–9	Classification of Metatarsophalangeal Joint Sprains (Turf Toe)—Clanton			
Type	Objective Findings	Pathologic Condition	Treatment	Return to Sports
I	No ecchymosis Minimal or no swelling Localized plantar or medial tenderness	Stretching of the capsuloligamentous complex	Ice/elevation NSAIDs Rigid insole Continued participation in athletics	Immediate
II	Diffuse tenderness Ecchymosis Pain, restriction of motion	Partial tear of the capsuloligamentous complex	Same as type I Restriction of athletic activity for 7-14 days, depending on clinical course	1-14 days
III	Severe tenderness to palpation Considerable ecchymosis and swelling Marked restriction of motion	Tear of the capsuloligamentous complex Compression injury of the articular surface	Same as type II Crutches and limited weight-bearing If MTP dislocated, reduction and immobilization initially with case Restriction of athletic activity	3-6 wk

MTP, metatarsophalangeal; NSAIDs, nonsteroidal anti-inflammatory drugs.
From Brotzman SB, Graves SG: In Griffin LY (ed): Orthopaedic Knowledge Update: Sports Medicine, Rosemont, IL, American Academy of Orthopaedic Surgeons, 1993.

on MRI when capsular tears and associated edema are demonstrated. Bone scan, CT, and MRI may be used to rule out sesamoid avascular necrosis, sesamoid fracture, sesamoid stress injury, hallux MTP joint arthrosis, metatarsal-sesamoid arthrosis, or stenosing flexor tenosynovitis.

TREATMENT

Treatment of first MTP joint sprains is based on symptoms. *Acute injuries* are treated with the RICE method, followed by a gentle ROM program and protected weight-bearing. *Chronic injuries* are treated with an ROM program and protected weight-bearing. The hallux MTP joint is supported by a variety of methods, including a walking cast, removable walking cast, rigid shoe modifications, rigid shoe inserts, stiff-soled shoes, and various taping methods (see Fig. 5-66). The joint is also protected by reducing activity levels, increasing rest intervals and duration, and avoiding rigid playing surfaces. Intra-articular steroids are of no benefit and may be detrimental to the joint.

Operative treatment is rare for isolated first MTP joint sprains. Occasionally, an associated condition is recognized and surgery becomes a treatment option (Table 5-10).

Prevention of turf toe includes the use of supportive footwear (with avoidance of an overly flexible shoe forefoot) and firm inserts and avoidance of hard playing surfaces (e.g., Astroturf) when possible.

Authors' Recommended Treatment

An acute turf toe injury is treated with the RICE method for several days, followed by a secondary evaluation that allows a subacute staging to better delineate the location and degree of injury. For **low-grade injuries** that do not involve significant capsular tears, the patient is instructed to perform gentle ROM. Motion is limited during athletic activity by taping or shoe modification. For **moderate and severe injuries**, including severe capsular tears and dorsal articular fractures, the initial treatment is modified by a brief period of casting with a solid walking cast or, alternatively, a removable walking boot. Once the swelling and pain subside, attention is focused on re-establishing ROM. Activity is resumed after pain-free ROM has been established.

TABLE 5–10	**Surgical Options for the First Metatarsophalangeal Joint**
Injury	**Surgical Treatment**
Intra-articular loose body	Joint débridement
Hallux rigidus	Joint débridement and exostectomy (cheilectomy)
Hallux arthrosis	Arthroplasty (not silicone), Keller procedure, or metatarsophalangeal arthrodesis
Sesamoid nonunion	Bone graft
Sesamoid arthrosis	Sesamoid excision
Stenosing flexor hallucis longus tenosynovitis	Flexor tunnel release
Hallux fracture or dislocation	Open reduction and internal fixation

Chronic turf toe is treated by activity and shoe modifications designed to limit ongoing injury. Shoe style, shoe inserts, playing surface, and taping are evaluated and adjusted to minimize pain and protect the MTP joint. NSAIDs and ice are used as adjuncts to reduce inflammation. Adequate rest and recovery must be scheduled with increased frequency and duration.

REHABILITATION FOR TURF TOE

Fundamental to the protocol is prevention of recurrent injury by limiting hallux MTP dorsiflexion with appropriate shoe wear, taping, or rigid shoe inserts. Taping is useful but is limited by time-related failure and the poor results associated with self-application. Off-the-shelf devices, such steel leaf plates and low-profile carbon fiber inserts, are readily available. Custom devices may be used for difficult sizes or specialty shoe wear. The phases of rehabilitation are variable in length and depend completely on re-establishment of ROM and resolution of pain. Flexibility is emphasized throughout the protocol.

REHABILITATION PROTOCOL | ***After Treatment of Turf Toe***
Casillas and Jacobs

PHASE 1: ACUTE PHASE—DAYS 0-5

- Rest, ice bath, contrast bath, whirlpool, and ultrasound for pain, inflammation, and joint stiffness
- Joint mobilization (see Fig. 5-67), followed by gentle passive and active ROM
- Isometrics around the MTP joint as pain allows
- Cross-training activities, such as water activities and cycling, for aerobic fitness
- Protective taping and shoe modifications for continued weight-bearing activities
- Modalities to decrease inflammation and joint stiffness
- Emphasis on increasing flexibility and ROM, with both passive and active methods and joint mobilization
- Progressive strengthening
  - Towel scrunches (see Fig. 5-71)
  - Toe pick-up activities (see Fig. 5-72)
  - Manual resistive hallux MTP dorsiflexion and plantar flexion (see Fig. 5-75)
  - Seated toe and ankle dorsiflexion with progression to standing (see Fig. 5-73)
  - Seated isolated toe dorsiflexion with progression to standing
  - Seated supination-pronation with progression to standing
- Balance activities, with progression of difficulty to include use of a BAPS board (see Fig. 5-74)
- Cross-training activities (slide board, water running, cycling) to maintain aerobic fitness

PHASE 3: RETURN-TO-SPORT PHASE—WEEK 7

- Continued use of protective inserts or taping
- Continued ROM and strength exercises
- Running, to progress within the limits of a pain-free schedule
- Monitored plyometric and cutting program, with progression of difficulty

Care should be taken to avoid reinjury during these activities.

Morton's Neuroma (Interdigital Neuroma)

CLINICAL BACKGROUND

The most common manifestation of an interdigital (Morton's) neuroma is pain between the third and fourth metatarsal heads (in the third interspace) (Fig. 5-79) that radiates to the third and fourth toes. Patients often describe it as a burning pain that intermittently "moves around." Usually, the pain is exacerbated by tight-fitting or high-heeled shoes or increased activity on the foot. The pain is often relieved by removing the shoe and rubbing the forefoot. Occasionally, these symptoms occur in the second interspace with radiation into the second and third toes. Seldom do neuromas occur in both interspaces simultaneously.

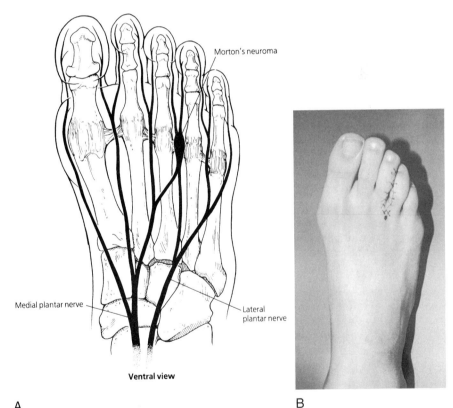

A

B

Figure 5–79   **A**, Morton's neuroma represents a proliferation of fibrous tissue surrounding the plantar nerve where the medial and lateral plantar branches approximate in the area between the third and the fourth metatarsal heads. The nerve is tethered proximally by the flexor digitorum brevis tendon and is stretched around the transverse metatarsal ligament as the toes naturally dorsiflex during ambulation. This repetitive trauma causes localized inflammation and irritation in the area of the third and fourth web space. **B**, Typical distribution of sensation affected by Morton's neuroma in the third interspace (although this has some variability). (**A**, From Mann RA, Coughlin MJ: Surgery of the Foot and Ankle, 6th ed. St Louis, CV Mosby, 1993, p 560.)

TABLE 5–11	Percentage of Preoperative Symptoms Noted by Patients with Morton's Neuroma	
Symptom	**Incidence (%)**
Plantar pain increased by walking	91
Relief of pain by resting	89
Plantar pain	77
Relief of pain by removing shoes	70
Pain radiating into toes	62
Burning pain	54
Aching or sharp pain	40
Numbness in toes or foot	40
Pain radiating up foot or leg	34
Cramping sensation	34

From Mann R, Coughlin M: Surgery of the Foot and Ankle. St Louis, CV Mosby, 1997.

Table 5-11 presents a list of the preoperative symptoms given by patients (percentage) with an interdigital neuroma in Mann's series (1997).

ANATOMY AND PATHOPHYSIOLOGY

The "classic" Morton neuroma is a lesion of the common digital nerve that supplies the third and fourth toes (see Fig. 5-79). It is not a true neuroma, but rather an irritated perineural fibrosis in which the nerve passes plantar to the transverse metatarsal ligament (Fig. 5-80).

It has been speculated that because the common digital nerve to the third interspace has branches from the medial and lateral plantar nerves (and thus increased thickness), the third interspace is the one most commonly involved. The occasional involvement of the second interspace may be a result of anatomic variation in the distribution of the common digital nerves.

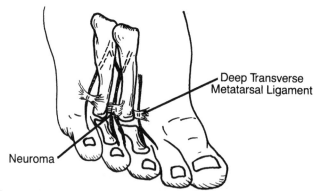

Figure 5–80 Interdigital neuroma. (From Mann RA, Coughlin MJ: Surgery of the Foot and Ankle, 6th ed. St Louis, CV Mosby, 1993.)

The incidence of interdigital neuroma is 8 to 10 times higher in females.

The mechanism is probably chronic hyperextension of the MTP joints (in high heels) with tethering and irritation of the nerve across the transverse metatarsal ligament, which results in an entrapment neuropathy.

DIAGNOSIS

The diagnosis of a Morton neuroma is clinical. There are no useful radiographic or electrodiagnostic tests. Serial examinations may be necessary to establish the correct diagnosis.

Examination

Direct palpation and palpation with a stripping motion (Fig. 5-81) of the interspace will usually reproduce the patient's pain. This maneuver, called "**Mulder's sign,**" often reproduces a clicking or popping sensation and pain in the third (or second) interspace. The examiner places the index finger and thumb proximal to the metatarsal heads in the interspace and, while pushing firmly into the interspace, "strips" distally to the end of the interspace; a click or pop that elicits pain (Mulder's click) is often felt.

Widening of the involved (third and fourth) toes may be noted on occasion as a result of the neuroma mass in the interspace. Subjective numbness of the involved toes is frequently noted, but sensory examination may reveal partial, complete, or no sensory deficit in the nerve's distribution (see Fig. 5-79).

A patient with Morton's neuroma does not have pain over the metatarsal heads.

Occasionally, the examination will be positive only after a vigorous workout or tight shoe wear. Because the patient's physical examination is often inconclusive, several serial examinations and ruling out of related pathology could be required.

Differential Diagnosis

Morton's neuroma may be mimicked by a number of other conditions. The following differential diagnoses should be considered to rule out an incorrect diagnosis of Morton's neuroma.

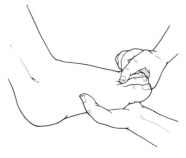

Figure 5–81 Mulder's sign. The examiner places the index finger and thumb proximal to the metatarsals in the interspace and, while pushing firmly, strips the interspace distally. A pop or click reproducing the patient's pain should be elicited. (Adapted from Coughlin MJ, Pinsonneault T: Operative treatment of interdigital neuroma. J Bone Joint Surg Am 83:1321, 2001.)

1. Neurogenic pain, tingling, or numbness
   - *Peripheral neuropathy* typically has more global numbness (entire foot or glove and stocking rather than in the interspace and its two toes) and causes numbness (not pain) unless early in the onset of neuropathy.
   - *Degenerative disk disease* often has accompanying motor, sensory, and reflex changes rather than numbness in a single interspace and its corresponding two toes.
   - *Tarsal tunnel syndrome* is associated with a positive Tinel sign over the tarsal tunnel (medial aspect of the ankle) and numbness limited to the **plantar** aspect of the foot (no dorsal foot numbness) (Figs. 5-82 and 5-83).
   - Lesions of the medial or lateral plantar nerves (see above).

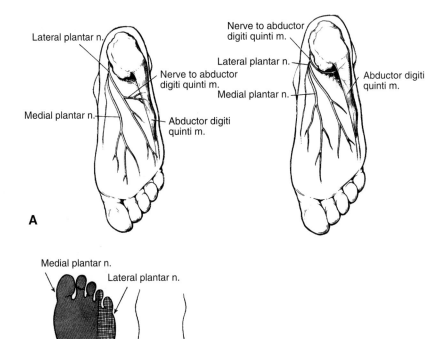

Figure 5–82 **A,** Distribution of the medial and lateral plantar nerves on the bottom of the foot. **B,** Distribution of symptoms (numbness) on the plantar aspect (bottom only) of the foot associated with tarsal tunnel syndrome. (**A**, *Left*, From Gray H: Anatomy: Descriptive and Surgical. Philadelphia, Henry C Tea, 1870, p 660; *Right*, modified from Mann RA, Coughlin MJ: Foot and Ankle Surgery, 6th ed. St Louis, CV Mosby, 1993. **B**, from Chapman MW: Operative Orthopaedics. Philadelphia, JB Lippincott, 1988.)

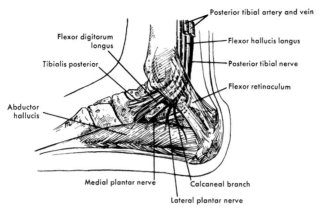

Figure 5–83   Tarsal tunnel syndrome. A Tinel sign reproduces the pain or paresthesias (or both) on palpation of the tibial nerve of the medial aspect of the ankle. The paresthesias occur in the distribution of the tibial nerve (plantar skin). It may involve the medial plantar nerve, the lateral plantar nerve, or both. (From Mann RA, Coughlin MJ: Surgery of the Foot and Ankle. St Louis, CV Mosby, 1993, p 554.)

2. MTP joint pathology
   - *Synovitis of the lesser MTP joint or joints* from rheumatoid arthritis or nonspecific synovitis is associated with tenderness over the metatarsal head or MTP joint rather than the interspace (see Fig. 5-55).
   - *Fat pad atrophy* or degeneration of the plantar fat pad or capsule has tenderness over the metatarsal head or MTP joint rather than the interspace.
   - *Subluxation or dislocation* of the lesser MTP joints is marked by tenderness over the metatarsal head or MTP joint rather than the interspace.
   - *Arthritis of the MTP joint* has tenderness over the metatarsal head or MTP joint rather than the interspace.
3. Plantar foot lesions
   - *Synovial cyst* is usually a tender mass but is not associated with numbness or tingling.
   - *Soft tissue tumors of the interspace*: ganglion, synovial cyst, lipoma, soft tissue neoplasm; usually a tender mass but no numbness or tingling.
   - *Abscess*. Plantar abscess foot. Usually a tender mass but no numbness or tingling.

TREATMENT OF MORTON'S NEUROMA

REHABILITATION PROTOCOL	*After Excision of Morton's Neuroma* Brotzman

- Maximal elevation of foot as much as possible for 72 hours
- Light, compressive, well-padded forefoot dressing in a wooden shoe for approximately 3 weeks
- Weight-bearing as tolerated with crutches for 1-14 days postoperatively
- Work on active ankle ROM exercises and stretching to avoid stiffening of the ankle
- At 3-4 weeks, begin using a wide, soft, comfortable, loosely laced tennis shoe, low-impact activities (e.g., bicycling)

REHABILITATION PROTOCOL	*Initial Nonoperative Treatment of Morton's Neuroma (Interdigital Neuroma)* Brotzman

SHOE MODIFICATION

- Use a soft, wide comfortable shoe with a *wide* toe box to allow the foot to spread out and relieve metatarsal pressure on the nerve. Women should go to men's tennis shoes because of the increased width in men's shoes.
- Wear low heels to avoid hyperextension of the MTP joints associated with high heels.
- Change the lacing pattern on shoes to avoid pressure across the forefoot.

PADS IN THE SHOE

- A metatarsal pad (Hapad) placed proximal to the involved metatarsal may relieve some pressure on the inflamed area. We put the Hapad in the right place (proximal to the metatarsal heads) by using a marker to mark the balls of the foot (Fig. 5-84) and then place the pad just proximal to the ink marks left by the metatarsal heads.

INJECTION OF THE INTERSPACE

- Injection of a small amount of 1% lidocaine *without* epinephrine (2-3 mL) and 1 mL of cortisone may be a useful diagnostic tool (Fig. 5-85). Relief of symptoms often indicates a painful neuroma. The physician should inject the medicine in the affected interspace.
- The use of injected corticosteroids is helpful. Greenfield and associates (1984) noted that 80% of injected neuromas had relief that lasted more than 2 years.

    Many physicians use NSAIDs for 2 weeks in an attempt to decrease inflammation.

    If the patient has continued symptoms despite shoe wear modification, padding, and cortisone injection, surgical resection of the Morton neuroma is indicated.

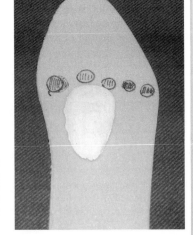

Figure 5–84 With the heel in the correct position in the orthotic, mark the metatarsal heads that you wish to pad (e.g., third and fourth) with a marker; then lower the foot onto the insert. This leaves a dark black circle on the insert. Place the Hapad just proximal to these circles.

REHABILITATION PROTOCOL: *Initial Nonoperative Treatment of Morton's Neuroma (Interdigital Neuroma)* Continued

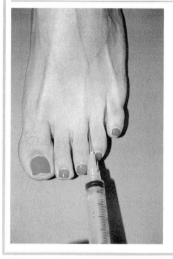

Figure 5–85   Area of injection of 1 mL of cortisone (e.g., 40 mg of methylprednisolone [Depo-Medrol]) and 1 mL of 1% lidocaine without epinephrine to decrease the size and irritation of a Morton neuroma.

Bibliography

PLANTAR FASCIITIS (HEEL PAIN)

Alvarez RG, Ogden JA, Jaahkola J, Cross GL: Symptom duration of plantar fasciitis and the effectiveness of orthotripsy. Foot Ankle 24:916, 2003.

Baxter DE, Thigpen CM: Heel pain: Operative results. Foot Ankle Int 5:16, 1984.

Berman DL: Diagnosing and treating heel injuries in runners. Physician Asst 3:331, 1986.

Buch M, Schoeller C, Goeble F, et al: Extracorporeal shock wave therapy for plantar fasciitis. BMJ 327:75, 2003.

Campbell JW, Inman VT: Treatment of plantar fascitis with UCBL insert. Clin Orthop 103:57, 1974.

DeMaio M, Paine R, Mangine RE, Drez D Jr: Plantar fasciitis. Orthopedics 10:1153, 1993.

Doxey GE: Calcaneal pain: A review of various disorders. J Orthop Sports Phys Ther 9:925, 1987.

Dreeban SM, Mann RA: Heel pain: Sorting through the differential diagnosis. J Musculoskel Med 9:21, 1992.

Erdemir A, Hamel AJ, Fauth AR, et al: Dynamic loading of the plantar aponeurosis in walking. J Bone Joint Surg Am 86:546, 2004.

Graham CE: Painful heel syndrome. J Musculoskel Med 3:42, 1986.

Jahss MH, Michelson JD, Desai P, et al: Investigations into the fat pads of the sole of the foot: Anatomy and histology. Foot Ankle Int 13:233, 1992.

James SL, Bates BT, Osternig LR: Injuries to runners. Am J Sports Med 6:40, 1978.

Josey RA, Marymont JV, Varner KE, et al: Immediate full weightbearing cast treatment of acute Achilles tendon ruptures: A long-term follow-up study. Foot Ankle Int 24:775, 2003.

Kosmahl EM, Kosmahl HE: Painful plantar heel, plantar fasciitis, and calcaneal spur: Etiology and treatment. J Orthop Sports Phys Ther 9:17, 1987.

Leach RE, Schepsis A: When hindfoot pain slows the athlete. J Musculoskel Med 9:82, 1992.

Leach RE, Seavey MS, Salter DK: Results of surgery in athletes with plantar fasciitis. Foot Ankle Int 7:156, 1986.

Miller RA, Decoster TA, Mizel MA: What's new in foot and ankle surgery? J Bone Joint Surg Am 87:90917, 2005.

Noyes FE, DeMaio M, Mangine RE: Heel pain. Orthopedics 16:1154, 1993.

Rask MR: Medial plantar neurapraxia (jogger's foot): Report of 3 cases. Clin Orthop 134:193, 1987.

Riddle DL, Pulisic M, Sparrow K: Impact of demographic and impairment related variables on disability associated with plantar fasciitis. Foot Ankle Int 25:311, 2004.

Riddle DL, Schappert SM: Volume of ambulatory care visits and patterns of care for patients diagnosed with plantar fasciitis: A national study of medical doctors. Foot Ankle Int 25:303, 2004.

Schepsis AA, Leach RE, Goryzca J: Plantar fasciitis. Clin Orthop 266:185, 1991.

Tanner SM, Harvey JS: How we manage plantar fasciitis. Physician Sports Med 16(8):39, 1988.

Tanz SS: Heel pain. Clin Orthop 28:169, 1963.

Wapner KL, Sharkey PF: The use of night splints for treatment of recalcitrant plantar fasciitis. Foot Ankle Int 12:135, 1991.

CHRONIC LATERAL INSTABILITY

Aydogan U, Glisson RR, Nunly JA: Biomechanical comparison of the Broström. Paper presented at the annual winter meeting of the AOFAS, March 13, 2004, San Francisco.

Hamilton WG: Foot and ankle injuries in dancers. Clin Sports Med 1:143, 1988.

Hamilton WG, Thompson FM, Snow SW: The modified Broström procedure for lateral instability. Foot Ankle 14:1, 1993.

POSTERIOR TIBIAL TENDON INSUFFICIENCY

Frey C, Shereff M, Greenidge N: Vascularity of the posterior tibial tendon. J Bone Joint Surg Am 6:884, 1990.

Holmes GB Jr, Mann RA: Possible epidemiological factors associated with rupture of the posterior tibial tendon. Foot Ankle 13(2):70, 1992.

Johnson K: Tibialis posterior tendon rupture. Clin Orthop 177:140, 1983.

Johnson KA, Strom DE: Tibialis posterior tendon dysfunction. Clin Orthop 239:206, 1989.

HALLUX RIGIDUS

Bingold AC, Collins DH: Hallux rigidus. J Bone Joint Surg Br 32:214, 1950.

Mann RA, Clanton TO: Hallux rigidus treatment by cheilectomy. J Bone Joint Surg Am 70:400, 1988.

Mann RA, Coughlin MJ, DuVries HL: Hallux rigidus: A review of the literature and a method of treatment. Clin Orthop 142:57, 1979.

McMaster MJ: The pathogenesis of hallux rigidus. J Bone Joint Surg Br 60:82, 1978.

Moberg E: A simple operation for hallux rigidus. Clin Orthop 142:55, 1979.

FIRST METATARSOPHALANGEAL JOINT PAIN (TURF TOE)

Bowers KD Jr, Martin RB: Turf-toe: A shoe-surface related football injury. Med Sci Sports Exerc 8:81, 1976.

Clanton TO: Athletic injuries to the soft tissues of the foot and ankle. In Coughlin MJ, Mann RA (eds): Surgery of the Foot and Ankle. St Louis, CV Mosby, 1999, p 1184.

Clanton TO, Butler JE, Eggert A: Injuries to the metatarsophalangeal joint in athletes. Foot Ankle 7:162, 1986.

Coker TP, Arnold JA, Weber DL: Traumatic lesions to the metatarsophalangeal joint of the great toe in athletes. Am J Sports Med 6:326, 1978.

MORTON'S NEUROMA

Greenfield J, Rea J Jr, Ilfeld FW: Morton's interdigital neuroma: Indications for treatment by local injections versus surgery. Clin Orthop 185:142, 1984.

Mann RA, Coughlin MJ: Surgery of the Foot and Ankle, 6th ed. St Louis, CV Mosby, 1993.

ACHILLES TENDON

Bruggeman NB, Turner NS: Wound complications after open Achilles repair. Paper presented at the annual winter meeting of the AOFAS, March 13, 2004, San Francisco.

Clain MR, Baxter DE: Achilles tendonitis. Foot Ankle 13:482, 1992.

Clement DB, Taunton JE, Smart GW: Achilles tendinitis and peritendinitis: Etiology and treatment. Am J Sports Med 12(3):179, 1984.

Gill SS, Gelbke MK, Mattson SL, et al: Fluoroscopically guided low volume peritendinous corticosteroid injection for Achilles tendinopathy: A safety study. J Bone Joint Surg Am 86:802, 2004.

Gorschewsky O, Pitzl M, Putz A, et al: Percutaneous versus open tendon Achilles repair. Foot Ankle Int 25:775, 2004.

Hugate R, Pennypacker J, Saunders M, Juliano P: The effects of intratendinous and retrocalcaneal intrabursal injections of corticosteroid on the biomechanical properties on rabbit Achilles tendons. J Bone Joint Surg Am 86:794, 2004.

James SL, Bates BT, Osternig LR: Injuries to runners. Am J Sports Med 6(2):40, 1978.

Lagergren C, Lindholm A: Vascular distribution of the Achilles tendon. Acta Chir Scand 116:491, 1959.

Leach RE, Schepsis AA, Takai H: Long-term results of surgical management of Achilles tendonitis. Clin Orthop 282:208, 1992.

Leitze Z, SElla EJ, Aversa JM: Endoscopic decompression of the retrocalcaneal space. J Bone Joint Surg Am 85:1488, 2003.

Marcus DS, Reicher MA, Kellerhouse LE: Achilles tendon injuries. J Comput Assist Tomogr 13:480, 1989.

Paolini JA, Appleyard RC, Nelson J, Murrell GA: Topical trinitrite treatment of chronic noninsertional Achilles tendinopathy: A randomized, double blind, placebo controlled trial. J Bone Joint Surg Am 86:916, 2004.

Puddu G, Ippolito E, Postachinni F: A classification of Achilles tendon disease. Am J Sports Med 4(4):145, 1976.

Schepsis AA, Leach RE: Surgical management of Achilles tendonitis. Am J Sports Med 15(4):308, 1987.

Scioli MW: Achilles tendonitis. Orthop Clin North Am 25:177, 1994.

6 The Arthritic Lower Extremity

HUGH CAMERON, MD • S. BRENT BROTZMAN, MD

The Arthritic Hip

Clinical Background

General Features of
Osteoarthritis

Primary Symptoms and Signs
of Osteoarthritis

Classification of Hip Arthritis

Diagnosis of Hip Arthritis

Treatment of Hip Arthritis

The Arthritic Knee

Clinical Background

Classification

Diagnosis

Radiographic Evaluation of the
Arthritic Knee

Treatment of Knee Arthritis

Total Knee Arthroplasty

Findings in Common Conditions of the Pelvis, Hip, and Thigh

OSTEOARTHRITIS OF THE HIP

- *Pain reproduced by passive internal rotation of the hip*
- Tenderness over the anterior hip capsule (variable)
- Restricted range of motion (ROM) (rotation is usually affected first)
- Pain reproduced by the Stinchfield test
- Abductor limp (with severe involvement)
- Functional leg-length discrepancy (if abduction contracture has developed)

POSTERIOR HIP DISLOCATION

- Motor vehicle accident or history of major trauma
- Hip held in a position of flexion, internal rotation, and adduction
- Possible concomitant sciatic nerve injury (weakness of dorsiflexion and plantar flexion of the ankle)

ANTERIOR HIP DISLOCATION

- Motor vehicle accident or history of major trauma
- Hip held in a position of mild flexion, abduction, and external rotation
- Possible associated femoral nerve injury (quadriceps weakness)

HIP FRACTURE

- Tenderness over the anterior hip capsule or the intertrochanteric region
- Limb externally rotated and shortened (displaced fracture)
- Stinchfield test painful or cannot be performed

Continued

Findings in Common Conditions of the Pelvis, Hip, and Thigh *Continued*

PELVIC FRACTURE OR DISRUPTION

- Tenderness of the pubic symphysis, pubic rami, iliac crest, or sacroiliac joint
- Pain in response to pelvic compression tests (lateral and anteroposterior [AP] pelvic compression tests, pubic symphysis stress test)
- Pain with the Patrick test or Gaenslen test (especially in fractures of the sacroiliac joint)

SACROILIAC JOINT DYSFUNCTION

- Tenderness over the sacroiliac joint
- Pain with the Patrick test or Gaenslen test (especially in the sacroiliac joint)

ENTRAPMENT OF THE LATERAL FEMORAL CUTANEOUS NERVE (MERALGIA PARESTHETICA)

- Altered sensation over the anterolateral aspect of the thigh (numbness, dysesthesias)
- Symptoms reproduced by pressure or percussion of the nerve just medial to the anterior superior iliac spine

PIRIFORMIS TENDINITIS

- Tenderness to deep palpation near the hook of the greater trochanter
- Pain reproduced by the piriformis test

GLUTEUS MAXIMUS TENDINITIS

- Tenderness at the gluteal fold at the inferior aspect of the gluteus maximus
- Pain reproduced by the Yeoman test

GLUTEUS MINIMUS TENDINITIS

- Tenderness just proximal to the greater trochanter
- Pain reproduced by resisted abduction of the hip

TROCHANTERIC BURSITIS

- Tenderness over the lateral aspect of the greater trochanter
- Popping or crepitation felt with flexion-extension of the hip (occasionally)
- Tight iliotibial tract revealed by the Ober test (variable)

QUADRICEPS STRAIN OR CONTUSION

- Tenderness and swelling of the involved area of the quadriceps
- Weakness of quadriceps contraction
- Restriction of knee flexion, especially when the hip is extended
- Palpable divot in the quadriceps (more severe injuries)
- Warmth and firmness in the quadriceps (impending myositis ossificans)

HAMSTRING STRAIN

- Localized tenderness and swelling at the site of injury
- Ecchymosis (frequently)
- Restricted knee extension and straight leg raises (SLRs) from posterior hamstring pain
- +Palpable divot in the injured hamstring (more severe injuries)
- Abnormal tripod sign

Modified from Reider B: The Orthopaedic Physical Examination. Philadelphia, WB Saunders, 1999.

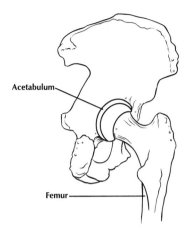

Figure 6-1

Osteoarthritis is the most prevalent joint disease in the United States, with an estimated 43 million people afflicted. A report by the Centers for Disease Control and Prevention indicated that patients with arthritis have substantially worse health-related quality of life than do those without it.

The Arthritic Hip

CLINICAL BACKGROUND

Arthritis of the hip (Fig. 6-1) can result from many causes, such as childhood sepsis, slipped capital epiphysis, and rheumatoid arthritis. About 30% of all patients with hip arthritis have a mild form of acetabular dysplasia (a shallow socket), and 30% have a retroverted socket. Both these conditions **reduce the contact area** of the femoral head in the acetabulum, which increases the pressure and makes wear more likely. Approximately 30% of patients have no obvious risk factors.

Arthritis of the hip is marked by progressive loss of articular cartilage with joint space narrowing and pain. **Stiffness** encourages the development of osteophyte formation (bone spurs), which in turn leads to further stiffness, thus making it difficult for the patient to put on socks and shoes. This process eventually leads to the general picture of shortening, adduction deformity, and external rotation of the hip, often with a fixed flexion contracture. Bone loss usually occurs slowly, but with avascular necrosis it occasionally occurs precipitously.

> ### Disorders of the Hip Joint for Which Total Hip Arthroplasty May Be Indicated
>
> Arthritis
>   Rheumatoid
>   Juvenile rheumatoid (Still's disease)
>   Pyogenic—resolved infection
> Ankylosing spondylitis

Continued

> ### *Disorders of the Hip Joint for Which Total Hip Arthroplasty May Be Indicated* *Continued*
>
> Avascular necrosis
>   After fracture or dislocation
>   Idiopathic
> Bone tumor
> Cassion's disease
> Degenerative joint disease
>   Osteoarthritis
> Developmental dysplasia of the hip
> Failed hip reconstruction
>   Cup arthroplasty
>   Femoral head prosthesis
>   Girdlestone procedure
>   Resurfacing arthroplasty
>   Total hip replacement
> Fracture or dislocation
>   Acetabulum
>   Proximal femur
> Fusion or pseudarthrosis of hip
> Gaucher's disease
> Hemoglobinopathies (sickle cell disease)
> Hemophilia
> Hereditary disorders
> Legg-Calvé-Perthes disease
> Osteomyelitis (remote, not active)
>   Hematogenous
>   Postoperative osteotomy
> Renal disease
>   Cortisone induced
>   Alcoholism
> Slipped capital femoral epiphysis
> Tuberculosis

GENERAL FEATURES OF OSTEOARTHRITIS*

- A heterogeneous group of conditions that share common pathologic and radiographic features
- Focal loss of articular cartilage in part of a synovial joint accompanied by hypertrophic reaction in the subchondral bone and joint margin
- Radiographic changes of joint space narrowing, subchondral sclerosis, cyst formation, and marginal osteophytes
- Common and age related, with identified patterns of involvement targeting the hands, hips, knees, and apophyseal joints of the spine
- Clinical findings often include joint pain with use, stiffness of joints after a period of inactivity, and lost ROM

---

*From Dieppe P: Osteoarthritis: Are we asking the wrong questions? Br J Rheumatol Aug 23(3):161, 1984.

PRIMARY SYMPTOMS AND SIGNS OF OSTEOARTHRITIS*

Symptoms

- Pain during activity
- Stiffness after inactivity (stiffness usually lasts less than 30 minutes)
- Loss of movement (difficulty with certain tasks)
- Feelings of insecurity or instability
- Functional limitations and handicap

Signs

- Tender spots around the joint margin
- Firm swellings of the joint margin
- Coarse crepitus (creaking or locking)
- Mild inflammation (cool effusions)
- Restricted, painful movements
- Joint "tightness"
- Instability (obvious bone or joint destruction)

CLASSIFICATION OF HIP ARTHRITIS

The radiographic appearance of hip osteoarthritis can be classified as (1) **concentric**, in which there is uniform loss of articular cartilage; (2) **downward and medial migration** of the femoral head; or (3) **upward** and **superolateral migration** of the femoral head. This is important if a corrective osteotomy is being considered but is otherwise of no significance.

DIAGNOSIS OF HIP ARTHRITIS

Hip pain can be simulated by referred pain from the spine, L3-4 sciatica, and stenosis of the internal iliac artery. Causes of referred pain must be ruled out. *The classic clinical test for hip arthritis is internal rotation of the hip in flexion.* With hip arthritis, this internal rotation will be limited and painful. The **differential diagnosis** includes hip dislocation, hip fracture, pelvic fracture or disruption, entrapment of the lateral femoral cutaneous nerve, tendinitis of the piriformis or the gluteus maximus or minimus tendons, trochanteric bursitis, L3-4 sciatica, spine-referred pain, internal iliac artery stenosis, and strain or contusion of the quadriceps or hamstring muscles.

Radiographic examination includes an AP view of the pelvis and AP and lateral views of the hip. **The lateral view must be a modified frog-leg lateral or Lauenstein.** A shoot-through lateral is of no value to the surgeon because it gives a distorted picture of the femur. Serologic investigations are seldom required. The only indication for further imaging studies such as bone scanning and magnetic resonance imaging is suspected avascular necrosis in the absence of radiologic findings.

TREATMENT OF HIP ARTHRITIS

Anti-inflammatories and analgesics are of some value (albeit limited). In general, nonsteroidal anti-inflammatory drugs (NSAIDs) act by reversibly inhibiting the

---

*From Dieppe P: Osteoarthritis: Are we asking the wrong questions? Br J Rheumatol Aug 23(3):161, 1984.

cyclooxygenase or lipoxygenase side of arachidonic acid metabolism, which effectively blocks the production of proinflammatory agents such as prostaglandins and leukotrienes. Also inhibited are the beneficial effects of prostaglandins, including protective effects on the gastric mucosal lining, renal blood flow, and sodium balance. Unlike aspirin, which has an irreversible antiplatelet effect persisting for the life of the platelet (10 to 12 days), NSAID bleeding times usually correct within 24 hours of discontinuation.

Dyspepsia (gastrointestinal upset) is the most common side effect of NSAIDs. Other potential side effects include gastrointestinal ulceration, renal toxicity, hepatotoxicity, and cardiac failure.

Contraindications to the use of NSAIDs include a history of gastrointestinal, renal, or hepatic disease or simultaneous anticoagulation therapy. The American College of Rheumatology recommends an annual complete blood count, liver function, and creatinine testing in patients with prolonged NSAID use. Hemograms and fecal occult blood testing are recommended both before initiating NSAIDs and regularly thereafter.

Because of its favorable side effect profile and equivalent efficacy in pain relief (Bradley et al., 1991), acetaminophen (Tylenol) has become accepted as a first-line analgesic agent by the orthopaedic and rheumatologic communities. The recommended dosage of acetaminophen is 650 mg every 4 to 6 hours as needed, to a maximum dosage of 4000 mg/day. A dose of 1000 mg three times a day is usually sufficient. **Neutraceuticals** such as chondroitin sulfate and glucosamine are popular but unproven.

Glucosamine and chondroitin sulfate are synergistic endogenous molecules in articular cartilage. Glucosamine is thought to stimulate chondrocyte and synoviocyte

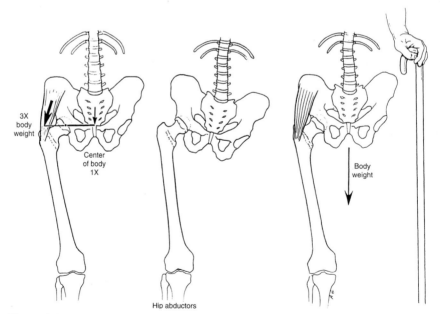

Figure 6-2 Use of a cane redirects the force across the hip. Without the cane, the resultant force across the hip is about three times body weight because the force of the abductors acts on the greater trochanter to offset body weight and levels the pelvis in single stance. (From Kyle RF: Fractures of the hip. In Gustilo RB, Kyle RF, Templeton D [eds]: Fractures and Dislocations. St Louis, CV Mosby, 1993.)

metabolism, and chondroitin sulfate is believed to inhibit degradative enzymes and prevent the formation of fibrin thrombi in periarticular tissues (Ghosh et al., 1992).

A minimum of 1 g of glucosamine and 1200 mg of chondroitin sulfate per day are the standard recommended doses. The average cost of this oral therapy is 50 dollars per month.

A **cane** in the opposite hand helps unload the hip significantly (Fig. 6-2). A properly fitted cane should reach the top of the patient's greater trochanter of the hip while wearing shoes. **Stretching** and strengthening exercises or joining a yoga class can be of surprising value in terms of regaining ROM because it may be stiffness (e.g., inability to put on shoes and socks) rather than pain that makes surgery necessary.

Exercises for the Arthritic Hip (NOT after Total Hip Replacement)

We use exercises that strengthen and stretch the muscles and capsule of the arthritic hip (see also Tables 6-1, 6-2, and 6-3) and incorporate motion and strength needed by the patient for daily functioning. **These exercises are for an arthritic hip,** *not after hip replacement.*

LEG ROTATIONS (FIG. 6-3)

1. Lying on your back, straighten your right leg and bend your left knee to take strain off your back.
2. Point your toes (right foot) up to the ceiling; then rotate the leg clockwise and hold for 10 seconds. Next rotate the foot counterclockwise, again pointing at the ceiling; then point inward toward the left side of the body.
   Number of repetitions: repeat for each leg, 10 times a set.
   Number of sets: 2 per day.

LEG RAISES (FIG. 6-4)

1. Stand next to a chair and lean on it for support.
2. Raise your left leg to the front as far as you can while keeping it straight.
3. Lower your left leg and repeat the exercise with your right leg.
4. Face the chair and, while leaning on it for support, lift your left leg out to the side as far as you comfortably can.
5. Lower your left leg and repeat the exercise with your right leg.
   Number of repetitions: 10-15.
   Number of sets: 2 per day.

KNEE CROSS-OVERS (FIG. 6-5)

1. Lie on your right side on a bed or the floor and rest your head on your right arm. For support, bend your left arm in front of your chest. Straighten your legs.
2. Bend your left knee and pull it toward your chest. Your left foot should have moved close to your right knee.

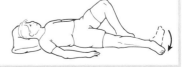

Figure 6-3   Leg rotations. The patient internally and externally rotates the hip while lying supine.

Continued

Exercises for the Arthritic Hip (NOT after Total Hip Replacement)   *Continued*

KNEE CROSS-OVERS—cont'd

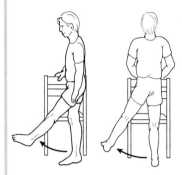

Figure 6-4   Leg raises.

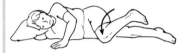

Figure 6-5   Knee cross-overs.

3. Cross your left knee over your right leg and down toward the bed or floor.
4. While keeping your left foot on your right knee, lift the left knee and return it to its starting position in step 2.
5. Roll onto your left side and repeat the exercise with your right leg.
  Number of repetitions: 10-15.
  Number of sets: 2 per day.

STRENGTHENING EXERCISES

Leg Scissors against Resistance (Fig. 6-6)

1. Loop elastic tubing over your ankles, calves, or thighs.
2. Lie on your back on a bed or the floor and extend your legs straight in front of you. Let your arms rest at your sides.
3. Spread your legs as far apart as you can against the resistance of the elastic tubing, and then bring them back together. (If your doctor permits, you may raise your legs slightly off the bed or floor before spreading them.)
  Number of repetitions: 5-10.
  Number of sets: 2-3 per day.

Straight Leg Lifts (Fig. 6-7)

1. Lie on your back. Keep both knees bent and your feet flat on the floor or bed. Let your arms rest at your sides.
2. Straighten your right leg, and then while keeping your knee straight, lift it as high as you can.

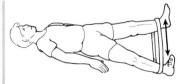

Figure 6-6   Leg scissors against resistance.

Exercises for the Arthritic Hip (NOT after Total Hip Replacement)   *Continued*

STRENGTHENING EXERCISES—cont'd

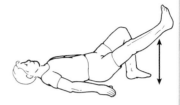

Figure 6-7   Straight leg raises.

3. Lower your leg slowly to the floor and bend your knee to return to the starting position.
4. Repeat the exercise with your left leg.
   Number of repetitions: 10-15.
   Number of sets: 2 per day.

Knee-to-Chest Lifts (Fig. 6-8)

1. Lie on your back. Keep both knees bent and your feet flat on the floor or bed. Let your arms rest at your sides.
2. Bend your right leg at the hip and bring your knee as close to your chest as you can.
3. Lower your leg slowly to its starting position, and relax.
4. Repeat the exercise with your left leg.
   Number of repetitions: 10.
   Number of sets: 2-3 per day.

Side Kicks (Fig. 6-9)

1. Lie on your right side while resting your head on your right arm. For support, bend your left arm in front of your chest and bend your right knee.
2. While keeping your upper (left) leg straight and in line with your body, lift it as high as you can. Make sure that your toes remain pointing forward.
3. Hold the position for a few seconds; then lower your leg slowly.
4. Turn on your left side and perform the side kicks with your right leg.
   Number of repetitions: 10-15.
   Number of sets: 2 per day.

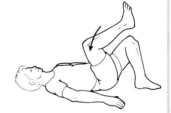

Figure 6-8   Knee-to-chest lifts.

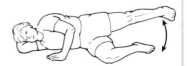

Figure 6-9   Side kicks.

Continued

Exercises for the Arthritic Hip (NOT after Total Hip Replacement)   *Continued*

STRENGTHENING EXERCISES—cont'd

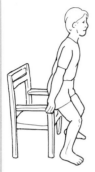

Figure 6-10   Thirty-degree mini-squat with the patient standing over a chair.

Minimal Sit-Downs (Flexing the Knees Only 30 Degrees) (Fig. 6-10)

1. Stand in front of a chair or up against the wall. Let your arms rest at your sides.
2. Bend your hips and knees and begin to lower yourself into a sitting position.
3. Stop when you are halfway into the chair, or 30 degrees of bend, and return to a standing position. Do not use your hands and arms to help lower and raise yourself. Do *not* bend the knees deeply. Thirty degrees should barely bend the knees (have your therapist show you 30 degrees of knee flexion).
   Number of repetitions: 10-15.
   Number of sets: 2 per day.

Note: Do not lower yourself to the point where you cannot use your leg muscles to stand up or so far that your knees hurt.
   From Eichner ER: Patient handout for the arthritic hip. Womens Health Orthop Ed 2(4):1, 1999.

TABLE 6–1	Suggested Exercise Plan for Patients with Osteoarthritis of the Hips*

Mild Symptoms	Moderate to Severe Symptoms (Pain on ROM)
Active ROM exercises	Active-assisted ROM exercises
Stretches for the hip flexor, adductor, iliotibial band, and gastrocnemius muscles and for the hamstring tendons	Stretches
	Isometric strengthening only when ROM is less painful
	Physical therapy modalities as needed
Strengthening (belt exercises, leg lifts, closed–kinetic chain exercises, standing on one foot, walking)	Unloaded ambulation (**Aquasizer**, **pool**, grocery cart, cane, walker). Start at a comfortable duration (1 min if necessary), once to several times a day, and gradually increase to 45 min. Then gradually

TABLE 6–1	Suggested Exercise Plan for Patients with Osteoarthritis the Hips*—cont'd

Mild Symptoms	Moderate to Severe Symptoms (Pain on ROM)
Aerobic conditioning (preferably walk 1 hr, 5 times a week) Aquatic therapy in warm water (not a hot tub) to "unload"	reload (shallower water, less pressure on cane) until fully loaded for 1 hr, 3-5 times per week

*Patients with mild symptoms receive one or two physical therapy visits. Patients with moderate to severe symptoms see a therapist daily for 1 to 2 weeks, then three times a week for 1 to 2 months, then once a week for 1 to 4 weeks, and then once a month for a total of approximately 6 months until they are advancing independently.

ROM, range of motion.

From Ike RW, Lampman RM, Castor CW: Arthritis and aerobic exercise: A review. Phys Sports Med 17(2):27, 1989.

TABLE 6–2	Exercise Devices Suitable for Patients with Arthritis

	Joints Stressed				
	Hip	Knee	Ankle	Shoulder	Spine
Stationary bicycle	+ +	+ +	+	−	+
Arm-crank ergometer	−	−	−	+ +	+ +
Rowing machine	−	−	−	+ +	+ +
Cross-country skiing machine	+	±	±	±	+
Climbing machine	+ +	+ +	+ +	+	+
Water running with limited-buoyancy vest	−	−	−	±	±

+ +, Greatly stressed; +, stressed; ±, somewhat stressed; −, not stressed.

From Ike W, Lampman RM, Castor W: Arthritis and aerobic exercise: A review. Physician Sports Med 17(2):27, 1989.

TABLE 6–3	Aerobic Conditioning Protocol for Patients with Arthritis (Low to Moderate Intensity on Bicycle Ergometer)

Frequency	Three times per week
Workload	Resistance that attains 70% of the maximal heart rate at
Structure	50 rpm in a stable class 1 or 2 patient
	Five exercise sessions separated by 1-min rest periods
Progression of *exercise time* initially	2 min (low intensity) 15 min (moderate intensity)
Rate of increase	2 minutes every 2 wk
Maximum	15 min/session (low intensity) 35 min/session (moderate intensity)

From Ike RW, Lampman RM, Castor CW: Arthritis and aerobic exercise: A review. Physician Sports Med 17(2):27, 1989.

Operative Options for Hip Arthritis

Osteotomies, such as pelvic and intertrochanteric osteotomy, were popular in the past, and they may still have a limited role in selected situation. **Fusion** still has a role, but in very early childhood only. **The mainstay of surgical treatment is total hip replacement** (Fig. 6-11). In general, for elderly patients with low activity demands, both the acetabular and the stem components can be cemented. For young, high-demand patients, the current trend is to use noncemented implants. These are only general guidelines. In revisions with poor-quality bone, the surgeon bases fixation choices on the intraoperative findings.

Weight-bearing restrictions are very different after arthroplasty with cemented and cementless hip devices. **Cement** is as strong as it will ever be 15 minutes after insertion. Some surgeons believe that some weight-bearing protection should be provided until the bone at the interface with the cement (which has been damaged by mechanical and thermal trauma) has reconstituted with the development of a peri-implant bone plate. This phenomenon takes 6 weeks. **Most surgeons, however, believe that the initial stability achieved with cement fixation is adequate to allow immediate full weight-bearing with a cane or walker.**

With a **noncemented hip prosthesis**, the initial fixation is press-fit, and maximal implant fixation is unlikely to be achieved until some tissue ongrowth or ingrowth into the implant has been established. Stability is usually adequate by 6 weeks. **However, maximal stability is probably not achieved until approximately 6 months with noncemented prostheses.** For these reasons, many surgeons advocate **toe-touch weight-bearing for the first 6 weeks**. Some believe that the initial stability achieved is adequate to allow weight-bearing as tolerated immediately after surgery.

SLRs can produce very large out-of-plane loads on the hip and should be avoided. Side leg lifting in the lying position also produces large loads on the hip. Even vigorous isometric contractions of the hip abductors should be practiced with caution, especially if a trochanteric osteotomy has been performed.

The initial rotational resistance of a noncemented hip may be low, and thus it may be **preferable to protect the hip from large rotational forces for 6 weeks**

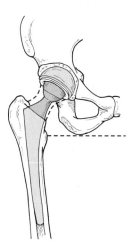

Figure 6-11 Total hip replacement.

or more. The most common rotational load occurs when arising from a sitting position, so pushing with hands from a chair is strongly recommended.

After full weight-bearing is established, it is essential that the patient continue to use a cane in the contralateral hand until the limp stops. This helps prevent the development of a **Trendelenburg gait**, which may be difficult to eradicate at a later date. In some difficult revisions in which implant or bone stability has been difficult to establish, a patient may be advised to continue to use a cane indefinitely. In general, when a patient gets up and walks away, forgetting about the cane, this is an indicator that the cane may be safely discarded.

Contraindications to Total Hip Arthroplasty

ABSOLUTE CONTRAINDICATIONS

1. Active infection in the joint, unless carrying out a revision as either an immediate exchange or an interval procedure
2. Systemic infection or sepsis
3. Neuropathic joint
4. Malignant tumors that do not allow adequate fixation of the components

RELATIVE CONTRAINDICATIONS

1. Localized infection, especially bladder, skin, chest, or other local regions
2. Absent or relative insufficiency of the abductor musculature
3. Progressive neurologic deficit
4. Any process rapidly destroying bone
5. Patients requiring extensive dental or urologic procedures, such as transurethral resection of the prostate, should have these procedures performed before total joint replacement

---

Rehabilitation after Total Hip Replacement

The protocols outlined here for rehabilitation after total hip replacement are general and should be tailored to specific patients. For example, **weight-bearing should be limited to toe-touch if an osteotomy of the femur has been performed for any reason**. Osteotomies can be required for **alignment correction**, either **angular** or **rotational**; **shortening**, such as a calcar episiotomy or subtrochanteric shortening; or **exposure**, such as a trochanteric osteotomy or slide, extended trochanteric osteotomy or slide, or a window. **Expansion osteotomies** allow the insertion of a larger prosthesis, and **reduction osteotomies** allow narrowing of the proximal end of the femur. In patients with any of these osteotomies, weight-bearing should be delayed until some union is present. This is obviously the decision of an operating surgeon. **These patients should also avoid SLR and side leg lifting until, in the opinion of the surgeon, it is safe to do so**.

Treatment may also have to be adjusted because of difficulty of **initial fixation**. In revision surgery, a stable press-fit of the acetabular component may be difficult to achieve, and thus multiple-screw fixation may be required. Under these circumstances, caution should be exercised in rehabilitation.

Treatment might also have to be adjusted because of **stability**. Revision of recurrent dislocations may require the use of an abduction brace to prevent adduction and flexion of more than 80 degrees for varying periods of up to 6 months. Similarly, leg shortening through a hip at the time of revision with or without a constrained socket should be protected for several months with an abduction brace until the soft tissues tighten up.

These considerations should be reviewed and integrated into a specific rehabilitation protocol tailored to the individual patient.

Postoperative Precautions after Total Hip Replacement

To avoid prosthesis dislocation (posteriorly with our posterior surgical approach), we give our patients the following handout and instruct them in the office on motions to avoid.

Patient Instructions after Total Hip Replacement (Posterior Surgical Approach)

Do Not Bend Over Too Far.
Do not let your hand pass your knee.
Use your reacher (Fig. 6-12).
Do Not Lean Over to Get Up.
Instead, slide the hips forward first and then come to standing (Fig. 6-13).

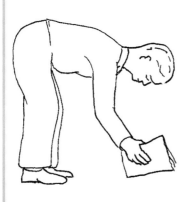

Figure 6-12

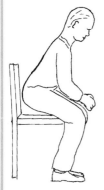

Figure 6-13

Patient Instructions after Total Hip Replacement (Posterior Surgical Approach)   *Continued*

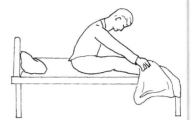

Figure 6-14

Do Not Pull Blankets Up Like This.
Use your reacher (Fig. 6-14).
Do Not Sit Low on a Toilet or Chair.
You must use a raised toilet seat.
Build up a low chair with pillows (Fig. 6-15).
Do Not Stand with Toes Turned In.
Do not let your knees roll inward while sitting (Fig. 6-16).
Do Not Cross Your Legs
While sitting, standing, or lying down (Fig. 6-17).

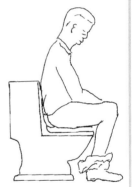

Figure 6-15

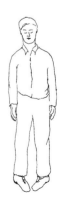

Figure 6-16

Continued

Patient Instructions after Total Hip Replacement (Posterior Surgical Approach) Continued

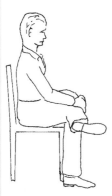

Figure 6-17

Do Not Lie Down without a Pillow between Your Legs.
You do not want to cross or turn your legs inward (Fig. 6-18).
   You have been instructed to **avoid**
   1. Crossing your legs or bringing them together—adduction.
   2. Bringing your knee too close to your chest—extreme hip flexion (you can bend until your hand gets to your knee).
   3. Turning your foot in toward the other leg (internal rotation).
   Listed below are several positions that could occur during your everyday activities. Remember to apply the above precautions.
   1. When sitting, sit with your knees comfortably apart.
   2. Avoid sitting in low chairs and, especially, overstuffed sofas or chairs.
   3. Do not lie on the involved side until cleared by your doctor.
   4. When lying on the uninvolved side, always have a large pillow or two small pillows between your knees. Have the knees in a slightly bent position.
   5. Continue to use your elevated commode seat after you have been discharged from the hospital, until cleared by the doctor (usually around 6-10 weeks).
   6. Do not cross legs while walking, especially when turning.
   7. Avoid bending past 80 degrees (e.g., touching your feet, pulling up your pants, picking up something off the floor, pulling up blankets while in bed).
   8. Sit in a slightly reclined position—avoid leaning forward when sitting on the commode. Do not let your shoulders get ahead of your hips when sitting or getting up.
   9. Avoid raising your knee higher than your hip when sitting in a chair.
   10. Do not try to get into a bathtub for a bath, unless using a tub chair.
   11. *Going up and down stairs:*
      Up—step up with uninvolved leg, keeping crutches on the step below until both feet are on the step above, and then bring both crutches on the step.
      Down—place crutches on the step below, step down with the involved leg, and then step down with the uninvolved leg.

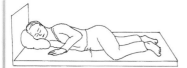

Figure 6-18

Patient Instructions after Total Hip Replacement (Posterior Surgical Approach)   *Continued*

12. Continue to use your crutches or walker until you return to see your doctor.
13. Avoid prolonged sitting for longer than 1 hour before standing and stretching.
14. You can return to driving 6 weeks after surgery only if you have good control over the involved leg and can move your extremity from the accelerator to the brake with little effort.
15. Place a nightstand on the same side of the bed as the uninvolved leg. Avoid twisting the trunk toward the involved side, which would be the same as turning the leg inward.
16. Try to lie flat in bed at least 15-30 minutes per day to prevent tightness in the front part of the hip.
17. If you find you have increased swelling in the involved leg after going home, try propping the foot up (remembering to lean back)—if swelling persists, contact your doctor. Also contact your doctor if calf tenderness develops. Remember that as long as you are touch weight-bearing only, the muscles are not acting to pump blood up the leg, so the leg is likely to swell somewhat until full weight-bearing is established. This swelling usually disappears during the night.

This precaution sheet is borrowed with permission from the www.orthovid.com patient instructional video series on postoperative total joint rehabilitation.

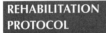

REHABILITATION PROTOCOL   *Postoperative Total Hip Replacement—Posterior Approach*
Cameron and Brotzman

GOALS

- Guard against dislocation of the implant.
- Gain functional strength.
- Strengthen the hip and knee musculature.
- Prevent bed rest hazards (e.g., thrombophlebitis, pulmonary embolism, decubitus ulcers, pneumonia).
- Teach independent transfers and ambulation with assistive devices.
- Obtain pain-free ROM within precaution limits.

Rehabilitation Considerations after Cemented and Cementless Techniques

- Cemented total hip:
  - Weight-bearing to tolerance with a walker immediately after surgery.

PREOPERATIVE INSTRUCTIONS

- Instruct on precautions for hip dislocation (handout).
- Transfer instructions:
  - In and out of bed.
  - Chair:
    - Depth-of-chair restrictions: avoid deep chairs. We also instruct patients to look at the ceiling as they sit down to minimize trunk flexion.
    - Sitting: avoid crossing the legs.
    - Rising from a chair: scoot to the edge of the chair, then rise.

Continued

REHABILITATION PROTOCOL: *Postoperative Total Hip Replacement—*
Posterior Approach *Continued*

PREOPERATIVE INSTRUCTIONS—cont'd

- Use of an elevated commode seat: an elevated seat is placed on the commode at a slant, with the higher part at the back, to aid in rising. Have an elevated seat sent to the house before surgery for installation.
- Ambulation: instruct on the use of any anticipated assistive device (walker).
- Exercises: demonstrate day 1 exercises (see following).

POSTOPERATIVE REGIMEN

- Out of bed in a stroke chair twice a day with assistance 1 or 2 days postoperatively. Do **NOT** use a low chair.
- Begin ambulation with an assistive device twice a day (walker) 1 or 2 days postoperatively with assistance from a therapist.

WEIGHT-BEARING STATUS

- *Cemented prosthesis:* weight-bearing as tolerated with a walker for at least 6 weeks; then use a cane in the contralateral hand for 4-6 months.
- *Cementless technique:* touch-down weight-bearing with a walker for 6-8 weeks (some authors recommend 12 weeks); then use a cane in the contralateral hand for 4-6 months. A wheelchair may be used for long distances with careful avoidance of excessive hip flexion of more than 80 degrees while in the wheelchair. The therapist must check to ensure that the foot rests are long enough. Place a triangular cushion on the wheelchair seat with the highest cushion point posterior to avoid excessive hip flexion.

ISOMETRIC EXERCISES (REVIEW RESTRICTIONS)

- Quadriceps sets: tighten the quadriceps by pushing the knee down and holding for a count of 4.
- Gluteal sets: squeeze the buttocks together and hold for a count of 4.
- Ankle pumps: pump the ankle up and down repeatedly.
- Isometric hip abduction with self-resistance while lying. Later, wrap a Thera-Band around the knees and perform abduction against the Thera-Band.
- Four-point exercise:
  - Bend the knee up while standing.
  - Straighten the knee.
  - Bend the knee back.
  - Return the foot to the starting position.
- Hip abduction-adduction (hold initially if the patient had a trochanteric osteotomy):
  - Supine position: abduct (slide the leg out to the side) and return the leg while keeping the toes pointed up. Make sure that the leg is not externally rotated or the gluteus medius will not be strengthened.
  - Standing position: move the leg out to the side and back. Do not lean over to the side.
  - Side-lying position (probably 5-6 weeks postoperatively): while lying on the side, the patient abducts the leg against gravity (Fig. 6-19). The patient should be turned 30 degrees toward prone to use the gluteus maximus and medius muscles. Most patients would otherwise tend to rotate toward the supine position, thus abducting with the tensor fasciae femoris.

REHABILITATION PROTOCOL: *Postoperative Total Hip Replacement—*
Posterior Approach *Continued*

Figure 6-19 Side-lying hip abduction. Post-operatively, while lying on the side, the patient lifts the involved extremity 8 to 10 inches away from the floor. The patient should turn the body 30 degrees toward prone and hold until the surgeon requests. There is the potential for loss of fixation of a trochanteric osteotomy with this exercise.

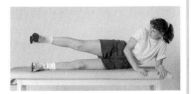

Cameron (1999) emphasizes that hip abductor strengthening is the most important single exercise that will allow the patient to return to ambulation without a limp. The type of surgical approach (e.g., trochanteric osteotomy) and implant fixation (e.g., cement) dictate the timing of initiating hip abduction exercises (see pp. 658 and 659).

- SLR (if not contraindicated): tighten the knee and lift the leg off the bed while keeping the knee straight. Flex the opposite knee to aid this exercise. SLRs are more important after total knee arthroplasty than after total hip arthroplasty. the surgeon may desire to withhold SLRs, depending on construct stability.

ROM AND STRETCHING EXERCISES

- 1 or 2 days postoperatively, begin daily *Thomas stretching* to avoid flexion contracture of the hip. Pull the **uninvolved** knee up to the chest while lying supine in bed. At the same time, **push the postoperative leg into extension against the bed**. The hip extension stretches the anterior capsule and hip flexors of the involved hip and aids with previous flexion contracture and avoidance of postoperative contracture. Perform this stretch 5-6 times per session, 6 times a day (Fig. 6-20).
- May begin stationary exercise bicycling with a high seat 4-7 days postoperatively. To mount the bicycle, the patient stands facing the side of the bicycle and places one hand on the center of the handle bars and the other on the seat. Place the uninvolved leg over the bar and onto the floor so that the seat is straddled. Protect the involved leg from full weight-bearing by putting pressure on the hands. With both hands on the handle bars and partial weight on the involved leg, place the uninvolved leg on the pedal. Stand on the uninvolved leg to sit on the seat. Then turn the pedals so that the involved leg can be placed on the pedal at the bottom of the arc.
  - Until successful completion of a full arc on the bicycle, the seat should be set as high as possible. Initially, most patients find it easier to pedal backward until they can complete a revolution. The seat may be progressively lowered to increase hip flexion within safe parameters.
  - Initially, the patient should ride the bicycle with minimal tension at 15 mph, 2-4 times a day. We leave a stationary bicycle on the hospital floor for use in the room. By 6-8 weeks, may increase the tension until fatigue occurs after approximately 10-15 minutes of riding.

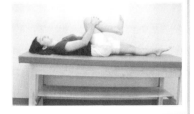

Figure 6-20 Thomas stretch. The patient lies supine in bed while holding the uninvolved knee flexed to the chest and the postoperative (left) leg perfectly straight, pressing down on the bed.

Continued

REHABILITATION PROTOCOL: *Postoperative Total Hip Replacement—*
Posterior Approach   *Continued*

ROM AND STRETCHING EXERCISES—cont'd

- May also perform extension stretching of the anterior capsule (to avoid a hip flexion contracture) by extending the involved leg while the uninvolved leg is mildly flexed at the hip and knee, supported by a walker **(the therapist stabilizes the walker)**. Slowly thrust the pelvis forward and the shoulders backward for a sustained stretch of the anterior capsule (Fig. 6-21).
- Observe and correct gait faults because many of these faults involve the patient's avoidance of stretching the anterior structures of the hip secondary to pain (see p. 669).

ABDUCTION PILLOW

- Keep an abduction pillow between the legs while in bed.

  Note: Many surgeons also use a knee immobilizer on the ipsilateral knee during the first week to avoid possible dislocation of the prosthesis. The knee immobilizer does not allow excessive hip or knee flexion. Use the abductor pillow while asleep or resting in bed for 5-6 weeks; it may then be safely discontinued.

BATHROOM REHABILITATION

- Permit bathroom privileges with assistance and an elevated commode seat.
- Teach bathroom transfers when the patient is ambulating 10-20 feet outside the room.
- Use an elevated commode seat at all times.

ASSISTIVE DEVICES

The occupational therapist brings devices these and instructs the patient on assisted activities of daily living:
- "Reacher" or "grabber" to help retrieve objects on the floor or assist with socks or stockings. Do not bend to put on slippers.
- Shoe horn and loosely fitting shoes or loafers.

TRANSFER INSTRUCTIONS

- Bed to chair:
  - Avoid leaning forward to get out of a chair or off the bed.
  - Slide the hips forward to the edge of the chair first; then come to standing.

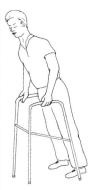

Figure 6-21 Extension stretch of the anterior capsule while the patient is standing. The therapist must stabilize the walker during stretching.

REHABILITATION PROTOCOL: *Postoperative Total Hip Replacement—*
Posterior Approach   *Continued*

TRANSFER INSTRUCTIONS

- Do not cross the legs when pivoting from the supine to the bedside position.
- A nurse or therapist assists until able to perform safe, secure transfers.
- Bathroom:
  - Use an elevated toilet seat with assistance.
  - Continue assistance until able to perform safe, secure transfers.

TRANSFER TO HOME

- Instruct the patient to travel in the back seat of a four-door sedan, sitting or reclining lengthwise across the seat and leaning on one or two pillows under the head and shoulders to avoid sitting in a deep seat.
- Avoid sitting in conventional fashion (hip flexed more than 90 degrees) to avoid posterior dislocation in the event of a sudden stop.
- Urge those without a four-door sedan to sit on two pillows with the seat reclined (minimize flexion of hip).
- Adhere to these principles for 6 weeks until soft tissue stabilization is achieved (Steinberg and Lotke, 1988).
- May begin driving 6 weeks postoperatively.
- Review hip precautions and instructions with the patient (see boxes).

EXERCISE PROGRESSION

- Hip abduction: progress exercises from isometric abduction against self-resistance to a Thera-Band wrapped around the knees. At 5-6 weeks, begin standing hip abduction exercises with pulleys, a sports cord, or weights. Also may perform side stepping with a sports cord around the hips, as well as lateral step-ups with a low step, if clinically safe.

Progress hip abduction exercises until the patient exhibits a normal gait with good abductor strength. Our progression for a postoperative cemented prosthesis with *no trochanteric osteotomy* generally follows the outline below.

1. Supine isometric abduction against a hand or bedrail (2 or 3 days).
2. Supine abduction, sliding the involved leg out and back.
3. Side-lying abduction with the involved leg on top and abduction against gravity.
4. Standing abduction, moving the leg out to the side and back (Fig. 6-22).
5. Thera-Band exercises, sports cord, and step-ups (5-6 weeks).

Perform *prone-lying extension exercises* of the hip to strengthen the gluteus maximus (Fig. 6-23). These exercises may be performed with the knee flexed (to isolate the hamstrings and gluteus maximus) and with the knee extended (to strengthen the hamstrings and gluteus maximus).

Note: This exercise progression is slower in certain patients (see pp. 658 and 659).

Initiate general strengthening exercises to enhance endurance, cardiovascular health, and general strengthening of all extremities.

INSTRUCTIONS FOR HOME

- Continue previous exercises (pp. 665 and 666) and ambulation activities.
- Continue to observe hip precautions.
- Install an elevated toilet seat in the home.
- Supply a walker for home.
- Review rehabilitation specific to the home situation (e.g., steps, stairwells, narrow doorways).
- Ensure that home physical therapy and/or home nursing care has been arranged.

REHABILITATION PROTOCOL: *Postoperative Total Hip Replacement—*
Posterior Approach Continued

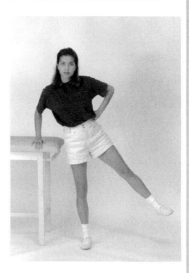

Figure 6-22 Standing abduction: moving the leg out to the side and back.

INSTRUCTIONS FOR HOME—cont'd

- Orient the family to the patient's needs, abilities, and limitations, and **review hip precautions with family members**.
- Reiterate avoidance of driving for 6 weeks (most cars have very low seats).
- Give the patient a prescription for prophylactic antibiotics, which may eventually be needed for dental or urologic procedure.

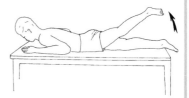

Figure 6-23 Prone-lying extension exercises of the hip are performed to strengthen the gluteus maximus. Lying prone, the patient lifts the leg 8 to 10 inches from the floor while keeping the knee locked.

Managing Problems after Total Hip Replacement

1. **Trendelenburg gait** (weak hip abductors):
   - Concentrate on hip abduction exercises to strengthen the abductors.
   - Evaluate for any leg-length discrepancy.
   - Have the patient stand on the involved leg while flexing the opposite (uninvolved) knee 30 degrees. If the opposite hip drops, have the patient try to lift and hold in an effort to re-educate and work the gluteus medius muscle (hip abductor).

2. **Flexion contracture** of the hip
   * **AVOID** placing pillows under the knee after surgery.
   * Walking backward helps stretch a flexion contracture. Perform a Thomas stretch (p. 665) 30 times a day (5 stretches 6 times per day). Pull the uninvolved knee to the chest while supine. Push the involved (postoperative) leg into extension against the bed. This stretches the anterior capsule and hip flexors of the involved leg.

Gait Faults

Gait faults should be watched for and corrected. Chandler and colleagues (1982) point out that most gait faults are either caused by or contribute to flexion deformities at the hip.

The **first** and **most common gait fault** occurs when the patient takes a large step with the involved leg and a short step with the uninvolved leg. The patient does this to avoid extension of the involved leg, which causes a stretching discomfort in the groin. The patient should be taught to **concentrate on taking longer strides with the uninvolved extremity**.

A **second common gait fault** occurs when the patient breaks the knee in late stance phase. Again, this is done to avoid extension of the hip. It is associated with flexion of the knee and early and excessive heel rise at late stance phase. The patient should be instructed to keep the heel on the ground in late stance phase.

A **third common gait fault** occurs when the patient flexes forward at the waist in mid and late stance. Once again, the patient is attempting to avoid hip extension. To correct this fault, teach the patient to thrust the pelvis forward and the shoulders backward during the mid and late stance phase of gait.

One additional fault, a limp, occasionally arises simply as a habit that can be difficult to break. A full-length mirror is a useful adjunct in gait training because it allows patients to observe themselves while walking toward it.

All these gait faults are correctable with observation and teaching.

Position of Postoperative Total Hip Instability
(Cameron)

* Posterior dislocation: flexion, adduction, and internal rotation will cause dislocation.
* Anterior dislocation: extension, adduction, and external rotation will cause dislocation.

IMPORTANT REHABILITATION POINTS

* **Going up stairs:** step up first with the uninvolved leg, keep the crutches on the step below until both feet are on the step above, and then bring both crutches up on the step. If available, hold the handrail.
* **Going down stairs:** place the crutches on the step below, step down with the involved leg, and then step down with the uninvolved leg. If possible, hold the rail.

Continued

Position of Postoperative Total Hip Instability Continued

IMPORTANT REHABILITATION POINTS—cont'd

- Stretching of the anterior hip structures can be gently achieved by having the patient hang the involved leg laterally off the table as the therapist stabilizes the pelvis (Fig. 6-24).

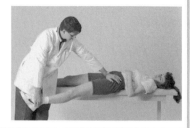

Figure 6-24 Therapist stretching the anterior hip structures.

Stair Training

The good go up to Heaven: the "good" extremity goes first upstairs.
The bad go down to Hell: the "bad" or involved extremity goes first downstairs.

RESTRAINTS OF THE HOME ENVIRONMENT AND ACTIVITIES OF DAILY LIVING

- Assess the home environment and activities of daily living for unique rehabilitation problems.
- Assess home equipment needs.
- Assess unique barriers to mobility.
- Institute a home exercise program that may be realistically performed.

CANE

We also advocate the long-term use of a cane in the contralateral hand to minimize daily forces across the hip arthroplasty and, it is hoped, to prolong implant longevity (see Fig. 6-2).

Deep Vein Thrombosis Prophylaxis for Total Joint Replacement

Thromboembolic disease is the most common cause of serious complications after total hip arthroplasty. The mortality caused by emboli in total hip arthroplasty patients who do not receive prophylactic medication is reported to be five times greater than that after abdominal and thoracic surgery. It is the most common cause of death occurring within 3 months of surgery. Kakkar and colleagues (1985) found that 29% of thrombi developed before postoperative day 12 and 23% between 12 and 24 days after surgery. *Thus, the risk for deep vein thrombosis (DVT) appears to be highest during the first 3 weeks after surgery.*

Numerous studies have shown clotting in the calf or thigh veins in up to 50% of patients after elective surgery; 80% to 90% of the thromboses occur in the limb that has undergone surgery. Calf thrombi alone are unlikely to produce clinically apparent

---

Deep Vein Thrombosis Prophylaxis for Total Joint Replacement   *Continued*

---

pulmonary emboli; they typically arise from larger, more proximal veins. Five percent to 23% of calf vein DVT propagates proximally.

Several factors increase the risk for thromboembolism:
- Prior episode of thromboembolism
- Previous venous surgery and varicose veins
- Previous orthopaedic surgery
- Advanced age
- Malignancy
- Congestive heart failure and chronic lower extremity swelling
- Immobilization
- Obesity
- Oral contraceptives and hormones
- Excessive blood loss and transfusion

Spinal anesthesia and epidural anesthesia carry a lower risk for DVT than general anesthesia does (13% versus 27%).

The best method of prophylaxis remains controversial. Much of the literature is difficult to interpret because of variability in reporting calf or thigh thrombi, clinical methods used to detect pulmonary embolism and DVT, and large variation in pharmacologic protocols. Multiple pharmacologic agents are available for prophylaxis, but data from comparison studies vary widely. The most commonly used agents are low-dose warfarin, low-dose heparin, adjusted-dose heparin, dextran, and aspirin. The duration of therapy is also a source of disagreement in the literature.

Most authors recommend early ambulation, leg elevation, and the use of graded-pressure stockings, but the effectiveness of these stockings is not well documented. External sequential pneumatic compression devices may decrease the overall incidence of DVT, but they are less effective in reducing the formation of more proximal thrombi. The choice of anticoagulation therapy is the physician's and is beyond the scope of this rehabilitation text.

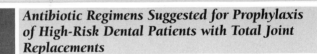

Antibiotic Regimens Suggested for Prophylaxis of High-Risk Dental Patients with Total Joint Replacements

PROPHYLACTIC ANTIBIOTICS FOR FUTURE DENTAL AND GENITOURINARY PROCEDURES (see p. 672)

To avoid possible hematogenous seeding of joint prostheses after transient bacteremia caused by invasive dental or urologic procedures, most orthopaedists recommend antibiotic prophylaxis. No conclusive research data have established the true risk for infection of joint replacements after dental-related bacteremia. Significant disagreement exists in the dental literature. Because of the catastrophic nature of a total joint infection, we advocate prophylactic antibiotic use for dental procedures, genitourinary procedures, or purulent skin infections. Concomitant gingival sulcus irrigation and mouth rinsing with chlorhexidine solution are recommended in potentially high-risk patients before periodontal procedures or extractions.

STANDARD REGIMENS

- Cephradine (Anspor or Velosef), 1 g orally 1 hour before dental procedure
- Cephalexin (Keflex), 1 g orally 1 hour before, 500 mg 6 hours later

Continued

Antibiotic Regimens Suggested for Prophylaxis for High-Risk Dental Patients with Total Joint Replacements Continued

- Cephalexin (Keflex), 2 g orally 1 hour before, 1 g 6 hours later
- Cephalexin (Keflex) 1 g orally 1 hr prior, 500 mg 4 hr later

ALLERGIC TO PENICILLIN OR CEPHALOSPORINS

- Clindamycin, 600 mg orally 1 hour before dental procedure
- Clindamycin, 300 mg orally 1 hour before dental procedure
- Clindamycin, 600 mg orally 1 hour before dental procedure, 600 mg 6 hours later
- Erythromycin, 500 mg orally 1 hour before dental procedure, 500 mg 4 hours later

From Little JW: Managing dental patients with joint prostheses. J Am Dent Assoc 125:1376, 1994.

Patients with Increased Risk for Postoperative Infection after Total Joint Replacement

PREDISPOSING CONDITIONS

- Rheumatoid arthritis
- Steroid use
- Use of other agents causing immunosuppression
- Insulin-dependent diabetes
- Hemophilia
- Hemoglobinopathies such as sickle cell disease

LOCAL FACTORS

- Complications associated with joint prosthesis
- Replacement of prosthesis
- Loose prosthesis
- History of previous infection

ACUTE INFECTION LOCATED AT DISTANT SITES

- Skin
- Other

Modified from Little JW: Managing dental patients with joint prostheses. J Am Dent Assoc 125:1376, 1994.

❙ The Arthritic Knee

CLINICAL BACKGROUND

Arthritis of the knee can be due to many causes, including congenital deformities (such as axial and rotatory deformity), trauma, and rheumatoid arthritis (Table 6-4). Medial compartment osteoarthritis develops in 80% of patients, and as the bone wears away, a **varus** or "bow-legged" deformity develops. Lateral compartment osteoarthritis resulting in a **valgus** or "knock-kneed" deformity develops in 5% to 10%. A small percentage of patients have rotatory deformities of the tibia that cause significant patellar maltracking or subluxation.

TABLE 6–4	Risk Factors for Osteoarthritis of the Knee
Established	**Controversial**
Obesity	Physical activity
Age	Genetics
Osteoarthritis at other sites	Smoking
Previous knee trauma or injury	Estrogen deficiency
Previous knee surgery	
Female (gender)	

CLASSIFICATION

Arthritic deformity of the knee is classified as varus or valgus (with or without symptomatic patellar involvement). **Patellofemoral arthritis** is common in an arthritic knee.

Articular surface damage has been variously classified, but the most useful categories are **minimal**, in which there is no radiologic narrowing; **mild**, in which there is loss of a third of the joint space; **moderate**, in which two thirds of the joint space has been lost; and **severe**, in which there is bone-on-bone contact.

DIAGNOSIS

To examine for arthritis of the knee, move the joint under load (e.g., to examine the medial compartment, a varus strain is applied to the knee and the knee is moved). Crepitus will be felt under the hand applying the varus strain and pain will be produced. Similarly, a valgus strain and load are applied to the lateral aspect of the joint. The knee should be examined for laxity of the collateral ligaments and, to some extent, the cruciate ligaments, although this is less important. The presence of any fixed flexion deformity (e.g., lack of passive extension of the knee) should be noted. The patellar position (central or subluxated) is important, as is the presence of a rotatory deformity of the tibia. When the patient stands, note any genu varum (bow-legged) or genu valgum (knock-kneed).

By the end of our history and examination of the arthritic knee we have obtained the following information:
1. Symptom location
   - Isolated (medial, lateral, or patellofemoral)
   - Diffuse
2. Type of symptoms
   - Swelling
   - Giving way, instability (ligament tear or weak quadriceps)
   - Diminished ROM
   - Mechanical (crepitance, locking, catching, pseudolocking)
3. Timing of onset
   - Acute
   - Insidious
4. Duration
5. Exacerbating factors
6. Previous intervention (e.g., NSAIDs, surgery) and the patient's response

TABLE 6-5	Findings Indicating the Presence of Knee Osteoarthritis	
Symptoms	**Signs**	**Radiography**
Pain with activity	Joint line or condylar tenderness	Subchondral sclerosis Intra-articular osseous debris (loose bodies, or joint mice)
Stiffness	Effusion Crepitation Decreased range of motion Angular deformity	Joint narrowing (unicompartmental) Joint irregularity Subchondral cysts Osteophytosis ("central or marginal")

RADIOGRAPHIC EVALUATION OF THE ARTHRITIC KNEE

Evaluation should always include a standing (weight-bearing) AP view of the knee. If surgery is contemplated, there should be a full-limb (3-foot) view to detect any deformities or problems above and below the standard radiographic views (e.g., a valgus deformity of the ankle). A lateral radiograph is required, as is a skyline view of the patella. **If the problem is on the lateral side of the joint, a standing posteroanterior view must be obtained with the knee in 30 degrees of flexion**. The reason for this is that the articular cartilage loss in the medial compartment is in the distal femur and central tibia, but articular cartilage loss in the lateral compartment is in the posterior femur and posterior tibia (Table 6-5).

TREATMENT OF KNEE ARTHRITIS

See "Rehabilitation Protocol."

Nonoperative

Treatment of early osteoarthritis of the knee may be very effective if conscientiously carried out. **Weight loss** should be strongly encouraged but not expected immediately. **Quadriceps strengthening** makes a surprising difference. Very strong quadriceps can considerably delay the necessity for surgery. If the patella is painful, extension exercises should be carried out only over the last 20 degrees of extension. Activities such as deep squatting, kneeling, and stair climbing that increase patellofemoral joint reaction forces increase pain. These activities should be avoided. If the patient starts with extremely weak muscles, electric stimulation may be used to begin the process. **Modalities** other than heat or cold have not been shown to be of value. **Hyaluronic acid injections** into the knee are of limited value. They appear to work best *before* bone-on-bone crepitus has occurred. Studies by independent researchers have found hyaluronic acid injections to be of "equal benefit" to NSAIDs (naproxyn [Naprosyn]). Petrella (2002) purports that hyaluronic acid intra-articular injection was of benefit. Careful review of the study actually reveals that injection of hyaluronate sodium (Synvisc, Provise, and Suplasyn) is no better than placebo. Similarly, **intra-articular steroid injections** have a very temporary and limited role.

Keating and associates (1993) found that of 85 patients with medial compartment arthritis of the knee, more than 75% had statistical improvement in their Hospital for Special Surgery pain scores at 12 months with the use of a lateral wedged insole in their shoe. For example, a 0.25-inch soft wedge or a 5-degree wedged insole placed laterally will reduce medial joint reactive forces from the medial joint line.

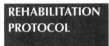

REHABILITATION PROTOCOL — *Nonoperative and Operative Treatment Algorithms for Patients with Arthritis of the Lower Extremity (Hip or Knee)*
Brotzman

TIER 1: NONOPERATIVE OPTIONS

- **Weight loss**!—successful weight loss (though difficult) dramatically improves pain in lower extremity arthritics and prolongs the longevity of total joint arthroplasties. The physician must be proactive and implement low-impact aerobic exercise (water aerobics, cycling, swimming) and direct the patient to a reputable weight loss center (e.g., Weight Watchers).
- Activity modification (Table 6-6):
  - Discontinue high-impact sports (e.g., running, tennis, basketball); change to low-impact **water-based** sports or cycling.
  - Avoid stair climbing, kneeling, squatting, and low chairs in patients with patellofemoral arthritis.
  - Change a hard surface at work to a soft one if possible, sit more than previously, and so on.
  - Perform water aerobics in a warm pool (*not* a hot tub) for aerobic exercise or strengthening.
- NSAIDs
  - We typically use cyclooxygenase-2 inhibitors (e.g., celecoxib [Celebrex]) with periodic liver and renal function tests.
  - Take the *minimal* effective dose, intermittent use if possible.
  - The potential long-term *complications* make long-term everyday use of NSAIDs less attractive:
    - Peptic ulcer disease
    - Renal effects
    - Gastrointestinal bleeding
    - Possible cardiac implications
- *Cane* in the *opposite* hand (see Fig. 6-2):
  - Greatly decreases stress on the arthritic joint, but for cosmesis considerations, many "young" or female arthritics will not use a cane.
- Viscosupplementation of the knee (e.g., hylan G-F 20 [Synvisc], hylauronate sodium [Hyalgan]):
  - Although some patients do respond well to serial injections, other studies have shown comparable efficacy only with Naprosyn.
- "Unloading" graphite braces for knee arthritis (not hip):
  - If the patient has unicompartmental knee involvement (e.g., medial), some benefit may be derived from a custom "unloader" brace.
    - Very expensive.
    - Most patients quickly quit wearing it secondary to bulkiness, inconvenience.

Continued

REHABILITATION PROTOCOL: *Nonoperative and Operative Treatment Algorithms for Patients with Arthritis of the Lower Extremity (Hip or Knee)* Continued

TIER 1: NONOPERATIVE OPTIONS—cont'd

TABLE 6–6	Suggested Exercise Plan for Patients with Osteoarthritis of the Knee
Mild Symptoms*	**Moderate to Severe Symptoms**
Active ROM exercises for the hip, knee, and ankle	Active-assisted ROM exercises for the hip, knee, and ankle
Physical therapy modalities as needed	Physical therapy modalities as needed
Knee sleeve if comfortable	Stretching of the quadriceps, hamstrings, adductors (Fig. 6-25), and gastrocnemius; may use ultrasound for the hamstrings if contraction is present
Quadriceps sets for the vastus medialis obliquus, especially with a prominent patellofemoral component of the symptoms	Quadriceps sets for the vastus medialis obliquus; start supine if there is a hamstring contracture and gradually work up to a sitting position
Advance to isometric progressive resistive exercises for the quadriceps, hamstrings, and hip adductors and abductors	Unloaded aerobic conditioning (pool, walker, grocery cart, cane); advance as described for the hip
Low-impact conditioning exercises. Avoid high patellofemoral compressive forces	Advance strengthening to isometric closed–kinetic chain exercises, such as wall sitting (not "slide" because this word implies repetitions, which are not usually well tolerated)
The authors are strong proponents of aquatic (unloading) exercise for mild, moderate, and severe arthritis (see Chapter 7)	Hip adductor and abductor strengthening
	Later, add straight leg raising progressive resistance exercise (2 pounds on the thigh)
	Later still, try lunges; however, lunges require great strength and excellent balance and coordination, and few patients are strong enough or can understand the importance of positioning. Lunges can therefore aggravate symptoms

*The program for mild symptoms is given in one or two physical therapy visits.
ROM, range of motion.
From Baum AL, Baum J: Coming to grips with depression in rheumatoid arthritis. J Musculoskel Med 15:36, 1998.

REHABILITATION PROTOCOL: *Nonoperative and Operative Treatment Algorithms for Patients with Arthritis of the Lower Extremity (Hip or Knee)* *Continued*

TIER 1: NONOPERATIVE OPTIONS—cont'd

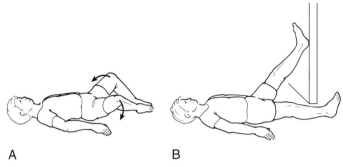

A   B

Figure 6-25   Stretching exercises help preserve or increase joint range of motion (ROM). **A**, In this example of a hip adductor stretch, the patient lies supine on a firm surface with the hips and knees bent and the feet flat. The patient then lets the knees fall apart while keeping the soles of the feet together until an inner thigh stretch is felt. **B**, To stretch the hamstrings, the patient lies on the floor near a doorway with one leg extending into the doorway. The patient slides forward while gently raising the other leg with the foot flat against the wall until a gentle stretch is felt behind the knee.

- Knee sleeve for proprioception (knee arthritis):
  - Some patients derive benefit from a light neoprene knee sleeve, which may improve proprioceptive feedback (indications are soft, but the braces are inexpensive with little if any possible complication).
- Chondroitin sulfate/glucosamine:
  - Moderately expensive ($40 per month).
  - Essentially no side effects or complications. If patients wish to try to derive great benefit, we have them continue. Otherwise, the patient is instructed to discontinue at 3 months if no benefit is noted.
- Physical therapy:
  - A brief course of therapy to teach a home program of hamstring and quadriceps strengthening, flexibility, ROM exercises, and aquatic therapy is *very* useful if patient compliance is good. Schedule follow-up visits to monitor compliance and progression.
- Intra-articular cortisone (knee, *not* hip):
  - Response to aspiration and injection is variable (2 weeks to 6 months).
  - Injections should be limited to three per year (potential articular cartilage softening/avascular necrosis). Warn patients of potential corticosteroid-related flare. Application of ice that evening can help avoid this problem.
  - We do use intra-articular cortisone in our clinic.
- Topical therapy:
  - We have found topical therapy to be largely ineffective.
  The Arthritis Foundation offers the following exercise programs for arthritic patients:
    - Aquatics—heated pool, 6-10 weeks, minimal joint stress, increased ROM.
    - Joint efforts—6-8 weeks, for patients with very limited mobility or the elderly.

Continued

REHABILITATION PROTOCOL: *Nonoperative and Operative Treatment Algorithms for Patients with Arthritis of the Lower Extremity (Hip or Knee)* *Continued*

TIER 1: NONOPERATIVE OPTIONS—cont'd

- PACE (People with Arthritis Can Exercise)—6-8 weeks, two levels of classes.
- PEP (Pool Exercise Program)—45-minute video that increases flexibility, strength, and endurance.

  Multiple brochures with information on arthritis are available. Call the Arthritis Foundation at 1-800-283-7800 or contact them at www.arthritis.org.

TIER 2: OPERATIVE OPTIONS FOR PATIENTS WITH SYMPTOMATIC ARTHRITIC KNEES

Arthroscopy

- With osteoarthritis, degenerating articular cartilage and synovial tissue release proinflammatory cytokines that induce chondrocytes to release lytic enzymes, thereby leading to degradation of type 2 collagen and proteoglycans.
- The "lavaging" effect of arthroscopy may dilute or "wash out" these inflammatory mediators, *although the effect is temporary*.
- Patients often have unrealistic expectations of arthroscopy for arthritis, so counseling on the palliative or temporary effect is needed.
- Microfracture may or may not offer some pain benefit. Drilling and abrasion chondroplasty seem to offer little benefit.
- Patients who benefit most from arthroscopy have mechanical symptoms (locking meniscus) of short duration (<6 months) with mild arthritis on radiographs.
- Patients with 3-6 months of unsuccessful supervised nonsurgical management, normal mechanical alignment, and mild to moderate arthritis on weight-bearing films are considered candidates for arthroscopic débridement.
- Patients with tibial spine pain, osteophyte formation, and lack of extension (flexion deformity) may benefit from arthroscopic notchplasty and osteophyte removal.
- Table 6-7 reviews the prognostic factors for arthroscopic débridement of an arthritic knee.
- Arthroscopic management of an arthritic knee should be considered palliative, temporary, and most effective in patients with concomitant mechanical findings (e.g., bucket-handle meniscal tear with a positive McMurray examination).

Surgery for Focal Cartilage Defects of the Femur (Cartilage Transfer or Chondrocyte Implantation) (Table 6-8)

Osteotomy

- *Varus* malalignment of the knee (bow-legged) in a younger, active patient with medial compartment arthritis is addressed with a valgus-producing, high tibial osteotomy.
- Mild *valgus* malalignment (<10 degrees of valgus) may be treated with a medial, high tibial closing wedge osteotomy. Patients with greater than 10 degrees of valgus undergo femoral osteotomy.
- Supracondylar femoral osteotomies do not interfere with subsequent total knee replacements. However, tibial osteotomies compromise total knee replacement results. For this reason, osteotomies are seldom performed in the United States. New opening wedge osteotomy techniques for the tibia purport not to alter the joint line for later total knee replacement.

REHABILITATION PROTOCOL: *Nonoperative and Operative Treatment Algorithms for Patients with Arthritis of the Lower Extremity (Hip or Knee)* Continued

TIER 2: OPERATIVE OPTIONS FOR PATIENTS WITH SYMPTOMATIC ARTHRITIC KNEES—cont'd

TABLE 6–7	Prognostic Factors for Arthroscopic Débridement of the Arthritic Knee		
History	Physical Examination	Radiographic Findings	Arthroscopic Findings
Good Prognosis			
Short duration	Medial tenderness	Unicompartmental	Outerbridge I or II changes
Associated trauma	Effusion	Normal alignment	Meniscal flap tear
First arthroscopy	Normal alignment	Minimal Fairbank changes	Chondral fracture or flap
Mechanical symptoms	Ligaments stable	Loose bodies Relevant osteophytes	Loose bodies Osteophytes at symptom site
Poor Prognosis			
Long duration	Lateral tenderness	Bi- or tri- compartmental	Outerbridge III or IV changes
Insidious onset	No effusion	Malalignment	Degenerative meniscus
Multiple procedures	Malalignment Varus, >10 degrees; valgus, >15 degrees	Significant Fairbank changes	Diffuse chondrosis
Pain at rest	Ligaments unstable	Irrelevant osteophytes	Osteophyte away from the symptom site
Litigation Work related			

From DiNubile N: Osteoarthritis of the knee—a special report. Physician Sports Med 2000.

Unicompartmental Knee Replacement

- More controversial, patient selection is critical.
- Ideal candidate:
  - Older than 60 years
  - Low-demand (sedentary)
  - Thin
  - Isolated unicompartmental arthritic involvement (Table 6-9)

TIER 3: OPTIONS FOR A SYMPTOMATIC ARTHRITIC KNEE

TOTAL Joint Replacement

- Total joint replacements work best in thin sedentary patients older than 65 years.
- A proportion of replacements "wear out" with time (osteolysis) and require revision. The revision rate is increased with obesity, high-impact activity, overuse, and so on.

Continued

TABLE 6–8	Surgical Treatment Options for Symptomatic Focal Cartilage Defects of Femur*		
Lesion	Treatment	Rehabilitation[†]	Comments
	Primary		
<2 cm²	Débridement and lavage	Straightforward	Provides short-term symptomatic relief
	Marrow stimulation techniques	Significant	Ideal for smaller lesions located on the femoral condyle; provides intermediate short-term relief; low cost
	Osteochondral autograft	Moderate	Relatively new procedure; probably as good as, if not better than marrow stimulation techniques; provides potentially long-term relief
>2 cm²	Débridement and lavage	Straightforward	Provides short-term symptomatic relief
	Marrow stimulation techniques	Significant	Has lower success rate for larger lesions; good choice for symptomatic relief in low-demand individuals; intermediate-term relief is possible; low cost
	Cartilage biopsy for future autologous chondrocyte implantation	Straightforward	Staged procedure
	Osteochondral autograft	Significant	With larger lesions, potential for donor site morbidity exists; results are variable
	Osteochondral allograft	Significant	Useful for larger lesions with significant bone stock loss; small concern for disease transmission and allograft availability; provides potentially long-term relief

Secondary

<2 cm²	Osteochondral autograft	Moderate	Relatively new procedure; probably as good as, if not better than marrow stimulation techniques; provides potentially long-term relief
	Autologous chondrocyte implantation	Significant	High success rate for return to activities; potentially long-term relief; relatively high cost
>2 cm²	Osteochondral autograft	Significant	With larger lesions, potential for donor site morbidity exists; results are variable
	Osteochondral allograft	Significant	Useful for larger lesions with significant bone stock loss; small concern for disease transmission and allograft availability; provides potentially long-term relief
	Autologous chondrocyte implantation	Significant	High success rate for return to activities; potentially long-term relief; relatively high cost

*Selection of the procedure depends on the patient's age, expectations, demand, activity level, coexisting pathology, and extent and location of disease. For rehabilitation after articular defect surgery, please see Chapter 4, Knee Injuries.

†Straightforward, early weight-bearing and return to activities within 4 weeks; moderate, short-term protected weight-bearing and return to activities within 12 weeks; significant, prolonged protected weight-bearing and significant delay until return to activities (6 to 8 months).

‡Follows failed primary treatment.

From Cole BJ: Arthritis of the knee—a special report. Physician Sports Med 28(5):1, 2000.

TABLE 6–9	Treatment Criteria for Unicompartmental Knee Arthritis			
	Unicompartmental Knee Arthroplasty	**High Tibial Osteotomy**	**Total Knee Arthroplasty**	
History	>60 yr old Sedentary Pain with weight-bearing Noninflammatory arthritis No patellofemoral symptoms	<60 yr old, ideally 50s Laborer Activity-related pain Noninflammatory arthritis No patellofemoral symptoms	>65 yr old Sedentary Degenerative traumatic or inflammatory arthritis	
Examination	ROM 5–90 degrees or better <15 degrees coronal deformity Intact ACL (controversial) Intact collateral ligaments, <200 pounds (90 kg)	Flexion >90 degrees Flexion contracture <15 degrees Competent MCL Heavier patients	Joint line tenderness Altered ROM (flexion contracture, etc.) Varus or valgus deformity	
Radiographs	Isolated unicompartmental disease Asymptomatic patellofemoral disease Acceptable No tibial or femoral bowing	Mild to moderate osteoarthritis Varus alignment	Multicompartmental disease Varus or valgus alignment	
Intraoperative findings	Contralateral compartment without eburnated bone and has normal meniscus No evidence of inflammatory process	Inspection of articular surface before osteotomy of no prognostic value	Multicompartmental articular degeneration	
Contraindications	Inflammatory arthritis Limited ROM Advanced patellofemoral disease or contralateral compartment disease Chondrocalcinosis (controversial) ACL deficiency (controversial)	Inflammatory arthritis Limited ROM Advanced patellofemoral disease Varus >10 degrees	Bony defects Acute infection Extensor mechanism disruption Severe recurvatum deformity Severe vascular disease	

ACL, anterior collateral ligament; MCL, medial collateral ligament; ROM, range of motion.
From Seigel JA, Marwin SE: The role of unicompartmental knee arthroplasty. Orthopaedics Special Ed 5(2):62, 1999.

Operative—Arthritic Knee

Arthroscopic débridement is of temporary value in that it simply cleans out the tags and meniscal tears and flushes fluid that contains pain-producing peptides from the joint. Cole and Harners' (1999) article on the evaluation and management of knee arthritis provides an excellent overview on arthroscopy in patients with knee arthritis.

Livesley et al. (1991) compared the results in 37 painful arthritic knees treated with arthroscopic lavage by one surgeon against those in 24 knees treated with physical therapy alone by a second surgeon. The results suggested that there was better pain relief in the lavage group at 1 year. Edelson et al. (1995) reported that lavage alone provided good or excellent results in 86% of their patients at 1 year and in 81% at 2 years according to the Hospital for Special Surgery scale.

Jackson and Rouse (1982) reported on the results of arthroscopic lavage alone versus lavage combined with débridement, with a 3-year follow-up. Of the 65 patients treated by lavage alone, 80% had initial improvement but only 45% maintained that improvement at follow-up. Of the 137 patients treated by lavage plus débridement, 88% showed initial improvement and 68% maintained improvement at follow-up. Gibson et al. (1992) demonstrated no statistically significant improvement with either method, even in the short term. Patients with flexion deformities associated with pain or discomfort and osteophyte formation around the tibial spines may benefit from osteophyte removal and notchplasty, as demonstrated by Puddu et al. (1994).

The efficacy of lavage with or without débridement is controversial, and randomized prospective controlled trials have not been performed. The literature suggests that arthroscopic lavage and débridement, when performed for appropriate indications, will provide improvement in pain relief for 50% to 70% of patients, with relief lasting from several months to several years. Drilling and abrasion arthroplasty do not appear to offer additional benefit. Arthroscopy is also a sensitive way to evaluate cartilage when contemplating osteotomy or unicompartmental knee arthroplasty because plain radiography and magnetic resonance imaging often underestimate the extent of osteoarthritis.

Several factors determine the prognosis after lavage and débridement. **Those who benefit most** have a history of mechanical symptoms, symptoms of short duration (<6 months), normal alignment, and only mild to moderate radiographic evidence of osteoarthritis. It is not uncommon for patients to have unrealistic expectations after arthroscopic débridement. Thus, it is important to counsel patients about the limited indications and palliative results.

Osteotomy of the Knee

In this mechanical load-shifting procedure, the mechanical axis of the knee is "shifted" from the worn compartment (usually medial) to the good compartment. Closing wedge osteotomies have an inherent disadvantage in that the tibiofibular joint must be disrupted with some degree of shortening and joint line alteration. *Because the joint line must remain "horizontal," in patients with osteoarthritis and a valgus deformity the osteotomy is performed through the supracondylar region of the femur; for varus deformity, it is performed through the proximal end of the tibia.* Contraindications to tibial osteotomy include panarthrosis (tricompartmental involvement), severe patellofemoral disease, severely restricted ROM (loss of more than 15 to 20 degrees of extension or flexion less than 90 degrees), and inflammatory arthritis. There are very few contraindications to a varus osteotomy other than damage to the medial compartment, whereas there are many ***contraindications to a tibial osteotomy***. The outcome after a valgus osteotomy depends on the varus thrust force. This force, however, can be detected only with the use of very sophisticated force plate analysis, of which there are very few available worldwide, and other indications must be used. The ***strength-to-weight ratio*** is extremely important because the older and heavier the patient, the less the indication. A straight tibial diaphysis will result in an oblique joint line. A pagoda-shaped or sloping surface of the tibial plateaus usually produces a bad result. Lateral subluxation of the tibia on the femur and flexion contracture of more than 7 degrees also produce a bad result.

No osteotomy will last indefinitely. **Supracondylar femoral osteotomies do not interfere with subsequent total knee replacement because the osteotomy is done above the level of the collateral ligaments. Tibial osteotomy will produce an inferior result with a total knee replacement because the osteotomy is done inside the collateral ligaments and patellar tendons and may produce a patella baja deformity**. Eventually, a total knee replacement will be required in these patients. For this reason, osteotomies are seldom performed in the United States, although they remain moderately popular in many places in the world. New "opening wedge" techniques with Puddu plate–type fixation are currently being evaluated. Their purported value is that the open wedge does not adversely affect the joint line in subsequent total knee replacement.

TOTAL KNEE ARTHROPLASTY

Many surgeons use identical routines after total knee replacement, whether the implants are cemented or noncemented. ***Their rationale is that the initial fixation of noncemented femoral and tibial components is in general so good that loosening is very uncommon***. The tibia is largely loaded in compression. The stability achieved with pegs, screws, and stems on modern implants is now adequate to allow full weight-bearing. However, if the bone is exquisitely soft, weight-bearing should be delayed. Progression to weight-bearing must therefore be based solely on the surgeon's discretion and intraoperative observations.

The guidelines for rehabilitation given here are general guidelines and should be tailored to individual patients. ***Concomitant osteotomies and significant structural bone grafting are indications for limited weight-bearing until healing has been achieved***. Similarly, if the bone is extremely osteoporotic, full weight-bearing is delayed until the peri-implant bone plate develops. Exposure problems requiring a tibial tubercle osteotomy or division of the quadriceps tendon may require that SLR be avoided until adequate healing has occurred, which typically takes 6 to 8 weeks.

Component design, fixation methods, bone quality, and operative techniques all affect perioperative rehabilitation. The implant choice no longer determines the rehabilitation method. It does not or should not make much difference whether the implant is unconstrained, semiconstrained, or fully constrained.

Postoperative return of 90 degrees of knee flexion is generally considered the minimal requirement for activities of daily living with involvement of one knee. However, if both knees are replaced, it is essential that one knee be capable of more than 105 degrees of knee bend to allow the patient to rise from a normal low toilet seat.

Continuous passive motion (CPM) may be initiated after surgery, but there is a certain increase in wound problems with it. Furthermore, if CPM is used for long periods, a fixed flexion contracture of the knee tends to develop. Therefore, if CPM is to be used, the patient must come off the machine for part of the day and work at achieving full extension. We limit aggressive or prolonged CPM use in patients with the potential for wound problems (such as those with diabetes or obesity).

Immediately after surgery, patients frequently have a flexion contracture because of hemarthrosis and irritation of the joint. These flexion contractures generally resolve with time and appropriate rehabilitation. However, patients who have been left with a fixed flexion contracture at the time of the surgery are frequently unable to achieve full extension. *It is therefore important that full extension be achieved in the operating room*.

Manipulation under anesthesia may occasionally be required. This is a very individual decision on the part of the surgeon. One author's (H.U.C.) preference is to carry out full manipulation under anesthesia with the use of a muscle relaxant if the patient has not achieved greater than 70 degrees of flexion by 1 week. **The usual area at which adhesions develop is the suprapatellar pouch**. Many surgeons rarely perform any manipulations under anesthesia and believe that the patient will be able to work through the motion loss. Late manipulation under anesthesia (after 4 weeks) requires great force and risks serious injury to the knee. Alternatively, arthroscopic lysis of adhesions in the suprapatellar pouch can be done with an arthroscopic obturator or a small periosteal elevator.

Reflex sympathetic dystrophy (RSD) of the knee is uncommon after total knee replacement and is usually diagnosed late. The hallmarks are chronic pain that is present 24 hours a day and allodynia or skin tenderness. Such patients generally fail to achieve reasonable ROM, and a flexion contracture also usually develops. If this is suspected, a lumbar sympathetic block may be of not only diagnostic but also of therapeutic value and should be carried out as soon as possible.

Total Knee Arthroplasty: Indications and Contraindications

Indications for total knee arthroplasty include disabling knee pain with functional impairment, radiographic evidence of significant arthritic involvement, and failed conservative measures, including ambulatory aids (cane), NSAIDs, and lifestyle modification (see p. 675).

CONTRAINDICATIONS TO TOTAL KNEE ARTHROPLASTY

Absolute

- Recent or current joint infection—unless carrying out an infected revision
- Sepsis or systemic infection
- Neuropathic arthropathy
- Painful solid knee fusion (painful healed knee fusions are usually due to RSD. RSD is not helped by additional surgery)

Relative Contraindications

- Severe osteoporosis
- Debilitated poor health
- Nonfunctioning extensor mechanism
- Painless, well-functioning arthrodesis
- Significant peripheral vascular disease

Classification of Tricompartmental Total Knee Implants

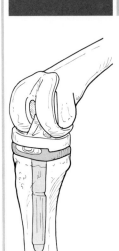

Figure 6-26 Total knee arthroplasty.

CONSTRAINT

Unconstrained (Fig. 6-26)

- Relies heavily on soft tissue integrity to provide joint stability
- Rarely used in total knee arthroplasty

Semiconstrained

- Most knee prostheses fall into this group
- With judicious soft tissue releases and proper implant selection, flexion contractures up to 45 degrees and angular deformities up to 25 degrees can be corrected

Fully Constrained

- Fully constrained in one or more planes of motion
- Because of restriction of motion in one or more planes of motion, implant stresses are very high, with a potentially higher incidence of loosening, excessive wear, and breakage
- Reserved for severe instability and severe deformity too large for semiconstrained implants

Goals of Rehabilitation after Total Knee Arthroplasty

- Prevent hazards of bed rest (e.g., DVT, pulmonary embolism, pressure ulcers).
- Assist with adequate and functional ROM.
  - Strengthen knee musculature.
  - Assist patient in achieving functional independent activities of daily living.
- Independent ambulation with an assistive device.

Perioperative Rehabilitation Considerations

Component design, fixation method, bone quality, and operative technique (osteotomy, extensor mechanism technique) will all affect perioperative rehabilitation. Implants can be posterior cruciate ligament (PCL) sacrificing, PCL sacrificing with substitution, or PCL retaining. See the box for advantages and disadvantages of these component designs.

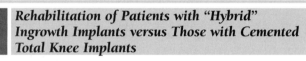

Rehabilitation of Patients with "Hybrid" Ingrowth Implants versus Those with Cemented Total Knee Implants

CEMENTED TOTAL KNEE ARTHROPLASTY

- Ability for weight-bearing as tolerated with a walker from 1 day after surgery

"HYBRID" OR INGROWTH TOTAL KNEE ARTHROPLASTY

- Touch-down weight-bearing only with a walker for the first 6 weeks
- Next 6 weeks, begin crutch walking with weight-bearing as tolerated
  Note: Surgeon's preference may be different. Many believe that because of compression with weight-bearing and good stability of the tibial implant, weight-bearing as tolerated with a walker is allowed immediately after surgery.

Posterior Cruciate Ligament—Sacrifice or Retain

ADVANTAGES OF PRESERVING THE POSTERIOR CRUCIATE LIGAMENT

- Potentially restores more normal knee kinematics, thereby resulting in more normal stair-climbing ability than in those with PCL-sacrificing knees

DISADVANTAGES OF PRESERVING THE POSTERIOR CRUCIATE LIGAMENT

- Excessive rollback of the femur on the tibia if too tight
- Preoperative joint line must be reproduced
- More difficult collateral ligament balancing
- More difficulty in correcting large flexion contractures

Fixation Methods for Total Knee Implants

CEMENTED

- Used for older, more sedentary patients

POROUS INGROWTH

- Theoretically, porous ingrowth fixation should not deteriorate with time (unlike cemented fixation) and is thus the ideal choice for younger or more active candidates

HYBRID TECHNIQUE

- Noncemented "ingrowth" femoral and patellar component with a cemented tibial component
- Frequently used because of reports in the literature of failure to achieve fixation with some of the original porous-coated tibial components

Continuous Passive Motion

There are conflicting data on the long-term effects of CPM on ROM, DVT, pulmonary embolism, and pain relief. Several studies have shown a shorter period of hospitalization with the use of CPM by decreasing the length of time required to achieve 90 degrees of flexion. However, an increased incidence of wound complications has also been reported. Reports vary on whether there is any long-term (1 year) improvement of postoperative flexion in patients using CPM versus those who do not.

Transcutaneous oxygen tension of the skin near the incision for total knee replacement has been shown to decrease significantly after the knee is flexed more than 40 degrees. Therefore, a CPM rate of 1 cycle per minute and maximal flexion limited to 40 degrees for the first 3 days are recommended.

If a CPM unit is used, the leg seldom comes out into full extension. Such a device must be removed several times a day so that the patient can work to prevent the development of a fixed flexion deformity.

Patient-Related Risk Factors for Postoperative Complications

- Chronic use of corticosteroids
- Smoking
- Obesity
- Malnutrition (albumin <3.5 and lymphocyte count <1500)
- Diabetes mellitus
- Immunosuppressive use (e.g., methotrexate)
- Hypovolemia
- Peripheral vascular disease

Deep Vein Thrombosis Prophylaxis

The incidence of DVT after total knee arthroplasty is much higher than originally suspected. Based on clinical detection, the DVT rate after total knee arthroplasty ranges from 1% to 10%. However, more sensitive techniques (radioactive fibringen scans) have revealed a much higher incidence (50% to 70%). Prophylactic treatment is indicated (p. 670).

Total Knee Arthroplasty Rehabilitation Outline

PREOPERATIVE PHYSICAL THERAPY

- Review transfers with the patient
  - Bed-to-chair transfers
  - Bathroom transfers
  - Tub transfers with a tub chair at home
- Teach postoperative knee exercises and give the patient a handout
- Teach ambulation with assistive device (walker): touch-down weight-bearing or weight-bearing as tolerated for total knee arthroplasty at the discretion of the surgeon
- Review precautions
  - To prevent possible dislocation, avoid hamstring exercises in a sitting position when using a posterior-stabilized prosthesis (cruciate sacrificing).

INPATIENT REHABILITATION GOALS

- 0-90 degrees ROM in the first 2 weeks before discharge from an inpatient (hospital or rehabilitation unit) setting
- Rapid return of quadriceps control and strength to enable the patient to ambulate without a knee immobilizer
- Safety during ambulation with a walker and transfers
- Rapid mobilization to minimize the risks associated with bed rest
  Because of tradeoffs between early restoration of knee ROM (especially flexion) and wound stability in the early postoperative period, different protocols may be used, according to surgeon preference.

REHABILITATION PROTOCOL

Total Knee Arthroplasty—"Accelerated" Postoperative Rehabilitation Protocol
Cameron and Brotzman

DAY 1

- Initiate isometric exercises (p. 655):
  - SLR
  - Quad sets
- Ambulate twice a day with a knee immobilizer, assistance, and a walker.
  NOTE: Use a knee immobilizer during ambulation until the patient is able to perform three SLRs in succession out of the immobilizer.
- Cemented prosthesis: Weight-bearing as tolerated with a walker.
- Noncemented prosthesis: Touch-down weight-bearing with a walker.
- Transfer out of bed and into a chair twice a day with the leg in full extension on a stool or another chair.

Continued

REHABILITATION PROTOCOL: *Total Knee Arthroplasty—"Accelerated" Postoperative Rehabilitation Protocol*　*Continued*

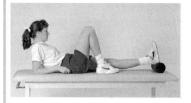

Figure 6-27　Passive range-of-motion exercises for knee extension. The patient places a towel under the foot. Use a slow, sustained push with the hands downward on the quadriceps.

- **CPM machine:**
  - Do not allow more than 40 degrees of flexion on settings until after 3 days.
  - Usually 1 cycle per minute.
  - Progress 5-10 degrees a day as tolerated.
  - Do not record passive ROM measurements from the CPM machine, but rather from the patient because these measurements may differ 5-10 degrees.
- Initiate active ROM and active-assisted ROM exercises.
- During sleep, replace the knee immobilizer and place a pillow under the ankle to help passive knee extension.

2 DAYS-2 WEEKS

- Continue isometric exercises throughout rehabilitation.
- Use vastus medialis obliquus biofeedback if the patient is having difficulty with quadriceps strengthening or control.
- Begin gentle passive ROM exercises for the knee:
  - Knee extension (Fig. 6-27)
  - Knee flexion
  - Heel slides
  - Wall slides
- Begin patellar mobilization techniques when the incision is stable (postoperative days 3-5) to avoid contracture.
- Perform active hip abduction and adduction exercises.
- Continue active and active-assisted knee ROM exercises.
- Continue and progress these exercises until 6 weeks after surgery. Assign home exercises and outpatient physical therapy 2-3 times per week.
- Provide discharge instructions. Plan discharge when ROM of the involved knee is 0-90 degrees and the patient can independently execute transfers and ambulation.

10 DAYS-3 WEEKS

- Continue previous exercises.
- Continue use of a walker until otherwise instructed by the physician.
- Ensure that home physical therapy and/or home nursing care has been arranged.
- Prescribe prophylactic antibiotics for possible eventual dental or urologic procedures.
- Do not permit driving for 4-6 weeks. The patient must have regained functional ROM and good quadriceps control and have passed physical therapy functional testing.

REHABILITATION PROTOCOL: *Total Knee Arthroplasty—"Accelerated" Postoperative Rehabilitation Protocol* Continued

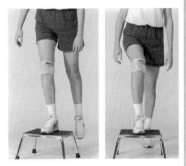

Figure 6-28 Four-inch-high step-ups for quadriceps strengthening.

- Provide a walker for home and equipment and supplies as needed.
- Orient the family to the patient's needs, abilities, and limitations.
- Review tub transfers:
  - Many patients lack sufficient strength, ROM, or agility to step over the tub for showering.
  - Place a tub chair as far back in the tub as possible, facing the faucets. The patient backs up to the tub, sits on the chair, and then lifts the leg over.
  - Tub mats and nonslip stickers for tub floor traction are also recommended.

6 WEEKS

- Begin weight-bearing as tolerated with an ambulatory aid if not already begun.
- Perform wall slides; progress to lunges.
- Perform quadriceps dips or step-ups (Fig. 6-28).

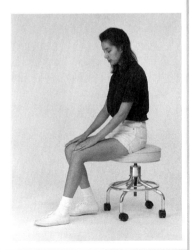

Figure 6-29 Lap stool exercises for hamstring strengthening.

REHABILITATION PROTOCOL: *Total Knee Arthroplasty—"Accelerated" Postoperative Rehabilitation Protocol* *Continued*

- Begin closed-chain knee exercises on a total gym and progress over a period of 4-5 weeks:
  - Bilateral lower extremities
  - Single-leg exercises
  - Incline
- Progress stationary bicycling.
- Perform lap stool exercises (hamstring strengthening) (Fig. 6-29).
- Cone walking: progress from 4- to 6- to 8-inch cones.
- Use McConnell taping of the patella to unload patellofemoral stress if patellofemoral symptoms occur with exercise.
- Continue home physical therapy exercises.

REHABILITATION PROTOCOL	***After Total Knee Arthroplasty*** Wilk

PHASE 1: IMMEDIATE POSTOPERATIVE PHASE—DAYS 1-10

Goals

- Active quadriceps muscle contraction
- Safe (isometric control), independent ambulation
- *Passive knee extension to 0 degrees*
- Knee flexion to 90 degrees or greater
- Control of swelling, inflammation, and bleeding

Days 1-2

Weight-Bearing

- Walker/two crutches, weight-bearing as tolerated

Continuous Passive Motion

- 0-40 degrees as tolerated if stable wound and no contraindications. Take the knee out of CPM several times a day and place in a knee immobilizer with pillows under the ankle (not the knee) to encourage passive knee extension (see p. 690).

Cryotherapy

- Commercial unit used

Deep Vein Thrombosis Prophylaxis

- Per physician

Exercises

- Ankle pumps with leg elevation
- Passive knee extension exercise
- SLR if not contraindicated (see p. 690)
- Quad sets
- Knee extension exercise (90-30 degrees)
- Knee flexion exercises (gentle)

REHABILITATION PROTOCOL: *After Total Knee Arthroplasty*

PHASE 1: IMMEDIATE POSTOPERATIVE PHASE—DAYS 1-10—cont'd

Days 4-10

Weight-Bearing

- As tolerated

Continuous Passive Motion

- 0-90 degrees as tolerated

Exercises

- Ankle pumps with leg elevation
- Passive knee extension stretch
- Active-assisted ROM knee flexion
- Quad sets
- SLR
- Hip abduction-adduction
- Knee extension exercise (90-0 degrees)
- Continue use of cryotherapy

Gait Training

- Continue safe ambulation
- Instruct in transfers

PHASE 2: MOTION PHASE—WEEKS 2-6

Criteria for Progression to Phase 2

- Leg control, able to perform SLRs
- Active ROM (0-90 degrees)
- Minimal pain and swelling
- Independent ambulation and transfers

Goals

- Improve ROM
- Enhance muscular strength and endurance
- Dynamic joint stability
- Diminish swelling and inflammation
- Establish return to functional activities
- Improve general health

Weeks 2-4

Weight-Bearing

- As tolerated with an assistive device

Continued

REHABILITATION PROTOCOL: *After Total Knee Arthroplasty* Continued

Exercises

- Quad sets
- Knee extension exercise (90-0 degrees)
- Terminal knee extension (45-0 degrees)
- SLR (flexion-extension)
- Hip abduction-adduction
- Hamstring curls
- Squats
- Stretching
  - Hamstrings, gastrocnemius, soleus, quadriceps
- Bicycle ROM stimulus
- Continue passive knee extension stretches
- Continue use of cryotherapy
- Discontinue use of TED (thromboembolic disease) hose at 2-3 weeks (with physician's approval)

Weeks 4-6

Exercises

- Continue all exercises listed above
- Initiate
  - Front and lateral step-ups (minimal height)
  - Front lunge
  - Pool program
  - Continue compression, ice, and elevation for swelling

PHASE 3: INTERMEDIATE PHASE—WEEKS 7-12

Criteria for Progression to Phase 3

- ROM (0-110 degrees)
- Voluntary quadriceps muscle control
- Independent ambulation
- Minimal pain and inflammation

Goals

- Progression of ROM (0-115 degrees and greater)
- Enhancement of strength and endurance
- Eccentric-concentric control of the limb
- Cardiovascular fitness
- Functional activity performance

Weeks 7-10

Exercises

- Continue all exercises listed in phase 2
- Initiate progressive walking program
- Initiate endurance pool program
- Return to functional activities
- Lunges, squats, step-ups (small 2-inch step to start)
- Emphasize eccentric-concentric knee control

REHABILITATION PROTOCOL: *After Total Knee Arthroplasty*   *Continued*

PHASE 4: ADVANCED ACTIVITY PHASE—WEEKS 14-26

Criteria for Progression to Phase 4

- Full, nonpainful ROM (0-115 degrees)
- Strength of 4+/5 or 85% of contralateral limb
- Minimal or no pain and swelling
- Satisfactory clinical examination

Goals

- Allow selected patients to return to advanced level of function (recreational sports)
- Maintain and improve strength and endurance of lower extremity
- Return to normal lifestyle

Exercises

- Quad sets
- SLR (flexion-extension)
- Hip abduction-adduction
- Squats
- Lateral step-ups
- Knee extension exercise (90-0 degrees)
- Bicycle for ROM stimulus and endurance
- Stretching
  - Knee extension to 0 degrees
  - Knee flexion to 105 degrees
- Initiate gradual golf, tennis, swimming, bicycle, walking program

---

Long-Term Activities Recommended after Total Joint Replacement

DeAndrade (1993) developed an evaluation scale of activities for patients with total joint replacements. Stress on the joint replacement should be minimized to avoid excessive wear and tear, which would reduce the longevity of the implant. The intensity of the exercise should be adjusted so that it is painless but still promotes cardiovascular fitness. Running and jumping should be avoided, and shoes should be well cushioned in the heel and insole. Joints should not be placed at the extremes of motion. Activity time should be built up gradually, with frequent rest periods between activity periods. Correct use of walking aids is encouraged to minimize stress on the joint replacement. The first long-term activity undertaken should be walking (Table 6-10).

Management of Rehabilitation Problems after Total Knee Arthroplasty

Recalcitrant Flexion Contracture (Difficulty Obtaining Full Knee Extension)

- Initiate backward walking.
- Perform passive extension with the patient lying prone and the knee off the table, with and without weight placed across the ankle (see Fig. 4-25). This should be avoided if contraindicated by the PCL status of the arthroplasty.

TABLE 6-10	Long-Term Activities Recommended after Total Hip or Knee Replacement			
Very Good, Highly Recommended	Good, Recommended	Needs Some Skill, Prior Significant Expertise	With Care, Ask Your Doctor	AVOID
Stationary bicycling	Bowling	Bicycling (street)	Aerobic exercise	Baseball
Ballroom dancing	Fencing	Canoeing	Calisthenics	Basketball
Square dancing	Rowing	Horseback riding	Jazz dancing	Football
Golf	Speed walking	Ice skating	Rock climbing	Softball
Stationary (Nordic- Trac) skiing	Table tennis		Inline skating	Handball
Swimming	Cross-country skiing		Nautilus exercises	Jogging
Walking			Downhill skiing	Racquetball/ squash
Weightlifting			Tennis—doubles	Lacrosse
			Step machines (for patients with hip replacements; not for those with knee replacements)	Soccer
				Tennis— singles
				Volleyball

From De Andrade RJ: Activities after replacement of the hip or knee. Orthop Special Ed 2(6):8, 1993.

- Eccentric extension. The therapist passively extends the leg and then holds the leg as the patient attempts to lower it slowly.
- With the patient standing, flex and extend the involved knee. A sports cord or rubber bands can be used for resistance.
- Use electric stimulation and vastus medialis oblique biofeedback for muscle re-education if the problem is active extension.
- Passive extension is also performed with a towel roll placed under the ankle and the patient pushing downward on the femur (or with weight on top of the femur) (see Fig. 6-27).

Delayed Knee Flexion

- Passive stretching into flexion by the therapist.
- Wall slides for gravity assistance.
- Stationary bicycle. If the patient lacks enough motion to bicycle with the saddle high, begin cycling backward, then forward, until able to make a revolution. Typically, this can be done first in a backward fashion.

Bibliography

HIP ARTHRITIS

Brady LP: Hip pain: Don't throw away the cane. Postgrad Med 83(8):89, 1988.

Cameron HU: The Cameron anterior osteotomy. In Bono JV, (ed): Total Hip Arthroplasty. New York, Springer-Verlag, 1999.

Centers for Disease Control and Prevention: Health-related quality of life among adults with arthritis: Behavioral risk factor surveillance system. MMWR Morb Mortal Wkly Rep 49(17):366, 2000.

Chandler DR, Glousman R, Hull D, et al: Prosthetic hip range of motion and impingement: The effects of head and neck geometry. Clin Orthop 166:284, 1982.

Collis DK: Total joint arthroplasty. In Frymoyer JW (ed): Orthopedic Knowledge Update, No. 4. Rosemont, IL, American Academy of Orthopaedic Surgeons, 1993.

DeAndrade RJ: Activities after replacement of the hip or knee. Orthop Special Ed 2(6):8, 1993.

Horne G, Rutherford A, Schemitsch E: Evaluation of hip pain following cemented total hip arthroplasty. Orthopedics 3:415, 1990.

Johnson R, Green JR, Charnley J: Pulmonary embolism and its prophylaxis following Charnley total hip replacement. J Arthroplasty Suppl 5:21, 1990.

Kakkar VV, Fok PJ, Murray WJ: Heparin and dihydroergotamine prophylaxis against thrombo-embolism of the hip arthroplasty. J Bone Joint Surg Br 67:538, 1985.

Little JW: Managing dental patients with joint prostheses. J Am Dent Assoc 125:1374, 1994.

Pellicci PM: Total joint arthroplasty. In Daniel DW, Pellicci PM, Winquist RA (eds): Orthopedic Knowledge Update, No. 3, Rosemont, IL, American Academy of Orthopaedic Surgeons, 1990.

Steinberg ME, Lotke PA: Postoperative management of total joint replacements. Orthop Clin North Am 19(4):19, 1988.

KNEE ARTHRITIS

Bradley JD, Brandt KD, Katz BP, et al: Comparison of an anti-inflammatory dose of ibuprofen, an analgesic dose of ibuprofen, and acetaminophen in the treatment of patients with osteoarthritis of the knee. N Engl J Med 325:87, 1991.

Chen PQ, Cheng CK, Shang HC, Wu JJ: Gait analysis after total knee replacement for degenerative arthritis. J Formos Med Assoc 90:160, 1991.

Cole BJ, Harner CD: Degenerative arthritis of the knee in active patients: Evaluation and management. J Am Acad Orthop Surg 7:389, 1999.

Colwell CW, Morris BA: The influence of continuous passive motion on the results of total knee arthroplasty. Clin Orthop 276:225, 1992.

Corsbie WJ, Nichol AC: Aided gait in rheumatoid arthritis following knee arthroplasty. Arch Phys Med Rehabil 71:191, 1990.

DeAndrade RJ: Activities after replacement of the hip or knee. Orthop Spec Ed 2(6):8, 1993.

Edelson R, Burks RT, Bloebaum RD: Short-term effects of knee washout for osteoarthritis. Am J Sports Med 23:345, 1995.

Fox JL, Poss P: The role of manipulation following total knee replacement. J Bone Joint Surg Am 63:357, 1981.

Ghosh P, Smith M, Wells C: Second-line agents in osteoarthritis. In Dixon JS, Furst DE (eds): Second-Line Agents in the Treatment of Rheumatic Diseases. New York, Marcel Dekker, 1992, p 363.

Gibson JN, White MD, Chapman VM, Strachan RK: Arthroscopic lavage and debridement for osteoarthritis of the knee. J Bone Joint Surg 74:534, 1992.

Jackson RW, Rouse DW: The results of partial arthroscopic meniscectomy in patients over 40 years of age. J Bone Joint Surg Br 64:481, 1982.

Keating EM, Faris PM, Ritter MA, Kane J: Use of lateral heel and sole wedges in the treatment of medial osteoarthritis of the knee. Orthop Rev 22:921, 1993.

Kozzin SC, Scott R: Current concepts: Unicondylar knee arthroplasty. J Bone Joint Surg Am 71:145, 1989.

Livesley PJ, Doherty M, Needoff M, Moulton A: Arthroscopic lavage of osteoarthritic knees. J Bone Joint Surg Br 73:922, 1991.

Maloney WJ, Schurman DJ, Hangen D: The influence of continuous passive motion on outcome in total knee arthroplasty. Clin Orthop 256:162, 1990.

McInnes J, Larson MG, Daltroy LH: A controlled evaluation of continuous passive motion in patients undergoing total knee arthroplasty. JAMA 268:1423, 1992.

Morrey BF: Primary osteoarthritis of the knee: A stepwise management plan. J Musculoskel Med 79, 1992.

Petrella RJ, DiSilvestro MD, Hildebrand C: Effects of hyaluronate sodium on pain and physical function-
    ing in osteoarthritis of the knee: A randomized, double-blind, placebo-controlled trial. Arch Intern
    Med 162:292, 2002.

Puddu G, Cipolla M, Cerullo C, Scala A: Arthroscopic treatment of the flexed arthritic knee in active
    middle-aged patients. Knee Surg Sports Traumatol Arthrosc 2(2):73, 1994.

Ritter MA, Campbell ED: Effect of range of motion on the success of a total knee arthroplasty.
    J Arthroplasty 2:95, 1987.

Ritter MA, Stringer EA: Predictive range of motion after total knee arthroplasty. Clin Orthop 143:115,
    1979.

Shoji H, Solomoni WM, Yoshino S: Factors affecting postoperative flexion in total knee arthroplasty.
    Orthopedics 13:643, 1990.

Steinberg ME, Lotke PA: Postoperative management of total joint replacements. Orthop Clin North Am
    19(4):19, 1988.

VanBaar ME, Assendelft WJ, Dekker J: Effectiveness of exercise therapy in patients with osteoarthritis of
    the hip or knee: A systematic review of randomized clinical trials. Arthritis Rheum 42:1361, 1999.

7

Special Topics

THOMAS CLANTON, MD • STAN L. JAMES, MD •
S. BRENT BROTZMAN, MD

Hamstring Injuries in Athletes

Thomas Clanton, MD • Kevin J. Coupe, MD •
S. Brent Brotzman, MD • Anna Williams, BS, MS, PT

CLINICAL BACKGROUND

Hamstring injuries are common in athletes and often become a troublesome chronic condition. The hamstring muscle group consists of three muscles: the **semimembranosus**, the **semitendinosus**, and the **biceps femoris** (long and short heads). These three muscles function during the early stance phase for knee support, during the late stance phase for propulsion of the limb, and during midswing to control momentum of the extremity. Injury to the hamstrings, whether partial or complete, typically occurs at the myotendinous junction where the eccentric force is concentrated.

Hamstring injuries are also notorious for reinjury, often because of inadequate rehabilitation and premature return to competition before complete recovery of the hamstring muscle group.

ANATOMY

The three muscles of the hamstring group, the semimembranosus, semitendinosus, and biceps femoris (long and short heads) (Fig. 7-1), originate as a tendinous mass from the ischial tuberosity of the pelvis, with the exception of the short head of the biceps femoris.

- The ischial tuberosity acts as a common point of attachment and may thus occasionally result in an avulsion fracture.
- This short head of the biceps femoris originates from the linea aspera along the distal end of the femur. This is the only hamstring muscle with a dual innervation.
- The semimembranosus, semitendinosus, and long head of the biceps femoris are innervated by the tibial branch of the sciatic nerve. The short head of the biceps femoris is innervated by the peroneal portion of the sciatic nerve.

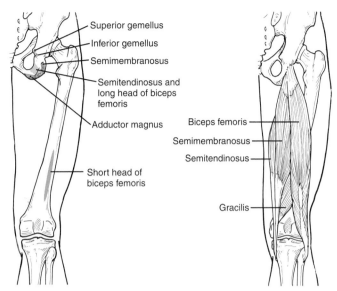

Figure 7-1 Origins of the hamstring tendons (*left*) and muscles of the hamstring group (*right*). (Adapted from Clanton TO, Coupe KJ: Hamstring strains in athletes: Diagnosis and treatment. J Am Acad Orthop Surg 6:237-248, 1998.)

- The semimembranosus and semitendinosus muscles course along the medial aspect of the femur to their separate medial attachments (Fig. 7-2). The semi-membranosus has multiple insertions at the posterior medial corner of the knee and is a significant contributor to knee stability. The semitendinosus joins with the gracilis and sartorius to form the pes anserinus attachment to the medial tibial metaphysis in close proximity to the distal insertion of the medial collateral ligament of the knee.

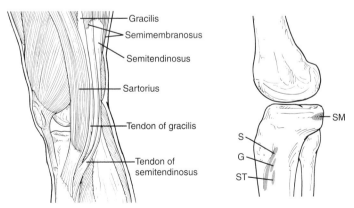

Figure 7-2 *Left,* Attachment of the semitendinosus with the pes anserinus at the proximal medial aspect of the tibia. *Right,* Insertions of the gracilis (G), sartorius (S), semimembranosus (SM), and semitendinosus (ST). (Adapted from Clanton TO, Coupe KJ: Hamstring strains in athletes: Diagnosis and treatment. J Am Acad Orthop Surg 6:237-248, 1998.)

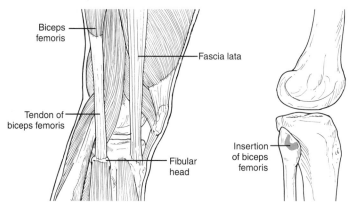

Biceps femoris

Fascia lata

Tendon of biceps femoris

Fibular head

Insertion of biceps femoris

Figure 7-3   Insertions of the long and short heads of the biceps femoris at the lateral aspect of the knee. (Adapted from Clanton TO, Coupe KJ: Hamstring strains in athletes: Diagnosis and treatment. J Am Acad Orthop Surg 6:237-248, 1998.)

- The biceps femoris attaches laterally as shown in Figure 7-3.
- The hamstring group is a two-joint muscle group, which means that the muscle crosses two joints. This is believed to make it more susceptible to strain. Clanton and Coupe (1998) describe the mechanism of injury as increased force generated during eccentric action of the muscle, as opposed to a concentric contraction. In the running cycle, the hamstring becomes vulnerable when the muscle group decelerates the extending knee during forward swing and also at take-off because of the sudden change in function of the muscle from stabilizing the knee in flexion to having to assist in paradoxical extension of the knee.

The most common site of injury to the hamstrings is the myotendinous junction, just as with most indirect muscle injuries.

MECHANISM OF INJURY

The two most common factors in hamstring injury are lack of adequate flexibility and strength imbalance in the hamstrings (decreased flexor-to-extensor ratio and right-to-left imbalance).

An imbalance may exist in the muscle strength of the hamstrings between the patient's limbs, and there may also be a decreased ratio between the flexor (hamstring) and the extensor (quadriceps) groups. A flexor-to-extensor strength ratio of less than 0.6 or a strength imbalance of 10% or more between the right and the left hamstrings has been proposed as a causative factor in hamstring injury. Numerous studies have used isokinetic dynamometry to suggest appropriate flexor-to-extensor ratios, extension torque ratios, and flexion torque ratios. Initially, a flexion-to-extension ratio of 0.5 to 0.6 was considered a standard for a number of years. It has become apparent that these ratios actually vary between male and female athletes, as well as among athletes in different sports and playing different positions in the same sport.

Right-to-left hamstring strength imbalance appears to increase the likelihood for hamstring injury in the lower extremity. In addition, a ratio of 50% to 65% for hamstring strength versus quadriceps strength (flexor-to-extensor ratio) is recommended to decrease the chance of hamstring injury.

Other controllable factors such as lack of adequate warm-up, lack of flexibility, overall conditioning, and muscle fatigue should all be corrected to minimize the chance of hamstring injury.

PREVENTION

Because strength imbalance, lack of adequate flexibility, lack of adequate warm-up, and overall conditioning play varying roles in the cause of hamstring injuries, a prevention regimen addressing these factors is very important. A preparticipation hamstring stretching regimen and warm-up algorithm are presented on page 706.

CLINICAL FINDINGS

Hamstring injuries are common in all athletes, especially those who participate in kicking, running, and jumping. Typically, an injury occurs during sprinting or high-speed exercises (e.g., the lead leg for a hurdler, a jumper's take-off leg). Avulsion fractures of the ischial tuberosity may also occur in other sports, including water skiing, weightlifting, dancing, and ice skating.

Most hamstring injuries occur acutely when the athlete experiences a sudden onset of pain in the posterior aspect of the thigh during strenuous exercises. These injuries most commonly occur during sprinting. Often, a history of inadequate warm-up or fatigue may be elicited.

The participant may describe an audible pop and pain that would not allow continued participation in the sport. In more severe injuries, the patient may report falling to the ground. Milder injuries are often described as a pull or tightness in the posterior aspect of the thigh during exercise that did not limit participation but subsequently "tightened up."

Avulsion fractures of the ischial tuberosity typically result from severe hip flexion while the knee is maintained in full extension.

CLINICAL EXAMINATION

A minor hamstring strain may produce no physical findings, whereas a severe tear may produce extensive bruising, swelling, tenderness, and possibly a palpable defect.

With an acute injury, the athlete may be lying on the ground grabbing the back of the thigh. This is not pathognomonic but is highly suggestive of a hamstring injury.

The entire length of the hamstring muscles should be palpated by the examiner. This is typically done with the patient lying prone and the knee flexed to 90 degrees (Fig. 7-4). Any extension of the knee may cause cramping or increased pain, which will limit the scope of the examination. The muscle is palpated while fully relaxed and then with mild tension. Palpation should also be done at the ischial tuberosity for any possible palpable bony avulsion. The position of maximal tolerance for a straight leg raise (SLR) should be documented because this is a useful guide for determining the initial severity of the injury and the probable response to rehabilitation.

Another useful guideline is restriction of passive extension of the knee with the hip flexed to 90 degrees (Fig. 7-5). In this position, active knee flexion will serve as an indicator of the amount of tension that can be generated before pain when compared with the contralateral, uninvolved leg.

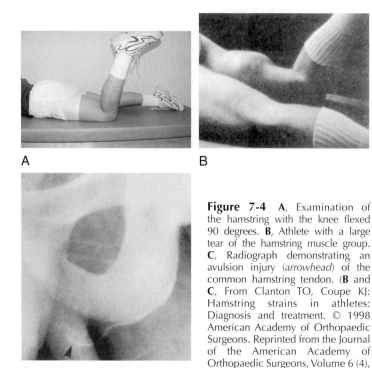

Figure 7-4 **A**, Examination of the hamstring with the knee flexed 90 degrees. **B**, Athlete with a large tear of the hamstring muscle group. **C**, Radiograph demonstrating an avulsion injury (*arrowhead*) of the common hamstring tendon. (**B** and **C**, From Clanton TO, Coupe KJ: Hamstring strains in athletes: Diagnosis and treatment. © 1998 American Academy of Orthopaedic Surgeons. Reprinted from the Journal of the American Academy of Orthopaedic Surgeons, Volume 6 (4), pp 237-248, with permission.)

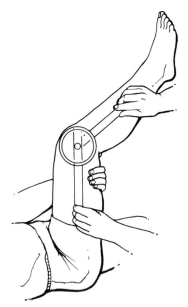

Figure 7-5 Measurement of restriction of passive knee extension after a hamstring injury. (From DeLee JC, Drez D Jr: Orthopaedic Sports Medicine: Principles and Practice. Philadelphia, WB Saunders, 1994.)

Rarely, the injury is dramatic and there is a large defect with an impressive palpable wad of muscle appearing in the posterior aspect of the thigh during contraction of the hamstrings.

CLASSIFICATION

Hamstring injuries are classified into three groups: mild (grade I), moderate (grade II), and severe (grade III) (Table 7-1).

- **Grade I** strain, or a "pulled muscle," signifies an overstretching of the muscle resulting in disruption of less than 5% of the structural integrity of the musculotendinous unit.
- **Grade II** represents a partial tear with a more significant injury but an incomplete rupture of the musculotendinous unit.
- **Grade III** represents a complete rupture of the muscle with severely torn, frayed ends similar to those seen in an Achilles tendon rupture.

Avulsion fractures may occur at the ischial tuberosity proximally or at the distal insertion at the knee.

Kujala and Orava (1993) further classified injuries of the *ischial apophysis* (growth plate). This classification includes apophysitis, adult tug lesions, a painful unfused apophysis, and acute and chronic avulsion of the apophysis. Very young patients have a much lower frequency of hamstring strains, in part because of the much greater flexibility in this age group and their greater susceptibility to injury of the apophyseal attachment of the hamstring than the myotendinous junction. Surgery is considered in patients with dislocation of the apophysis (bony avulsion) of more than 2 cm.

RADIOGRAPHIC STUDIES

Currently, there is *little indication* for detailed radiographic studies of acute hamstring injuries.

TABLE 7–1	Signs and Symptoms of Muscle Strains	
Severity	**Symptoms**	**Signs**
Mild (first degree)	Local pain, mild pain on passive stretch and active contraction of the involved muscle, minor disability	Mild spasm, swelling, ecchymosis; local tenderness; minor loss of function and strength
Moderate (second degree)	Local pain, moderate pain on passive stretch and active contraction of the involved muscle, moderate disability	Moderate spasm, swelling, ecchymosis; local tenderness; impaired muscle function and strength
Severe (third degree)	Severe pain, disability	Severe spasm, swelling, ecchymosis, hematoma, tenderness, loss of muscle function; palpable defect may be present

From Andrews JR, Harrelson GL: Physical Rehabilitation of the Injured Athlete. Philadelphia, WB Saunders, 1991, p 344.

The information provided by magnetic resonance imaging (MRI) typically does not change the course of treatment.

MRI should be used infrequently. On MRI, acute injuries typically appear as high signal intensity on T2-weighted images as a result of hemorrhage or edema within the muscle belly. Chronic muscle injuries are less predictable in appearance.

Plain radiographs are of little value unless an avulsion fracture of the ischial tuberosity is suspected. Because *bony avulsions with more than 2 cm of displacement are surgically repaired*, plain films of the pelvis (anteroposterior view of the pelvis that includes the ischial tuberosity) should be taken if an avulsion fracture of the ischial tuberosity is suspected.

Chronic myositis ossificans may be shown on plain radiographs but is very uncommon. The discovery of calcification or ossification of the soft tissues of the thigh on plain radiographs should raise the examiner's suspicion for other pathology (e.g., neoplasm) and initiate a more extensive investigation and work-up.

AVOIDING HAMSTRING INJURIES

Because of the chronicity of hamstring injuries, emphasis at our institution is placed on prevention of the injury. Because the most common factors cited in hamstring injury are *lack of flexibility* and *strength imbalance* (hamstring to quadriceps, right to left leg), we emphasize these areas in our exercises.

In prepractice regimens for collegiate and high-school athletes, the following stretches are used.

Hamstring Stretching Regimen

Single-Leg Hamstring Stretch

Lie supine with both legs flat on the table. Loop a towel around the foot and hold the ends of the towel with your hands. Keep the knee straight and the foot in dorsiflexion (pointing toward the ceiling). Pull the leg up toward the ceiling. Pull until you feel a stretch in back of the leg and sustain the stretch for 30 seconds. Relax the leg and repeat (Fig. 7-6).

Straddle Groin and Hamstring Stretch

Sit on the floor with both legs straddled (Fig. 7-7). Keep the knees straight with the kneecap facing the ceiling and the feet in dorsiflexion (pointing toward the ceiling). Be sure to keep your back straight and bend forward at the hips. First reach straight

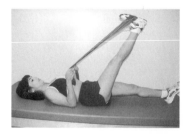

Figure 7-6   Single-leg hamstring stretch.

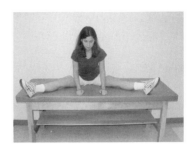

Figure 7-7   Straddle groin and hamstring stretch.

forward until you feel a stretch in the hamstring and sustain the stretch for 30 seconds. Relax and reach to the right until a stretch is felt and hold for 30 seconds. Relax and reach to the left.

Side-Straddle and Hamstring Stretch

Sit on the floor with the injured leg straight, the kneecap facing the ceiling, and the foot pointing toward the ceiling. The uninvolved leg is relaxed with the knee bent. Bend forward at the hips while keeping your back straight. Reach for the injured leg's ankle until a hamstring stretch is felt, and then sustain the stretch for 30 seconds (Fig. 7-8). Relax and repeat.

Pelvic-Tilt Hamstring Stretch

Sit on the edge of the chair with the injured leg resting straight. The uninjured leg is bent at 90 degrees (Fig. 7-9). With your back straight, bend forward at the hips. Rest your hands on your thighs for support. Lean forward until you feel a stretch and then hold for 30 seconds. Relax and repeat.

Hamstring Strengthening Regimen for Prevention of Injury

Hamstring strengthening exercises are also used to improve the quadriceps-to-hamstring ratio and any asymmetry between the hamstrings of the right and left legs. Strong, symmetrical hamstrings should be less prone to injury.

Isometric Hamstring Curls

Sit on the floor with the uninjured leg straight. The involved leg is bent with the heel on the floor. Push the heel into the floor, and then pull toward the buttocks to

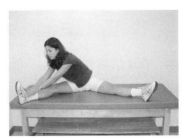

Figure 7-8   Side-straddle groin and hamstring stretch.

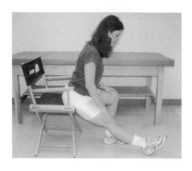

Figure 7-9 Hamstring stretch with anterior pelvic tilt.

tighten the hamstring muscle (Fig. 7-10). Hold the contraction for 5 seconds. Relax. Begin with one set of 12 to 15 and progress to perform two to three sets of 12 to 15 repetitions.

Prone Hamstring Curls

Place an ankle weight on the involved leg. Lie prone and place a pillow under the involved knee if needed. With the foot in position, as shown in the Figure 7-11, bring the heel toward the buttocks in a slow, controlled manner. Begin with one set of 12 to 15 repetitions and progress to two to three sets of 12 to 15 repetitions.

Standing Hamstring Curls

Place an ankle weight on the involved leg. Stand with your feet shoulder-width apart. Holding on to a support, curl the heel toward the buttocks in a slow, controlled manner. Be sure to maintain proper knee alignment with the uninvolved leg. Begin with one set of 12 to 15 repetitions and progress to two to three sets of 12 to 15 repetitions (Fig. 7-12).

Hamstring Curl Machine

The exercise can be performed on a prone or a standing hamstring machine. The weight will be at the ankle. Curl the leg against resistance by bringing the heel toward the buttocks. Begin with one set of 12 to 15 repetitions and progress to two to three sets of 12 to 15 repetitions.

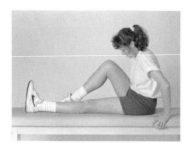

Figure 7-10 Isometric hamstring exercise. The patient pushes down against the bed with the left (involved) leg.

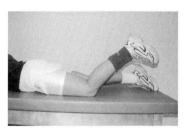

A

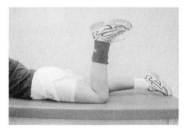

Figure 7-11 **A** and **B**, Prone hamstring curls with weight.

B

Seated Walking

Sit on a rolling stool with wheels. Begin walking forward while sitting on the stool (Fig. 7-13).

TREATMENT OF HAMSTRING INJURIES

Treatment of hamstring injuries is directed toward restoration of strength and flexibility of the muscle group. This is critical for appropriate muscle regeneration and prevention of reinjury. A shortened, scarred, hamstring muscle is more susceptible to strain.

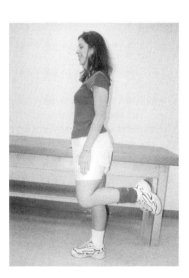

Figure 7-12   Standing hamstring curls.

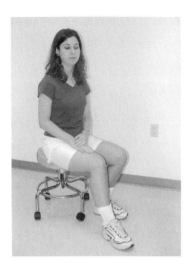

Figure 7-13   Seated walking on a stool with wheels.

Days 1 through 5 after Hamstring Injury

For the first 3 to 5 days after injury, the main goal of treatment is control of hemorrhage, swelling, and pain. The familiar RICE (rest, ice, compression, elevation) regimen is used during this period. Any range of motion (ROM) is gently increased, and strengthening exercises are gradually progressed with resumption of activities. Several days to weeks may be necessary, depending on the extent of injury, the level of competition, and the upcoming activities anticipated for the athlete. The two competing processes that the physician has to manage are muscle regeneration and production of connective scar tissue.

The goal is to maximize muscle regeneration and minimize dense, restrictive scar formation.

- **Rest**. Jarvinen and Lehto (1993) have shown that a *relatively short period of immobilization is advantageous* in limiting the extent of dense connective tissue scar at the site of injury. The absolute optimal time of mobilization has not been defined, but *less than 1 week of relative immobilization is typically recommended* in the literature.

   Early controlled mobilization guided by pain tolerance is begun after 1 to 5 days of immobilization. This will allow better regeneration and alignment of the injured muscle fiber.

   In the laboratory setting, weakened muscle is able to regain its normal capacity for energy absorption at around 7 days. Until this time is reached, the muscle is more susceptible to further injury.

   Acutely, crutches or occasionally bed rest may be warranted for a severe grade II or grade III hamstring injury, but *complete immobilization* of the knee or hip *is not indicated*. Crutches are weaned from two crutches to one crutch and then discontinued when the patient is able to ambulate without a limp or alteration in gait. Early motion is important but is progressed in controlled fashion.

- **Ice**. Ice should be applied to the hamstring immediately in an effort to delay and decrease inflammation and edema. The physiologic effects of ice are beneficial in the healing process and allow more rapid return to athletics.

Ice should be applied to the hamstring in a plastic bag that is wrapped directly over the posterior aspect of the thigh with an elastic bandage. We typically apply the ice for 20 to 30 minutes and reapply it two to four times a day or as frequently as every 2 hours for the first 48 to 72 hours.

- **Compression**. Gentle compression is achieved with a firm compressive bandage placed around the thigh. No studies have documented any efficacy of compression alone for treatment of muscle injury.
- **Elevation**. In an effort to reduce edema and allow return of fluid to the heart, the athlete elevates the extremity *above the heart* two to three times a day whenever possible. We do not recommend bed rest for hamstring injuries.
- **Anti-inflammatory medication**. The only controversy with regard to the use of anti-inflammatory agents is the timing of administration. Almekinders (1993) recommends the use of anti-inflammatory drugs immediately after injury and discontinuation in 3 to 5 days. Other research indicates that anti-inflammatories interfere with chemotaxis of cells necessary for laying down new muscle fibers, therefore possibly inhibiting the healing response. These studies suggest delaying the administration of anti-inflammatories for 2 to 4 days.

We use anti-inflammatories beginning on day 3 and discontinue on day 6.

GENERAL TREATMENT AND REHABILITATION GOALS

Treatment is directed toward restoration of both strength and flexibility to this muscle unit. Even in the early period after injury, attention is turned to initiating gentle muscle action to prevent atrophy and promote healing.

- Because motion is initially limited and painful, *isometric exercises* involving submaximal isometric contraction are initiated first (e.g., two to three sets of five repetitions, 5-second contraction, varying by 15- to 20-degree increments). Care should be taken to limit tension to the injured muscle to avoid reinjury during this period.
- With improvement in motion and pain, the isometric exercises are replaced by *isotonic exercises with light weights*. The weights can be increased daily in 1-pound increments. This program uses concentric contractions with no pain. Eccentric muscle activity is avoided to prevent increased tension in the muscle unit.
- When the athlete is pain free throughout the prone hamstring exercise program, a *high-speed, low-resistance isokinetic exercise program* is begun. Machines that create only concentric contractions are used. Isokinetic exercises are advanced as tolerated to include higher resistance and slower speeds.
- Pool walking and stationary bicycling with no resistance are also used in the early stages because they allow pain-free motion with controlled resistance. Hamstring curls in the water are likewise beneficial in the early postinjury phase. This is eventually progressed to running in place in the water with a supportive vest in the deep end of the pool, as well as swimming with a gentle flutter kick and the use of a kick board.
- Well-leg exercise and upper body exercises are also used throughout for aerobic conditioning.
- When the patient has a normal gait with minimal tenderness and improved muscle strength, a walking program on the track is initiated with eventual progression to a walk/jog program.

- Isokinetic testing is performed to gain useful information on strength, balance, and the degree of persistent deficit in hamstring strength. The final decision is based on clinical parameters and the athlete's progress and functional activities.

Stretching after Injury

Stretching to avoid loss of flexibility is an important component of the postinjury treatment regimen. Gentle active stretching is used initially, with progression to passive static stretching as pain allows. Worrell (1994) emphasized the advantage of hamstring stretching in an anterior pelvic tilt (see Fig. 7-9) and minimized the advantage of proprioceptive neuromuscular facilitation (PNF) stretching over static stretching. The former generally requires an assistant trained in the technique, such as a therapist or athletic trainer. Others prefer this method for gaining and maintaining flexibility.

OPERATIVE INDICATIONS

Surgery is typically considered only after a complete hamstring avulsion from the ischial tuberosity with a bony avulsion displacement of 2 cm or more.

Distal hamstring injuries are typically present in combination with more serious injuries, such as biceps femoris tendon ruptures associated with injuries to the posterolateral corner of the knee.

Distal avulsions are treated like proximal avulsions when they occur in isolation (rarely occur).

Readiness for Return to Competition

Isokinetic testing is used to confirm restoration of muscle strength imbalances to appropriate ratios.

REHABILITATION PROTOCOL	***Treatment of Hamstring Strain*** Modified Clanton, Coupe, Williams, and Brotzman Protocol		
	TIME FRAME	**GOALS**	**TREATMENT**
Phase 1: Acute	3-5 days	• Control pain and edema	• RICE regimen
	1-5 days	• Limit hemorrhage and Inflammation	• Immobilization (brief in extension), nonsteroidal anti-inflammatory drugs (NSAIDs)
	After 5 days	• Prevent muscle fiber adhesions	• *Pain-free passive ROM* (gentle stretching). Sit on a firm surface with a sock on the foot. Place a towel around the foot as though the foot were in a sling. Gently pull the towel to bring the heel toward the buttocks. Hold for 3-5 seconds and slowly return to the starting position (Fig. 7-14)

REHABILITATION PROTOCOL: ***Treatment of Hamstring Strain*** *Continued*

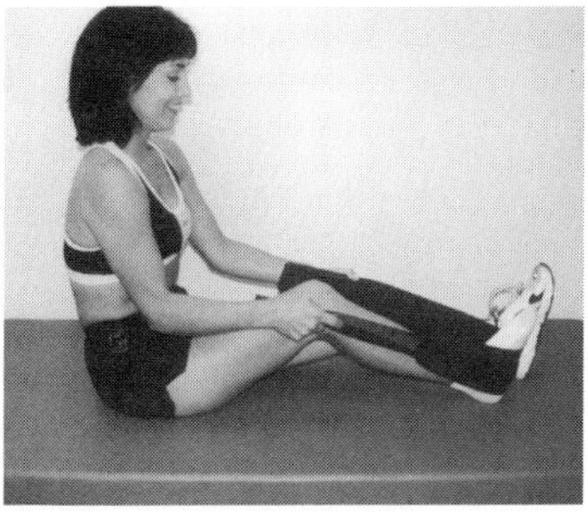

Figure 7-14 Pain-free passive range of motion (gentle stretching) of the hamstrings.

	TIME FRAME	GOALS	TREATMENT
			• *Heel slides.* Sit on a firm surface with a sock on the foot or a towel under the heel. Gently flex the knee with the foot approaching the buttocks, and then return to the starting position (Fig. 7-15) • *Wall slides.* Lie on a firm surface with the feet resting on the wall. Slowly begin to walk the feet down the wall while gently increasing knee flexion. At the end range, slowly begin returning to the starting position (Fig. 7-16) • *Hamstring stretch.* Sit on a firm surface with a small bolster or towel roll under the ankle. Place a 3- to 5- pound weight on the top of the thigh to allow a passive stretch of the hamstring muscle (Fig. 7-17)
	Up to 1 wk	• Normal gait	• Crutches
Phase 2: Subacute	Day 3 to >3 wk	• Control pain and edema	• Ice, compression, and electric stimulation
		• Full active ROM	• Pain-free pool activities
		• Alignment of collagen	• Pain-free passive and active ROM
		• Increase collagen strength	• *Pain-free submaximal isometrics*

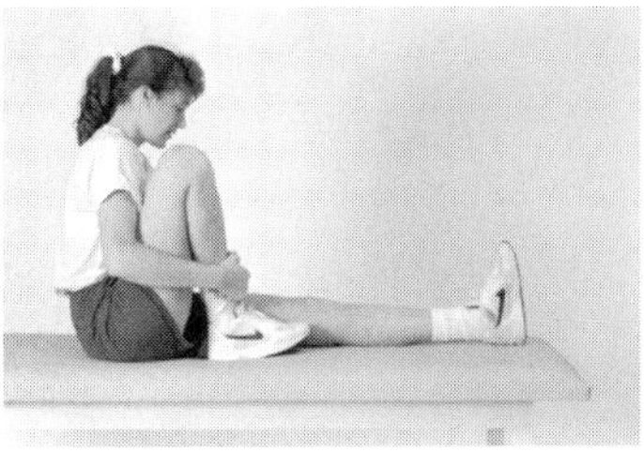

Figure 7-15 Heel slides on a table.

Continued

REHABILITATION PROTOCOL: *Treatment of Hamstring Strain*   *Continued*

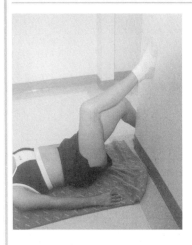

Figure 7-16   Wall slides.

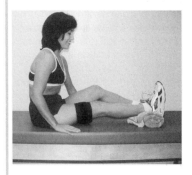

Figure 7-17   Hamstring stretch.

TIME FRAME	GOALS	TREATMENT
		• Sit on a firm surface with the involved leg in slight flexion and the heel on the mat. Push the heel into the firm surface and then pull toward the buttocks (Fig. 7-18). It is important to note that no actual movement of the extremity occurs—only a hamstring muscle contraction. Hold the contraction for 5 seconds and then relax. Also perform stationary bicycling
	• Maintain cardiovascular conditioning	• Well-leg stationary bike, swimming with pull buoys, upper body exercise
Phase 3: Remodeling	1-6 wk • Achieve phase 2 goals	• Ice and compression

REHABILITATION PROTOCOL: *Treatment of Hamstring Strain* *Continued*

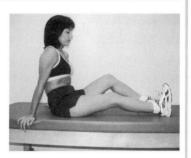

Figure 7-18 Pain-free submaximal isometric hamstring exercise.

TIME FRAME	GOALS	TREATMENT
	• Control pain and edema • Increase collagen strength	• Ice and electric stimulation • *Prone concentric isotonic exercises.* Lie prone on a firm surface with a pillow under the hips to increase hip flexion. Place a cuff weight on the involved leg and flex the leg to bring the heel toward the buttocks. Perform the flexion movement slowly, and then return the leg to the starting position (Fig. 7-19) • *Standing concentric isotonic exercises.* Stand near a table or wall for support. Place a cuff weight on the involved leg. While keeping the knees aligned, flex the involved leg to bring the heel toward the buttocks in a slow, controlled manner. Return the leg to the starting position (Fig. 7-20) • *Isokinetic exercise.* Must be performed at a facility with the proper equipment. Lie prone on the table with a stabilizing strap placed across the hips. The involved leg will also have a stabilizing strap placed across the thigh. The ankle is strapped into the movable arm. The therapist then programs the computer to perform the movement at a certain speed and angle* (Fig. 7-21)

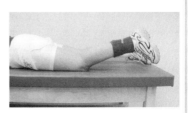

Figure 7-19 Prone concentric isotonic exercise.

Continued

REHABILITATION PROTOCOL: *Treatment of Hamstring Strain*   *Continued*

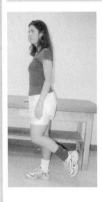

Figure 7-20   Standing concentric isotonic hamstring exercise.

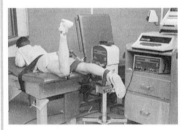

Figure 7-21   Isokinetic exercise for the hamstring. (From Andrews JR, Harrelson GL, Wilk KE: Physical Rehabilitation of the Injured Athlete, 2nd ed. Philadelphia, WB Saunders, 1998.)

TIME FRAME	GOALS	TREATMENT
		• *Rolling stool.* Sit on a rolling stool and propel forward. Begin by using both legs simultaneously and progress to alternating the lower extremities. To advance further, propel with only one extremity (Fig. 7-22)

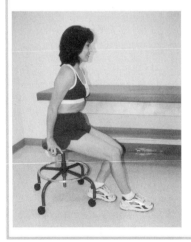

Figure 7-22   Seated walking on a stool with wheels, eventual propulsion with one extremity.

REHABILITATION PROTOCOL: *Treatment of Hamstring Strain*   *Continued*

TIME FRAME	GOALS	TREATMENT
	• Increase hamstring flexibility	• Moist heat or exercise before pelvis-tilt hamstring stretching
	• Increase eccentric loading	• *Prone eccentric exercise.* Performed the same as for concentric exercise, except quickly flex the lower extremity and return to the starting position in a very slow, controlled manner. Also jump rope (Fig. 7-23)
		• *Standing eccentric isotonic exercise.* Same for as the standing concentric exercise, except flex the lower extremity *quickly* and return to the starting position in a very slow, controlled manner
Phase 4: Func-tional	2 wk-6 mo	• Return to sport without reinjury
		• Walk/jog, jog/sprint, sport-specific skills and drills (slideboard, lateral drills)
	• Increase hamstring flexibility	• *Pelvic-tilt hamstring stretching.* Sit on the edge of the chair with the spine in neutral position. The involved leg is straight, with the heel resting on the floor and the toes in dorsiflexion. The uninvolved leg is resting in a comfortable position with the hip and knee flexed 90 degrees. While keeping the spine straight, lean forward, bending at the hips. A stretch will be felt along the posterior aspect of the leg (Fig. 7-24)

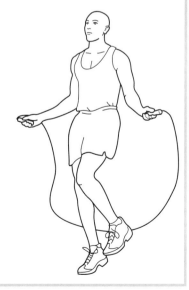

Figure 7-23   Jumping rope.

Continued

REHABILITATION PROTOCOL: *Treatment of Hamstring Strain*   *Continued*

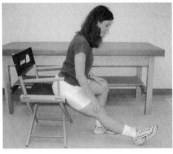

Figure 7-24   Pelvic-tilt hamstring stretch.

TIME FRAME	GOALS	TREATMENT
		• *Supine hamstring stretch.* Sit on a firm surface.Place a towel around the sole of the foot. While keeping the knee straight and the toes dorsiflexed, pull the towel toward the chest. The foot will raise as if doing an SLR. Hold the stretch for 30 seconds. Return to the starting position (Fig. 7-25)
	• Increase hamstring strength • Control pain	• *Prone concentric and eccentric exercises.* Heat, ice, and modalities; NSAIDs as needed
Phase 5: Return to Competition	3 wk-6 mo	• Avoid reinjury	• Maintenance stretching and strengthening

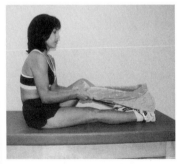

Figure 7-25   Supine hamstring stretch.

*Concentric high speeds at first, proceeding to eccentric low speeds.

Quadriceps Strains and Contusions

Steven J. Meyers, MD • S. Brent Brotzman, MD

IMPORTANT REHABILITATION POINTS FOR QUADRICEPS INJURIES

- Acute thigh injuries are common and represent approximately 10% of all sports injuries.
- Differentiating between a quadriceps **strain** or **tear** (indirect mechanism) and a **contusion** (direct trauma mechanism) is important for appropriate treatment.
- **Quadriceps contusions** result from a **direct blow** to the anterior aspect of the thigh by a knee or helmet.
- **Quadriceps tears or strains** are typically caused by **indirect trauma**. The patient complains of a feeling of a "pulled" muscle, and the mechanism often involves missing a soccer ball and striking the ground violently with forced stretching of the contracting quadriceps muscle.

QUADRICEPS STRAIN OR TEAR (INDIRECT MECHANISM)

- **Risk factors** for quadriceps strains (or tears) include inadequate stretching, inadequate warm-up before vigorous exercise, and muscle imbalance of the lower extremity.
- **Prevention** of quadriceps injuries involves quadriceps stretching before activity (Fig. 7-26) and institution of proper warm-up before vigorous play. Muscle imbalances (e.g., large quadriceps and atrophic hamstrings) are corrected in off-season training.

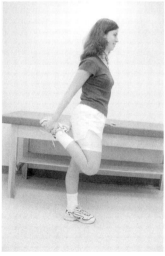 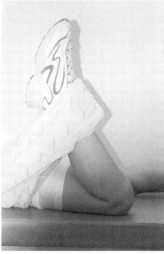

A   B

Figure 7-26   **A**, Standing quadriceps stretch. **B**, Single-leg quadriceps stretch. A towel is used to stretch the quadriceps muscle gradually. In later stages of rehabilitation, the proprioceptive neuro-muscular facilitation contract-relax technique can be used to increase range of motion.

- The patient typically complains of a "pulled" thigh.
- Examination generally reveals tenderness on palpation of the rectus femoris (strain) or defect (tear). It is usually found in the muscle belly.
- Because the rectus femoris is the only quadriceps that crosses the hip joint, extending the hip with the knee flexed causes more discomfort than flexing the hip with the knee extended. This **extended hip maneuver** causes pain because of isolation of the rectus femoris.
- Look for a muscle defect (tear) on this maneuver or on quadriceps contraction.

REHABILITATION PROTOCOL *Treatment of Quadriceps Strains (or Tears)*

ACUTE PHASE

- RICE
- NSAIDs if not contraindicated
- Crutches in a touch-down or partial weight-bearing (painless) fashion
- Hold all lower extremity athletic participation
- *Avoid SLR in early rehabilitation because of increased stress on the torn rectus femoris*

INTERMEDIATE PHASE (USUALLY 3-10 DAYS AFTER INJURY)

Goals

- Regain normal gait
- Regain normal knee and hip motion
- Usually the intermediate phase begins 3-10 days after injury, depending on severity

Exercises

- Initiate a *gentle* quadriceps (see Fig. 7-26) and hamstring (Fig. 7-27) stretching program
- PNF patterns

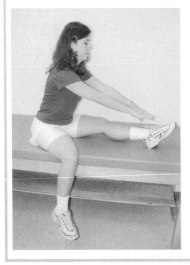

Figure 7-27 Single hamstring stretch.

REHABILITATION PROTOCOL: *Treatment of Quadriceps Strains (or Tears)*   *Continued*

INTERMEDIATE PHASE (USUALLY 3-10 DAYS AFTER INJURY)—cont'd

- Aquatic rehabilitation program in deep water with a flotation belt
- Cycling with no resistance

RETURN-OF-FUNCTION PHASE

- Terminal knee extension exercises
- Increase the aquatic program (deep-water running [DWR])
- Begin knee extension with light weights, progress
- SLR, quad sets progressing to progressive resistance exercises (PREs) with a 1- to 5-pound weight on the ankle
- Increase low-impact exercises to progress endurance and strength
  - Progress bicycle resistance and intensity of workout
  - Elliptical trainer
  - Thera-Bands for hip flexion, extension, abduction, adduction
  - Walking progression to jogging (painless)
  - 30-degree mini-squats (painless)
  - Initiate sport-specific drills and agility training
  - Isokinetic equipment (at higher speeds) with the patient supine
  Note: Even quadriceps tears with palpable defects typically respond to this conservative regimen. Persistent defects are common but rarely, if ever require surgery or cause loss of function.
  Initiate a pre-activity quad stretching program and an appropriate warm-up regimen with return to sports.

CRITERIA FOR RETURN TO PLAY

- Quadriceps flexibility equal bilaterally
- Asymptomatic with functional drills at full effort
- Quadriceps strength 85% to 90% (via isokinetic testing) of the contralateral quadriceps

---

QUADRICEPS CONTUSIONS (DIRECT BLOW [HELMET] MECHANISM)

- Severity ranges from a mild bruise to a large, deep hematoma requiring months to heal.
- Rarely, compartment syndrome of the thigh or an artery injury occurs (be aware).
- Attempt to avoid the development of myositis ossificans.
- Jackson and Feagin (1973) functionally classify thigh contusions into **mild, moderate,** or **severe.** The classification is designated **24 to 48 hours after the injury** to observe the edema and hematoma, which should have stabilized at that point (Table 7-2).
- **Cryotherapy (icing) to reduce edema and bleeding is key in the early stages of this injury** (Table 7-3).
- **Normal knee flexion is typically the slowest parameter to return after thigh contusions. For this reason, Jackson and Feagin's protocol recommends placing the knee and hip in flexion (120 degrees at the knee) for the first 24 hours only** (Fig. 7-28).
- Aronen and colleagues (1990) place the knee in immediate passive flexion to 120 degrees, apply ice within 10 minutes of the injury, and maintain the ice for 24 hours. The passive flexion places the quadriceps under tension and may lessen

TABLE 7–2	Clinical Grading of the Severity of Quadriceps Contusion*			
Contusion Severity	Knee Range of Motion	Gait	Physical Findings	Can Do Deep Knee Bend?
Mild	>90 degrees	Normal	Mild tenderness	Yes
Moderate	45-90 degrees	Antalgic	Enlarged, tender thigh	No
Severe	<45 degrees	Severe limp	Greatly swollen thigh, pain with quadriceps contraction	No

*Severity is graded 24 to 48 hours after injury.

From Kaeding CC, Sanka WA, Fisher RA: Quadriceps strains and contusions: Decisions that promote rapid recovery. Physician Sports Med 23:59, 1995.

TABLE 7–3	Management of Quadriceps Contusions Immediately after Injury
Time after Injury	Treatment
Immediately	Knee immobilization in 120 degrees of flexion
First 24 hr	Knee bracing in 120 degrees of flexion, crutches, then discontinue brace
After 24 hr	Crutches, high-voltage galvanic stimulation, ice, quadriceps stretching exercises
Return to play	Protective pad over the injury site for rest of the season

intramuscular bleeding. This maximizes stretching of the quadriceps and decreases flexion loss.

• Other authors use simultaneous cryotherapy with frequent 20-minute intervals of knee flexion.
• *Do not* aspirate or inject cortisone or enzymes.
• **Avoid heat, massage, or ultrasound of thigh contusions initially, which intensifies swelling and the inflammatory reaction**.
• A special thigh pad manufactured from foam-covered plastic is worn when patients return to contact sport. The pad is secured to the thigh to avoid migration (Fig. 7-29).

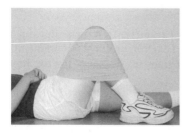

Figure 7-28 After an acute quadriceps contusion, the athlete's knee is passively flexed and immobilized in 120 degrees of flexion with an elastic wrap.

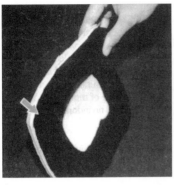
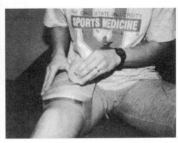

A   B

Figure 7-29 A special pad worn after a quadriceps contusion can help prevent reinjury in patients who play contact sports. **A,** An appropriate thigh pad consists of a rigid foam-covered plastic shell with a thick, ring-shaped foam pad (*arrow*) inside it. It should be of appropriate size and shape to cover and protect the injured site and be comfortable for athletic participation. **B,** The injured area should be centered in the ring-shaped pad, and the pad must be secured to the thigh so that it does not migrate. (From Kaeding CC, Sanko WA, Fisher RA: Quadriceps strains and contusions: Decisions that promote rapid recovery. Physician Sports Med 23:59-64, 1995.)

Criteria for Return to Play after Thigh Contusion

- Injured area appropriately protected in contact sports (thigh pad)
- Full, symmetrical quadriceps flexibility
- Eighty-five percent to 90% strength, power, and time to peak torque on isokinetic and dynamometer testing when compared with the uninvolved quadriceps
- Nontender to palpation of the injured quadriceps

REHABILITATION PROTOCOL	*Quadriceps Contusion*		
	PHASE 1	**PHASE 2**	**PHASE 3**
Purpose	• Limit the hemorrhage	• Restoration of pain-free motion	• Functional rehabilitation; strength and endurance
Modalities	• High-voltage galvanic stimulation • *Rest:* weight-bearing to tolerance, *crutch ambulation* if limp present; frequent ice; ice massage for 10 minutes; cold-pack/cool whirlpool, 20 minutes	• Ice or cool whirlpool, 15-20 minutes; pain-free isometric quadriceps exercises, 15-20 minutes; supine and prone active flexion; well-leg gravity-assisted motion; static cycling, minimum resistance; *discard:* (1) crutches when ROM >90 degrees, no limp,	• Always pain-free: static cycling with increasing resistance; Cybex; swim; walk; jog (pool and surface); run

Continued

REHABILITATION PROTOCOL: *Quadriceps Contusion*   *Continued*

	PHASE 1	**PHASE 2**	**PHASE 3**
	• *Compression:* elastic wrap on entire thigh (occasional use: long-leg support hose, confirm taping)	good quadriceps control, and pain-free with flexed weight-bearing gait; (2) elastic wrap when thigh girth reduced to equivalent of uninjured thigh; initiate pain-free quadriceps stretching several times a day (see Fig. 7-26)	
	• *Elevation:* in class and in barracks, hip and knee flexed to tolerance; isometric quadriceps contracture, 10 repetitions; immobilize the knee in 120 degrees of flexion for 24 hours (hinged leg brace)		
Advance to Next Phase When	• Comfortable; pain-active free at rest; stabilized thigh	• >120 degrees pain-free motion; equal thigh girth bilaterally	• Full active ROM; full squat; pain-free in all activities; wear with **thick thigh pad** 3-6 months for all contact sports

Modified from Ryan JB, Wheeler JH, Hopinkson WJ, et al: Quadriceps contusions: West Point update. Am J Sports Med 19:299-304, 1991.

Groin Pain

S. Brent Brotzman, MD

BACKGROUND

- Groin pain is a broad, confusing "garbage can" type of term that means different things to different people. Patients may say "I pulled my groin" (groin strain), "I got kicked in the groin" (testicle), or "I have a lump in my groin" (lower abdominal wall).
- The key to this diagnostically challenging problem is a very thorough history-taking and examination.
- In our institution, we first try to accurately establish whether this is an **acute injury** (usually musculoskeletal) or a **chronic** symptom (often nonmusculo-skeletal in origin).

- Second, we attempt to establish the correct **anatomic area** being described as the groin (e.g., hip adductors [medial], hip, testicle, lower abdominal wall).
- The commonly accepted **definition of a groin strain** focuses on injury to the hip adductors and includes the iliopsoas, rectus femoris, and sartorius musculotendinous units (Fig. 7-30). An accurate area of anatomic pain must be delineated by the examiner (e.g., adductor origin or testicular pain with radiation).

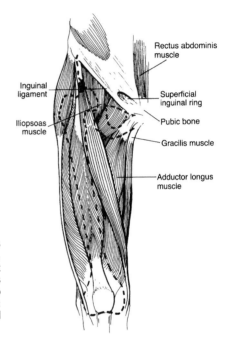

Figure labels: Rectus abdominis muscle; Inguinal ligament; Iliopsoas muscle; Superficial inguinal ring; Pubic bone; Gracilis muscle; Adductor longus muscle

Figure 7-30 Among the musculotendinous injuries of the thigh that can cause groin pain, adductor longus muscle injuries are most common. Any injury to the iliopsoas, rectus femoris, sartorius, or gracilis muscle can also produce groin pain. (From DeLee JC, Drez D Jr: Orthopaedic Sports Medicine: Principles and Practice. Philadelphia, WB Saunders, 1994.)

Differential Diagnosis of Groin Pain: Using a "How to Approach Groin Pain" Mnemonic

How	Hip/pelvis
To	Thigh
Approach	Abdomen
Groin	Genitalia
Pain	Pain (referred)

Hip/Pelvis

    Stress fracture of the femoral neck*

    Pubic ramus fracture*

    Osteitis pubis*

Continued on following page

Legg-Calvé-Perthes disease*

Slipped capital femoral epiphysis*

Avulsion fracture about the pelvis*

Snapping hip*

Acetabular labral tear*

Bursitis (iliopectineal,* trochanteric)

Avascular necrosis

Osteoarthritis

Synovitis or capsulitis

Thigh

Muscle strains

Adductor longus*

Rectus femoris*

Iliopsoas*

Sartorius*

Gracilis*

Femoral hernia

Lymphadenopathy

Abdomen

Lower abdominal wall

Strain of the rectus abdominis*

Inguinal hernia*

Ilioinguinal nerve entrapment*

Sports hernia (hockey player's syndrome)*

Abdominal organ conditions

Abdominal aortic aneurysm

Appendicitis

Diverticulosis, diverticulitis

Inflammatory bowel disease

Pelvic inflammatory disease

Ovarian cyst

Ectopic pregnancy

Continued on following page

> **Genitalia**
>> Prostatitis
>> Epididymitis
>> Hydrocele/varicocele
>> Testicular torsion
>> Testicular neoplasm
>> Urinary tract infection
>
> **Pain (Referred)**
>> Herniated disk
>> Renal lithiasis
>> Spondyloarthropathy

*Common sports-related musculoskeletal cause.
From Lacroix VJ: A complete approach to groin pain. Physician Sports Med 28:66-86, 2000.

HISTORY

Careful history-taking is required to avoid missing a potentially catastrophic problem (e.g., stress fracture of the femoral neck).

Acute (Traumatic) Injuries

- Mechanism of injury (e.g., change of direction, pivoting)
- Hear or feel a pop?
- Swelling or bruising noted? If so, location?
- Previous groin injury?
- Recent change in training regimen?

Chronic Injuries or Those with No Clear-Cut Traumatic, Musculoskeletal Mechanism

- Pain at rest or at night (neoplasm possible)
- Does the pain radiate (e.g., to the back, thigh, hip, scrotum, or perineum)?
- What alleviates the pain (e.g., physical therapy, rest, NSAIDs)?
- Associated numbness (look for a dermatomal pattern emanating from the back)
- Pain on coughing or sneezing, which increases intra-abdominal pressure (hernia or low back disk)
- Can the patient reproduce the pain with exertion or certain movements?
- Fever or chills (possible infection or neoplasm)
- Activities that cause the pain
- Recent weight loss (neoplasm)
- Urinary symptoms such as dysuria, urgency, frequency, hematuria (possible sexually transmitted disease, urinary tract infection, stones)
- Bowel symptoms such as blood in stool, mucus, diarrhea (Crohn's disease, ulcerative colitis)

Risk Factors for Groin Injuries

Contact sports
Obesity
Poor muscle conditioning
Inflexibility
Sports that require quick starts

EXAMINATION

- Examination should include the groin, hip area, back, genitourinary system, and lower abdominal wall.
- See Tables 7-4 and 7-5 for examination and potential causes of groin pain.
- If the patient's complaint is anatomically hip rather than groin pain, the differential diagnosis can include a number of possible causes of hip pain in athletes.

Differential Diagnosis of Hip Pain in Athletes

Hip dislocation

Hip subluxation with or without acetabulum or labrum injury

Osteochondritis dissecans

Acetabulum or pelvis fracture or stress fracture

Femoral neck fracture or stress fracture

Anterior superior iliac spine avulsion (sartorius or rectus femoris origin)

Iliac spine contusion (hip pointer)

Adductor muscle strain

Osteitis pubis

Inguinal hernia

Lateral femoral cutaneous nerve entrapment or injury (meralgia paresthetica)

Femoral artery or nerve injury

Idiopathic avascular necrosis of the femoral head

Idiopathic chondrolysis

Slipped capital femoral epiphysis

Legg-Calvé-Perthes disease

Metabolic disorders

Continued on following page

Sickle cell disease

Inflammatory disease

Lumbar disk disease

Neoplastic abnormalities of the pelvis, acetabulum, or femur

Piriformis syndrome

From Lacroix VJ: A complete approach to groin pain. Physician Sports Med 28:66-86, 2000.

TABLE 7–4	Physical Examination of the Groin (Fig. 7-31)	
Patient's Position	**Procedure**	**Details**
Standing	Observe posture, gait, limb alignment, muscle wasting, ability to sit and stand up, swelling	Have the patient point to the area of pain and the pattern of radiation Have the patient reproduce painful movements
	Examine the low back: active ROM	Forward flexion, side bending, extension
	Examine the hip: active ROM	Trendelenburg's sign (hip adductor strength), ability to squat and duck-walk
	Examine the hernia	Palpate the inguinal region (have the patient cough or strain down)
Supine	Examine the abdomen	Palpate for abdominal aortic aneurysm, pain, rebound, guarding, hernia, pulses, nodes Test for costovertebral angle tenderness (renal area) When appropriate, perform a rectal examination to palpate the prostate and rule out occult blood
	Examine male genitalia	Palpate for a testicular mass, varicocele, or tender epididymis
	Pelvic examination in women, if appropriate	Look for purulent vaginal discharge of pelvic inflammatory disease and bluish cervix of pregnancy (ectopic) Palpate for tender cervix or adnexa, ovarian mass
	Examine low back, sciatic nerve roots	Perform SLR, test for Laségue sign and Bragard sign (dorsiflexion of ankle)
	Examine hip motion	Evaluate flexion, external rotation, **internal rotation,** abduction, adduction, joint play, quadrant tests; **any groin pain with internal rotation?** Perform passive SLR, Thomas, and rectus femoris stretch tests

Continued

TABLE 7–4	Physical Examination of the Groin (Fig. 7-31)—cont'd	
Patient's Position	**Procedure**	**Details**
	Palpate pelvic structures	Palpate symphysis, pubic rami, iliac crests, adductor insertions, ASIS, PSIS, ischial tuberosities
	Examine sacroiliac joints	Perform Patrick (flexion, abduction, external rotation, extension [FABERE]) test, palpate sacroiliac joint
	Look for leg-length discrepancy	Verify grossly and determine true length by measuring from ASIS to lateral malleoli
Prone	Examine hip motion	Evaluate extension as well as internal and external rotation
		Perform Ely and femoral nerve stretch tests
Side-lying	Examine iliotibial band	Perform Ober test
Sitting	Evaluate muscle strength	Test hip flexion (L2, L3), hip extension (L5, S1, S2), abduction (L4, L5, S1), adduction (L3, L4)
	Test reflexes	Assess patellar tendon (L4)
	Test sensation	Assess lower abdomen (T12), groin (L1), medial thigh (L2), anterior quadriceps (L3)

From Lacroix VJ: A complete approach to groin pain. Physician Sports Med 28:66, 2000.

ASIS, anterior superior iliac spine; PSIS, posterior superior iliac spine; ROM, range of motion; SLR, straight-leg raises.

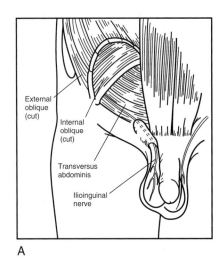

A

External oblique (cut)

Internal oblique (cut)

Transversus abdominis

Ilioinguinal nerve

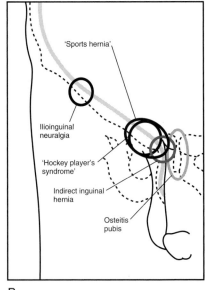

'Sports hernia'

Ilioinguinal neuralgia

'Hockey player's syndrome'

Indirect inguinal hernia

Osteitis pubis

B

Figure 7-31, cont'd
For Legend see opposite page.

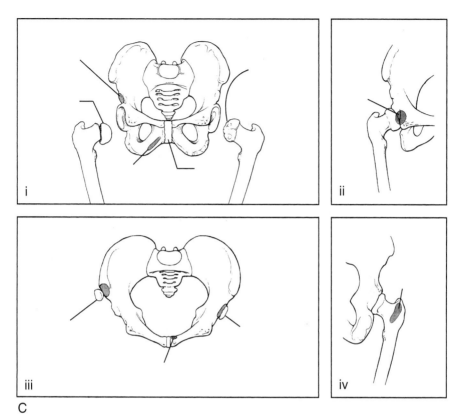

C

Figure 7-31   **A**, Direct trauma, intense abdominal muscle training, or inflammatory conditions can lead to entrapment of the ilioinguinal nerve, which innervates the lowest portions of the transversus abdominis and internal oblique muscles and the skin overlying the inguinal ligament. The nerve transmits sensation from the base of the penis, scrotum (or labium major), and part of the medial aspect of the thigh. Patients describe a burning or shooting pain in these areas. Hip hyperextension may exacerbate it. Treatment usually consists of injecting anesthetics or corticosteroids. **B**, Typical sites of pain in a "sports hernia," "hockey player's syndrome," and other conditions that cause pain in the same general anatomic region. **C**, Anterior (**i**, **ii**), superior (**iii**), and posterior (**iv**) views of the pelvis depict anatomy relevant to various sports-related causes of groin pain. **A** and **B**, From Lacroix VJ: A complete approach to groin pain. Physician Sports Med 28:32-37, 2000; **C**, from Swain R, Snodgrass S: Managing groin pain even when the cause is not obvious. Physician Sports Med 23:54-62, 1995;

Continued

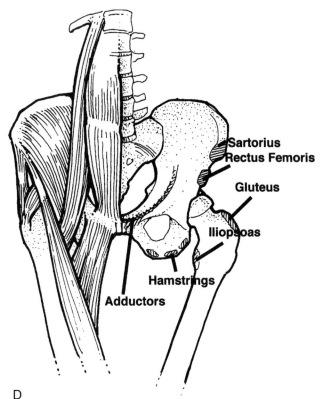

D

Figure 7-31, cont'd   **D**, Locations of several major muscle origins and insertions of the pelvis and proximal end of the femur. Avulsion injuries have been reported at each of these sites. (**D**, from Anderson K, Strickland SM, Warren R: Hip and groin injuries in athletes. Am J Sports Med 29:521-533, 2001.)

TABLE 7–5	Potential Causes of Groin Pain: Key Features and Treatments	
Causes	**Key Features**	**Treatment Options**
Musculoskeletal		
Abdominal muscle tear	Localized tenderness to palpation, pain with activation of rectus abdominis	Relative rest, analgesics
Adductor tendinitis	Tenderness over involved tendon, pain with resisted adduction of lower extremity	NSAIDs, rest, physical therapy

Modified from Ruane JJ, Rossi TA: When groin pain is more than just a strain. Physician Sports Med 26(4):78, 1998.

TABLE 7–5	Potential Causes of Groin Pain: Key Features and Treatments—cont'd	

Causes	Key Features	Treatment Options
Avascular necrosis of femoral head	Radiation of pain into groin with internal rotation of hip, decreased hip ROM	Recommend MRI *Mild*: conservative measures, possible core decompression *Severe*: total hip replacement, **needs orthopaedic hip specialty consultation**
Avulsion fracture	Pain on palpation of injury site, pain with stretch of involved muscle, radiograph positive, felt a pop when "turning on speed"	Relative rest, ice, NSAIDs, possibly crutches; evaluate for ORIF of fragment if >1-cm displacement
Bursitis	Pain over site of bursa	Injection of cortisone, anesthetic, or both; avoid injections around nerves (e.g., sciatic)
Conjoined tendon dehiscence	Pain with Valsalva maneuver	Surgical referral (general surgeon)
Herniated nucleus purposus	Positive dural or sciatic tension signs	Physical therapy or appropriate referral (spine specialist)
Legg-Calvé-Perthes disease	Irritable hip with pain on rotation, positive radiographs, pediatric (usually ages 5-8 yr)	Pediatric orthopaedic surgeon referral
Muscle strain	Acute pain over proximal muscles of medial thigh region, swelling, occasional bruising	Rest; avoidance of aggravating activities; initial ice, with heat after 48 hr; hip spica wrap; NSAIDs for 7-10 days See section on treatment
Myositis ossificans	Pain and decreased ROM in involved muscle; palpable mass within substance of muscle, radiograph shows calcification; often history of blow (helmet) to area	Moderately aggressive active or passive ROM exercises; wrap thigh with knee in maximum flexion for first24 hr; NSAIDs used sparingly for 2 days after trauma
Nerve entrapment	Burning or shooting pain in distribution of nerve; altered light-touch sensation in medial groin; pain exacerbated by hyperextension at hip joint, possibly radiating; tenderness near superior iliac spine	Possible infiltration of site with local anesthetic, topical cream (e.g., capsaicin)
Osteitis pubis	Pain around abdomen, groin, hip, or thigh, increased by resisted adduction of thigh; tender on palpation of pubis symphysis; radiograph positive for sclerosis irregularity; osteolysis at pubis symphysis; bone scan positive	Relative rest; initial ice and NSAIDs; possibly crutches; later, stretching exercises

Continued

TABLE 7–5	Potential Causes of Groin Pain: Key Features and Treatments—cont'd	
Causes	**Key Features**	**Treatment Options**
Osteoarthritis	Groin pain with hip motion, especially internal rotation	Non-narcotic analgesics or NSAIDs; hip replacement for intractable pain See Chapter 6, The Arthritic Lower Extremity
Pubic instability	Excess motion at pubic symphysis; pain in pubis, groin, or lower abdomen	Physical therapy, NSAIDs, compression shorts
Referred pain from knee or spine	Hip ROM and palpation response normal	Identify true source of referred pain
Seronegative spondyloarth-ropathy	Signs of systemic illness, other joint involvement	Refer to rheumatologist
Slipped capital femoral epiphysis†	Inguinal pain with hip movement; insidious development in ages 8-15 yr; walking with limp, holding leg in external rotation	Discontinue athletic activity; refer to orthopaedic surgeon for probable pinning, TDWB with crutches
Stress fracture Pubic ramus	Chronic ache or pain in groin, buttock, and thighs	Relative rest, avoid aggravating activities, PWB with crutches
Femoral neck*	Chronic ache or pain in groin, buttock, and thighs or pain with decreased hip ROM (internal rotation in flexion)	Refer to orthopaedist if radiographs or bone scan shows lesion; TDWB with crutches and cessation of all weight-bearing activities until orthopaedic consultation
Nonmusculoskeletal		
Genital swelling or inflammation		
Epididymitis	Tenderness over superior aspect of testes	Antibiotics if appropriate or refer to urologist
Hydrocele	Pain in lower spermatic cord region	Refer to urologist
Varicocele	Rubbery, elongated mass around spermatic cord	Refer to urologist
Hernia	Recurrent episodes of pain, palpable mass made more prominent with coughing or straining, discomfort elicited by abdominal wall tension	Refer for surgical evaluation and treatment (general surgeon)
Lymphadeno-pathy	Palpable lymph nodes just below inguinal ligaments; fever, chills, discharge	Antibiotics, work-up; also rule out underlying sexually transmitted disease
Ovarian cyst	Groin or perineal pain	Refer to gynecologist
PID	Fever, chills, purulent discharge plus chandelier sign, "PID shuffle"	Refer to gynecologist

TABLE 7–5	Potential Causes of Groin Pain: Key Features and Treatments—cont'd	

Causes	Key Features	Treatment Options
Postpartum symphysis separation	Recent vaginal delivery with no previous history of groin pain	Physical therapy, relative rest, analgesics
Prostatitis	Dysuria, purulent discharge	Antibiotics, NSAIDs
Renal lithiasis	Intense pain that radiates to scrotum	Pain control, increased fluids until stone passes; hospitalization sometimes necessary
Testicular neoplasm	Hard mass palpated on testicle; may not be tender	Refer to urologist
Testicular torsion or rupture†	Severe pain in scrotum; nausea, vomiting; testes hard on palpation or not palpable	Refer immediately to urologist
Urinary tract infection	Burning with urination, itching, frequent urination	Short course of antibiotics

*Non–weight-bearing until orthopaedic evaluation to avoid fracture.
†Emergency immediate referral.
MRI, magnetic resonance imaging; NSAIDs, nonsteroidal anti-inflammatory drugs; ORIF, open reduction and internal fixation; PID, pelvic inflammatory disease; PWB, partial weight-bearing; TDWB, touch-down weight-bearing.

Urgent Hip/Groin Diagnoses That Require Immediate Attention and Appropriate Treatment

- Hip dislocation
- Neurovascular injury (Fig. 7-32)
- Hip fracture
  - Acetabulum
  - Femoral neck
  - Femur
- Septic hip (infected)
- Slipped capital femoral epiphysis
- Sickle cell crisis
- Testicular torsion or rupture
- Incarcerated hernia
Special attention should be given to
- Legg-Calvé-Perthes disease
- Neoplasm
- Avascular necrosis
- Idiopathic chondrolysis
- Femoral neck stress fracture

Continued

Urgent Hip/Groin Diagnoses That Require Immediate Attention and Appropriate
Treatment   *Continued*

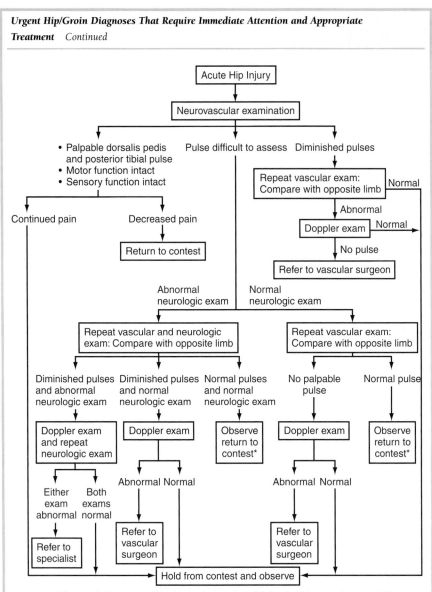

* The on-field physician decides whether the athlete should return to competition based on the athlete's symptoms.

Figure 7-32   Neurovascular evaluation of an athlete who has hip pain during an athletic event. (From Lacroix VJ: A complete approach to groin pain. Physician Sports Med 28:32-37, 2000.)

REHABILITATION PROTOCOL

After Groin (Adductor) Strain
Brotzman

PHASE 1: IMMEDIATE POSTINJURY PHASE

Activity

- Relative rest from athletic injury until the patient is asymptomatic and the rehabilitation protocol is complete
- Avoidance of lateral movements, pivoting, twisting, reverse of direction
- Initiation of the PRICE regimen (protection, rest, ice, compression, elevation above the heart)

Crutches

- Use of crutches weight-bearing as tolerated until the patient walks with a normal, nonantalgic gait

Modalities

- Cryotherapy after exercise
- Pulsed ultrasound
- Electric stimulation

Exercises

- DWR in pool
- Stationary bicycling with no resistance
- Active ROM exercises of the hip
  - Flexion, extension, abduction, gentle adduction
- Isometric exercises
  - Hip adduction
  - Hip abduction
  - Hip flexion
  - Hip extension
- SLR, quad sets

PHASE 2: INTERMEDIATE PHASE

Criteria for Progression to Phase 2

- Minimal to no pain on gentle groin stretching
- Good, painless gait
- Swelling minimal

Progressive Resistance Exercises (1- to 5-Pound Weight)

- Hip abduction, adduction, flexion, extension
- SLR

Continue modalities (ultrasound, moist heat)

Proprioceptive exercises

- Initiate *gentle* groin stretches
  - Wall groin stretch (Fig. 7-33)
  - Groin stretch (Fig. 7-34)
  - Straddle groin and hamstring stretch (see Fig. 7-7)
  - Side-straddle groin/hamstring stretch (see Fig. 7-8). (Note: long 10- to 15-second stretches with no bobbing)
- Hamstring stretches

Continued

REHABILITATION PROTOCOL: *After Groin (Adductor) Strain*   *Continued*

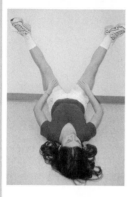

Figure 7-33   Wall groin stretch.

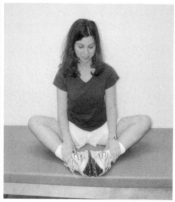

Figure 7-34   Groin stretch.

PHASE 2: INTERMEDIATE PHASE—cont'd

- Passive rectus femoris stretch (Fig. 7-35)
- Passive hip flexor stretch (Fig. 7-36)
  - Progress stationary bicycling resistance
  - DWR in pool (see the section on aquatic therapy)
  - PNF patterns

PHASE 3: ADVANCED PHASE

- Continue above stretches
- Concentric and eccentric hip abduction and adduction with Thera-Band
- Function drills after warmed up and fully stretched
  - Cariocas
  - Slideboard
  - Jogging/running
  - Box drill
- Protective wrapping or commercial hip spica-type protection (Fig. 7-37)

Criteria for Return to Sports

- Equal muscular strength of the adductors, abductors, flexors, extensors on manual muscle testing
- Full, pain-free ROM

REHABILITATION PROTOCOL: *After Groin (Adductor) Strain*   *Continued*

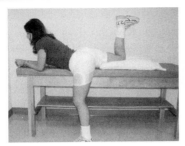

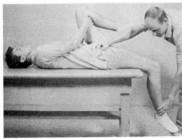

A   B

Figure 7-35   **A**, Passive rectus femoris stretch. The amount of passive stretch can be modified by the amount of hip extension, which is based on the athlete's tolerance to stretch. It can be used in conjunction with cryotherapy techniques. **B**, Manual rectus femoris stretch can be used to stretch the muscle and also to determine its length. (**B**, From Andrews JR, Harrelson GL, Wilk KE: Physical Rehabilitation of the Injured Athlete, 2nd ed. Philadelphia, WB Saunders, 1998.)

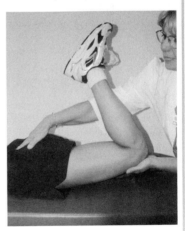

Figure 7-36   Passive hip flexor stretch.

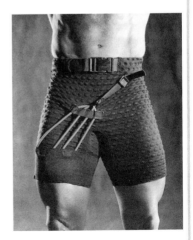

Figure 7-37   Commercial hip spica brace for groin injury. (From Kinetic Innovation, 1-887-272-2376.)

Continued

REHABILITATION PROTOCOL: *After Groin (Adductor) Strain*   *Continued*

PHASE 3: ADVANCED PHASE—cont'd

- Ability to perform all sport-specific functional drills at full speed without pain
- Athlete must develop a rigorous pre- and post-sporting activity groin stretching program for the remainder of the season

Modified from Andrews JR, Harrelson GL, Wilk KE: Physical Rehabilitation of the Injured Athlete. Philadelphia, WB Saunders, 1998.

Aquatic Therapy for the Injured Athlete

Teresa Triche, M Ed

IMPORTANT REHABILITATION POINTS FOR AQUATIC THERAPY TRAINING

- As athletes train harder, compete more often, and take less time to taper (at advancing ages), overuse injuries become more frequent.
- Elite athletes are under time constraints (often self-imposed) for injury rehabilitation.
- Research has demonstrated that 6 weeks of inactivity may result in significant loss of cardiovascular fitness (as much as 14% to 16% of maximal oxygen consumption). Even 3 weeks of inactivity causes significant cardiovascular fitness loss.
- Aquatic therapy allows "active rest" that avoids high impact to the injured extremity (e.g., stress fractures of the foot) yet maintains
  - Cardiovascular fitness.
  - Flexibility
  - Speed
  - Balance and proprioception
  - Coordination
  - Strength
- Exercises performed against the water's resistance almost always elicit concentric muscle contractions. Eccentric contractions may be elicited for the lower extremity if the water is shallow enough to minimize buoyancy (e.g., lunges in hip-deep water elicit eccentric quadriceps contraction).

  In general, heart rates during deep-water exercise will be approximately 17 beats per minute (bpm) lower than comparable exercise on land. Training heart rates should be established in the water rather than applying land-based heart rates. Because of the physiologic changes incurred while immersed, it is recommended that the athlete train at a heart rate 17 to 20 bpm lower than on land.
- The rate of perceived exertion (RPE) by the athlete is often unreliable because of the effects of skill and comfort on perceived exertion.
- Warm-up and cool-down are essential and should be done in the pool.
- The fundamental guidelines for cardiovascular training should be incorporated into the program design: 25 minutes five times per week at a minimum, with longer training periods for elite athletes.
- Exercises should *not* be done in hot tub temperatures (100°F to 103°F).

- Therapy pools serving an orthopaedic population are typically 90°F to 94°F. The Arthritis Foundation requires that pool temperature for its approved courses be at least 84°F to 86°F.
- Thein and Brody (1998) recommend that elite athletes undergoing intense training train in water between 26°C and 28°C to prevent heat-related complications. Warm water increases cardiovascular demands above those of the exercise done. The athlete should be kept well hydrated.
- Before resuming land-based impact activities, the athlete is placed through a battery of sport-specific tests in shallow water to assess readiness for impact. Athletes should be able to complete the test without pain, swelling, or significant soreness.
- On initiation of a land-based impact program, the water-based program is continued on alternate days.
- We typically use AquaJogger equipment (e.g., flotation belt, dumbbells, AquaRunners). This equipment is available at www.aquajogger.com or 1-800-922-9544.
- VO_2max, referred to in the following section, is the maximal amount of oxygen that can be taken in by the body, delivered to the muscles, and used.

DEEP-WATER RUNNING—BACKGROUND

Individuals who perform land-based training exercises, such as running or jogging, may be required to discontinue that activity if an injury occurs. One treatment for running-related injuries is to simply decrease or discontinue running for 4 to 6 weeks. Runners fear that such a break will lead to a decrease in fitness or an increase in body weight (BW), and few are willing to endure long periods of inactivity. It is well known that the cessation of activity results in significant loss of functional capacity. A 4- to 6-week period of inactivity will lead to a 14% to 16% reduction in VO_2max over the 4- to 6-week period. Thus, we use aquatic-based therapy for "active rest" from an injury. The goal is to maintain cardiovascular endurance, mobility, strength, and flexibility while "resting" the injury.

Many athletic organizations today, from those in high schools to those representing the professional athlete, are recognizing the benefits of including an aquatic rehabilitation component when an injury is sustained. **DWR** has become the newest form of aquatic therapy for injured athletes. It has been accepted as a popular and effective form of cardiovascular conditioning for both rehabilitation and training. It is becoming popular among runners as a training exercise during periods of injury because there is less musculoskeletal stress than with normal running. Runners are also replacing part of their existing training program with DWR to reduce overuse injuries. DWR enables the athlete to continue in an activity that is specific to running without incurring the possible harmful effects of weight-bearing work.

DWR consists of simulated running in the deep end of the pool aided by a flotation device (vest or belt) that maintains the head above water. The athlete may be held in one location by a tether cord, essentially running in place, or may actually run through the water the length or width of the pool.

- During DWR, the body is tilted slightly forward approximately 5 degrees past the vertical, with the spine in neutral position. The bend should occur at the hips, not the waist.
- The head is held comfortably out of the water, facing forward; avoid neck extension.
- Arm action is the same as for land running, with the primary movement occurring at the shoulder and the hands relaxed but lightly closed.

- Ankles should perform both dorsiflexion and plantar flexion.
- Hip flexion should reach about 60 to 80 degrees.
- No contact is made with the bottom of the pool, thus eliminating impact.
- This form of running in water closely follows the pattern used on land. However, the center of gravity on land is at the hips. In water, the center of buoyancy is at the lungs. To get used to this change, the athlete must retrain the body to use the abdominal muscles to maintain the correct vertical posture.

The athletic community has been attracted to DWR as a way to maintain cardio-vascular conditioning while recovering from injury. The literature has shown that DWR can duplicate the sport-specific activity of running, and with 4 to 6 weeks of DWR, there is a drop in VO$_2$max of 5% to 7%. DWR allows runners to put in miles without incurring the impact of land-based training. In addition, land-based runners who water-train maximize speed gains—and these gains can transfer to land performance.

Water's buoyancy virtually eliminates the effects of gravity; because 90% of BW is supported in deep water, impact is reduced and greater flexibility is created. Water acts as a cushion for the body's weight-bearing joints by reducing stress on muscles, tendons, and ligaments. The depth of the water directly affects the amount of impact transferred through the musculoskeletal system. Moving deeper in the water decreases the impact for a given exercise. Moving to the shallower end of the pool increases the load on the body. The use of variable depths is very helpful when recovering from an injury, after a hard training session, or to partially unload the body.

Exercise intensity is an important component of any program. Conventional exercise prescription for DWR has relied on heart rate and subjective rating of perceived exertion. ***Three methods are useful for grading exercise intensity*** and maximizing physiologic responses during deep-water exercise: ***heart rate, RPE, and cadence. The American College of Sports Medicine's Guidelines for Graded Exercise Testing and Exercise Prescription (1986) suggest that for a training effect, one should exercise at a level between 55% and 90% of one's maximal heart rate.*** This method is most applicable when one wishes to train at a constant rate, that is, the target heart rate. Most authors suggest that it is important for alternative training to be conducted at or close to actual training intensities.

HEART RATES

In the aquatic environment, the heart rate can be affected by the water's temperature, compression, reduced gravity, partial pressure, and the dive reflex. It is recommended that a 6-second heart rate count be used in the water. Heart rate levels in the water tend to be lower than those attained on land. If an aquatic exercise heart rate is to be used to measure intensity, 13 or 17 bpm should be taken from the minimal and maximal training thresholds. The physiologic changes that occur when the athlete is submerged up to the neck in water will cause the heart rate to be 10% to 15% lower than for similar effort on land.

In other words, because of the physiologic changes incurred while immersed in water, it is recommended that athletes train at a heart rate that is 17 to 20 bpm lower than they do on land. The RPE is often unreliable because of the effects of skill and comfort on perceived exertion.

RATE OF PERCEIVED EXERTION

The most commonly used scale of perceived exertion is the **Borg scale**, a 15-point scale with verbal descriptions ranging from very, very light to very, very hard (Table 7-6).

TABLE 7–6	Borg Scale of Perceived Exertion
6	
7	Very, very light
8	
9	Very light
10	
11	Fairly light
12	
13	Somewhat hard
14	
15	Hard
16	
17	Very hard
18	
19	Very, very hard
20	

In DWR, however, the **Brennan scale** is very popular (Table 7-7). It is a 5-point scale designed for DWR, with verbal descriptions ranging from very light to very hard. The intensity level is subjectively determined by the participant in this method. The Brennan scale facilitates the incorporation of both speed and distance work into the athlete's workout.

CADENCE

Another form of monitoring intensity is counting cadence (Table 7-8). Brennan (1990) has the athlete count the number of times that the right knee comes forward and up. That count is taken on the last 30 seconds of each interval. Doubling the count gives the cycles per minute (cpm).

TABLE 7–7	How Hard Are You Working in the Pool? Brennan Rate of Perceived Exertion

	Rate of Perceived Exertion				
	1 Very Light	2 Light	3 Somewhat Hard	4 Hard	5 Very Hard
Cadence (cycles/min)	60	60-70	70-80	80-90	90+
Dry-land equivalent	Brisk walk	Easy jog	Brisk jog	Race pace	Track

Level 1	Light jog or recovery run
Level 2	Long steady run
Level 3	5- to 10-km road race pace
Level 4	400- to 800-m track speed
Level 5	Sprinting (100- to 200-m track speed)

Note: Cycles per minute are approximate numbers for a well-conditioned athlete. Substitute the cadence numbers that are appropriate for your training level.

TABLE 7–8	Deep-Water Running Cadence Chart	
RPE	Water Tempo (cpm)	Land-Based Equivalent (min/mile)
1	Very light (50)	Slow walk (>21)
2	Light (50-60)	Medium-paced walk (15-20)
3	Somewhat hard (60-75)	Fast walk/jog (<15)
4	Hard (75-85)	Run (5-10)
5	Very hard (>85)	Very hard run (<5)

cpm, cycles per min; double the number of times your right knee comes forward and up; this count is taken on the last 30 seconds of each interval; RPE, rating of perceived exertion.

Wilder and associates (1993, 1994) discovered a high correlation between cadence, an environment-specific measure, and heart rate during DWR. In their study, they found that a quantitative, objective measure (cadence) could be used to predict a cardiovascular response to a particular workout for DWR and concluded that cadence can be used as a measure for exercise prescription for DWR.

Heart rates are used primarily during long runs, or prolonged periods of exercise at a specific rate (target heart rate). RPE exertion and cadence are most often used for interval sessions. RPE is most useful in group settings, whereas cadence is most appropriate for individual sessions (Wilder and Brennan, 1993).

David Brennan, M.Ed, assistant clinical professor in the department of physical medicine and rehabilitation at Baylor College of Medicine in Houston, recommends that people new to aquatic running initially be taught at low speeds, for example, under 65 cpm. Participants can then increase speed gradually. Most distance runners tend to peak at 85 to 95 cpm.

Patients with lower extremity injuries start in deep water. A 6-week program includes DWR with incorporation of all the training methods used in a land-based program. Long runs, interval training, and strength runs can be incorporated into a training schedule. Resistive equipment can be introduced at about week 3.

After 6 weeks, the athlete can be moved from deep water to chest level, which is about 25% loading. After several weeks, the athlete can be moved to waist level, which is about 50% loading. The belt is kept on to further reduce the impact. To begin progressing to land, the belt is removed to increase the loading effect and transfer to land.

Indications for Aquatic Therapy

An athlete with any of (but not limited to) the following conditions may benefit from aquatic therapy:
- Inability to train for a specific sport on land in a normal training environment
- Poor proximal stability and core weakness
- Weakness and deconditioning
- Pain
- Limited ROM
- Muscle spasm
- Limited weight-bearing or non–weight-bearing

Indications for Aquatic Therapy   *Continued*

- Gait deviations
- Limited functional ability
- Abnormal tone
- Impaired sensation
- Decreased lung capacity
- Spatial-perceptual problems
- Uncoordination
- Decreased aerobic fitness
- Weight reduction
- Depression
- Impaired circulation
- Edema (especially in the extremities)
- Decreased ability to relax
- Decreased self-image secondary to being unable to perform normal activities

From Harvey G: "Why Water?" Sports Med Update. HealthSouth Patient Education Handout. Birmingham, AL, HealthSouth, 1996.

Aquatic Therapy for Orthopaedic Patients

Orthopaedic conditions that may benefit from aquatic therapy include, but are not limited to the following:

- Sports injuries: non–weight-bearing or partial weight-bearing sport-specific training and rehabilitation
- Muscle and connective tissue injuries, e.g., sprains, strains, contusions, tears, tendinitis, bursitis
- Multiple traumatic injuries
- Joint injuries: presurgical, postsurgical, and nonsurgical
- Joint replacements: total hip, total knee, and total shoulder
- Fractures: open reduction and internal fixation, external fixation, nonrepaired fractures, casted fractures (removable casts or casts that can be covered), instrumentation removal, and bone grafts
- Spine injuries (cervical, thoracic, or lumbar): acute injury, chronic injury, exacerbation, strain, sprain, spasm, herniated disks, stenosis, spondylosis, spondylolisthesis, fracture and compression fracture, conservative care (nonsurgical or presurgical), and postsurgical status (e.g., fusion, diskectomy, laminectomy)
- Arthritis
- Fibromyalgia
- Lupus
- Ankylosing spondylitis
- Reflex sympathetic dystrophy
- Parkinson's disease
- Spina bifida
- Guillain-Barré syndrome
- Upper motor neuron lesions
- Peripheral neuropathy

From Harvey G: "Why Water?" Sports Med Update. HealthSouth Patient Education Handout. Birmingham, AL, HealthSouth, 1996.

Precautions for Aquatic Therapy

- Medically controlled seizure disorders.
- Diabetes. (Determine the severity, method of control, and related symptoms. Instruct the patient to take medication properly and to eat and hydrate before exercising in the pool.)
- Cardiac involvement. (Determine the type of involvement and whether medically controlled. Instruct the patient to take medication as prescribed. If the patient carries nitroglycerin or other emergency medication, it should be accessible in the pool area.)
- Pulmonary problems or disorders (e.g., chronic obstructive pulmonary disease, asthma). (A portable oxygen unit can be used poolside when necessary. Inhalers should be readily accessible from the poolside.)
- Neurologic deficits or problems. (Patients may require hands-on treatment.)
- Fear or apprehension of the water. (Determine the patient's swimming ability and comfort level in water. If the patient is fearful, make a special effort to slowly progress, give extra attention, and do not enter deep water. Keep the patient next to the edge of the pool, and stay with the patient in the water. Either assist the patient or avoid activities that require the feet to float off of the bottom of the pool. **Monitor closely**.)
- Lung capacity of 1.5 L or less. (The patient may have to be treated in shallow water or in the supine position, with the lungs gradually immersed over time to build up tolerance to hydrostatic pressure.)
- Autonomic dysreflexia. (The patient may require hands-on treatment and additional staff.)
- Behavioral problems (depression, magnified pain behavior, combative behavior, inappropriate sexual behavior, or other disruptive behavior). (The patient may require special scheduling or additional staff.)
- Tracheotomies. (If proper precautions can be taken so that no water enters the stoma, the patient may be treated.)
- Open wounds, surgical incisions, or skin conditions. (If a wound, incision, or skin lesion is not actively bleeding or oozing, it may be covered with an occlusive dressing to avoid contact with the water. Warm water increases circulation and will exacerbate bleeding, oozing, blistering, or boils.)
- External fixators. (If the pin holes are not oozing or bleeding, the patient can get into the pool. The pin hole sites can be covered with an occlusive dressing, but this is usually unnecessary if proper pin care is done before and after aquatic therapy.)
- Colostomy stomas. (Caps or plugs are available to fit a stoma and prevent water contamination. If the patient does not have a cap or plug, the stoma can be covered with an occlusive dressing.)
- Indwelling catheters. (The bag can be emptied, clamped, and taped to the patient's leg.)
- Subclavian catheters and heparin locks. (These can also be covered with an occlusive dressing, and they cannot leak. Use a sterile cotton applicator to apply a generous painting of tincture of benzene onto the skin where the edges of the dressing meet the skin. Apply the dressing so that benzene is underneath it and extends beyond all edges as well. Also, smaller pieces of dressing overlapping each other are more adhesive and create a tighter seal. If an edge is peeling up, it will leak. Reapply and cut a strip of occlusive dressing to reinforce the edge. This same technique works well to cover incisions or anything with the dressing.)
- Incontinence of bowel or urine. (If the patient is on a successful bowel program and is able to eliminate on a regulated basis, treatment can be successfully completed in the pool without accident. However, the patient must successfully eliminate before each pool session to ensure that an accident does not occur. Waterproof adult diapers may be purchased as a precaution.)

Precautions for Aquatic Therapy   *Continued*

- Orthostatic hypotension. (Monitor all patients exiting the pool and hot tub. A healthy, young person can experience orthostatic hypotension and fall unconscious without much warning.)
- Hypersensitivity—tactile or temperature. (Water increases tactile stimulation. This can often be used to desensitize the athlete, but monitor the patient closely for nontolerance.)
- Medically controlled hypertension. (Obtain the results of the last blood pressure reading from the patient. If the patient is unsure of the reading, a resting test may reveal that that the blood pressure is not under control. If the resting blood pressure remains higher than 165/95 after three tests, the patient should be referred back to the physician treating the hypertension and not be allowed to exercise in warm water until the blood pressure is brought within reasonable limits.)
- Low blood pressure. (There are no standards to limit participation; however, monitor closely, especially for orthostatic hypotension.)

From Harvey G: "Why Water?" Sports Med Update. HealthSouth Patient Education Handout. Birmingham, AL, HealthSouth, 1996.

Contraindications to Aquatic Therapy

The following contraindicate safe treatment for the athlete or for other patients in the pool:
- Fever (exercise in warm water will increase fever)
- Incontinence of bowel (and possibly urine)
- Open wounds, incisions, or skin lesions that are oozing or bleeding and cannot be covered with an occlusive dressing
- Blistering
- Boils close to rupture
- Infectious processes such as hepatitis A (fecal-oral–contracted diseases), strep throat and other communicable diseases, vaginal or urinary infection untreated by antibiotic or treated for less than 24 hours, staphylococcus infection that will be exposed through a wound or other infectious processes where skin lesions are present. (Blood-borne pathogens cannot be spread through the water unless blood contaminates the water.)
- Skin infections
- Uncontrolled seizure disorder (the light, reflection, and acoustics in a pool can trigger auras)
- Uncorrected cardiac problems
- Impaired vital capacity with intolerance to the water pressure even in modified positions
- Acute lung infection (tuberculosis)
- Catheters or intravenous lines that cannot be clamped or covered with an occlusive dressing
- Tracheotomies
- No internal protection during the menstrual cycle
- Excessively high or low blood pressure
- Extreme fear
- Inappropriate or disruptive behavior

From Harvey G: "Why Water?" Sports Med Update. HealthSouth Patient Education Handout. Birmingham, Alabama, HealthSouth, 1996.

REHABILITATION PROTOCOL	*Deep-Water Training for the Athlete with a Lower Extremity Injury* Triche

WEEK 1

Goals

- Introduce the athlete to DWR.
- Maintain cardiovascular fitness.
- Perform specific exercises in relation to the injury.
- Proceed as tolerated.

Begin by introducing the athlete to the correct form used in DWR (Figs. 7-38 and 7-39).

20-40 min of steady-pace RPE at 1 or 2 (see Tables 7-2 and 7-3); begin with three or four times a week.

Perform ROM exercises in relation to the injury.

Example: ankle injury:

- Ankle flexion and extension
- Foot circles, inversion, and eversion

WEEKS 2-3

Goals

- Introduce the athlete to "cadence" with interval training (see the section on aquatic therapy).
- Maintain cardiovascular fitness.
- Increase sets and repetitions of ROM exercises in relation to the injury.
- Proceed as tolerated; if not well tolerated, repeat week 1.

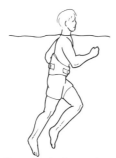 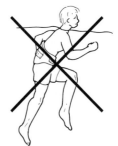

Correct body alignment   Incorrect body alignment

Figure 7-38 Correct posture for deep-water running. The key to any safe, effective exercise or movement is correct body alignment. Initially, as you adjust to the buoyancy, you may find yourself hunching over in the water. It is common when you first get in the water to lean forward at the waist as you adjust to a new center of gravity. To adapt to this new environment and attain the correct body position, lean back slightly and try a small flutter kick with your feet directly under you. Checklist for vertical body alignment:

- Head up
- Chest lifted
- Shoulders positioned directly above the hips
- Abdominals tight (do not hold your breath)
- Buttocks squeezed together and slightly tucked under (pelvic tilt)

(Adapted from Aquajogger Handbook: The New Wave of Fitness. Eugene, OR, Excel Sports Science, 1998.)

REHABILITATION PROTOCOL: *Deep-Water Training for the Athlete with a Lower Extremity Injury   Continued*

Figure 7-39   Correct form for deep-water running. The desired running form in water is almost identical to the running form on land. Maintain a vertical posture with your head tall and your chest lifted; coordinate arm and leg movements as in running.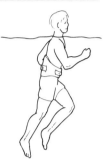
- Push down with a flat foot as though you are stomping on grapes, and then lift your heel toward your buttocks as you cycle through.
- Cup your hands and swing your arm from the shoulder in a relaxed, pendulum-like action with the elbow about 3 inches out from your side.
- Avoid hunching your shoulders, bending at the hips, or reaching out too far in front of the body with the lower part of your leg.

(Adapted from Aquajogger Handbook: The New Wave of Fitness. Eugene, OR, Excel Sports Science, 1998.)

WEEKS 2-3—cont'd

Teach the athlete how to count "cadence."
Begin with 2 days/wk of intervals:
- Repeats of 2- to 4-min RPE of 3-4 with a 30-second recovery (depending on the fitness level of the athlete; (increase recovery time if needed)
- 2 days/wk of easy running at an RPE of 2 (30-45 minutes)

ROM Exercises

- *Example*: stress fracture.

WEEK 4

Goals

- Add resistive equipment as tolerated (gloves, delta bells, AquaRunners).
- Maintain cardiovascular fitness.

Athlete continues with interval training (specific to the sport and fitness level) two times a week.

Example: training sprinters is different from training marathon runners—marathon runners might perform low-intensity, long-duration cardiovascular exercise and maintain the workload at 70% to 80% maximal oxygen consumption. A sprinter would work at peak oxygen consumption, with intermittent jogging for recovery.
- Sprinters: 1-2 minutes (10 times) at RPE 4-5 (15- to 30-second rest)
- Marathoners: 3-5 minutes (6-8 times) at RPE 4 (30- to 60-second rest)

Easy running (30-45 minutes) two times a week with resistive equipment (as tolerated).

Example: I add AquaRunners (foot flotation) for my athletes with stress fractures to increase the workload.

Continue with ROM exercise.

WEEKS 5-6

Goals

- Sport-specific training.
- Increase cardiovascular conditioning.
- Resistive equipment continued (as tolerated).

Athletes are trained in the water specifically to their sport.

Example: marathoners:
- 1 day/wk: long run; run in the water at RPE of 2-3 for 1-2 hours (depending on the fitness level and timing of the training)
- 1 day/wk: interval training at RPE of 4-5 with 30-second recovery

Continued

REHABILITATION PROTOCOL: *Deep-Water Training for the Athlete with a Lower Extremity Injury*   *Continued*

WEEKS 5-6—cont'd

- 1 day/wk: strength run; a steady run of 20-40 minutes at RPE of 3 (can also do 2 × 20-minute runs with a 1-minute rest between)
- 2 days/wk: easy running in water; 30-60 minutes at RPE of 2

Use the easy days between the hard training sessions to give the body a chance to recover. The hard-easy system of training works best.

INTRODUCTION TO LAND EXERCISES: LOADING

After 6 weeks of DWR, there are two options for introduction to loading.

Option 1

- The athlete starts with 1 day/wk on land at a slow, easy jog on a soft surface (10-15 minutes) as tolerated. The other days are a continuation of weeks 5-6.

Progression of Land Exercises

- Each week, add another day of land running; can increase the time by 5 minutes. Continue all interval training in the water.
- Continue until the athlete is back running; then keep the athlete in the water 1-2 days/wk until the end of the season so that injury does not recur.

Option 2

- One or 2 days/wk bring the athlete to chest-deep water.
- Keep the flotation belt on. Have the athlete run in the water for 10-15 minutes (as tolerated). Continue the DWR on the other days.

Other commonly used water aerobic exercises are illustrated in Figures 7-40 to 7-43.

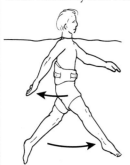

Figure 7-40   Cross-country ski position for deep-water running. Scissor straight arms and legs forward and back. Keep your limbs fairly straight and work out of the shoulders and hips. Your trunk should remain stable and the abdominals and buttocks tight.
- Cup your hands and point your toes for increased resistance.
- Work both sides of the body with equal force.

(Adapted from Aquajogger Handbook: The New Wave of Fitness. Eugene, OR, Excel Sports Science, 1998.)

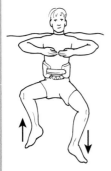

Figure 7-41   Sumo wrestler position for deep-water exercise. Stand tall and outwardly rotate your hips with your legs turned out and your feet flexed. Alternate pushing each leg down with the foot flat for maximum surface area. Breast-stroke with your arms.
- Make sure that you maintain a strong neutral spine, which is achieved by keeping your back and neck vertical and relaxed.
- Sumo legs will work well with many different arm moves; experiment with a variety of upper body exercises.

(Adapted from Aquajogger Handbook: The New Wave of Fitness. Eugene, OR, Excel Sports Science, 1998.)

REHABILITATION PROTOCOL: *Deep-Water Training for the Athlete with a Lower Extremity Injury   Continued*

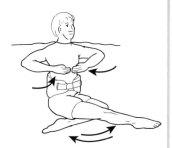

Figure 7-42 Sit kicks for deep-water exercise. Visualize sitting in a chair with your legs resting on the seat and your spine against the back of the chair. Keep your thighs level with your hips. Kick out from the knee; then pull your heel back to your bottom. Breast-stroke, scull, or scoop the water in toward your chest.
• Point your toes to increase resistance.
• Stay tall and keep your abdominal muscles tight.
(Adapted from Aquajogger Handbook: The New Wave of Fitness. Eugene, OR, Excel Sports Science, 1998.)

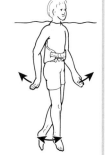

Figure 7-43 Flutter kick for deep-water exercise. Stand tall and flutter your legs while focusing on pushing your thighs forward and keeping your ankles and knees relaxed. This is a small but strengthening exercise that is great for toning the buttocks.
• Flutter kick is an excellent leg exercise to mix and match with different arm movements. Try biceps curls, figure-of-eights at your side, or breast-stroke.
• Keep your kicks small and powerful.
(Adapted from Aquajogger Handbook: The New Wave of Fitness. Eugene, OR, Excel Sports Science, 1998.)

Running Injuries

Stan L. James, MD

BACKGROUND INFORMATION

The incidence of injuries in serious runners (>20 miles a week) in a given year is approximately 34% to 65%. *The most common causes of running injuries are training errors.* The most significant training errors involve duration (high mileage), frequency, and intensity, along with rapid changes or transitions in the program. Anatomic and biomechanical factors, shoes, surfaces, gender, age, experience, and running terrain are also contributory factors (Table 7-9). A history of previous injury is also a significant risk factor for reinjury. It is interesting that through the years no correlation has been established between a specific anatomic or biomechanical variation and a specific running injury.

The most frequent injuries in runners include
• Anterior knee pain with extensor mechanism problems (Fig. 7-44)
• Iliotibial band syndrome (Fig. 7-45)
• Achilles tendinopathy
• Medial tibial stress syndrome
• Plantar fasciitis
• Stress fractures (Table 7-10)

TABLE 7–9	**Risk Factors for Running Injuries**	
Characteristics of Runners	**Characteristics of Running**	**Characteristics of the Running Environment**
Age	Distance	Terrain
Gender	Speed	Surface
Structural abnormalities	Stability of pattern	Climate
Body build	Form	Time of day
Experience	Stretching, weight training, warm-up, cool-down	Shoes
Individual susceptibility		
Past injury		

Tissues in these areas are subjected to repetitive force several times BW while running and are therefore more susceptible to injury. In distance running, the injuries are generally due to excessive, repetitive use of various tissues in which their stress/strain characteristics for sustained use are exceeded and a degenerative process or chronic overuse syndrome results. The musculoskeletal system is tremendously adaptable to changes in stress but does require time to accommodate. Its response to stress is either a desirable physiologic, anabolic, regenerative response or an undesirable, pathologic, catabolic, degenerative response, depending on the level and duration of stress. Training within the physiologic window of stress or subthreshold level with small incremental increases in stress (training) results in increased tissue strength with a desirable training effect and avoids injury. To achieve this goal, a carefully designed training program becomes essential.

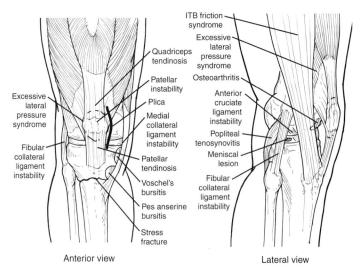

Figure 7-44   Sites in the knee frequently affected in runners. ITB, iliotibial band.

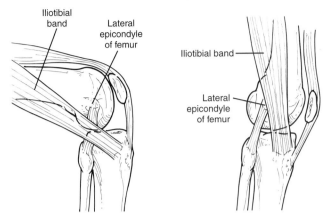

Figure 7-45   As the knee moves from flexion to extension, the **iliotibial band (ITB)** passes from behind to in front of the lateral femoral epicondyle. The pain experienced by runners with ITB friction syndrome is caused by the tight band rubbing over the bony prominence of the lateral epicondyle. This pain is manifested as lateral pain and tenderness palpated at the ITB insertion just distal to the lateral joint line. (Adapted from Dugas R: Causes and treatment of common overuse injuries in runners. J Musculoskel Med 17[2]:72-79, 1991.)

TREATMENT OF RUNNERS' INJURIES

This treatment protocol is applicable to virtually all running injuries and provides a logical, consistent guide for the treating physician.

The Training Program

Most running injuries are related to the training program, and therefore analysis of training is essential. Experienced runners are as likely to make the same mistakes as beginning runners. *The most common errors* are high mileage and a sudden change or transition in the program. To a lesser extent, shoes, surfaces, terrain, and anatomic factors play a role. An optimal program, doing the least training while maximizing the runner's capability, is ideal. A training program should consist of hard, or quality, days with interspersed easy days essential for recovery. A hard, or quality, day is one of appropriate incremental increase, whereas an easy day is one that does not detract

TABLE 7–10	Most Common Problems in Runners (*N* = 232)
Knee pain	29%
Shin splints	13%
Achilles tendinitis	11%
Plantar fasciitis	7%
Stress fractures	6%
Iliotibial tract tendinitis	5%

From James SL, Bates BT, Oslering LR: Injuries to runners. Am J Sports Med 6:40, 1978.

from the training benefits of a quality day. Most runners can safely tolerate 3 quality days in a 7- to 10-day period. The increase in weekly mileage should be no more than 5% to 10%. Maximal training benefits for distance running can be achieved at approximately 80 to 90 km per week. *It is better to be slightly "undertrained" and still running than injured as a result of overtraining.*

A customized training program for an individual runner at a level below "the line" at which injury or illness becomes a serious risk is desirable. This is where good coaching, appropriate goals, and common sense become essential. Too often, injury occurs when emphasis is placed on training the aerobic system while disregarding the ability of the musculoskeletal system to accommodate to the imposed repetitive stress, and training is therefore disrupted.

If injury occurs, reducing training is more acceptable than ceasing training, although cessation may be necessary in some circumstances. Aerobic conditioning should be maintained by cross-training with no- or low-impact activities such as running in water with a flotation device (see the aquatic therapy section), biking, and the use of steppers and elliptical trainers.

BIOMECHANICAL AND ANATOMIC FACTORS

No specific anatomic or biomechanical variation correlates with a specific condition or injury, but biomechanics do play a role. *The most important aspect of the examination is to evaluate the entire lower extremity and not just concentrate on the area of injury.* The lower extremity functions as a kinetic chain, and disruption at any given area can affect function throughout.

The running stride is divided into an active and passive absorption phase and a generation phase (Fig. 7-46). The purpose of the **active absorption phase**

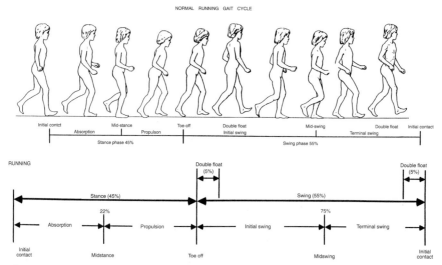

Figure 7-46   Normal running gait cycle. (From Mann RA, Coughlin MJ: Surgery of the Foot and Ankle, 6th ed. St Louis, CV Mosby, 1993, p 28.)

is initially to decelerate the rapidly forward-swinging recovery leg with eccentric hamstring activity, first absorbing and then transferring the energy to the extending hip, which places the hamstrings under considerable stress. **Passive absorption** begins at foot-strike, with absorption of the shock of ground reaction force (GRF) resulting in a force 2.5 to 3 times BW and up to 10 times BW when running downhill. This initial shock is attenuated by the surface, the shoe, and the heel pad, but not to a great extent. Subsequently, GRF is actively absorbed by muscles and tendons as it increases to midsupport with a relative shortening of the extremity. This is accomplished by hip and knee flexion, ankle dorsiflexion, and subtalar pronation accompanied by eccentric contraction of the hip abductors, quadriceps, and gastrosoleus muscles, along with stretching of the quadriceps and patellar tendon, Achilles tendon, and plantar fascia. *At this point, the GRF with running may be as much as five times BW.* The stretched tendons absorb energy, store it as potential energy, and then return 90% of it later in the generation or propulsive phase as kinetic energy, with the remaining 10% creating heat in the tendon.

During the **generation phase** in the second half of support, concentric muscle contraction and joint extension cause a relative lengthening of the extremity, and the stored potential energy is returned as kinetic energy, with the tendons significantly assisting the now concentrically contracting muscles. Peak forces maximize at the sites of chronic injury (Scott and Winter, 1990). Forces in the patellofemoral joint (estimated at 7 to 11.1 times BW), the patellar tendon (4.7 to 6.9 times BW), the Achilles tendon (6 to 8 times BW), and the plantar fascia (1.3 to 2.9 times BW) predispose the tissues to potential injury from repetitive overuse—particularly if combined with even a minor anatomic or functional variation.

Examination of the entire lower extremity becomes essential (Fig. 7-47) when the extremity is viewed as a kinetic chain whose normal function is dependent on the proper sequential function of each segment. Therefore, concentrating on only the area of complaint may overlook the underlying cause of the problem (e.g., anterior knee pain related to compensatory foot pronation).

The examination evaluates (Fig. 7-48)
- Bilateral lower extremity length
- Alignment of the extremity in the frontal and sagittal planes
- Hip motion
- Muscle strength and flexibility
- Extensor mechanism dynamics
- Leg-heel alignment
- Heel-forefoot alignment
- Subtalar motion
- Shoe inspection

A basic video analysis of the runner's gait is also helpful and can be accomplished with an inexpensive camcorder in the office.

SHOES

Most shoe manufacturers have three general classifications of running shoes: (1) motion control for control of compensatory pronation, (2) support for a "normal"-type foot, and (3) cushion for the more rigid, higher-arched foot. These are merely general guidelines, with selection still largely being a factor of what fits, feels good, and has worked in the past. Much emphasis has been placed on the role of shoes in shock absorption at foot-strike, and shoes are of some benefit but provide little, if any attenuation of force when the force is maximal at midsupport. This does not mean that shoes are of no importance in protecting the runner, perhaps just not as much as was once thought.

RUNNER ENCOUNTER SHEET

Name_____   Date_____

Age_____   Sex_____   Weight_____   Height_____

1. Decribe how your injury occurred and where you are hurting.
_____
_____
_____

2. How long ago did you notice your first symptoms?
_____
_____

3. Pain is present
   _____ At all times
   _____ During running
   _____ During walking
   _____ After running
   _____ At rest

4. If pain during running starts:
   _____ Midrun
   _____ Late run
   _____ After run
   _____ Start of run

5. Pain is _____improving _____worsening _____unchanged

6. Present running mileage
   _____ miles per day
   _____ miles per week

7. How many days a week do you run?_____

8. Mileage before injury
   _____ miles per day
   _____ miles per week

9. What surface do you run on?
   _____ Grass   _____ Indoor track
   _____ Concrete   _____ Hills
   _____ Asphalt   _____ Street with slope or pitch
   _____ Cinder   _____ Other

10. Have you recently
    _____ Increased your distance   _____ Increased hill running   _____ Increased workout intensity
    _____ Gained significant weight   _____ Changed shoes   _____ Started interval training
    _____ Changed surfaces

11. Do you stretch
    _____ Before run
    _____ After run

12. List and describe other running injuries in the past year
_____
_____
_____

A

Figure 7-47   Runner's encounter form.

Continued

Shoes can be modified for certain specific conditions, such as leg-length discrepancy; a difference in configuration, function, or size of the feet; and decompression of areas of pressure by changing the upper configuration or midsole and heel wedge stiffness.

Inspect the shoes that have been worn for running for a while for excessive wear or distortion, particularly the heel wedge and heel counters.

13. Describe pain
   ____ Burning   ____ Sharp
   ____ Aching   ____ Dull
   ____ Cramping   ____ Pins and needles

14. On a scale of 1 to 10 (10 worst pain you've ever had)
    rate your pain ____ at rest ____ during activity

15. How many miles do you run on each pair of shoes before changing? (approximate)

16. Do your shoes wear out in more than one area
    ____   inner toe
    ____   outer toe
    ____   inner heel
    ____   outer heel
    ____   other Describe _____

Other notes:

B

Figure 7-47, cont'd   Runner's encounter form.

RUNNER EXAM SHEET

Standing exam
Increased Q angle ______
Genu valgum ______
Genu varum ______
Normal knee align ______
Tibial torsion ______
Foot Pronation ______
(pes planus) ______
Foot Supination ______
(pes cavus) ______
Pelvic obliquity ______
Scoliosis ______
Obesity ______

Sitting exam **Supine exam**
Patellar maltracking ______
Patellar crepitance ______
Motor strength ______
Hip extension ______
flexion ______
Knee flexion ______
extension ______
Ankle ______
inversion ______
eversion ______
DF ______
PF ______
Muscle imbalance(s) ______
______
______
forefoot alignment ______
hindfoot alignment ______

Leg length
discrepancy of ______
shorter leg is L or R ______
ROM
hip ______
knee ______
ankle ______
subtalar ______
INFLEXIBILITY
Hip ______
Hamstring ______
Quad ______
Iliotibial band (Ober's) ______

meniscal
pathology ______
patellofemoral ______

Gait assessment **Asymetric arm motion** ______
Antalgic gait ______ Excessive pelvic tilt ______
Pronator ______ Supinator ______ neutral ______

Areas of point tenderness
______
______
______

Shoes
____new ____very worn
type of shoe ______
wear pattern
____medial toe box
____lateral toe box
____medial hindfoot
____lateral hindfoot

Miscellaneous
pathology ______
______
______
knee effusion ______
ligament
exam knee ______
Generalized
ligamentous
laxity ______
forefoot alignment ______
hindfoot alignment ______
excess callosities ______
______
______
______

______
______
______
______
______

Figure 7-48 Runner's examination sheet.

Patterns of Wear for Running Shoes

Severe compensatory pronation frequently overruns (i.e., wears down) the heel counter medially, and cavus-type feet distort (i.e., wear down) the heel counter laterally.

Distorted shoes must be replaced as needed. A poorly padded heel counter may apply pressure to the Achilles insertion site. Outsole wear patterns may indicate an anatomic or functional problem, with the area of wear representing abnormal application of force (e.g., a plantar-flexed first ray will display wear under the first metatarsophalangeal joint). Temperature changes may affect the midsole and heel wedge stiffness and thus alter shoe function.

A relatively inflexible midsole in a shoe may be associated with Achilles tendinopathy by functionally increasing the forefoot lever arm and applying more stress to the Achilles tendon.

A shoe that still "looks good" may have lost many of its protective qualities, with most midsole material having a life of approximately 300 miles.

We recommend new shoes in a serious runner every 300 miles.

A running shoe should possess an adequate toe box; a well-molded, substantial, properly aligned and padded heel counter; protection from the laces; a flexible midsole with appropriate cushion; and adequate heel height in relation to the midsole.

ORTHOTICS

Orthotic inserts have been used for a number of running-related conditions with reportedly satisfactory results, but significant data on their efficacy and precise function are soft. Theoretically, the purpose of orthotic inserts is to promote more normal, efficient subtalar and midtarsal motion, which in turn will result in more normal function of the proximal kinetic segments of the lower extremity and therefore reduce injury. Empirically, a well-fabricated orthotic insert does appear useful in many conditions. I have found orthotics to be most successful for plantar fasciitis (consider a lateral forefoot post with plantar fasciitis) and medial tibial stress syndrome. Other conditions reportedly helped by orthotics are patellofemoral disorders, Achilles tendinopathy, and leg-length discrepancy. The past few years have seen a plethora of orthotic inserts on the market ranging from a variety of off-the-shelf inserts to expensive "customized" types mostly of the semirigid variety. *Theoretically, a less rigid accommodative insert is applicable to a more rigid cavus-type (high arch) foot, which requires more cushion and less control, whereas a more rigid insert is indicated for a more unstable foot, with compensatory pronation benefiting from more control.*

A trial of a less expensive off-the-shelf insert to see whether there is a benefit may be a reasonable approach before prescribing a more expensive custom insert. When prescribing a custom orthotic, be certain to understand and fulfill the fabricator's requests for measurements and cast molds. A poorly fabricated orthotic is a waste of time and money. The insert should be as light as possible. The foot of a runner is the worst location to apply additional weight.

MEDICATIONS

Medications such as aspirin, acetaminophen, and NSAIDs are useful in reducing minor pain and inflammation, but they do not substitute for ceasing the abusive activity or taking steps to correct the offending condition. The use of narcotics to continue running or the injection of analgesics cannot be condoned. Excessive or prolonged use of NSAIDs can have significant side effects, even at the recommended reduced dose when purchased over the counter.

The literature cautions against indiscriminate use of oral or injectable steroids. One condition in which steroid injection may have reasonable success is acute iliotibial band friction syndrome with injection deep to the iliotibial band over the prominence of the lateral femoral condyle. Injection directly into tendons should be avoided and injection into peritendinous tissues done with caution.

NEVER inject cortisone into or around the Achilles tendon or posterior tibial tendon because it can result in weakening and rupture of the tendon.

SURGERY

An earnest, conservative rehabilitation program is generally effective for most running-related conditions. Surgery should be considered only after failure of a conservative program, as long as it does not lead to unnecessary delay for well-indicated surgery; nonetheless, many serious runners can be impetuous in electing surgery as an anticipated "quick fix." The indications for surgery are the same as for any athletically active person. If surgery is elected, all options should be explained in detail, and with some conditions, the patient should be cautioned that despite well-planned and executed surgery, the odds for return to running may not be good.

PHYSICAL THERAPY AND REHABILITATION

Treatment of runners must be a coordinated effort on the part of the physician, therapist/trainer, coach, and runner.

The goal of a rehabilitation program for runners after injury or surgery is restoration of flexibility, ROM, muscle strength, balance, and endurance of the entire lower extremity with return to uninterrupted running.

As a general rule, closed-chain exercise, including concentric and eccentric muscle activity, is preferable for runners. Isolated, concentric, open-chain exercises may induce strength changes in ROM not present in running, as well as muscle imbalance. Specific rehabilitation regimens for a given condition are covered elsewhere in the book under the condition.

Stretching for flexibility (Figs. 7-49 and 7-50) should be an integral part of not only the rehabilitation program but also the daily training program (see each section). Though important for all runners regardless of age, it becomes even more significant with aging because tendons become less extensible and joints tend to lose flexibility.

The vague complaint of the extremity "not feeling right" may be due to muscle imbalance secondary to weakness or contracture. Runners frequently have chronic hamstring and gastrocnemius-soleus muscle contractures resulting in recurrent or chronic muscle or tendon strains with imbalance. This can lead to alterations in stride and predispose tissues to excessive stress.

A tip for hamstring strains, chronic or acute, is to run uphill or up stairs, which places less strain on the hamstrings just before foot-strike when the hamstrings are simultaneously decelerating the forward-swinging leg and extending the hip.

A program should be designed to simulate as close as possible the normal muscle and joint function of running. Frequently, so much emphasis is placed on the injured area that the rest of the body is ignored. Total body fitness should be included, and cross-training techniques such as running in water can be beneficial, as well as recondition the injured area.

Once the runner is ready to return to running after missing training, the following guidelines may be helpful. If left to their own judgment, most will return too fast and either delay recovery or be reinjured.

RETURN TO RUNNING

This program is a "guide" for return to running after a significant **absence of 4 weeks or more from training** (Table 7-11). The purpose is to condition the musculoskeletal system; it is not intended to be a significant aerobic conditioning program,

RUNNER'S FLEXIBILITY PROGRAM

1. Back stretch: Lie on your back with both knees bent. Pull one or both knees up to your chest and hold for 5 seconds. Repeat.

2. Hip abductor stretch: Stand with your feet together. Move your hips sideways, while your torso moves in the opposite direction. You will feel a stretch on the outside of your hip. Hold for 5 seconds. Place your hands on your hips or grasp a stationary object for support.

3. Iliotibial band stretch: Cross one leg over in front of the other leg. Bend the knee of the back leg slightly. Move your hips sideways toward the side with the bent knee. You will feel a stretch on the outside of the bent knee. Hold for 5 seconds.

4. Hamstring stretch: Sit on the floor with your legs straight in front of you. Reach for your toes until you feel a stretch in the back of your thighs. Hold for 5 seconds.

5. Quad stretch: Stand facing a stationary object for support. Bend one knee as far as possible, reach back, and grasp the foot. Pull the heel toward your buttocks until you feel a stretch in the front of the thigh. Hold this position for 5 seconds. Do not arch back.

6. Heel cord stretch: Stand facing a stationary object with your feet apart and your toes turned in slightly. Place your hands on the object and lean forward until you feel a stretch in the calf of your leg. Hold for 5 seconds. Do not bend your knees or allow your heels to come off the floor.

7. Soleus stretch: Assume the same position as in number 6. Place one foot in front of the other foot and bend both knees. Lean forward, keeping the heel of the front foot on the ground. You should feel a stretch in the lower calf of the front leg. Hold for 5 seconds.

Figure 7-49 Runner's flexibility program.

which can be accomplished with low- or no-impact cross-training. The running pace should be no faster than 7 minutes per mile and the walking done briskly. The program is based on time, not distance. A rest day should be scheduled every 7 to 10 days. The schedule can be varied to meet individual situations. If need be, the runner may hold at a given level longer, drop back a level, or in some instances, skip a level if progressing well. Discomfort may be experienced, but it should be transient and certainly not accumulate. Include general strength training, specific prescribed exercises for rehabilitation, and stretching for flexibility.

ILIOTIBIAL BAND STRETCHING PROGRAM

Each exercise is to be done____times per day,____repetitions of each exercise. Hold all stretches for 5 seconds.

1. Hip Abductor Stretch

Stand with legs straight, feet together. Bend at waist toward side opposite leg to be stretched. Unaffected knee may be bent.

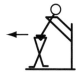

2. Iliotibial Band Stretch

Stand with knees straight; cross leg to be stretched behind other as far a possible. Stretch to side of leg in front.

3. Iliotibial Band Stretch

Same stance as exercise number 2. Slightly bend back knee. Move trunk toward unaffected side and hips toward affected side. Stretch will be felt along outside of bent knee.

4. Iliotibial band/Hamstring Stretch

Stand with knees straight. Cross legs so that affected knee rests against back of unaffected leg. Turn trunk away from affected side as far as possible, reaching and attempting to touch heel of affected leg.

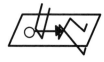

5. Iliotibial Band Stretch

Lie on unaffected side with your back a few inches from table edge. Bend unaffected hip to maintain balance. Straighten affected knee and place leg over edge of table so leg hangs straight. Let gravity pull leg down, causing the stretch.

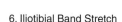

6. Iliotibial Band Stretch

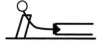

Lie on affected side with knee locked and leg in a straight line with trunk; bend upper knee with your hands placed directly under shoulders to bear the weight of the trunk. Push up, extending your arms as far as possible. Affected leg must be kept straight to get maximum stretch in hip.

Figure 7-50   Iliotibial band stretching program. (Modified from Lutter LD: Form used in the Physical Therapy Department at St. Anthony Orthopaedic Clinic and the University of Minnesota, St. Paul.)

TABLE 7–11	Runner's Guide for Return to Running after an Absence of 4 Weeks or More from Training

Week	Schedule
1	Walk 30 min, alternating 1 min normal and 1 min fast
2	Walk 30 min, alternating 1.5 min normal and 1.5 min fast. If doing well, jog easily instead of walking fast
3	Alternate walking 1 min and jogging 2 min × 7. The next day, run easy 5 min and walk 1 min × 3
4	Alternate walking 1 min and jogging 3 min × 7. The next day, run 5 min and walk 1 min × 4
5	Run continuously 20 min. The next day, run 5 min and walk 1 min × 5
6	Run continuously 20 min. The next day, run 10 min and walk 1 min × 3
7	Run continuously 20 min one day and 35 min the next
8	Run continuously 20 min one day and 40 min the next
9	If doing well, resume a training schedule, increasing the duration, intensity, and frequency appropriately
	The key is to avoid reinjury

From James SL, Bates BT, Oslering LR: Injuries to runners. Am J Sports Med 6:40, 1978.

For Return to Running after Missed Training
James

The following protocol is a conservative guide that can be varied depending on individual situations.

Absence from training for
- 1 week or less—reduce training 60% for 3 days, 30% for the next 3 days, and then resume normal training, but monitor closely.
- 1-2 weeks—reduce training 60% the first 5 days, 30% the second 5 days, and then resume appropriate training.
- 2-3 weeks—reduce training 60% the first 5 days, 40% the second 5 days, 20% the third 5 days, and then resume appropriate training.
- 4 weeks or more—see Table 7-11.

Nirschl Pain Phase Scale for Athletes' Overuse Injuries

Phase 1. Stiffness or mild soreness after activity. Pain is usually gone within 24 hours.

Phase 2. Stiffness or mild soreness before activity that is relieved by warm-up. Symptoms are not present during activity but return after and last up to 48 hours.

Phase 3. Stiffness or mild soreness before a specific sport or occupational activity. Pain is partially relieved by warm-up. It is minimally present during activity but does not cause the athlete to alter activity.

Phase 4. Similar to but more intense than phase 3 pain. Phase 4 pain causes athlete to alter performance of the activity. Mild pain may also be noticed with activities of daily living.

Continued

Nirschl Pain Phase Scale for Athletes' Overuse Injuries Continued

Phase 5. Significant (moderate or greater) pain before, during, and after activity that causes alteration of activity. Pain occurs with activities of daily living but does not cause a major change in them.

Phase 6. Phase 5 pain that persists even with complete rest. Phase 6 pain disrupts simple activities of daily living and prohibits doing household chores.

Phase 7. Phase 6 pain that also consistently disrupts sleep. Pain is aching in nature and intensifies with activity.

From O'Connor FG, Nirschl RP: Five step treatment for overuse injuries. Physician Sports Med 20(10):128, 1992.

General Treatment Guidelines for Overuse Injuries in Runners
Brotzman

First, establish the correct diagnosis and pathoanatomy.

1. Discontinue or decrease running, depending on the severity
2. Cross-train with nonimpact cardiovascular exercise (DWR exercise with an AquaJogger belt [www.aquajogger.com], bicycling, swimming, elliptical trainer)
3. Ice
4. NSAIDs
5. Initiate stretching exercises for the area of tightness (e.g., iliotibial band, hamstrings, quadriceps)
6. Patient education on avoiding training errors in the future (e.g., too rapid a progression)
7. Conservative correction of underlying biomechanical malalignment (e.g., orthotics for pronators, McConnell taping or Palumbo bracing for patellofemoral malalignment, heel-lift for leg-length discrepancy)
8. Education on appropriate running shoes and less than 300 miles per pair
9. Address and treat any underlying metabolic contributors to overuse injury (e.g., address amenorrhea, obesity, calcium or protein deficiency, osteoporosis, eating disorders)
10. Surgery only as a last resort for injuries failing conservative measures and time
11. Gradual resumption of running as described by James rather than the overzealous return attempted by all runners if not supervised
12. Alteration of the surface to grass, cinder, or a cushioned track. Avoid running on a road with a slope; avoid hill running
13. No cortisone injections except for iliotibial band tendinitis
14. Improve overall fitness and resistance to breakdown or overuse by sport-specific agility, speed, and skill drills such as plyometrics, eccentric strengthening, and coordinating and strengthening antagonistic muscles and supporting muscles

Shin Splints in Runners

Mark M. Casillas, MD • Margaret Jacobs, PT

Shin splints is a nonspecific term typically used to describe exertional leg pain. Though common in runners, this condition is probably overdiagnosed. A number of specific conditions are known to also cause exercise-induced leg pain. It is appropriate to identify a specific etiology whenever possible.

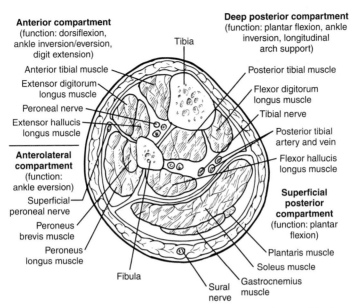

Anterior compartment
(function: dorsiflexion,
ankle inversion/eversion,
digit extension)

Anterior tibial muscle

Extensor digitorum
longus muscle

Peroneal nerve

Extensor hallucis
longus muscle

**Anterolateral
compartment**
(function:
ankle eversion)

Superficial
peroneal nerve

Peroneus
brevis muscle

Peroneus
longus muscle

Tibia

Fibula

Sural
nerve

Deep posterior compartment
(function: plantar flexion, ankle
inversion, longitudinal
arch support)

Posterior tibial muscle

Flexor digitorum
longus muscle

Tibial nerve

Posterior tibial
artery and vein

Flexor hallucis
longus muscle

**Superficial
posterior
compartment**
(function: plantar
flexion)

Plantaris muscle

Soleus muscle

Gastrocnemius
muscle

Figure 7-51 Cross-section through the midportion of the leg. Note the crural fascia and the four fascial compartments.

RELEVANT ANATOMY

The leg bones (tibia and fibula) serve as the origin for the extrinsic muscles of the foot and ankle. The muscles of the leg are surrounded and divided by the crural fascia. The resulting compartments (anterior, lateral, superficial posterior, and deep posterior) are unyielding with regard to volume and are prone to the development of increased pressure (Fig. 7-51). The anterior compartment contains the extensor muscles, including the anterior tibial, the extensor digitorum longus, and the extensor hallucis longus muscles. The posterior medial border of the tibia serves as the origin for the posterior tibial muscle, the flexor digitorum longus muscle, the soleus muscle, and the deep crural fascia.

ETIOLOGY

Anterior shin splints are related to dysfunction of the anterior leg compartment or its contiguous structures. **Medial tibial stress syndrome** is the clinical entity that most likely represents medial shin splints. The exercise-induced pain associated with medial tibial stress syndrome tends to involve the distal two thirds of the leg. The etiology of anterior shin splints is not completely understood; overuse or chronic injury of the anterior compartment muscles, fascia, and bony and periosteal attachments is most commonly implicated. The most likely cause of medial tibial stress syndrome is traction periostitis of the soleus or flexor digitorum longus muscle origins. Increased heel eversion is a suggested risk factor.

TABLE 7–12	Differential Diagnosis of Shin Splints
Differential Diagnosis	**Significant Findings**
Anterior shin splints	Exercise-induced leg pain, tender at the anterior compartment, normal radiograph and bone scan
Medial tibial stress syndrome (medial shin splints)	Exercise-induced leg pain, tender at the posterior-medial tibial border, normal radiograph, linear uptake on bone scan
Tibial stress fracture	Exertional pain at the tibia; point-tender tibia; pain with three-point stress; abnormal radiograph, fusiform uptake on bone scan, abnormal CT or MRI
Fibular stress fracture	Exertional pain at the fibula; pronation or valgus alignment; point-tender fibula; abnormal radiograph, bone scan, CT, or MRI
Acute compartment syndrome	Leg pain secondary to trauma, tender compartments, pain with passive motion, decreased sensation, elevated compartment pressures, paresthesias
Chronic exertional compartment syndrome	Exertional leg pain, no acute trauma, tender compartments, muscle herniation, decreased sensation after exertion, elevated postexertion compartment pressures, paresthesias
Congenital anomaly	Exertional leg pain, no acute trauma, anomalous muscle such as accessory soleus, symptoms similar to those of chronic exertional compartment syndrome, accessory muscle identified on MRI
Tumor	Night pain; abnormal radiograph, bone scan, CT, or MRI

DIAGNOSIS

A diagnosis of shin splints is suggested by a history of exercise-induced pain at the distal two thirds of the leg (Table 7-12). **The pain is localized to the anterior compartment in anterior shin splints and to the distal two thirds of the posterior medial tibial border in medial tibial stress syndrome** (Fig. 7-52). The pain is brought on by activity such as prolonged walking or running, and it is relieved by decreased activity. The condition is never associated with neurologic or vascular symptoms or findings.

Radiographic Examination

Radiographs are negative in this condition, but it should be remembered that they are also negative for the first weeks of a developing stress fracture. Therefore, a bone scan is used to differentiate between a stress fracture and shin splints. Longitudinal uptake along the posterior medial border of the distal end of the tibia is consistent with medial tibial stress syndrome, whereas focal or linear uptake is diagnostic of a stress fracture (Fig. 7-53). Compartment syndrome, spinal claudication, vascular claudication, anomalous muscle, infection, and tumor must be ruled out.

TREATMENT

Perhaps the most efficient approach to managing shin splints is prevention. Lower-impact conditioning and cross-training appear to reduce the incidence of shin splints.

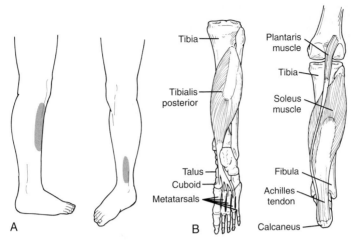

Figure 7-52 **A**, Pain is localized to the anterior compartment for anterior shin splints (*left*) or to the distal two thirds of the posterior medial tibial border for medial tibial stress syndrome (*right*). **B**, Posterior views of the attachments of the posterior tibial muscle (*left*) and the soleus muscle (*right*). (Adapted from Fick DS, Albright JP, Murray BP: Relieving painful "shin splints." Physician Sports Med 20[12]:105-111, 1992; McKeag DB, Dolan C: Overuse syndromes of the lower extremity. Physician Sports Med 17[7]:108-112, 1989.)

The acute exertional pain associated with shin splints is treated with the RICE regimen until symptoms subside. An increase in rest intervals and duration is also beneficial to both types of shin splints. Running is prohibited until the patient is free of pain.

Anterior shin splints are treated by aggressive warm-up and stretching, with particular attention directed to the gastrosoleus–Achilles tendon complex (Fig. 7-54). Anterior symptoms may also respond to decreased shoe weight and level running surfaces. **Medial tibial stress syndrome** is treated in similar fashion. Medial symptoms may also respond to antipronation taping and orthotics (Figs. 7-55 and 7-56) and running on a nonbanked, firm surface.

Surgery is never indicated for anterior shin splints. For recalcitrant medial tibial stress syndrome, deep posterior compartment fasciotomy with release of the soleus muscle origin off the posterior medial tibial cortex has been suggested.

The most important aspect of treatment is appropriate diagnosis. Radiographs and bone scans are obtained in all patients to rule out stress fracture. Once the diagnosis of shin splints is established, running is stopped until the exercise-related pain has resolved. Stretching and conditioning are emphasized throughout a comprehensive rehabilitation program. Antipronation orthotics are fitted if taping reduces symptoms.

Figure 7-53 **A** and **B**, Bone scans diagnostic of a right-sided posteromedial stress fracture. **C**, Lateral plain film of the tibia revealing an ominous focal transverse radiolucent line (stress fracture). (**A** and **B**, From Hutchinson MR, Cahoon S, Atkins T: Chronic leg pain. Physician Sports Med 26[7]:37-46, 1998; **C**, from Mann RA, Coughlin MJ: Surgery of the Foot and Ankle. St Louis, CV Mosby, 1999.)

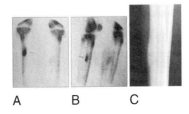

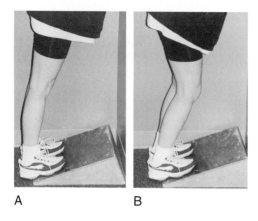

Figure 7-54 **A**, Gastrocnemius stretching on an inclined box with the knee extended. **B**, The soleus is stretched more effectively by flexing the knee and relaxing the gastrocnemius muscle.

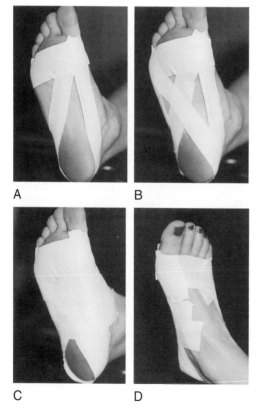

Figure 7-55 **A-D**, Antipronation taping.

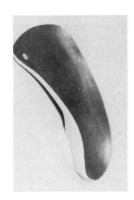

Figure 7-56 Orthotic for correction of pes planus. Pes planus feet have decreased "shock absorption" at the subtalar joint during high-impact activities because the subtalar joint is already everted at heel-strike. This precludes the usual shock absorption of the normal subtalar joint. Orthotics place the foot in a more subtalar neutral position.

Any underlying biomechanical, anatomic, or nutritional precipitating causes should also be treated.

Fundamental to the rehabilitation protocol is the patient's self-discipline to avoid running until the exercise-related pain has completely resolved. The phases of rehabilitation are variable in length and depend completely on resolution of pain with weight-bearing and eventually with running. Flexibility is emphasized throughout the protocol, with particular attention paid to the gastrosoleus–Achilles tendon complex for anterior shin splints and the soleus for medial tibial stress syndrome.

REHABILITATION PROTOCOL	*Shin Splints* Casillas and Jacobs

0-3 DAYS: ACUTE PHASE

This phase is defined by the initial date of treatment through the resolution of weight-bearing pain. Relative rest (no running), ice massage, and whirlpool are used for acute pain.
- Ultrasound therapy is considered if the bone scan demonstrates no bony involvement.
- Nonimpact activities are begun and are advanced as pain allows:
  - Gastrocnemius and soleus stretching
  - Isometrics
  - Seated towel scrunches
  - Cycling
  - Water activities (DWR) with an AquaJogger belt and swimming

DAY 4-WEEK 6: SUBACUTE PHASE

This phase begins with the resolution of weight-bearing pain and ends with the resolution of activity-related pain.
- Modalities to decrease inflammation are continued.
- Emphasis remains on improving flexibility.
- Isometrics are progressed to Thera-Band exercises.
- Towel scrunches are progressed from a seated to a standing position.
- Balance activities are begun with progression of difficulty to include the biomechanical ankle platform system (BAPS).
- Aerobic fitness is maintained with cross-training activities such as a slideboard, water running, and cycling.

Continued

REHABILITATION PROTOCOL: *Shin Splints* *Continued*

WEEK 7: RETURN-TO-SPORT PHASE
- Running commences once all activity-related pain has resolved.
- Warm-up and stretching are emphasized.
- Running is allowed to progress within the limits of a pain-free schedule. See James' protocol for gradual return to running (p. 763).
- Patients are to initially avoid running on uneven surfaces.
- If the patient is using an oval track, each direction should be used in an equal fashion (i.e., change direction).
- Attention is directed to first re-establishing distance, followed by re-establishing speed.
- Antipronation orthotics are fitted for patients with medial tibial stress syndrome or if warranted by a successful trial of low-dye taping.

Return to Play after a Concussion

S. Brent Brotzman, MD • Jenna Deacon Costella, MA, ATC • Mark Bohling, MS, ATC

BACKGROUND

A **concussion** is a clinical syndrome characterized by immediate and transient impairment of neural function, including alteration of consciousness, disturbance of vision, and loss of equilibrium as a result of mechanical injury.
- Less than 10% of concussions result in loss of consciousness (Cantu 1996).
- Common symptoms of concussions include headache, dizziness, confusion, tinnitus, blurred vision, and nausea.
- Simple neuropsychological tests are routinely used to assess an athlete suspected of having a concussion. The athlete is asked orientation questions such as
  - What field are we playing on?
  - Which team scored last?
  - What quarter is it?
  - Did our team win last week?
  - What team did we play last week?

Sideline Neurologic Evaluation for a Concussion

HISTORY
- Mechanism or description of how the injury occurred.
- Loss of consciousness? Duration?
- Amnesia? Duration?
- Headache? Duration?
- Associated symptoms? Duration?
- Sensation intact?
- Numbness?
- Extremity movement?
- Neck pain?

Sideline Neurologic Evaluation for a Concussion   Continued

PHYSICAL EXAMINATION

- Appearance (alert, dazed, unconscious)
- Mental status (person, place, time)
- Eyes (pupils, visual fields, equal ocular movements, fundi—if an ophthalmoscope is available)
- Cranial nerves
- Sensation (light touch, sharp)
- Motor (strength, movement)
- Reflexes
- Cognition (serial 7s, score, school, president)
- Arm extension
- Toe signs
- Cerebellar function (finger-to-nose, Romberg sign)
- Gait

FUNCTIONAL TESTS BEFORE RETURN TO PLAY

- Running, jumping, cutting
- Sport-specific skills
- Return-to-play criteria after a concussion is a controversial topic. The goal is to avoid exposing the athlete to an increased risk for injury.
- **Prevention of second-impact syndrome is of utmost importance**.
- **Second-impact syndrome** occurs when a player sustains a (minor) second head injury before the symptoms of a previous concussion have cleared. This syndrome results in brain swelling, which follows vascular engorgement caused by autoregulation of cerebral blood flow (Fig. 7-57). Vascular engorgement leads to a massive increase in intracranial pressure, and **death frequently follows**.
- Whether it takes days, weeks, or months to reach an asymptomatic state, the athlete must *never* be allowed to practice or compete while postconcussion syndrome is present.
- Because the additive effects of repeated head blows can be manifested as boxing's "punch-drunk syndrome," the number of concussions that an athlete is allowed to sustain should be very limited. The athlete should be rapidly, safely disqualified from further competition in high-risk sports.
- Football, hockey, and soccer players and wrestlers are at greatest risk for concussion. High-school football players face a 20% risk each season; high-school hockey players have a 10% risk.
- Cantu (1986) uses a scale that applies the *duration* of loss of consciousness and post-traumatic amnesia to differentiate mild, moderate, and severe concussions (Table 7-13). Other commonly used scales include the Colorado Guidelines for Management of Concussion in Sports (Table 7-14) and the American Academy of Neurology (AAN) guidelines.
- We use the Colorado or the AAN guidelines in our practice because "up to 5 minutes of loss of consciousness" in Cantu's classification is considered only a grade 2 injury. We consider this a grade 3 injury.
- **Evaluation and treatment of a concussion** should include survey of the **ABCs** (airway, breathing, circulation). If the patient has any neck pain or neurocervical symptoms, use cervical spine precautions for transportation. If the patient is unconscious, assume a cervical spine injury and use cervical spine precautions.
- *Do not remove the helmet* if a cervical spine injury is suspected. Instead, cut (detach) the plastic mounting clips on the facemask with trainer's angels.
- Airway protection should take precedence.

Continued

Sideline Neurologic Evaluation for a Concussion   *Continued*

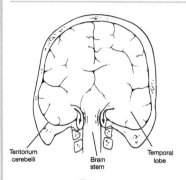

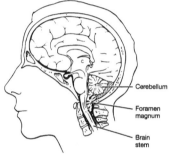

Figure 7-57   In **second-impact syndrome**, vascular engorgement within the cranium increases intracranial pressure, which leads to herniation of the uncus of the temporal lobe (*arrows*) below the tentorium in this frontal section (**A**) or to herniation of the cerebellar tonsils (*arrows*) through the foramen magnum in this midsagittal section (**B**). These changes compromise the brainstem, and coma and respiratory failure develop rapidly. The *shaded areas* of the brainstem represent the areas of compression. (From Cantu RC: Neurologic athletic injuries. Clin Sports Med 17:37-45, 1998.)

TABLE 7–13	Concussion Classification Systems and Return-to-Play Recommendations (Cantu)

Severity	First Concussion	Second Concussion	Third Concussion
Grade 1 (mild): No loss of consciousness; post-traumatic amnesia <30 min	May return to play if asymptomatic	May return in 2 wk if asymptomatic at that time for 1 wk	Terminate season; may return next year if asymptomatic
Grade 2 (moderate): Loss of consciousness <5 min or post-traumatic amnesia >30 min	Return after asymptomatic for 1 wk	Wait at least 1 mo; may return then if asymptomatic for 1 wk; consider terminating season	Terminate season; may return next year if asymptomatic
Grade 3 (severe): Loss of consciousness >5 min or post-traumatic amnesia >24 hr	Wait at least 1 mo; may return then if asymptomatic for 1 wk	Terminate season; may return next year if asymptomatic	

From Cantu RC: Guidelines for return to sports after cerebral concussion. Physican Sports Med 14(10):75, 1986.

TABLE 7–14	Colorado Guidelines to Return to Contact Sports after Cerebral Concussion (Authors' Choice)		
Severity	First Concussion	Second Concussion	Third Concussion
Grade 1 (mild): Confusion without amnesia; no loss of consciousness	May return to play if asymptomatic for at least 20 min	Terminate contest or practice for the day	Terminate season; may return in 3 mo if asymptomatic
Grade 2 (moderate): Confusion with amnesia; no loss of consciousness	Terminate contest/ practice; may return if asymptomatic for at least 1 wk	Consider terminating season but may return if asymptomatic for 1 mo	Terminate season; may return to play next season if asymptomatic
Grade 3 (severe): Loss of consciousness	May return after 1 mo if asymptomatic for 2 wk at that time; may resume conditioning sooner if asymptomatic for 2 wk	Terminate season; discourage any return to contact sports	

From Roos R: Guidelines for managing concussion in sports: A persistent headache. 24(2):67, 1996.

- When assessing an athlete with a suspected concussion, the examiner should consider and document
  - Time and place of injury
  - Mechanism of injury
  - Presence of duration of loss of consciousness
  - Postinjury behavior
  - Presence of convulsions after injury
  - Past medical history
  - Medication use

SIDELINE EVALUATION AFTER CONCUSSION

- ABCs (airway, breathing and circulation).
- Evaluate for loss of consciousness.
- Cervical spine assessment.
- Assess cranial nerves, coordination, and motor function.
- Assess cognitive function.

- Evaluate short-term and long-term memory (e.g., detailed questions about recent events, three-word memory, serial 7s).
- Frequent reassessment of the injured player to determine whether the symptoms are continuing or deteriorating.
- Any loss of consciousness should result in transport of the athlete to a hospital for further evaluation and work-up (computed tomography [CT] scan, neurologic consultation).
- Prolonged loss of consciousness should also result in immediate transportation to the hospital under cervical spine precautions. Perform CT or MRI to rule out an acute epidural or subdural hemorrhage.
- **Athletes who are symptomatic after a head injury are not to participate in collision or contact sports until** *all* **cerebral symptoms have** *subsided* **for** *at least 1 week*.
- Athletes who have sustained a concussion should be re-evaluated by a physician in a clinical setting within a few days of injury and again before they are allowed to return to participation.
- If an athlete with a concussion is sent home after the game, it should be in the care of a responsible adult provided with instruction and a head injury instruction sheet (Fig. 7-58).

HEAD INJURY INSTRUCTION SHEET

Date: _____

_____ has suffered a head injury. Although the athlete is currently alert, conscious and shows no signs or symptoms of serious brain injury, a potentially catastrophic result can still occur, leading to permanent neurological deficit or even death. Occassionly, following even the mildest head injuries, blood will slowly accumulate, causing compression of the brain hours or even days after the initial injury. Thus, the following guidelines should be followed in conjunction with the physician's or the athletic trainer's advice.

1. The injured athlete should never be alone for the first 24 hours after the injury.
2. The athlete should be awakened every two hours in the evening to establish arousability and alertness.
3. The following signs mandate immediate emergency room evaluation:

   - Blood or watery fluid emanating (coming out) from ears or nose
   - Unequal or dilated pupils
   - Weakness or clumsiness in arms or legs
   - Slurred or garbled speech
   - Asymmetry of the face
   - Increased swelling along the scalp
   - Hard to arouse, irritable or stuporous (reduced sensibilty)

4. The following symptoms (complaints) mandate immediate emergency room evaluation

   - Change in mental status (inability to concentrate or understand directions, alteration of alertness or consciousness)
   - Double or blurred vision
   - Severe headache
   - Increased incoordination (clumsiness) or weakness
   - Vomiting
   - Loss of memory
   - Difficulty with speech

Please realize the above are only guidelines to assist you. If a sign or symptom develops that is new and is not mentioned above, err on the side of safety and have the athlete evaluated by a physician immediately.

Figure 7-58   Head injury instruction sheet.

Osteoporosis: Evaluation, Management, and Exercise

S. Brent Brotzman, MD

BACKGROUND

- In the United States, 20 million people, predominantly postmenopausal women, have osteoporosis.
- Osteoporosis leads to more than 1.5 million fractures each year.
- One of every two women older than 50 years will have an osteoporosis-related fracture.
- One in every three men older than 75 years will be affected by osteoporosis.
- *The current goal for management of women who are at risk for or have osteoporosis is avoidance of fracture by preventing bone loss and increasing bone mass.*

DEFINITION OF OSTEOPOROSIS

- Osteoporosis is a disease characterized by **low bone mass**, microarchitectural deterioration of bone tissue leading to bone fragility, and consequent increase in fracture risk.
- Osteoporosis reflects inadequate accumulation of bone tissue during growth and maturation, excessive losses thereafter, or both.
- Fractures of the wrist, spine, and hip occur most commonly. Fractures of the ribs, humerus, and pelvis are not uncommon.
- Two categories of osteoporosis exist: **primary** and **secondary** osteoporosis.

Primary Osteoporosis

- The most common form of osteoporosis.
- Includes postmenopausal osteoporosis (**type 1**) and age-associated osteoporosis (**type 2**), formerly termed *senile* osteoporosis.

Secondary Osteoporosis

- Loss of bone is caused by an identifiable agent or disease process such as an inflammatory disorder, bone marrow cellularity disorder, and corticosteroid use.

Possible Secondary Causes of Osteoporosis

- Long-term use of corticosteroids
- Antiseizure medication (e.g., phenytoin)
- Gonadotropin hormones (for treatment of endometriosis)
- Excessive use of aluminum-containing antacids
- Excessive thyroid hormone medication
- Certain anticancer drugs

Continued

Possible Secondary Causes of Osteoporosis   *Continued*

- Inflammatory disorders treated with steroids (rheumatoid arthritis, asthma, and lupus)
- Hypogonadism (inadequate function of the gonads)
- Hyperparathyroidism
- Cushing's syndrome (overactive adrenal glands)
- Turner's or Kleinfelter's syndrome
- Low sex hormone levels
- In women: a result of excessive exercise (amenorrhea) or eating disorders that decrease estrogen production or premature menopause
- In men: a result of decreased testosterone production
- Blood or bone marrow disorders (myeloma)
- Organ transplantation (immunosuppressive agents such as cyclosporine or steroids)
- Chronic kidney, liver, lung, or gastrointestinal disorders
- Breast or prostate cancer (if treatment lowers estrogen levels)
- Spinal cord injury with paralysis of the lower limbs
- Multiple sclerosis (if steroids are used or walking is impaired)

RISK FACTORS FOR DEVELOPMENT OF OSTEOPOROSIS

 National Osteoporosis Foundation Physician Guidelines for Risk Factors for Osteoporotic Fracture

- Current cigarette smoking
- Low body weight (<127 pounds)
- Alcoholism
- Estrogen deficiency
- Prolonged amenorrhea (>1 year)
- Early menopause (<45 years) or bilateral ovariectomy
- Lifelong low calcium intake
- Recurrent falls
- Poor health/fragility
- Inadequate physical activity
- Impaired eyesight

PREVENTION OF OSTEOPOROSIS

- Prevention of osteoporosis begins in childhood with adequate calcium and vitamin D intake and continues throughout life (Fig. 7-59).
- Prevention is of great importance because of limited therapeutic alternatives for reversing loss of bone mass.
- **Osteomalacia**, which may masquerade as osteoporosis, must be excluded if risk factors exist.

Preventive Measures

- Adequate weight-bearing physical activity for 3-4 hr/wk
- Avoid low body weight or excessive thinness (<127 pounds)
- Avoid excess alcohol intake
- Lifelong appropriate calcium and vitamin D intake
- Avoidance of bone-leaching medicines if possible
- Maximal accumulation of bone during skeletal growth and maturation and reducing or eliminating bone loss after the skeleton matures

---

PATIENT EDUCATION HANDOUT

RISK FACTORS YOU CAN CHANGE

HORMONE LEVELS
Early menopause, occurring naturally or surgically (for example, surgical removal of the ovaries), can increase a woman's likelihood of developing osteoporosis. If you fall into this category, hormone supplements are available. It is important to discuss your bone health and hormone therapy with your physician.

DIET
Inadequate calcium and vitamin D intake is harmful to bone health. Excessive consumption of other nutrients, such as protein and sodium, can decrease calcium absorption.

EXERCISE
Maintaining a physically active lifestyle throughout life is important. Individuals who are inactive, immobilized, or bedridden for a long time, are at risk for osteoporosis.

LIFESTYLE CHOICES
Smoking and excessive alcohol consumption are bad for the skeleton. Women who smoke have lower estrogen levels than non-smokers and go through menopause earlier. Excessive alcohol use increases the risk of bone loss and fractures, due to both poor nutrition and increased risk of falling.

RISK FACTORS YOU CANNOT CHANGE

GENDER
Women are more likely to develop osteoporosis than men, because they have lighter, thinner bones, and lose bone mass rapidly after menopause.

AGE
The longer you live, the greater the likelihood of developing osteoporosis. Although all of us lose some bone tissue as we age, the amount and rate of loss varies widely in different individuals.

HEREDITY
Susceptibility to osteoporosis is in part due to heredity. Young women whose mothers and fathers have had fractures tend to have lower bone mass.

BODY SIZE
Small-boned, thin women and men are more at risk than larger, big-boned persons, but bigger bone size is no guarantee that you will not get osteoporosis.

ETHNICITY
Caucasians and those of Asian descent are at higher risk of developing osteoporosis than individuals of African-American descent, however, anyone may be at risk.

Figure 7-59 Patient education handout for osteoporosis. (From Brown EF, Evans RM, Cole HM, Coble YE [eds]: Managing Osteoporosis: Part 3, AMA Continuing Medical Education Program. Chicago, AMA Press, 2000.)

EVALUATION AND TREATMENT OF OSTEOPOROSIS

- Patients at increased risk for fracture may be identified on the basis of **clinical factors** (e.g., previous fracture, smoker) and through **bone mineral density (BMD) testing** (Table 7-15).
- The National Osteoporosis Foundation has identified the following **key risk factors** for osteoporosis (with a **recommendation that BMD** *tests be done on these patients*):
  - History of fracture as an adult
  - History of fracture in first-degree relative
  - Current cigarette smoking
  - Low body weight or thin (**<127** pounds)
- Drug therapy is considered if the BMD T-score is below −1.5 and concomitant risk factors are present (e.g., smoker).
- Patients with a BMD T-score below −2 should undergo drug therapy.
- Because of the strong correlation between BMD testing results and fracture risk, the World Health Organization diagnostic categories are based on BMD measurements.

Bone Mineral Density Parameters for Osteoporosis

Normal: bone density on BMD testing no lower than 1 SD below the mean for "young normal" adult women (T-score higher than −1).

Low bone mass (osteopenia): bone density on BMD testing between 1 and 2.5 SD below the mean for "young normal" adult women (T-score between −1 and −2.5).

Osteoporosis: bone density on BMD testing 2.5 SD below the "young normal" adult mean (T-score −2.5 or lower); women in this group who have already experienced one or more fractures are deemed to have severe or "established" osteoporosis; as a general rule, for every SD below the normal, the fracture risk doubles.

TABLE 7–15	Bone Mineral Density Testing Recommendations
Who Should Have a BMD Test?	**Main Risk Factors**
Postmenopausal women younger than 65 yr with one or more risk factors	Low BMD (T-score less than −1.5)
All postmenopausal women older than 65 yr	History of fracture—personal or first-degree relative
Postmenopausal women with fractures	Cigarette smoker
Women considering therapy for osteoporosis	Low body weight (<127 pounds)

Guidelines are based on data for white postmenopausal females.

Recommendations based on National Osteoporosis Foundation—"Guide to Prevention and Treatment of Osteoporosis." For more information contact the NOF at 202-223-2226 or at http://www.nof.org.

TABLE 7–16	Adequate Calcium Intake Guidelines
Life Stage Group	**Estimated Adequate Daily Calcium Intake (mg)**
Infants	
Birth-6 mo	210
6-12 mo	270
Young children (1-3 yr)	500
Older children (4-8 yr)	800
Adolescents and young adults (9-18 yr)	1300
Men and women (19-50 yr)	1000
(51 yr and older)	1200

Note: Pregnancy and lactation needs are the same as for nonpregnant women (i.e., 1300 mg for adolescents/young adults and 1000 mg for those 19 and older).

Adapted from Standing Committee on the Scientific Evaluation of Dietary Reference Intakes. Food and Nutrition Board, Institute of Medicine. Washington, DC, National Academy Press, 1997.

VITAMINS AND MEDICATIONS FOR OSTEOPOROSIS

Calcium

Patient Education Handout on Calcium

- **Calcium supplements.** Although food sources of calcium are preferred, sometimes it is necessary to use a calcium supplement to meet your daily calcium requirement. The amount of supplement you need depends on how much calcium is in your diet (Table 7-16).

    Many brands of calcium supplements are on the shelves in supermarkets, health food stores, and pharmacies (Table 7-17). The most expensive brand is not necessarily the best. The most common calcium supplements are calcium carbonate and calcium citrate (there are others). *Calcium carbonate*, the most popular

TABLE 7–17	Some Commonly Used Calcium Supplements		
Type	**Trade Name**	**Strength per Tablet (mg)**	**Elemental Calcium (mg)***
Calcium carbonate	Alka-Mints	850	340
	Caltrate	1600	600
	Os-Cal	625 or 1250	250 or 500
	Rolaids	550	220
	Titralac	420	168
	Titralac Liquid	1000	400
	Tums/Tums E-X	500 or 750	200 or 300
	Tums Ultra/Tums 500	1000 or 1250	400 or 500
Calcium citrate	Citracal Liquitabs	2376	500
	Citracal	950	200
	Citracal Caplets + D	1500	315 + 200 IU vitamin D

*Amount of usable calcium.

calcium supplement, has the highest percentage of calcium and the lowest unit cost. Both calcium carbonate and *calcium citrate* are easily absorbed and used by the body. Calcium carbonate should be taken with meals, whereas calcium citrate can be taken with or without.

- **Tips on taking calcium supplements:**
  - Look for the amount of "elemental" calcium that the supplement provides (this can be found by reading the label on the calcium supplement package). *Elemental refers to the amount of usable calcium in the mineral*. Figure out how much you will need to take to reach your daily requirement.
  - The supplement must meet *"dissolution" requirements*, which means that it will dissolve in the stomach (necessary for absorption). Look for labels that say "passed dissolution test" or "USP dissolution tested." If you are not sure about your supplement, you can test it yourself by placing the tablet in a small glass of vinegar or warm water. Stir it occasionally; after 30 minutes the tablet should dissolve. If not, it is probably not dissolving in your stomach either and is not being absorbed.
  - *Avoid calcium from unrefined oyster shell, bone meal, or dolomite*. These forms may contain higher amounts of lead and other toxic metals. Also, *avoid* using aluminum-containing antacids, which contain no calcium.
  - Calcium is absorbed better if 500 mg or less is taken at any one time.
  - Certain calcium preparations may cause side effects, such as constipation or gas. It may help to drink more fluids and eat more fiber. You may need to try different calcium supplements until you find one that works for you.
  - *Do not take more than 2000 mg of elemental calcium per day*.
  - Individuals with a personal or family history of kidney stones should talk to their physician before increasing their calcium intake. Calcium rarely causes kidney stones in people with normal kidney function.
  - Talk to your physician or pharmacist about possible interactions between calcium supplements and prescription and over-the-counter medications. For example, when calcium is taken with the antibiotic tetracycline, absorption of the tetracycline is reduced.
  - Because calcium can interfere with iron absorption, *iron supplements should not be taken at the same time as calcium carbonate supplements*. This does not happen if the iron supplement is taken with vitamin C or calcium citrate.

Vitamin D

- Recommend daily intake: 400 to 800 IU daily.
- Avoid higher doses to avoid vitamin D toxicity.
- The elderly may benefit from higher calcium intake (1200 mg) and higher vitamin D intake (up to 800 IU daily).

Patient Education Handout on Vitamin D

- Vitamin D plays a major role in calcium absorption and bone health. Vitamin D has been called the "key" that opens the intestinal wall "door" so that calcium can leave the intestine and enter the blood stream. Vitamin D also helps absorb calcium in the kidneys that might otherwise be lost in urine.
- Vitamin D is formed naturally in the body after skin exposure to *sunlight*. Fifteen minutes of sun each day is plenty of time for you to make and store all the

vitamin D you need. Remember that sunscreen will block the body's ability to manufacture vitamin D.
- The ability to make vitamin D in the skin decreases with age, so an older person may have to take a vitamin D supplement.
- Studies have shown that the elderly benefit from higher vitamin D (up to 800 IU) and calcium intake (1200 mg) daily.
- *Food sources* of vitamin D are vitamin D–fortified dairy products, egg yolk, saltwater fish, and liver. Some calcium supplements and many multivitamins contain vitamin D.
- Experts recommend a daily intake of 400 to 800 IU of vitamin D for bone health. Do not take more than 800 IU unless your physician prescribes it. Massive doses of vitamin D can be harmful.

OSTEOPOROSIS TREATMENT CONSIDERATIONS

A suggested algorithm for the evaluation and management of osteoporotic fracture risk is shown in Figure 7-60 (see also Tables 7-18 to 7-21).

Secondary Osteoporosis

- Possible causes of secondary osteoporosis (p. 775) should be considered in patients newly diagnosed osteoporosis
- A *z-score* may be helpful in determining the presence of secondary osteoporosis. A *z-score* is similar in concept to the *T-score* (p. 778), except with the z-score the BMD is compared with that of an **age-matched control group**, *not* a young healthy control group. A **low z-score** may reflect bone loss not attributable to age alone and suggests the possibility of secondary osteoporosis. **A z-score of −1.5 should arouse clinical suspicion of secondary osteoporosis.**
- National Osteoporosis Foundation guidelines suggest that women suspected of having **secondary osteoporosis** should undergo **initial laboratory evaluation** consisting of a *complete blood count*, *chemistry profile*, and *urinary calcium* test. After clinical evaluation, additional tests may be required, including
  - Serum thyrotropin
  - Protein electrophoresis
  - Parathyroid hormone
  - Urine cortisol
  - Vitamin D metabolites

Serial Bone Mineral Density Measurements

- Measurements from peripheral skeletal sites are *not* useful for serial BMD determination.
- For technical reasons, BMD measurements should, whenever possible, be done on the same machine.
- The usual intervals for serial BMD measurements are every 1 to 2 years. However, some situations dictate more frequent intervals (e.g., significant BMD loss because of steroid therapy may be detected within 6 months).

ALGORITHM FOR EVALUATION OF OSTEOPOROTIC FRACTURE RISK

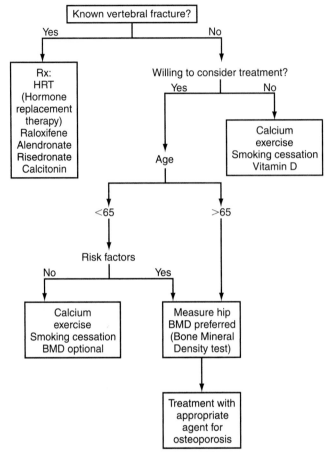

Figure 7-60   Algorithm for evaluation of osteoporotic fracture risk. (Modified from National Osteoporosis Foundation: Physician's Guide to Prevention and Treatment of Osteoporosis. Copyright 1998 National Osteoporosis Foundation, Washington, DC. For information on ordering single or bulk copies of the NOF guidelines, contact the National Osteoporosis Foundation, Professional Education Order Fulfillment, 1150 17th Street, NW, Suite 500, Washington, DC 20036.)

Prevention of Falls in Osteoporotic Patients

Elimination of environmental hazards is an easily modifiable risk factor for geriatric patients. The American College of Rheumatology recommends
- Night lights in bathrooms and hallways
- Nonskid soles for shoes
- Nonslip mats under rugs
- Grab bars for tub, shower, and toilet areas
- Rising cautiously from a supine position
- Sturdy stairway rails
- Flashlight kept by the bedside

TABLE 7-18	Osteoporosis Treatment Options
Option	**Comments**
Calcium	Increases spine BMD and reduces risk for fractures (vertebral and nonvertebral)
	Recommended intake for adults, 1000-1500 mg/day
	Preferred sources are dietary; supplements should have USP designation
Vitamin D	Essential for calcium absorption
	Maximally effective dosage is thought to be 400-1000 IU/day
Exercise	Resistance and impact exercises are probably the most beneficial to bone
	May promote attainment of high peak bone mass during childhood and adolescence
	May slow down decline in BMD if performed later in life, provided that calcium and vitamin D intake is adequate
Bisphosphonates (etidronate, alendronate [Fosamax], risedronate [Actonel])	Increase BMD at the spine and hip; reduce risk for vertebral fractures by 30% to 50%
	Reduce risk for nonvertebral osteoporotic fractures, including those caused by glucocorticoid-induced osteoporosis (alendronate and risedronate)
	Safety in children and young adults has not been evaluated
Hormone replacement therapy (including SERMs).	Established treatment of osteoporosis
	Observational data point to reduced hip fracture risk
	Trial data indicate reduced risk for vertebral fracture
	Approved by FDA for treatment and prevention of osteoporosis; reduces vertebral fracture risk by 36% (raloxifene, a SERM)
	Maintains bone mass in postmenopausal women; effect on fracture risk unclear (tamoxifen, a SERM)
Salmon calcitonin	Has positive effects on BMD at the lumbar spine
	Fracture risk data unclear
Phytoestrogens	Have weak estrogen-like effects
	Have positive effects on BMD at the lumbar spine
Other interventions	Physical therapy helps strengthen and improve balance
	Hip protectors may absorb or deflect impact of a fall

BMD, bone mineral density; FDA, U.S. Food and Drug Administration; SERM, selective estrogen receptor modulator; USP, *United States Pharmacopeia.*

From Brown EF, Evans RM, Cole HM, Coble YE (eds): Managing Osteoporosis: Part 3, AMA Continuing Medical Education Program. Chicago, AMA Press, 2000.

Exercise Treatment for Patients with Osteoporosis

How Exercise Builds Bone

Although the evidence that exercise prevents and combats osteoporosis is substantial, how it does so is far from clear. Both mechanical and hormonal processes appear to be involved. One explanation of the way bone responds to exercise is the "error strain distribution hypothesis."

According to this theory, bone cells sense the mechanical strain induced by weight-bearing or resistance exercise. The cells then communicate load imbalances with

TABLE 7–19	Pharmacologic Options for Managing Osteoporosis		
Drug	**Indications**	**Daily Dose**	**Comments**
HRT	Prevention and treatment	Conjugated equine estrogen, 0.625 mg; estropipate, 0.625 mg; micronized estradiol, 0.5 mg; transdermal estradiol, 0.05 mg	Benefits of cardioprotection and reduction of hot flashes must be weighed against risk for a modest increase in breast cancer risk and DVT; combining estrogen with progesterone reduces the problem of cyclic bleeding
Alendronate (Fosamax)	Prevention and treatment	5 mg for prevention; 10 mg for treatment	A bisphosphonate that specifically inhibits osteoclast-mediated bone resorption; an alternative for women who are not candidates for HRT or in whom HRT is ineffective; reduces the incidence of fracture at the spine, hip, and wrist by 50%; esophageal irritation can be reduced by taking the drug with a full glass of water on rising in the morning and avoiding the supine position and other medicine, food, and beverages for a half hour afterward.
Calcitonin	Treatment	200 IU	A polypeptide hormone that down-regulates osteoclastic activity; an alternative for women in whom HRT is unsuitable or in whom HRT or alendronate has been ineffective; less effective than these other agents; delivered as a nasal spray (a subcutaneous form is available but used rarely)
Raloxifene (Evista)	Prevention	60 mg	A selective estrogen receptor modulator; reduces the incidence of vertebral fracture by 40% to 50%; cannot be used to treat menopausal symptoms; incidence of DVT similar to that observed with estrogen; no estrogenic effect on uterus

DVT, deep venous thrombosis; HRT, hormone replacement therapy.
From Brown EF, Evans RM, Cole HM, Coble YE (eds): Managing Osteoporosis: Part 3, AMA Continuing Medical Education Program.

TABLE 7-20	Summary of Risks and Benefits of Osteoporosis Therapy				
	Estrogen	Raloxifene	Intranasal Calcitonin	Alendronate	Risedronate
Evidence supports reduction of spinal fractures	Yes	Yes	Yes	Yes	Yes
Evidence supports reduction of nonspinal fractures	Yes	No	No	Yes	Yes
Experience with long-term use	Large epidemiologic studies over decades	Randomized trial 3 yr	Randomized trial 5 yr	Randomized trial 4 yr	Randomized trial 3 yr
Administration	Orally: once daily any time	Orally: once daily any time	Intranasally: once daily any time	Once daily in AM, 30 min before eating, with water, while upright	Once daily in AM, 30-60 min before eating, with water, while upright
Specific adverse effects	Breast tenderness, vaginal bleeding, thromboembolic disorders	Increased risk for venous thrombosis, hot flushes, leg cramps	Nasal irritation	Dyspepsia, esophagitis; avoid in patients with esophageal disorders	Dyspepsia

Continued

TABLE 7–20	Summary of Risks and Benefits of Osteoporosis Therapy—cont'd				
	Estrogen	**Raloxifene**	**Intranasal Calcitonin**	**Alendronate**	**Risedronate**
Effect on cardiovascular mortality	Possibly decreased; unconfirmed by randomized trials	No final outcome data	None	None	None
Breast cancer	Increased, but probably very small increase in cancer risk	Possibly decreased risk for estrogen receptor–positive breast cancer	None	None	None
Endometrial cancer	Increased if unopposed estrogen used	None	None	None	None
Dementia, Alzheimer's disease	Epidemiologic studies suggest decreased incidence	Perhaps	None	None	None

From Brown EF, Evans RM, Cole HM, Coble YE (ed): Managing Osteoporosis: Part 3, AMA Continuing Medical Education Program. Chicago, AMA Press, 2000.

TABLE 7–21 Preparations of Estrogen and Progestin for Estrogen Therapy

Trade Name	Generic Name	Minimum Dose for Preventive Therapy (mg)	Upper-End Dose (mg)	FDA-Approved Labeling for Prevention of Osteoporosis	Comments
Premarin Cenestin	Conjugated equine estrogens	0.3 0.625	1.25 0.625-0.9	Prevention	Usual dose 0.625 mg, but 2.5 mg sometimes necessary to control hot flushes in young women
Ogen, Ortho-Est	Estropipate	0.625	1.25	Prevention	2.5 mg sometimes necessary to control hot flushes in young women
Estratab	Esterified estrogen	0.3	2.5	Prevention	Derived from plant (estrone, equilin) sterol precursors
Estratest, Estratest H.S.	Esterified estrogens and methyltestosterone	0.625-1.25 1.25-2.5	1.25/2.5	No indication for osteoporosis	Contains androgens
Estrace	Micronized estradiol	0.5	2.0	Prevention	0.5 mg effective for bone preservation
Transdermal estrogen Alora Climara Estraderm Vivelle	Estradiol	0.05-0.1 0.025		No indication Prevention Prevention Prevention	Patches applied once or twice a week, depending on manufacturer

Continued

TABLE 7–21   Preparations of Estrogen and Progestin for Estrogen Therapy—cont'd

Trade Name	Generic Name	Minimum Dose for Preventive Therapy (mg)	Upper-End Dose (mg)	FDA-Approved Labeling for Prevention of Osteoporosis	Comments
Transdermal estradiol/ progesterone					
CombiPatch	Estradiol and norethindrone	0.62 or 81 and 2.7-4.8		No indication for osteoporosis	Patch applied twice a week
Prempro	Conjugated equine estrogens/MPA	0.625/2.5 or 5		Prevention	If excessive bleeding, may consider increasing MPA dose to 5 mg
Premphase	Ethinyl estradiol	0.625/5		Prevention	
Femhrt 1/5	Norethindrone	0.005/1		Prevention	
Progestins					
Prometrium	Micronized progesterone MPA	100 (daily dose) 200 (cyclic dose)		No indication for osteoporosis	Does not attenuate lipid effects of estrogen
Provera Cycrin		5 or 10 (cyclic dose)			
Amen Aygestin	Norethindrone	2.5 (daily dose) 2.5-10		No indication for osteoporosis	

From Brown EF, Evans RM, Cole HM, Coble YE (ed): Managing Osteoporosis: Part 3, AMA Continuing Medical Education Program. Chicago, AMA Press, 2000. FDA, U.S. Food and Drug Administration; MPA, medroxyprogesterone acetate.

each other on a local level. In vitro, mechanical strain causes a cellular influx of calcium ions, followed by the production of prostaglandin and nitric oxide, increased enzyme activity, and the release of growth hormones; these changes may trigger bone remodeling. The theory suggests that such changes also occur in vivo.

Exercise Prescription (Impact Training)

- For general health reasons, walking or weight-bearing exercise should raise the heart rate enough to prove aerobic conditioning.
- Patients should walk (or perform comparable exercise) 15 to 20 minutes three to four times a week. No available studies have shown that longer duration or increased frequency improves the effect on osteoporosis. Overuse injuries (e.g., stress fractures) can occur with overtraining and lack of appropriate rest intervals.
- Patients should increase their exercise gradually—1 minute every other session—until they reach their target length of workout.
- Brisk walking is almost always the weight-bearing exercise of choice for osteoporosis unless contraindicated (e.g., arthritic lower extremities, cardiovascular limitations).
- *Do not* use the incline on the treadmill.
- Low-impact aerobics may be suitable for most patients, but high-impact aerobic exercises place too much stress on already weakened bone and should be avoided.
- **Avoid running** (five times BW at heel-strike) in patients with osteoporosis.
- **Avoid rowing machines**, which cause **vertebral compression fractures** in those at risk.
- Patients who do not have osteoporosis (or medical contraindications) may perform some high-impact exercises to help avoid osteoporosis.
- Counsel young female patients that excessive exercise and consuming fewer calories than required for vigorous training will cause significant bone loss (**athletic amenorrhea**).
- The "**female athlete triad**" describes a complex consisting of the deleterious interplay of menstrual irregularity (amenorrhea), eating disorder, and premature osteoporosis, as seen in some vigorous female athletes.
- Bone mineral loss in young female athletes with athletic amenorrhea of greater than 6 months' duration resembles that seen after menopause.

Resistance Training for Osteoporosis

The other component of an exercise prescription for osteoporosis, resistance training, should involve all major muscle groups so that it will affect the bones of the upper part of the body as well as the legs. Movements should be slow and controlled, with loads set to induce desired muscle fatigue after 10 to 15 repetitions. Good form is critical (use a trainer or coach initially). Start slowly with a gradual increase in exercise. the following is a list of recommended exercises and the muscle groups that they affect.

Resistance Training Exercises

- Hip extension—gluteal, hamstring, and low back
- Lumbar extension—low back (**avoid lumbar flexion**)
- Leg press—gluteal, quadriceps, and hamstring
- Pullover—latissimus dorsi, shoulders, trapezius, and abdominals

- Torso arm or rowing—latissimus dorsi, shoulders, and biceps
- Arm cross—chest and shoulders
- Chest press—chest, shoulders, and triceps

Ideally, such exercise should initially be supervised and done on machines in a fitness center. Perform resistance exercises every third day.

Patient Education Handout on Exercise

Exercise is important throughout life to build and maintain strong bones and muscles. Bones are similar to muscles in that they respond to exercise by becoming stronger and denser. Just as muscles get flabby if you do not use them, bones lose density if they are not used. People who are bedridden often have low bone density because they cannot get up and move about.

Two types of exercise that are best for bone health are **weight-bearing** and **resistance exercises**. Weight-bearing means that your feet and legs are bearing your weight. Jogging, walking, stair climbing, and dancing are examples of weight-bearing.

Much of the information from this section was derived from the American Medical Association's continuing medical education program, Managing Osteoporosis—Part 3.

Additional resources for osteoporosis patient information include

- **National Osteoporosis Foundation (NOF)**
  1232 22nd Street NW
  Washington, DC 20037-1292
  202-223-2226
  http://www.nof.org
- **National Institutes of Health**
  Osteoporosis and Related Bone Diseases—National Resource Center
  1232 22nd Street NW
  Washington, DC 20037-1292
  800-624-BONE
  http://www.osteo.org
- **American Academy of Orthopedic Surgeons**
  6300 North River Road
  Rosemont, IL 60018-4262
  800-346-AAOS
  http://www.aaos.org
- **American College of Rheumatology**
  1800 Century Place, Suite 250
  Atlanta, GA 30345
  404-633-3777
  http://www.rheumatology.com

Bibliography

HAMSTRING INJURIES IN ATHLETES

Almekinders LC: Anti-inflammatory treatment of muscular injuries in sports. Sports Med 15:139-145, 1993.

Burkett LN: Causative factors in hamstring strains. Med Sci Sports 2:39-42, 1970.

Burkett LN: Investigation into hamstring strains: The case of the hybrid muscle. J Sports Med 3:228-231, 1976.

Clanton TO, Coupe KJ: JAAOS hamstring strains in athletes: Diagnosis and treatment. J Am Acad Orthop Surg 6:237-248, 1998.

Grace TG: Muscle imbalance and extremity injury: A perplexing relationship. Sports Med 2:77-82, 1985.
Heiser TM, Weber J, Sullivan G, et al: Prophylaxis and management of hamstring muscle injuries in intercollegiate football players. Am J Sports Med 12:368-370, 1984.
Jarvinen JJ, Lehto MU: The effects of early mobilization and immobilization on the healing process following muscle injuries. Sports Med 15(2):78-89, 1993.
Kujala UM, Orava S: Ischial apophysis injuries in athletes. Sports Med 16:290-294, 1993.
Liemohn W: Factors related to hamstring strains. J Sports Med 18:71-76, 1978.
Orava S, Kujala UM: Rupture of the ischial origin of the hamstring muscles. Am J Sports Med 23:702-705, 1995.
Safran MR, Garret WE Jr, Seaber AV, et al: The role of warmup in muscular injury prevention. Am J Sports Med 16:123-129, 1988.
Sallay PI, Friedman RL, Coogan PG, Garrett WE: Hamstring muscle injuries among water skiers: Functional outcome and prevention. Am J Sports Med 24:130-136, 1996.
Stafford MG, Grana WA: Hamstring quadriceps ratios in college football players: A high-velocity evaluation. Am J Sports Med 12:209-211, 1984.
Worrell TW: Factors associated with hamstring injuries: An approach to treatment and preventative measures. Sports Med 17:338-345, 1994.
Zarins B, Ciullo JV: Acute muscle and tendon injuries in athletes. Clin Sports Med 2:167-182, 1983.

QUADRICEPS STRAINS AND CONTUSIONS

Aronen JG, Chronister RD: Quadriceps contusions: Hastening the return to play. Physician Sports Med 20(7):130-136, 1992.
Aronen JG, Chronister RD, Ove PN, et al: Quadriceps contusions: Minimizing the length of time before return to full athletic activities with early mobilization in 120°of knee flexion. Paper presented at 16th Annual Meeting of the American Orthopaedic Society for Sports Medicine, July 16-17, 1990, Sun Valley, Idaho.
Brewer BJ: Mechanism of injury to the musculotendinous unit. Instr Course Lect 17:354-358, 1960.
Garrett WE Jr: Strains and sprains in athletes. Postgrad Med 73:200-209, 1983.
Garrett WE Jr, Safran MR, Seaber AV, et al: Biomechanical comparison of stimulated and nonstimulated skeletal muscle pulled to failure. Am J Sports Med 15:448-454, 1987.
Jackson DW, Feagin JA: Quadriceps contusions in young athletes: Relation of severity of injury to treatment and prognosis. J Bone Joint Surg Am 55:95-105, 1973.
Kaeding CC, Sanko WA, Fisher RA: Quadriceps strains and contusions: Decisions that promote rapid recovery. Physician Sports Med 23:59, 1995.
Klafs CE, Arnheim DD: Modern Principles of Athletic Training: The Science of Sports Injury Prevention and Management, 4th ed. St Louis, CV Mosby, 1977, pp 370-372.
Martinez SF, Steingard MA, Steingard PM: Thigh compartment syndrome: A limb-threatening emergency. Physician Sports Med 21(3):94-104, 1993.
Novak PJ, Bach BR Jr, Schwartz JC: Diagnosing acute thigh compartment syndrome. Physician Sports Med 20(11):100-107, 1992.
Ryan JB, Wheeler JH, Hopkinson WJ, et al: Quadriceps contusions: West Point update. Am J Sports Med 19:299-304, 1991.
Winternitz WA Jr, Metheny JA, Wear LC: Acute compartment syndrome of the thigh in sports-related injuries not associated with femoral fractures. Am J Sports Med 20:476-477, 1992.
Zarins B, Ciullo JV: Acute muscle and tendon injuries in athletes. Clin Sports Med 2:167-182, 1983.

GROIN AND HIP PAIN

Anderson K, Strickland SM, Warren R: Hip and groin injuries in athletes. Am J Sports Med 29:521-530, 2001.
Lacroix VJ: A complete approach to groin pain. Physician Sports Med 28:32-37, 2000.
Swain R, Snodgrass S: Managing groin pain, even when the cause is not obvious. Physician Sports Med 23:54-62, 1995.

AQUATIC THERAPY FOR THE INJURED ATHLETE

American College of Sports Medicine: Guidelines for Graded Exercise Testing and Exercise Prescription. Philadelphia, Lee & Febiger, 1986.
Aquajogger Handbook: The New Wave in Fitness. Eugene, OR, Excel Sports Science, 1998.
Aquatic Fitness Professional Manual. Nokomis, FL, Aquatic Exercise Association, 1998.
Arnheim D: Modern Principles of Athletic Training. St Louis, St Louis Mirror/Mosby College, 1985.
Bates A, Hanson N: Aquatic Exercise Therapy. Philadelphia, WB Saunders, 1996.

Becker B, Cole A (eds): Comprehensive Aquatic Therapy. Newton, MA, Butterworth-Heinemann, 1997.

Borg GV: Psychophysical basis of perceived exertion. Med Sci Sports Exerc 14:377-387, 1982.

Brennan D, Wilder R: Aquarunning: An instructor's manual. Houston, Houston International Running Center, 1990.

Bushman B, Flynn MG, Andres FF: Effect of 4 weeks of deep water run training on running performance. Med Sci Sports Exerc 29:694-699, 1997.

Coyle EF, Martin WH, Sinacor DR, et al: Time course of loss adaptations after stopping prolonged intense endurance training. J Appl Physiol 57:1857-1864, 1984.

Eyestone E, Fellingham G, Fisher G: Effect of water running and cycling on maximal oxygen consumption and 2-mile run performance. Am J Sports Med 21:41-44, 1993.

Hickson R, Foster C, Pollock M, et al: Reduced training intensities and loss of aerobic power, endurance, and cardiac growth. J Appl Physiol 58:492-499, 1985.

Huey L, Forester R: The Complete Waterpower Workout Book. New York, Random House, 1993.

HYDRO-FIT News: Special Report: Wave Run Field Rest Study, Summer 1996.

Quinn T, Sedory D, Fisher B: Psychological effects of deepwater running following a land-based training program. Res Q Exerc Sport 64:386-389, 1994.

Ritchie S, Hopkins W: The intensity of exercise in deepwater running. Am J Sports Med 12:27-29, 1991.

Samuelson C: Aquatic one-on-one rehab with athletes. AKWA Lett April/May 2000, p 36.

Thein JW, Brody LT: Aquatic-based rehabilitation and training for the elite athlete. J Orthop Sports Phys Ther 27: 32-42, 1998.

Town G, Bradley S: Maximal metabolic responses of deep and shallow water running in trained runners. Med Sci Sports Exerc 23:238-241, 1991.

Wilder RP, Brennan DK: Physiologic responses to deep water running in athletes. Sports Med 16:374-380, 1993.

Wilder RP, Brennan DK: Aqua running for athletic rehabilitation. In Buschbacher LP, Braddom R (eds): State of the Art Reviews in Physical Medicine and Rehabilitation. Philadelphia, Hanley & Belfus, 1994.

Wilder RP, Brennan DK: Techniques in aqua running. In Becker B, Cole A (eds): Comprehensive Aquatic Therapy. Boston, Butterworth-Heinemann, 1997, pp 123-134.

Wilder RP, Brennan DK, Schotte D: A standard measure for exercise prescription for aqua running. Am J Sports Med 21:45-48, 1993.

RUNNING INJURIES

Fadale PD, Wiggins ME: Corticosteroid injections: Their use and abuse. J Am Acad Orthop Surg 2: 133-140, 1994.

James SL: Running injuries of the knee. Instr Course Lect 47:407-417, 1998.

James SL, Bates BT, Osternig LR: Injuries to runners. Am J Sports Med 6:40-50, 1978.

Leadbetter WB: Cell-matrix response in tendon injury. Clin Sports Med 11:533-578, 1992.

Nigg BM, Nurse MA, Stefanyshyn DJ: Shoe inserts and orthotics for sport and physical activities. Med Sci Sports Exerc Suppl 31:S421-S428, 1999.

Novachek TF: Running injuries: A biomechanical approach. Instr Course Lect 47:397-406, 1998.

Novachek TF, Trost JP: Running: Injury Mechanisms and Training Strategies. Instructional Videotape. St Paul, MN, Gillette Children's Specialty Healthcare Foundation, 1997.

Scott SH, Winter DA: Internal forces of chronic running injury sites. Med Sci Sports Exerc 22:357-369, 1990.

CONCUSSIONS: RETURN TO PLAY

Cantu RC: Guidelines for return to sports after cerebral concussion. Phys Sports Med 14(10):75-83, 1986.

Cantu RC: Second impact syndrome: Immediate management. Phys Sports Med 20(9):55-66, 1992.

Cantu RC: Head injuries in sport. Br J Sports Med 30:289-296, 1996.

Colorado Medical Society Sports Medicine Committee: Guidelines for the Management of Concussions in Sports. Denver, Colorado Medical Society, 1991.

Kelly JP, Nichols JS, Filley CM, et al: Concussion in sports: Guidelines for the prevention of catastrophic outcome. JAMA 266:2867-2869, 1991.

Kelly JP, Rosenberg J: Practice parameter: The management of concussion in sport (summary statement). Neurology 48:581-585, 1997.

Nelson WE, Jane JA, Gieck JH: Minor head injury in sports: A new system of classification and management. Phys Sports Med 12(3):103-107, 1984.

Roberts WO: Who plays? Who sits? Managing concussions on the sidelines. Phys Sports Med 20(6): 66-69, 1992.

Roos, R: Guidelines for managing concussion in sports: A persistent headache. Phys Sports Med 24(10): 67-74, 1996.

Saunders RL, Harbaugh RE: The second impact in catastrophic contact: Sports head trauma. JAMA 252: 538-539, 1984.

Torg JS: Athletic Injuries to the Head, Neck and Face. Philadelphia, Lea & Febiger, 1982.

Wildberger JE, Maroon JC: Head injuries in athletes. Clin Sports Med 8:1-9, 1989.

OSTEOPOROSIS

Brown EF, Evans RM, Cole HM, Coble YE (eds): Managing Osteoporosis: Part 3, AMA Continuing Medical Education Program. Chicago, AMA Press, 2000.

Lanyon LE: Using functional loading to influence bone mass and architecture: Objectives, mechanisms, and relationship with estrogen of the mechanically adaptive process in bone. Bone 18(Suppl 1):37S-43S, 1996.

Munnings F: Osteoporosis: What is the role of exercise? Phys Sports Med 20(6):127, 1992.

Shimegi S, Yanagita M, Okano H, et al: Physical exercise increases bone mineral density in postmenopausal women. Endocr J 41:49-56, 1994.

INDEX

Note: Page numbers followed by the letter f refer to figures; those followed by the letter t refer to tables.

Thera-Band strengthening exercises
(*Continued*)
anterior, 288-289, 298-299
multidirectional, 326
posterior, 316-317
of elbow, 151f, 152f
Therapeutic exercises
after ACL reconstruction
D'Amato and Bach protocol for, 425,
426, 427, 428
Wilk protocol for, 429, 431, 433, 433f,
434, 435, 436, 438
after ankle sprains, 558-559, 559f,
560-561, 560f, 563-564, 563f, 564f
after MCL injury, Reider and Mroczek
protocol for, 473, 474
after meniscal repair, D'Amato and Bach
protocol for, 484, 485
after PCL reconstruction
D'Amato and Bach protocol for,
454-455, 456
with ACL reconstruction, 465, 466, 467,
468
with biceps tenodesis, 462, 463, 464
with two-tunnel graft technique, 458,
459, 460, 461, 461f
for patellar excess pressure syndromes,
507, 508, 509
after distal and/or proximal realignment
procedures, 513, 514, 515
after first-time lateral dislocation, 509, 510
after lateral reticular release, 511, 512, 513
Thermal capsulorrhaphy, for multidirectional
shoulder instability, 323-328
Thigh. *See also* Groin *entries.*
musculotendinous injuries of, 725f
Thigh pad, for quadriceps contusions, 722,
723f
Thomas stretch, 665, 665f
Thompson squeeze test, of Achilles tendon
rupture, 605
Thoracic outlet syndrome, 175
Thromboembolic disease, prophylaxis for
after total hip arthroplasty, 670-671
after total knee arthroplasty, 689
Thrower's elbow, pathologic mechanism of,
118, 119f. *See also* Overhead throwing
athlete, elbow injuries in.
Thrower's shoulder, pathology of, 176-186.
See also Overhead throwing athlete,
shoulder in.
Thrower's Ten program
for elbow injuries, 122
for rotator cuff tendinitis, 236, 238f-239f

Throwing
peel-back mechanism of, 179, 181f
return to, isokinetic criteria for, 234t
six phases of, 232, 233, 233f
Thumb. *See also* Finger(s).
base of, fracture of, 45
carpometacarpal joint of
arthritis of, 2, 66, 97
arthroplasty for, 66-67
extensor pollicis longus of, injury to, 31
flexor pollicis longus of, injury to, 15-18,
16f-18f, 19-20
gamekeeper's, 3, 49-52, 50f, 51f
metacarpophalangeal joint of, injuries to
ulnar collateral ligament of, 49-52,
50f, 51f
skier's, 3, 49-52, 50f, 51f
Thumb spica cast
for Bennett fractures, 71-72, 72f
for scaphoid fractures, 71-72, 72f
Thumb spica splint
for Bennett fracture, 45
for de Quervain's tenosynovitis, 98
for extensor pollicis longus laceration, 31
for intersection syndrome, 101
Tibial fixation methods, for hamstring ACL
graft, 397, 398f
Tibial osteotomy
contraindications to, 684
for unicompartmental knee arthritis, 682t
Tibial stress fracture, 766t
Tibial stress syndrome, medial, 765, 766,
766t
treatment of, 767, 768f, 769f
Tibial tendon, posterior. *See* Posterior tibial
tendon (PTT).
Tibial tunnel placement, anterior, ACL graft
impingement due to, 402, 402f
Tibiotalar shuck test, of syndesmotic ankle
ligaments, 552, 552f
Tinel's sign (percussion test), 156
in carpal tunnel syndrome, 54, 55t
Tingling, in carpal tunnel syndrome, 53
Toe
drawer sign of, 617-618, 618f
turf, 632-638. *See also* Turf toe.
Toe dorsiflexion, for hallux rigidus, 629, 630f
Toe pick-ups, for hallux rigidus, 628, 629f
Toe raises, for ankle sprains, 560f
Too-many-toes sign, in posterior tibial tendon
insufficiency, 609-610, 610f
Topical therapy, for arthritic knee, 677
Torsion, testicular, groin pain due to, 735t
Total elbow arthroplasty, 170